A Reference Guide to Fetal and Neonatal Risk

DRUGS IN PREGNANCY AND LACTATION

second edition

A Reference Guide to Fetal and Neonatal Risk

DRUGS IN PREGNANCY AND LACTATION

second edition

Gerald G. Briggs, B.Pharm.
Clinical Pharmacist, Women's Hospital
Memorial Hospital of Long Beach, California
Assistant Clinical Professor of Pharmacy University of California, San Francisco
Assistant Clinical Professor of Pharmacy University of Southern California,
Los Angeles

Roger K. Freeman, M.D.
Medical Director, Women's Hospital
Memorial Hospital of Long Beach, California
Professor of Obstetrics and Gynecology University of California, Irvine

Sumner J. Yaffe, M.D.
Director, Center for Research for Mothers and Children
National Institute of Child Health and Human Development
National Institutes of Health Bethesda, Maryland

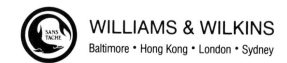

WILLIAMS & WILKINS
Baltimore • Hong Kong • London • Sydney

Editor: Carol-Lynn Brown
Associate Editor: Brian K. Smith
Copy Editor: Maryalice Ditzler
Design: Bob Och
Cover Design: Carmella M. Clifford
Production: Anne G. Seitz

Accurate indications, adverse reactions, and dosage schedules for drugs are provided in this book, but it is possible that they may change. The reader is urged to review the package information data of the manufacturers of the medications mentioned.

Made in the United States of America

First Edition, 1983

Library of Congress Cataloging-in-Publication Data

Briggs, Gerald G.
   Drugs in pregnancy and lactation.

   Rev. ed. of: Drugs in pregnancy and lactation/Gerald G. Briggs . . . [et al.]. c1983.
   Includes bibliographies and index.
   1. Fetus—Effect of drugs on. 2. Infants (Newborn)—Effect of drugs on. 3. Milk, Human—Contamination. 4. Pregnancy, Complications of. I. Freeman, Roger K., 1935–■■■. II. Yaffe, Sumner, J., 1923–■■■. III. Title. [DNLM: 1. Drug Therapy—adverse effects. 2. Fetus—drug effects. 3. Infant, Newborn—drug effects. 4. Lactation—drug effects. 5. Milk, Human—drug effects. 6. Pregnancy—drug effects. WQ210 B854d]RG627.6.D79B75 1986   618.3'2071   85-24122 ISBN 0-683-01058-1

88 89 90 91   10 9 8 7 6

Foreword

This book was written to be used by the clinician who deals with pregnant patients. Every day in an obstetrical, pediatric, or other medical practice, one encounters frequent questions about the use of drugs in pregnancy and lactation. These questions may involve the use of a drug for therapy of an associated condition, an inquiry about some drug a patient has already taken and then decides to ask about, or the determination if an untoward pregnancy outcome or an adverse effect observed in the infant was caused by the consumption of some therapeutic agent by the patient. Other health professionals, such as nurses and pharmacists, also are often confronted with questions concerning drug usage in the pregnant or breast-feeding woman.

Of course, this book of necessity lacks absolute answers on most drugs in question because experience in humans is not easy to gather. One seldom knows, even when the drug history is thought to be realistic, whether there is an actual cause-effect relationship between a specific drug and an adverse pregnancy outcome. Because the answers are generally inconclusive, physicians caring for pregnant patients should counsel their patients accordingly either when answering a question about some drug already ingested or when explaining the cost/benefit ratio to a patient who is being considered for some specific drug therapy.

For the breast-feeding patient, the risks from a particular drug are usually much clearer, although there are frequent examples where the risk must be inferred from related drugs. Unfortunately, many drugs have not been studied during nursing so the effects on the infant, if any, are completely unknown. A good rule to follow is if the drug can safely be given directly to the infant, it is generally safe to give to the mother during lactation.

This book allows the clinician to have at his or her fingertips an up-to-date summary of available data on specific drugs. It is easy to read and organized in a logical manner to save the busy clinician time.

Roger K. Freeman, M.D.
Medical Director
Women's Hospital
Memorial Hospital Medical Center
Long Beach, California
Professor of Obstetrics and Gynecology
University of California, Irvine

Preface *to the second edition*

Writing this edition of *Drugs in Pregnancy and Lactation. A Reference Guide to Fetal and Neonatal Risk* has been an enjoyable experience. The response to the first edition has been very encouraging, with many readers suggesting new areas to cover and different ways to handle the available information. Their thoughtful suggestions and criticisms have been helpful, and we have incorporated many of their ideas into this book. For example, the monographs on vitamins, gold, and bromocriptine resulted from questions and comments from various health professionals.

The amount of new information concerning drug effects on the fetus and newborn continues to grow at an accelerating pace. A similar increase is also noticeable for data on the excretion of drugs into breast milk. Whether or not this greater awareness will result in fewer exposures to chemicals during these two critical periods of life is debatable. We seem to be a society bent on chemical consumption and one that has never heeded a wise, but unknown author, who said "... life is not a drug-deficiency state." Fortunately, however, we are still able to say that most drugs, with some notable exceptions, do not pose an observable danger to the fetus or the newborn.

We have made few changes in the format for this edition. The tables have been removed and the data put into text. We believe this will allow easier interpretation and greater readability. We have also added page numbers to each index entry to simplify the process of finding a monograph.

As with any book, numerous people, whose names do not appear on the cover, have helped put this book together, and to them we offer a sincere thank you. Foremost among these have been the Library and Drug Information staffs at Memorial Hospital of Long Beach. The support of our Librarian, Mrs Frances I. Lyon and her staff, David Downing, Darryl Gaskin, Mori Lou Higa, and Emi I. Wong, continues to be a source of assistance without which this book would never have been written. We are again indebted to Drs Byron Schweigert and Phil Towne of the Drug Information Service for their constructive comments and expertise and to their secretary, Deena Munguia. Our thanks also go to Kay Brittingham of Waverly Press for the programs she wrote that enabled us to place this edition in computer files. A special thank you to my daughter, Leslee, for the many hours of computer time she willingly invested to put the monographs into readable form. Finally, to my wife, Susan, whose patience and understanding has been twice tested, goes my gratitude for making an impossible task possible.

GGB

Preface *to the first edition*

We have always been amazed by the number of drugs and chemicals the fetus is exposed to during its nine-month sojourn in the womb. Perhaps just as surprising is the realization that in spite of this chemical bath, the vast majority of newborns enter the world with the correct number of parts, all functioning properly. Teratology and, to a lesser extent, drugs in breast milk are and have been a major topic of interest and worry to the pregnant woman, to her relatives, and to the health professionals who care for her and her child. Over the past decade, we have been frequently confronted with questions concerning this area from physicians, nurses, pharmacists, patients, and the lay public. Almost all of the health professionals wanted more information on a specific drug than they could find in available reviews. Spurred on by this continued interest, we gradually accumulated a large number of primary references on drugs and the fetus. As we accumulated the references, we summarized the experiences contained in these reports into brief monographs to facilitate answering future questions. From this background, the idea to publish our monographs emerged in 1979. The breast milk sections were added due to the number of inquiries on this subject and its close relationship to drug effects on the developing fetus. Unfortunately, the passage of many drugs into breast milk has not been studied, and the cryptic "No data available" appears often. Individuals wishing to contribute to this area of knowledge have many opportunities to do so.

We have attempted to include all of the pertinent articles on a specific drug. On a few occasions, due to a large number of references, we have resorted to the use of a recent review (e.g., Coumarin Derivatives). The use of reviews has been kept to a minimum since we believe one of the values of our work lies in the citation of the available literature so that readers can arrive at their own conclusions as to the risk a particular drug poses to the fetus or newborn. Although we frequently used case reports as our only source of information, knowledgeable readers will be painfully aware that most reports of this type are biased in several aspects: for example, their lack of reporting the total drug exposure history and its timing; the fact that they are retrospective and must rely on the memory of the patient at a very depressing moment; and their lack of reporting nonteratogenic exposures so that results are weighted toward the negative side; their omission of important factors such as the reason for taking the drug, the relevant family history, and the general state of the mother's health. Inclusion of these data would certainly make evaluation of the literature easier.

There is frequent use of one reference source (Heinonen OP, Slone D, Shapiro S. *Birth Defects and Drugs in Pregnancy*. Littleton:Publishing Sciences Group, 1977) in our work. This prospective study often provided the only available information on some drugs. We extend our apologies in advance to authors whose work we inadvertently omitted. In any work of this magnitude, some important citations will be overlooked. Also, many drugs have not been included due to time and space limitations. We have attempted, however, to include those agents and classes of agents that have generated the most inquiries in our experience. With your assistance and the blessings of time, in future editions, we hope to eliminate these shortcomings. We wish to express our sincere thank you to the many people who assisted us in putting this book together, including: Dr William E. Smith, Administrator of the Pharmacy Department at Memorial Hospital; Mrs Frances Lyon, Librarian at Memorial and her staff, Emi Kosaka, Lisa Ginsbarg, Mori Higa, Ellen Phillips, and David Downing; Dr Byron Schweigert, Director of the Drug Information Service at Memorial and his staff, Dr Philip Towne and Barbara Matthias; all of the manufacturers who responded to our pleas for information on their products and especially to Dr John J. Whalen, Director of Professional Information at Merck Sharp and Dohme, who probably answered more of our letters than he cares to remember; the personnel at Auto-Type Word Processing Center, in particular Ms Irene Mendoza, Office Manager, for their typing of the manuscript; Susan and Leslee Briggs for the many hours they spent assembling the Index. Finally, and most important, our special thanks to our families, Susan and Leslee, and Kathleen and Derek, who have suffered through our long hours away from home, late dinners, cancelled vacations, and irritable husbands/fathers over the past three years.

GGB
TWB

Contributors *to the second edition*

Thomas W. Bodendorfer, Pharm D, Clinical Coordinator of Pharmacy Services, The Crawford W. Long Memorial Hospital of Emory University, Atlanta, Georgia

Larry Sonnenschein, Pharm D, Hermosa Beach, California

Introduction

Sumner J. Yaffe, M.D.

The birth of a normal infant is the expectation of the parents when pregnancy is considered. Normality is not limited to the time of birth but includes the achievement of full potential in adulthood. Today, advances in medical knowledge and delivery have made this aspiration more readily achievable than ever before. However, there is a threat to the fulfillment of the prospective parents' dreams resulting from the very advances that contributed to better health. Indeed, modern technology poses a risk to the fetus and lactating infant from the drugs used in obstetric practice and from the increasing numbers of chemicals in the environment. New social, cultural, and ecologic conditions have modified the experiences of today's pregnant woman.

Studies are needed to clarify their specific impact and to facilitate the development of prevention and/or curative strategies. This knowledge must be transferred rapidly to all interested parties—physicians, midwives, nurses, mothers-to-be, and the public at large—as an informed individual will be more inclined to seek and follow medical advice.

Every day physicians and midwives usher newborns into the world with the full expectation that their advice and prescribed medications will be adhered to by the new mothers and will result in healthy infants. In addition, if they so wish, new mothers are ready to nurse their babies.

Special responsibilities are vested in the partnership between the pregnant woman and her physician. The physician has the responsibility to provide all the medical knowledge and skills available to him. The pregnant woman is expected to follow the physician's advice and prescriptions.

This has been the established arrangement since physicians began attending childbirth. The primary difference between those early times and today is what is expected of the physician. Hippocrates, Soranus, Aetios, and Avicenna, whose time ranged from the fourth century before the common era through the first millenium AD, maintained highly authoritative positions within their communities and provided their ministrations in a categorical fashion.

Soranus of Ephesus (1), representing the consumate thinking of the time (second century AD), wrote in a threatening autocratic manner, "Even if a woman transgresses some or all of the rules mentioned (re: administration of drugs, sternutatives, pungent substances, and drunkenness, especially during the first trimester) and yet miscarriage of the fetus does not take place, let no one assume that the fetus has not been injured at all. For it has been harmed: it is weakened, becomes retarded in growth, less well nourished, and in general, more easily injured and susceptible to harmful agents; it becomes misshapen and of ignoble soul."

Drugs in Pregnancy

Today's physician does not have the authoritative luxury of yesterday's practitioner. In particular, the present-day obstetrician has suffered a diminution of confidence because of the thalidomide catastrophe.

In 1941 Gregg (2) demonstrated that rubella infection in the mother could result in anatomic malformation in the fetus. This raised the concept that environment could affect fetal outcome. In spite of this, physicians continued to practice their profession with little concern to the empirical observations.

Because of its sedative and hypnotic effects, physicians administered thalidomide to the pregnant woman for her discomfort. Thalidomide had been evaluated for safety in several animal species, had been given a clean bill of health, and had come to be regarded as a good pharmacologic agent. Yet the catastrophic and distinct embryopathic effects resulting from thalidomide administration to the human mother during early pregnancy are well-known.

It is important to note that even though thalidomide induces a distinct cluster of anatomic defects that are virtually pathognomonic for this agent, it required several years of thalidomide use and the birth of many thousands of grossly malformed infants before the cause and effect relationship between thalidomide administration in early pregnancy and its harmful effects was recognized. This serves to emphasize the difficulties that exist in incriminating drugs and chemicals that are harmful when administered during pregnancy. Hopefully, we will never have another drug prescribed for use during pregnancy whose teratogenicity is as potent as thalidomide (about one-third of women taking this agent during the first trimester gave birth to infants with birth defects).

Concern about the safety of foreign compounds administered to pregnant women has been increasingly evident since thalidomide. It was the direct response to this misadventure which led to the promulgation of the drug regulations of 1962 in the United States. According to these regulations, a drug must be demonstrated to be safe and effective for the conditions of use prescribed in its labeling. The regulations concerning this requirement state that a drug should be investigated for the conditions of use specified in the labeling, including dosage levels and patient populations for whom the drug is intended. In addition, appropriate information must be provided in the labeling in cases in which the drug is prescribed. The intent of the regulations is not only to ensure adequate labeling information for the safe and effective administration of the drug by the physician but also to ensure that marketed drugs have an acceptable benefit-to-risk ratio for their intended uses.

It is clear that any drug or chemical substance administered to the mother is able to cross the placenta to some extent unless it is destroyed or altered during passage. Placental transport of maternal substrates to the fetus and of substances from the fetus to the mother is established at about the fifth week of fetal life. Substances of low molecular weight diffuse freely across the placenta, driven primarily by the concentration gradient. It is important to note, therefore, that almost every substance used for therapeutic purposes can and does pass from the mother to the fetus. Of greater importance is whether the rate and extent of transfer are sufficient to result in significant concentrations within the fetus. We must discard the concept that there is a placental barrier.

Experiments with animals have provided considerable information concerning the teratogenic effects of drugs. Unfortunately, these experimental findings cannot be extrapolated from species to species, or even from strain to strain within the same species, much less from animals to humans. Research in this area and the prediction of toxicity in the human are further hampered by a lack of specificity between cause and effect.

Traditionally, teratogenic effects of drugs have been noted as anatomic malformations. It is clear that these are dose and time related and that the fetus is at great risk during the first three months of gestation. However, it is possible for drugs and chemicals to exert their effects upon the fetus at other times during pregnancy. Functional and behavioral changes are much more difficult to identify as to cause and effect. Consequently, they are rarely recognized. A heightened awareness on the part of health providers and recipients will make this task easier.

This was also understood by Hippocrates who, in the Corpus (3), maintained that the second trimester was a safe stage of fetal development for the administration of drugs. In the Aphorisms, that collection of short medical truths, he prescribed, "Drugs may be administered to pregnant women from the fourth to the seventh month of gestation. After that period, the dose should be less."

The mechanisms of teratogenic agents are poorly understood, particularly in the human. Drugs may affect maternal tissues with indirect effects upon the fetus or they may have a direct effect on the embryonic cells and result in specific abnormalities. Drugs may affect the nutrition of the fetus by interfering with the passage of nutrients across the placenta. Alterations in placental metabolism influence the development of the fetus since placental integrity is a determinant of fetal growth.

Administration of a drug to a pregnant woman presents a unique problem for the physician. Not only must maternal pharmacologic mechanisms be taken into consideration when prescribing a drug but also the fetus must always be kept in mind as a potential recipient of the drug.

Recognition of the fact that drugs administered during pregnancy can affect the fetus should lead to decreased drug consumption. Nonetheless, studies conducted in the past few years indicate drug consumption during pregnancy is increasing. This may be due to several reasons. Most people in the Western world are unaware of their drug and chemical exposure. Many are uninformed as to the potentially harmful effects of drugs on the fetus. Also, there are some who feel that many individuals in modern society are overly concerned with their own comfort.

Whatever the reasons, exposure to drugs, both prescribed and over the counter, among mothers-to-be continues unabated throughout pregnancy. It is possible that this exposure to drugs and chemicals may be responsible for the large numbers of birth defects which are seen in the newborn infant and in later development.

It is crucial that concern also be given to events beyond the narrow limits of congenital anatomic malformations; evidence exists that intellectual, social, and functional development also can be adversely affected. There are examples that toxic manifestations of intrauterine exposure to environmental agents may be subtle, unexpected, and delayed.

Concern for the delayed effects of drugs, following intrauterine exposure, was first raised following the tragic discovery that female fetuses exposed to diethylstilbestrol (DES) are at an increased risk for adenocarcinoma of the vagina. This type of malignancy is not discovered until after puberty. Additional clinical findings indicate that male offspring were not spared from the effects of the drug. Some have abnormalities of the reproductive system such as epididymal cysts, hypo-trophic testes, capsular induration, and pathologic semen.

The concept of long-term latency has been confirmed by investigations con-ducted in the research laboratories. Researchers found that when the widely used hypnotic-sedative agent phenobarbital was administered to pregnant rats it resulted in the birth of offspring who were significantly smaller than normal and who experienced delays in vaginal opening. Sixty percent of the females offspring of these animals were infertile (4).

Investigators in a laboratory at Children's Hospital of Philadelphia reported their research results with male animals (5). They found lower-than-normal testosterone levels in the brains and bloodstreams of male rats whose mothers were given low doses of phenobarbital late in pregnancy. Even at 120 days of age, these male rats showed abnormal testosterone synthesis. It is felt by the investigators that phenobarbital, encountered in fetal life, may alter brain programming which results in permanent changes in sexual function. Phenobarbital is an old drug that is widely prescribed. It is also a component of many multiingredient pharmaceuticals whose use does not abate during pregnancy. The clinical significance of these experiments in animals is admittedly unknown, but the striking effects upon reproductive function warrant careful scrutiny of the safety of these agents during human pregnancy before prescribing them.

The physician is confronted with two imperatives in treating the pregnant woman: alleviate maternal suffering and do not harm the fetus. Until now the emphasis has been on the amelioration of suffering, but the time has come to concentrate on not harming the fetus. The simple equation to be applied here is weighing the thera-peutic benefits of the drug to the mother against its risk potential to the developing fetus.

When one considers that more than 1.2 billion drug prescriptions are written each year, that there is unlimited self-administration of over-the-counter drugs, and that approximately 500 new pharmaceutical products are introduced annually, the need for prudency in the administration of pharmaceuticals has reached a critical point. Pregnancy is a symptom-producing event. Pregnancy has the potential of causing women to increase their intake of drugs and chemicals, with the potential being that the fetus will be nurtured in a sea of drugs.

In today's society the physician cannot stand alone in the therapeutic decision-making process. It now has become the responsibility of each woman of child-bearing age to carefully consider her use of drugs. In a pregnant woman, the decision to administer a drug should be made only after a collaborative appraisal between the woman and her physician of the benefits-to-risk ratio.

Breast Feeding and Drugs

Between 1930 and the late 1960's there was a dramatic decline in the percentage of American mothers who breast-fed their babies. This was accompanied by a reduction in the length of breast-feeding for those who did nurse. The incidence of breast-feeding declined from approximately 80% of the children born between 1926 and 1930 to 49% of children born some 25 years later. For children born between 1966 and 1970, 28% were breast-fed. As data have become available for the decade of the seventies, it is clear the decline has been reversed (6). By 1975, the percentage of first born who were breast-fed rose to 37. At the present time in the United States, it appears (from a number of surveys) that more than 50% of babies discharged from the hospital are breast-fed and the number is increasing.

Any number of hypotheses can be made regarding the decline and recent increase in breast-feeding in this country. A fair amount of credit can be given to the biomedical research of the past 15 years which has demonstrated the benefits of breast-feeding.

Breast-feeding is known to possess nutritional and immunologic properties superior to those found in infant formulas (6–9). The American Academy of Pediatrics has published a position paper emphasizing a return to breast-feeding as the best nutritional mode for infants for the first six months of age (6). In addition to those qualities, some studies also suggest significant psychologic benefits for both the mother and the infant in breast-feeding.

The upswing in breast-feeding, together with a markedly increased concern about health needs on the part of parents, has led to increased questioning of the physician, pharmacist, and other health professionals about the safety and potential toxicity of drugs and chemicals that may be excreted in breast milk. Answers to these questions are not very apparent. Our knowledge concerning the long- and short-term effects and safety of maternally ingested drugs on the suckling infant is meager. We know more now than Soranus did in 150 AD when he admonished wet nurses to refrain from the use of drugs and alcohol lest it have an adverse effect on the nursing infant. We must know more! The knowledge to be acquired should be specific with respect to dose administered to the mother and amount excreted in breast milk and absorbed by the suckling infant. In addition, effects on the infant should be determined (both acute and chronic).

It would be easy to recommend that the medicated mother not nurse, but it is likely that this recommendation would be ignored by the mother in discomfort and may well offend many health providers as well as their patients on both psychosocial and physiologic grounds.

It must be emphasized that virtually all investigations concerned with milk secretion and synthesis have been carried out in animals. The difficulty in studying human lactation employing histologic techniques and the administration of radio-active isotopes is obvious. There are considerable differences in the composition of milk in different species. Some of these differences in composition would obviously bring about changes in drug elimination. Of great importance in this regard are the differences in the pH of human milk (pH usually >7.0) as contrasted to the pH of cow's milk (pH usually <6.8) in which drug excretion has been extensively studied.

Human milk is a suspension of fat and protein in a carbohydrate-mineral solution. A nursing mother easily makes 600 ml of milk per day containing sufficient protein, fat, and carbohydrate to meet the nutritional demands of the developing infant. Milk proteins are fully synthesized from substrates delivered from the maternal circulation. The major proteins are casein and lactalbumin. The role of these proteins in the delivery of drugs into milk has not yet been completely elucidated. Drug excretion into milk may be accomplished by binding to the proteins or on to the surface of the milk fat globule.

There also exists the possibility for drug binding to the lipid as well as to the protein components of the milk fat globule. It is also possible that lipid-soluble drugs may be sequestered within the milk fat globule. In addition to lipids and protein, carbohydrate is entirely synthesized within the breast. All of these nutrients achieve a concentration in human milk that is sufficient for the needs of the human infant for the first six months of life.

The transport of drugs into breast milk from maternal tissues and plasma may proceed by a number of different routes. In general, however, the mechanisms that determine the concentration of a drug in breast milk are similar to those existing elsewhere within the organism. Drugs traverse membranes primarily by passive diffusion and the concentration achieved will be dependent not only on the concentration gradient but also on the intrinsic lipid solubility of the drug and its degree of ionization as well as binding to protein and other cellular constituents.

A number of reviews (10–12) give tables of the concentration of drugs in breast milk. Many times these tables also give the milk/plasma ratio. Most of the values from which the tables are derived consist of a single measurement of the drug concentration. Important information such as the maternal dose, the frequency of dose, the time from drug administration to sampling, the frequency of nursing, and the length of lactation is not given.

What these concentrations mean to the physician concerned about the infant is that the drug is present in the milk. This fact is apparent since, with few exceptions, all drugs that are present in the maternal circulation will be transferred into milk. Because the drug in the nursing infant's blood or urine is not measured, we have little information about the amount that is actually absorbed by the infant from the milk and, therefore, have no way of determining the possible pharmacologic effect on the infant. In fact, a critical examination of the tables that have been published reveals that much of the information was gathered decades ago when analytical methodology was not as sensitive as it is today. Since the discipline of pharmacokinetics was not developed until recently, many of the studies quoted in the tables in the review articles do not look precisely at the time relationship between drug administration and disposition.

Certain things are clear with regard to drugs administered during lactation. It is clear that physicians will have to become aware of the results of animal studies in this area and of the potential risk of maternal drug ingestion to the suckling infant. It is clear that a great many other drugs employed at this time need to be thoroughly studied in order to assess their safety during lactation. It is clear that if the mother needs the drugs for therapeutic purposes, then she should consider not nursing. The ultimate decision must be individualized according to the specific illness and the therapeutic modality. It is clear that nursing should be avoided following the administration of radioactive pharmaceuticals that are usually given to the mother for diagnostic purposes.

The situation with the excretion of drugs into human breast milk might well be considered analogous to the prethalidomide era when the effects on the fetus from maternally ingested drugs were recognized only as a result of a catastrophe. Objective evaluation of the efficacy and safety of drugs in breast milk must be undertaken. Until such data are available, the physician should always weigh the risk/benefit ratio when prescribing any maternal medication. It is also obligatory upon the nursing mother to become aware of the same factors and apply a measure of self-control before ingesting over-the-counter drugs. As stated before, it is quite evident that nearly all drugs will be present in breast milk following maternal ingestion. It is prudent to minimize maternal exposure, although very few drugs are currently known to be hazardous to the suckling child. If, after examining the benefit/risk factor, the physician decides that maternal medication is necessary, drug exposure to the infant may be minimized by scheduling the maternal dose just after a nursing period. More often than not, drugs are prescribed to the nursing mother for the relief of symptoms that do not require drug therapy. It is probable if the mothers were apprised by the physician of the potential risk to the infant, most would endure the symptoms rather than take the drug and discontinue breast-feeding.

Conclusions

We have two basic situations being dealt with throughout this book: 1) risk potential to the fetus of maternal drugs ingested during the course of pregnancy and 2) risk potential to the infant of drugs taken by the mother while nursing.

The obvious solution to fetal and nursing infant risk avoidance is maternal abstinence. However, from a pragmatic standpoint, that would be impossible to implement. Another solution is to disseminate knowledge, in an authoritative manner, to all those involved in the pregnancy and breast-feeding processes: physician, mother, midwife, nurse, father, and pharmacist.

This book helps fill a communication/information gap. We have carefully evaluated the research literature, animal and human, applied and clinical. We have established a risk factor for each of the more than 500 drugs, in keeping with the Food and Drug Administration guidelines, which may be administered during pregnancy and lactation. We feel that this book will be helpful to all concerned parties in developing the benefit/risk decision.

This is but a beginning. It is our fervent hope that the information gained from the use of this book will cause the concerned parties to be more trenchant in their future decision-making, either before prescribing or before ingesting drugs during pregnancy and lactation.

References

1. Soranus. *Gynecology* (translation). Baltimore:The Johns Hopkins University Press, 1956.
2. Gregg NM. Congenital cataract following German measles in the mother. Trans Ophthalmol Soc Aust 1941;3:35–41.
3. Chadwick J, Mann WN. *The Medical Works of Hippocrates*. Springfield, IL:Charles C Thomas, 1935.
4. Gupta C, Sondwane BR, Yaffe SJ, Shapiro BH. Phenobarbital exposure in utero: alterations in female reproductive functions in rats. Science 1980;208:508–10.
5. Gupta C, Yaffe SJ, Shapiro BH. Prenatal exposure to phenobarbital permanently decreases testosterone and causes reproductive dysfunction. Science 1982;216:640–2.
6. Nutrition Committee of the Canadian Pediatric Society and the Committee on Nutrition of the American Academy of Pediatrics. Breast feeding. Pediatrics 1978;62:591–601.
7. Fomon SJ. *Infant Nutrition*, ed 2. Philadelphia:WB Saunders, 1974:360–70.
8. Jelliffe DB, Jelliffe EFP. Breast is best: modern meanings. N Engl J Med 1977;297:912–5.
9. Applebaum RM. The obstetricians approach to the breasts and breast feeding. J Reprod Med 1975;14:98–116.
10. Knowles JA. Excretion of drugs in milk: a review. J Pediatr 1965;66:1068–82.
11. Hervada AR, Feit E, Sagrames R. Drugs in breast milk. Perinat Care 1978;2:19–25.
12. O'Brien TE. Excretion of drugs in human milk. Am J Hosp Pharm 1974;31:844–854.

Instructions for Use of the Reference Guide

The Reference Guide is arranged so that the user can quickly locate a monograph. If the American generic name is known, go directly to the monographs, which are listed in alphabetical order. If only the trade or foreign name is known, refer to the Index for the appropriate American generic name. Foreign trade names have been included in the Index. To the best of our knowledge, all trade and foreign generic names are correct as shown, but since these may change, the reader should check other reference sources if there is any question as to the identity of an individual drug. Combination products are generally not listed in the Index. The user should refer to the manufacturer's product information for the specific ingredients and then use the Reference Guide as for single entities.

Each monograph contains six parts:
- —Generic Name (United States)
- —Pharmacologic Class
- —Risk Factor
- —Fetal Risk Summary
- —Breast Feeding Summary
- —References (omitted from some monographs)

Fetal Risk Summary

The Fetal Risk Summary is a brief review of the literature concerning the drug. The intent of the Summary is to provide clinicians and other individuals with sufficient data to counsel patients and to arrive at conclusions on the risk/benefit ratio a particular drug poses for the fetus. Since few absolutes are possible in the area of human teratology, the reader must carefully weigh the evidence, or lack thereof, before utilizing any drug in a pregnant woman. Animal datum has been excluded from most monographs unless it contributes significantly, in our opinion, to the total information. Readers who require more details than are presented should refer to the specific references listed at the end of the monograph.

Breast Feeding Summary

The Breast Feeding Summary is a brief review of the literature concerning the passage of the drug into human breast milk and the effects, if any, on the nursing infant. In many studies of drugs in breast milk, infants were not allowed to breast-feed. Readers should pay close attention to this distinction (i.e., excretion into milk vs effects on the nursing infant) when using a Summary. Those who require more details than are presented should refer to the specific references listed at the end of the monograph.

Risk Factors

Risk Factors (A, B, C, D, X) have been assigned to all drugs, based on the level of risk the drug poses to the fetus. Risk Factors are designed to help the reader quickly classify a drug for use during pregnancy. They do not refer to breast-feeding risk. Because they tend to oversimplify a complex topic, they should always be used in conjunction with the Fetal Risk Summary. The definitions used for the Factors are the same as those put forth by the Food and Drug Administration (Federal Register 1980;44:37434–67). Since most drugs have not yet been given a letter rating by their manufacturers, the Risk Factor assignments were usually made by the authors. If the manufacturer rated its product in its professional literature, the Risk Factor on the monograph will be shown with a subscript M (e.g., C_M). If the manufacturer and the authors differed in their assignment of a Risk Factor, our Risk Factor is marked with an asterisk and the manufacturer's rating is shown at the end of the Fetal Risk Summary. Other Risk Factors marked with an asterisk (e.g., sulfonamides, morphine, etc) are drugs that present different risks to the fetus depending on when or for how long they are used. In these cases, a second Risk Factor will be found with a short explanation at the end of the Fetal Risk Summary. We hope this will increase the usefulness of these ratings. The definitions used for the Risk Factors are presented below.

Category A: Controlled studies in women fail to demonstrate a risk to the fetus in the first trimester (and there is no evidence of a risk in later trimesters), and the possibility of fetal harm appears remote.

Category B: Either animal-reproduction studies have not demonstrated a fetal risk, but there are no controlled studies in pregnant women or animal reproduction studies have shown an adverse effect (other than a decrease in fertility) that was not confirmed in controlled studies in women in the first trimester (and there is no evidence of a risk in later trimesters).

Category C: Either studies in animals have revealed adverse effects on the fetus (teratogenic or embryocidal or other) and there are no controlled studies in woman or studies in women and animals are not available. Drugs should be given only if the potential benefit justifies the potential risk to the fetus.

Category D: There is positive evidence of human fetal risk, but the benefits from use in pregnant women may be acceptable despite the risk (e.g., if the drug is needed in a life-threatening situation or for a serious disease for which safer drugs cannot be used or are ineffective).

Category X: Studies in animals or human beings have demonstrated fetal abnormalities or there is evidence of fetal risk based on human experience or both, and the risk of the use of the drug in pregnant women clearly outweighs any possible benefit. The drug is contraindicated in women who are or may become pregnant.

Contents

Name: **ACEBUTOLOL**

Class: **Sympatholytic (β-Adrenergic Blocker)**   Risk Factor: **B$_M$**

Fetal Risk Summary

Acebutolol, a cardioselective β-adrenergic blocking agent, has been used for the treatment of hypertension occurring during pregnancy (1–4). No fetal malformations attributable to acebutolol have been observed, but experience with the drug during the 1st trimester is lacking. In a study comparing three β-blockers, the mean birth weights of 56 newborns were slightly lower than those of 38 pindolol-exposed infants but higher than those of 31 offspring of atenolol-treated mothers (3,160 g vs 3,375 g vs 2,745 g) (2). It is not known if these differences were due to the degree of maternal hypertension, the potency of the drugs used, or a combination of these and other factors.

Acebutolol crosses the placenta, producing maternal:cord ratios of 0.8 (3). The corresponding ratio for the metabolite, N-acetylacebutolol, was 0.6. Newborn serum levels of acebutolol and the metabolite were <5–244 and 17–663 ng/ml, respectively (3).

In 10 newborns who had been exposed to acebutolol near term, blood pressure and heart rate were significantly lower than in similar infants who had been exposed to methyldopa (4). The hemodynamic differences were still evident 3 days after birth. Measurements were not made after this point, so it is not known how long the β-blockade persisted. Mean blood glucose levels were not significantly lower than in similar infants exposed to methyldopa, but transient hypoglycemia was present 3 hours after birth in four full-term newborns (4). The mean half-life of acebutolol in the serum of newborns has been calculated to be 10.1 hours, but the half-life based on urinary excretion was 15.6 hours (4). Therefore, newborn infants of women consuming the drug near delivery should be closely observed for signs and symptoms of β-blockade. Long-term effects of *in utero* exposure to β-blockers have not been studied but warrant evaluation.

Breast Feeding Summary

Acebutolol and its metabolite, N-acetylacebutolol, are excreted into breast milk (3). Milk:plasma ratios for the two compounds were 7.1 and 12.2, respectively. Absorption of both compounds has been demonstrated in infants who were breast-fed, but no adverse effects were mentioned (3). However, infants breast-fed by mothers taking acebutolol should be closely observed for hypotension, bradycardia, and other signs or symptoms of β-blockade. Long-term effects of exposure to β-blockers from milk have not been studied but warrant evaluation.

References

1. Dubois D, Petitcolas J, Temperville B, Klepper A. Beta blockers and high-risk pregnancies. Int J Biol Res Pregnancy 1980;1:141–5.

2. Dubois D, Petitcolas J, Temperville B, Klepper A, Catherine Ph. Treatment of hypertension in pregnancy with β-adrenoceptor antagonists. Br J Clin Pharmacol 1982;13(Suppl):375S–8S.
3. Bianchetti G, Dubruc C, Vert P, Boutroy MJ, Morselli PL. Placental transfer and pharmacokinetics of acebutolol in newborn infants. Clin Pharmacol Ther 1981;29:233–4 (Abstr.).
4. Dumez Y, Tchobroutsky C, Hornych H, Amiel-Tison C. Neonatal effects of maternal administration of acebutolol. Br Med J 1981;283:1077–9.

Name: **ACETAMINOPHEN**

Class: **Analgesic/Antipyretic**   Risk Factor: **B**

Fetal Risk Summary

Acetaminophen is routinely used during all stages of pregnancy for pain relief and to lower elevated body temperature. The drug crosses the placenta (1). In therapeutic doses, it is apparently safe for short-term use. However, continuous, high daily dosage in one mother probably caused severe anemia (hemolytic?) in her and fatal kidney disease in her newborn (2).

Theoretically, acetaminophen could cause severe liver damage in the fetus if a toxic dose was consumed by the mother, especially early in pregnancy (3). However, such damage was not observed in two separate cases of acute overdosage occurring in the 2nd and 3rd trimesters (4, 5). One woman at 36 weeks gestation consumed a single dose of 22.5 g of acetaminophen that produced a toxic blood level of 200 μg/ml (4). She delivered a normal infant approximately 6 weeks later. In the second case, a woman at 20 weeks gestation consumed a total of 25 g in two doses over a 10-hour interval (5). She gave birth at 41 weeks to a normal infant with an occipital cephalohematoma due to birth position. At 24 hours after birth, this infant developed jaundice, which responded to phototherapy, but did not show evidence of persistent liver damage. The jaundice was thought to have been due to the cephalohematoma. In both of these instances, protection against serious liver damage may have been due to the prompt administration of acetylcysteine.

The Collaborative Perinatal Project monitored 50,282 mother-child pairs, 226 of which had 1st trimester exposure to acetaminophen (6). Although no evidence was found to suggest a relationship to large categories of major or minor malformations, a possible association, based on three cases, with congenital dislocation of the hip was found (7). The statistical significance of this association is unknown, and independent confirmation is required. For use anytime pregnancy, 781 exposures were recorded. As with the qualifications expressed for 1st trimester exposure, possible associations with congenital dislocation of the hip (eight cases) and clubfoot (six cases) were found (9). A 1982 report described craniofacial and digital anomalies in an infant exposed *in utero* to large daily doses of acetaminophen and propoxyphene throughout pregnancy (10). The infant also exhibited withdrawal symptoms due to the propoxyphene (see also Propoxyphene). The authors speculated with caution that the combination of propoxyphene with other drugs, such as acetaminophen, might have been teratogenic. In a study examining 6,509 women with live births, acetaminophen with or without codeine was used by 697 (11%) during the 1st trimester (11). No evidence of a relationship with malformations was observed.

Unlike aspirin, acetaminophen does not affect platelet function, and there is no increased risk of hemorrhage if the drug is given to the mother at term (12, 13). In a study examining intracranial hemorrhage in premature infants, the incidence of bleeding after exposure of the fetus to acetaminophen close to birth was no different than that in nonexposed controls (see also Aspirin) (14).

Breast Feeding Summary

Acetaminophen is excreted into breast milk in low concentrations (15–17). No reports of adverse effects in nursing infants have been located. Unpublished data obtained from one manufacturer showed that following an oral dose of 650 mg, an average milk level of 11 μg/ml occurred (15). Timing of the samples was not provided. Following ingestion of a single analgesic combination tablet containing 324 mg of phenacetin, average milk levels of acetaminophen, the active metabolite, were 0.89 μg/ml (16). Milk:plasma ratios at 1 and 12 hours were 0.91 and 1.42; the milk half-life was 4.7 hours compared to 3.0 hours in the serum. Repeated doses at 4-hour intervals were expected to result in a steady-state concentration of 2.69 μg/ml. In three lactating women, a mean milk:plasma ratio of 0.76 was reported following a single oral dose of 500 mg of acetaminophen (17). In this case, the mean serum and milk half-lives were 2.7 and 2.6 hours, respectively. Peak milk concentrations of 4.2 μg/ml occurred at 2 hours. The American Academy of Pediatrics considers acetaminophen compatible with breast feeding (18).

References

1. Levy G, Garretson LK, Soda DM. Evidence of placental transfer of acetaminophen. Pediatrics 1975;55:895.
2. Char VC, Chandra R, Fletcher AB, Avery GB. Polyhydramnios and neonatal renal failure—a possible association with maternal acetaminophen ingestion. J Pediatr 1975;86:638–9.
3. Rollins DE, Von Bahr C, Glaumann H, Moldens P, Rane H. Acetaminophen: potentially toxic metabolite formed by human fetal and adult liver microsomes and isolated fetal liver cells. Science 1979;205:1414–6.
4. Byer AJ, Taylor TR, Semmer JR. Acetaminophen overdose in the third trimester of pregnancy. JAMA 1982;247:3114–5.
5. Stokes IM. Paracetamol overdose in the second trimester of pregnancy. Case report. Br J Obstet Gynaecol 1984;91:286–8.
6. Heinonen OP, Slone D, Shapiro S. Birth Defects and Drugs in Pregnancy. Littleton:Publishing Sciences Group, 1977:286–95.
7. Ibid, 471.
8. Ibid, 434.
9. Ibid, 484.
10. Golden NL, King KC, Sokol RJ. Propoxyphene and acetaminophen: possible effects on the fetus. Clin Pediatr 1982;21:752–4.
11. Aselton P, Jick H, Milunsky A, Hunter JR, Stergachis A. First-trimester drug use and congenital disorders. Obstet Gynecol 1985;65:451–5.
12. Pearson H. Comparative effects of aspirin and acetaminophen on hemostasis. Pediatrics 1978;62(Suppl):926–9.
13. Rudolph AM. Effects of aspirin and acetaminophen in pregnancy and in the newborn. Arch Intern Med 1981;141:358–63.
14. Rumack CM, Guggenheim MA, Rumack BH, Peterson RG, Johnson ML, Braithwaite WR. Neonatal intracranial hemorrhage and maternal use of aspirin. Obstet Gynecol 1981;58(Suppl):52S–6S.
15. Personal communication. McNeil Laboratories, Madison, WI, 1979.
16. Findlay JWA, DeAngelis RL, Kearney MF, Welch RM, Findlay JM. Analgesic drugs in breast milk and plasma. Clin Pharmacol Ther 1981;29:625–33.
17. Bitzen PO, Gustafsson B, Jostell KG, Melander A, Wahlin-Boll E. Excretion of paracetamol in human breast milk. Eur J Clin Pharmacol 1981;20:123–5.
18. Committee on Drugs, American Academy of Pediatrics. The transfer of drugs and other chemicals into human breast milk. Pediatrics 1983;72:375–83.

Name: **ACETAZOLAMIDE**

Class: **Carbonic Anhydrase Inhibitor**   Risk Factor: **C**

Fetal Risk Summary

Despite widespread usage, no reports linking the use of acetazolamide with congenital defects have been located. A single case of a neonatal sacrococcygeal teratoma has been described (1). The mother received 750 mg daily for glaucoma during the 1st and 2nd trimesters. A relationship between the drug and carcinogenic effects in the fetus has not been supported by other reports. Retrospective surveys on the use of acetazolamide during gestation have not demonstrated an increased fetal risk (2, 3). The Collaborative Perinatal Project monitored 50,282 mother-child pairs, 12 of which had 1st trimester exposure to acetazolamide (4). For use anytime during pregnancy, 1024 exposures were recorded (5). In neither case was evidence found to suggest a relationship to large categories of major or minor malformations or with individual defects.

Breast Feeding Summary

No data available.

References

1. Worsham GF, Beckman EN, Mitchell EH. Sacrococcygeal teratoma in a neonate. Association with maternal use of acetazolamide. JAMA 1978;240:251–2.
2. Favre-Tissot M, Broussole P, Robert JM, Dumont L: An original clinical study of the pharmacologic-teratogenic relationship. Ann Med Psychol (Paris) 1967:389.
3. McBride WG. The teratogenic action of drugs. Med J Aust 1963;2:689–93.
4. Heinonen OP, Slone D, Shapiro S. *Birth Defects and Drugs in Pregnancy*. Littleton:Publishing Sciences Group, 1977:372.
5. *Ibid*, 441.

Name: **ACETOHEXAMIDE**

Class: **Oral Hypoglycemic**   Risk Factor: **D**

Fetal Risk Summary

Acetohexamide is a sulfonylurea drug used for the treatment of adult-onset diabetes mellitus. It is not indicated for the pregnant diabetic. When administered near term, acetohexamide crosses the placenta and may persist in the neonatal serum for several days (1). One mother, who took 1 g/day throughout pregnancy, delivered an infant whose serum level was 4.4 mg/100 ml at 10 hours of life (1). Prolonged symptomatic hypoglycemia due to hyperinsulinism lasted for 5 days. If administered during pregnancy, acetohexamide should be stopped at least 48 hours before delivery to avoid this complication (2).

Although acetohexamide is teratogenic in animals, an increased incidence of congenital defects other than those expected in diabetes mellitus has not been found with acetohexamide (see also Chlorpropamide, Tolbutamide) (3–5). Maternal diabetes is known to increase the rate of malformations by 2- to 4-fold, but the mechanisms are not understood (see also Insulin). In spite of the lack of evidence for acetohexamide teratogenicity, the drug should not be used in pregnancy since it will not provide good control for diabetics whose disease cannot be controlled by diet alone (2). The manufacturer recommends the drug not be used in pregnancy (6).

Breast Feeding Summary

No data available (see Tolbutamide).

References

1. Kemball ML, McIver C, Milnar RDG, Nourse CH, Schiff D, Tiernan JR. Neonatal hypoglycaemia in infants of diabetic mothers given sulphonylurea drugs in pregnancy. Arch Dis Child 1970;45:696–701.
2. Friend JR. Diabetes. Clin Obstet Gynaecol 1981;8:353–82.
3. Malins JM, Cooke AM, Pyke DA, Fitzgerald MG. Sulphonylurea drugs in pregnancy. Br Med J 1964;2:187.
4. Adam PAJ, Schwartz R. Diagnosis and treatment: should oral hypoglycemic agents be used in pediatric and pregnant patients? Pediatrics 1968;42:819–23.
5. Dignan PSJ. Teratogenic risk and counseling in diabetes. Clin Obstet Gynecol 1981;24:149–59.
6. Product information. Dymelor. Eli Lilly & Co, Indianapolis, 1985.

Name: **ACETOPHENAZINE**

Class: **Tranquilizer**   Risk Factor: **C**

Fetal Risk Summary

Acetophenazine is a piperazine phenothiazine in the same group as prochlorperazine (see Prochlorperazine). Phenothiazines readily cross the placenta (1). No specific information on the use of acetophenazine in pregnancy has been located. Although occasional reports have attempted to link various phenothiazine compounds with congenital malformations, the bulk of the evidence indicates that these drugs are safe for the mother and the fetus (see also Chlorpromazine).

Breast Feeding Summary

No data available.

References

1. Moya F, Thorndike V. Passage of drugs across the placenta. Am J Obstet Gynecol 1962;84:1778–98.

Name: **ACETYLCHOLINE**

Class: **Parasympathomimetic (Cholinergic)**   Risk Factor: **C**

Fetal Risk Summary

Acetylcholine is used primarily in the eye. No reports of its use in pregnancy have been located. As a quaternary ammonium compound, it is ionized at physiologic pH, and transplacental passage in significant amounts would not be expected.

Breast Feeding Summary

No data available.

Name: **ACETYLDIGITOXIN**

Class: **Cardiac Glycoside**   Risk Factor: **C**

Fetal Risk Summary

See Digitalis.

Breast Feeding Summary

See Digitalis.

Name: **ACYCLOVIR**

Class: **Antiviral**   Risk Factor: **C$_M$**

Fetal Risk Summary

Acyclovir has been used intravenously (IV) in two women during the 3rd trimester for the treatment of disseminated herpes simplex (1, 2). In the first case, acyclovir, 7.5 mg/kg IV, was given every 8 hours for 20 doses with the last dose given shortly after delivery (1). The second patient received two courses of therapy, 5 mg/kg IV every 8 hours, for a total of 30 doses (2). Neither infant exhibited any toxicity from exposure to the antiviral agent.

Acyclovir applied topically may produce low levels of the drug in maternal serum, urine, and vaginal secretions (3). Although the antiviral agent has been used topically during pregnancy for the treatment of genital herpes, no published reports of these cases have yet appeared. The manufacturer is currently monitoring a group of these women during pregnancy, and data will be available when they deliver (4). They are also aware of two women treated topically during the 3rd trimester in England who delivered normal infants (4).

Breast Feeding Summary

No data available.

References

1. Lagrew DC Jr, Furlow TG, Hager WD, Yarrish RL. Disseminated herpes simplex virus infection in pregnancy. JAMA 1984;252:2058–9.
2. Grover L, Kane J, Kravitz J, Cruz A. Systemic acyclovir in pregnancy: a case report. Obstet Gynecol 1985;65:284–7.
3. Product information. Zovirax. Burroughs-Wellcome, Research Triangle Park, NC, 1985.
4. Burroughs-Wellcome, Research Triangle Park, NC, July 11, 1985. Personal communication.

Name: **ALBUTEROL**

Class: **Sympathomimetic (Adrenergic)**   Risk Factor: **C$_M$**

Fetal Risk Summary

Albuterol is a β-sympathomimetic used to prevent premature labor (see also Terbutaline and Ritodrine) (1–12). In an *in vitro* experiment using perfused human placentas, 2.8% of infused drug crossed to the fetal side (13).

No reports linking the use of albuterol to congenital anomalies have been located. In one patient, albuterol was infused continuously for 17 weeks via a catheter placed in the right subclavian vein (10, 14, 15). A normal male infant was delivered within a few hours of stopping the drug. A 1982 report described the use of albuterol in two women with incompetent cervix from the 14th week of gestation to near term (16). Both patients delivered normal infants.

Adverse reactions observed in the fetus and mother following albuterol treatment are secondary to the cardiovascular and metabolic effects of the drug. Albuterol may cause maternal and fetal tachycardia (1–3, 12, 17). Fetal rates may exceed 160 beats/min. Major decreases in maternal blood pressure have been reported with both systolic and diastolic values dropping more than 30 mm Hg (2, 4, 6). Fetal distress following maternal hypotension was not mentioned. One study observed a maximum decrease in diastolic pressure of 24 mm Hg (34% decrease) but a rise in systolic pressure (17). Other maternal adverse effects associated with albuterol have been acute congestive heart failure, pulmonary edema, and death (18–26).

Like all β-mimetics, albuterol may cause transient fetal and maternal hyperglycemia followed by an increase in serum insulin (4, 27–30). Cord blood levels of insulin are about twice those of untreated controls and are not dependent on the duration of exposure, gestational age, or birth weight (29, 30). These effects are more pronounced in diabetic patients, especially in juvenile diabetics, with the occurrence of significant increases in glycogenolysis and lipolysis (17, 31, 32). Maternal blood glucose should be closely monitored, and neonatal hypoglycemia can be prevented with adequate doses of glucose.

Albuterol decreases the incidence of neonatal respiratory distress syndrome similar to other β-mimetics (33, 34). Long-term evaluation of infants exposed to *in utero* β-mimetics has been reported but not specifically for albuterol (35, 36). No harmful effects in the infants were observed.

Breast Feeding Summary

No data available.

References

1. Liggins GC, Vaughan GS. Intravenous infusion of salbutamol in the management of premature labor. J Obstet Gynaecol Br Commonw 1973;80:29–33.
2. Korda AR, Lynerum RC, Jones WR. The treatment of premature labor with intravenous administered salbutamol. Med J Aust 1974;1:744–6.
3. Hastwell G. Salbutamol aerosol in premature labour. Lancet 1975;2:1212–3.
4. Hastwell GB, Halloway CP, Taylor TLO. A study of 208 patients in premature labor treated with orally administered salbutamol. Med J Aust 1978;1:465–9.
5. Hastwell G, Lambert BE. A comparison of salbutamol and ritodrine when used to inhibit premature labour complicated by ante-partum haemorrhage. Curr Med Res Opin 1979;5:785–9.

6. Ng KH, Sen DK. Hypotension with intravenous salbutamol in premature labour. Br Med J 1974;3:257.

7. Pincus R. Salbutamol infusion for premature labour—the Australian trials experience. Aust NZ Obstet Gynaecol 1981;21:1–4.

8. Gummerus M. The management of premature labor with salbutamol. Acta Obstet Gynecol Scand 1981;60:375–7.

9. Crowhurst JA. Salbutamol, obstetrics and anaesthesia: a review and case discussion. Anaesth Intensive Care 1980;8:39–43.

10. Lind T, Godfrey KA, Gerrard J, Bryson MR. Continuous salbutamol infusion over 17 weeks to pre-empt premature labour. Lancet 1980;2:1165–6.

11. Kuhn RJP, Speirs AL, Pepperell RJ, Eggers TR, Doyle LW, Hutchison A. Betamethasone, albuterol, and threatened premature delivery: benefits and risks. Study of 469 pregnancies. Obstet Gynecol 1982;60:403–8.

12. Eggers TR, Doyle LW, Pepperell RJ. Premature labour. Med J Aust 1979;1:213–6.

13. Sodha RJ, Schneider H. Transplacental transfer of β-adrenergic drugs studied by an in vitro perfusion method of an isolated human placental lobule. Am J Obstet Gynecol 1983;147:303–10.

14. Boylan P, O'Discoll K. Long-term salbutamol or successful Shirodkar suture? Lancet 1980;2:1374.

15. Addis GJ. Long-term salbutamol infusion to prevent premature labor. Lancet 1981;1:42–3.

16. Edmonds DK, Letchworth AT. Prophylactic oral salbutamol to prevent premature labour. Lancet 1982;1:1310–1.

17. Wager J, Fredholm B, Lunell NO, Persson B. Metabolic and circulatory effects of intravenous and oral salbutamol in late pregnancy in diabetic and non-diabetic women. Acta Obstet Gynecol Scand 1982; Suppl 108:41–6.

18. Whitehead MI, Mander AM, Hertogs K, Williams RM, Pettingale KW. Acute congestive cardiac failure in a hypertensive woman receiving salbutamol for premature labour. Br Med J 1980;280:1221–2.

19. Poole-Wilson PA. Cardiac failure in a hypertensive woman receiving salbutamol for premature labour. Br Med J 1980;281:226.

20. Fogarty AJ. *Ibid*.

21. Davies PDO. *Ibid*, 226–7.

22. Robertson M, Davies AE. *Ibid*, 227.

23. Crowley P. *Ibid*.

24. Whitehead MI, Mandere AM, Pettingale KW. *Ibid*.

25. Davies AE, Robertson MJS. Pulmonary oedema after the administration of intravenous salbutamol and ergometrine—case report. Br J Obstet Gynaecol 1980;87:539–41.

26. Milliez, Blot Ph, Sureau C. A case report of maternal death associated with mimetics and methasone administration in premature labor. Eur J Obstet Gynaecol Reprod Biol 1980;11:95–100.

27. Thomas DJB, Dove AF, Alberti KGMM. Metabolic effects of salbutamol infusion during premature labour. Br J Obstet Gynaecol 1977;84:497–9.

28. Wager J, Lunell NO, Nadal M, Ostman J. Glucose tolerance following oral salbutamol treatment in late pregnancy. Acta Obstet Gynecol Scand 1981;60:291–4.

29. Lunell NO, Joelsson I, Larsson A, Persson B. The immediate effect of a β-adrenergic agonist (salbutamol) on carbohydrate and lipid metabolism during the third trimester of pregnancy. Acta Obstet Gynecol Scand 1977;56:475–8.

30. Procianoy RS, Pinheiro CEA. Neonatal hyperinsulinism after short-term maternal sympathomimetic therapy. J Pediatr 1982;101:612–4.

31. Barnett AH, Stubbs SM, Mander AM. Management of premature labour in diabetic pregnancy. Diabetologia 1980;188:365–8.

32. Wager J, Fredholm BB, Lunell NO, Persson B. Metabolic and circulatory effects of oral salbutamol in the third trimester of pregnancy in diabetic and non-diabetic women. Br J Obstet Gynaecol 1981;88:352–61.

33. Hastwell GB. Apgar scores, respiratory distress syndrome and salbutamol. Med J Aust 1980;1:174–5.

34. Hastwell G. Salbutamol and respiratory distress syndrome. Lancet 1977;2:354.

35. Wallace RL, Caldwell DL, Ansbacher R, Otterson WN. Inhibition of premature labor by terbutaline. Obstet Gynecol 1978;51:387–92.

36. Freysz H, Willard D, Lehr A, Messer J, Boog G. A long term evaluation of infants who received a β-mimetic drug while in utero. J Perinat Med 1977;5:94–9.

Name: **ALPHAPRODINE**

Class: **Narcotic Analgesic**   Risk Factor: C_M*

Fetal Risk Summary

No reports linking the use of alphaprodine with congenital defects have been located. Characteristic of all narcotics used in labor, alphaprodine may produce respiratory depression in the newborn (1–8). Tissue pO_2 and pCO_2 were determined in nine women in active labor at term given intravenous alphaprodine, 0.4 mg/kg (prepregnancy weight) (9). Peak decreases in $tcpO_2$ occurred at 5 minutes postinjection with peak increases of $tcpCO_2$ occurring at 20 minutes. Both changes were statistically significant variations from baseline values. The fetal heart rate fell from a mean predose rate of 139 beats/min to 132 beats/min at 20 minutes, a significant change, with a consistent loss of variability occurring at 25 minutes. No adverse effects in the mother or fetus were noted.

In a group of 40 women treated with alphaprodine during labor, sinusoidal fetal heart rate patterns were observed in 17 fetuses (42.5%) (10). The pattern occurred about 19 minutes after administration of the narcotic and persisted for about 60 minutes. No apparent harm resulted from the abnormal patterns.

Suppression of collagen-induced platelet aggregation has been demonstrated, but specific data were not given (11). Abnormal bleeding following use of this drug has not been reported even though the magnitude of platelet dysfunction was comparable to that found in hemorrhagic states.

[* Risk Factor D if used for prolonged periods or in high doses at term.]

Breast Feeding Summary

No data available.

References

1. Smith EJ, Nagyfy SF. A report on comparative studies of new drugs used for obstetrical analgesia. Am J Obstet Gynecol 1949;58:695–702.
2. Hapke FB, Barnes AC. The obstetric use and effect on fetal respiration of Nisentil. Am J Obstet Gynecol 1949;58:799–801.
3. Kane WM. The results of Nisentil in 1,000 obstetrical cases. Am J Obstet Gynecol 1953;65:1020–6.
4. Backner DD, Foldes FF, Gordon EH. The combined use of alphaprodine (Nisentil) hydrochloride and levallorphan (Lorfan) tartrate for analgesia in obstetrics. Am J Obstet Gynecol 1957;74:271–82.
5. Gillan JS, Hunter GW, Darner CB, Thompson GR. Meperidine hydrochloride and alphaprodine hydrochloride as obstetric analgesic agents; a double-blind study. Am J Obstet Gynecol 1958;75:1105–10.
6. Roberts H, Kuck MAC. Use of alphaprodine and levallorphan during labour. Can Med Assoc J 1960;83:1088–93.
7. Burnett RG, White CA. Alphaprodine for continuous intravenous obstetric analgesia. Obstet Gynecol 1966;27:472–7.
8. Anthinarayanan PR, Mangurten HH. Unusually prolonged action of maternal alphaprodine causing fetal depression. Q Pediatr Bull 1977;3(Winter):14–6.
9. Miller FC, Mueller E, McCart D. Maternal and fetal response to alphaprodine during labor. A preliminary study. J Reprod Med 1982;27:439–42.
10. Gray JH, Cudmore DW, Luther ER, Martin TR, Gardner AJ. Sinusoidal fetal heart rate pattern associated with alphaprodine administration. Obstet Gynecol 1978;52:678–81.
11. Corby DG, Schulman I. The effects of antenatal drug administration on aggregation of platelets of newborn infants. J Pediatr 1971;79:307–13.

Name: **AMANTADINE**

Class: **Antiviral/Antiparkinsonism** Risk Factor: C_M

Fetal Risk Summary

A cardiovascular defect (single ventricle with pulmonary atresia) has been reported in an infant exposed to amantadine during the 1st trimester (1). The mother was taking 100 mg/day for a Parkinson-like movement disorder. The relationship between the drug and the defect is unknown. Amantadine is embryotoxic and teratogenic in animals in high doses (1, 2). Theoretically, amantadine may be a human teratogen, but the absence of reports may have more to do with the probable infrequency of use in pregnant patients than to its teratogenic potency (3).

Breast Feeding Summary

Amantadine is excreted into breast milk in low concentrations. Although no reports of adverse effects in nursing infants have been located, the manufacturer recommends the drug be used with caution in nursing mothers because of the potential for urinary retention, vomiting, and skin rash (2, 4).

References

1. Nora JJ, Nora AH, Way GL. Cardiovascular maldevelopment associated with maternal exposure to amantadine. Lancet 1975;2:607.
2. Product Information. Symmetrel. Du Pont Pharmaceuticals, 1985.
3. Coulson AS. Amantadine and teratogenesis. Lancet 1975;2:1044.
4. Committee on Drugs, American Academy of Pediatrics. The transfer of drugs and other chemicals into human breast milk. Pediatrics 1983;72:375–83.

Name: **AMBENONIUM**

Class: **Parasympathomimetic (Cholinergic)** Risk Factor: **C**

Fetal Risk Summary

Ambenonium is a quaternary ammonium chloride with anticholinesterase activity that is used in the treatment of myasthenia gravis. It has been used in pregnancy, but too little data are available to analyze (1, 2). Because it is ionized at physiologic pH, it would not be expected to cross the placenta in significant amounts. McNall and Jafarnia (1) have cautioned that intravenous anticholinesterases should not be used in pregnancy for fear of inducing premature labor.

Breast Feeding Summary

Because it is ionized at physiologic pH, ambenonium would not be expected to be excreted into breast milk (3).

References

1. McNall PG, Jafarnia MR. Management of myasthenia gravis in the obstetrical patient. Am J Obstet Gynecol 1965;92:518–25.
2. Heinonen OP, Slone D, Shapiro S. *Birth Defects and Drugs in Pregnancy*. Littleton: Publishing Sciences Group, 1977:345–56.
3. Wilson JT. Pharmacokinetics of drug excretion. In Wilson JT, ed. *Drugs in Breast Milk*. Balgowlah, Australia: ADIS Press, 1981:17.

Name: **AMIKACIN**

Class: **Antibiotic**   Risk Factor: **C**

Fetal Risk Summary

Amikacin is an aminoglycoside antibiotic. The drug rapidly crosses the placenta into the fetal circulation and amniotic fluid (1–4). Studies in patients undergoing elective abortions in the 1st and 2nd trimesters indicate that amikacin is distributed to most fetal tissues except the brain and cerebrospinal fluid (1, 3). The highest fetal concentrations were found in the kidneys and urine. At term, cord serum levels were ½ to ⅓ of maternal serum levels while measurable amniotic fluid levels did not appear until almost 5 hours postinjection (2).

No reports linking the use of amikacin to congenital defects have been located. Ototoxicity, which is known to occur after amikacin therapy, has not been reported as an effect of *in utero* exposure. However, eighth cranial nerve toxicity in the fetus is well known following exposure to other aminoglycosides (see Kanamycin and Streptomycin) and may potentially occur with amikacin.

Breast Feeding Summary

Amikacin is excreted into breast milk in low concentrations. Following 100- and 200-mg intramuscular doses, only traces of amikacin could be found over 6 hours in two of four patients (2, 5). Since oral absorption of this antibiotic is poor, ototoxicity in the infant would not be expected. However, three potential problems exist for the nursing infant: modification of bowel flora, direct effects on the infant, and interference with the interpretation of culture results if a fever work-up is required.

References

1. Bernard B, Abate M, Ballard C, Wehrle P. Maternal-fetal pharmacology of BB-K8. Antimicrob Agents Chemother 14th Ann Conf, Abstr 71, 1974.
2. Matsuda C, Mori C, Maruno M, Shiwakura T. A study of amikacin in the obstetrics field. Jpn J Antibiot 1974;27:633–6.
3. Bernard B, Abate M, Thielen P, Attar H, Ballard C, Wehrle P. Maternal-fetal pharmacological activity of amikacin. J Infect Dis 1977;135:925–31.
4. Flores-Mercado F, Garcia-Mercado J, Estopier-Jauregin C, Galindo-Hernandez E, Diaz-Gonzalez C. Clinical pharmacology of amikacin sulphate: blood, urinary and tissue concentrations in the terminal stage of pregnancy. J Int Med Res 1977;5;292–4.
5. Yuasa M. A study of amikacin in obstetrics and gynecology. Jpn J Antibiot 1974;27;377–81.

Name: **AMILORIDE**

Class: **Diuretic**   Risk Factor: **B$_M$**

Fetal Risk Summary

Amiloride is a potassium-conserving diuretic. Animal studies have not shown adverse effects in the fetus (1). Only one report of fetal exposure to amiloride has been located. In this case, a malformed fetus was discovered following voluntary abortion in a patient with renovascular hypertension (2). The patient had been treated during the 1st trimester with amiloride, propranolol, and captopril. The left leg of the fetus ended at mid-thigh without distal development, and no obvious skull formation was noted above the brain tissue. The authors attributed the defects to captopril.

Breast Feeding Summary

No data available.

References

1. Product Information. Midamor. Merck, Sharp and Dohme, 1985.
2. Duminy PC, Burger PT. Fetal abnormality associated with the use of captopril during pregnancy. S Afr Med J 1981;60:805.

Name: **AMINOCAPROIC ACID**

Class: **Hemostatic**   Risk Factor: **C**

Fetal Risk Summary

Aminocaproic acid was used during the 2nd trimester in a patient with subarachnoid hemorrhage due to multiple intracranial aneurysms (1). The drug was given over 3 days preceding surgery (dosage not given). No fetal toxicity was observed.

Breast Feeding Summary

No data available.

References

1. Willoughby JS. Sodium nitroprusside, pregnancy and multiple intracranial aneurysms. Anaesth Intensive Care 1984;12:358–60.

Name: **AMINOGLUTETHIMIDE**

Class: **Anticonvulsant/Antisteroidogenic**   Risk Factor: D_M

Fetal Risk Summary

Aminoglutethimide when given throughout pregnancy has been suspected of causing virilization (1, 2). No adverse effect was seen when exposure was limited to the 1st and early 2nd trimesters (3, 4). Virilization may be due to inhibition of adrenocortical function.

Breast Feeding Summary

No data available.

References

1. Iffy L, Ansell JS, Bryant FS, Hermann WL. Nonadrenal female pseudohermaphroditism: an unusual case of fetal masculinization. Obstet Gynecol 1965;26;59–65.
2. Marek J, Horky K. Aminoglutethimide administration in pregnancy. Lancet 1970;2:1312–3.
3. Le Maire WJ, Cleveland WW, Bejar RL, Marsh JM, Fishman L. Aminoglutethimide: a possible cause of pseudohermaphroditism in females. Am J Dis Child 1972;124:421–3.
4. Hanson TJ, Ballonoff LB, Northcutt RC. Aminoglutethimide and pregnancy. JAMA 1974;230:963–4.

Name: **AMINOPHYLLINE**

Class: **Spasmolytic/Vasodilator**   Risk Factor: **C**

Fetal Risk Summary

See Theophylline.

Breast Feeding Summary

See Theophylline.

Name: **AMINOPTERIN**

Class: **Antineoplastic**   Risk Factor: **X**

Fetal Risk Summary

Aminopterin is an antimetabolite antineoplastic agent. It is structurally similar to and has been replaced by methotrexate (amethopterin). Several reports have described fetal anomalies when the drug was used as an unsuccessful abortifacient (1–8). The malformations included:

Meningocephalocele	Cleft lip/palate
Cranial anomalies	Low-set ears

Abnormal positioning of extremities	Hypoplasia of thumb and fibula
Short forearms	Brachycephaly
Hydrocephaly	Anencephaply
Talipes	Clubfoot
Incomplete skull ossification	Syndactyly
	Hypognathia or retrognathia

Use of aminopterin in the 2nd and 3rd trimesters has not been associated with congenital defects (8). Long-term studies of growth and mental development in offspring exposed to aminopterin during the 2nd trimester, the period of neuroblast multiplication, have not been conducted (9).

Breast Feeding Summary

No data available.

References

1. Meltzer HJ. Congenital anomalies due to attempted abortion with 4-aminopteroglutamic acid. JAMA 1956;161:1253.
2. Warkany J, Beaudry PH, Hornstein S. Attempted abortion with aminopterin (4-amino-pteroylglutamic acid). Am J Dis Child 1959;97:274–81.
3. Shaw EB, Steinbach HL. Aminopterin-induced fetal malformation. Am J Dis Child 1968;115:477–82.
4. Brandner M, Nussle D. Foetopathic due a l'aminopterine avec stenose cogenitale de l'espace medullaire des os tubulaires ongs. Ann Radiol 1969;12:705–10.
5. Shaw EB. Fetal damage due to maternal aminopterin ingestion: follow-up at age 9 years. Am J Dis Child 1972;124:93–4.
6. Reich EW, Cox RP, Becker MH, Genieser NB, McCarthy JG, Converse JM. Recognition in adult patients of malformations induced by folic-acid antagonists. Birth Defects 1978;14:139–60.
7. Shaw EB, Rees EL. Fetal damage due to aminopterin ingestion: follow-up at 17 ½ years of age. Am J Dis Child 1980;134:1172–3.
8. Nicholson HO. Cytotoxic drugs in pregnancy; review of reported cases. J Obstet Gynaecol Br Commonw 1968;75:307–12.
9. Dobbing J. Pregnancy and leukemia. Lancet 1977;1:1155.

Name: *para*-AMINOSALICYLIC ACID

Class: **Antitubercular**   Risk Factor: **C**

Fetal Risk Summary

The Collaborative Perinatal Project monitored 50,282 mother-child pairs, 43 of which had 1st trimester exposure to *para*-aminosalicylic acid (1). Congenital defects were found in five infants. This incidence (11.6%) was nearly twice the expected frequency. No major category of malformations or individual defects was identified. An increased malformation rate for ear and limb and hypospadias have been reported for 123 patients taking 7–14 g of *para*-aminosalicylic acid per day with other antitubercular drugs (2). An increased risk of congenital defects has not been found in other studies (3–5).

Breast Feeding Summary

No data available.

References

1. Heinonen OP, Slone D, Shapiro S. *Birth Defects and Drugs in Pregnancy*. Littleton:Publishing Sciences Group, 1977:299.
2. Varpela E. On the effect exerted by first line tuberculosis medicines on the foetus. Acta Tuberc Scand 1964;35:53–69.
3. Lowe CR. Congenital defects among children born to women under supervision or treatment for pulmonary tuberculosis. Br J Prev Soc Med 1964;18:14–6.
4. Wilson EA, Thelin TJ, Ditts PV. Tuberculosis complicated by pregnancy. Am J Obstet Gynecol 1973;115;526–9.
5. Scheinhorn DJ, Angelillo VA. Antituberculosis therapy in pregnancy. Risk to the fetus. West J Med 1977;127;195–8.

Name: **AMIODARONE**

Class: **Antiarrhythmic** Risk Factor: **C**

Fetal Risk Summary

Amiodarone is an antiarrhythmic agent used for difficult or resistant cases of arrhythmias. The drug contains about 75 mg of iodine per 200-mg dose (1–3).

Experience in pregnancy is limited. Only four women who carried their infants to term are known to have been treated during gestation (1–3). In each of these cases, drug levels of amiodarone and its metabolite, desethylamiodarone, were determined in cord and maternal serum at delivery. Cord serum levels of the active drug and the metabolite (activity unknown) were 0.07–0.2 and 0.15–0.26 μg/ml, respectively. These levels represented cord:maternal ratios of 0.10–0.15 and 0.19–0.29, respectively (1–3).

Treatment intervals during pregnancy have ranged from 3 weeks to the entire gestational period. In one woman, amiodarone was begun at 34 weeks gestation when quinidine therapy failed (1). After an initial dose of 800 mg/day for 1 week, the dose was decreased to 400 mg/day and continued at this level until delivery at 41 weeks gestation. The healthy infant had bradycardia during labor induction (104–120 beats/min) and during the first 48 hours after birth. No other adverse effects were observed. In a second case, a woman was treated during the 37th–39th weeks of pregnancy with daily doses of 600, 400, and 200 mg, each for 1 week (2). No bradycardia or other abnormalities were noted in the newborn. A 1985 report described two women, one treated during the final 17 weeks of pregnancy and one throughout gestation (3). Doses varied from 200 to 800 mg/day, and both patients received diuretics and other medications. Bradycardia (100–120 beats/min) was observed in the fetus of one woman. Both newborns were normal with no apparent ill effects from the exposure. Newborn bradycardia was not mentioned.

Investigators using amiodarone during pregnancy have been concerned about the effects of the iodine contained in each dose on the fetal thyroid gland (see Potassium Iodide for fetal effects of iodine) (1–3). However, none of the four newborns had goiter, and all had normal thyroid function tests. Other abnormalities associated with amiodarone, such as corneal defects, were also absent.

Following chronic administration, amiodarone has a very long elimination half-life of 14–58 days (4). Therefore, the drug must be stopped several months before conception to avoid exposure in early gestation. Although no adverse effects other than transient bradycardia have been observed, the drug should be used with caution during pregnancy due to the limited data available. Newborns exposed to amiodarone *in utero* should have thyroid function studies performed because of the large proportion of iodine contained in each dose.

Breast Feeding Summary

Amiodarone is excreted into breast milk (1, 2). The drug contains about 75 mg of iodine per 200-mg dose (1–3). One woman, consuming 400 mg/day, had milk levels of amiodarone and its metabolite, desethylamiodarone (activity unknown), determined at varying times between 9–63 days after delivery (1). Levels of the two substances in milk were highly variable during any 24-hour period. Peak levels of amiodarone and the metabolite ranged from 3.6–16.4 and 1.3–6.5 μg/ml. The milk:plasma ratio of the active drug at 9 weeks postpartum ranged from 2.3 to 9.1 and that of desethylamiodarone from 0.8 to 3.8. The authors calculated that the nursing infant received about 1.4–1.5 mg/kg/day of active drug. Plasma levels of amiodarone in the infant remained constant at 0.4 μg/ml (about 25% of maternal plasma) from birth to 63 days. In a second case, a mother taking 200 mg/day did not breast-feed her infant, but milk levels of the drug and the metabolite on the 2nd and 3rd days after delivery ranged from 0.5–1.8 and 0.4–0.8 μg/ml, respectively (2).

Although no adverse effects were observed in the one breast-fed infant, relatively large amounts of the drug and its metabolite are available through the milk. Amiodarone, after chronic administration, has a very long elimination half-life of 14–58 days in adults (4). Data in pediatric patients suggest a more rapid elimination, but the half-life in newborns has not been determined. The effects of chronic neonatal exposure to this drug are unknown. Because of this uncertainty and also due to the high proportion of iodine contained in each dose (see also Potassium Iodide), breast-feeding is not recommended if the mother is currently taking amiodarone or has taken it chronically within the past several months.

References

1. McKenna WJ, Harris L, Rowland E, Whitelaw A, Storey G, Holt D. Amiodarone therapy during pregnancy. Am J Cardiol 1983;51:1231–3.
2. Pitcher D, Leather HM, Storey GAC, Holt DW. Amiodarone in pregnancy. Lancet 1983;1:597–8.
3. Robson DJ, Jeeva Raj MV, Storey GAC, Holt DW. Use of amiodarone during pregnancy. Postgrad Med J 1985;61:75–7.
4. Sloskey GE. Amiodarone: a unique antiarrhythmic agent. Clin Pharm 1983;2:330–40.

Name: **AMITRIPTYLINE**

Class: **Antidepressant**   Risk Factor: **D**

Fetal Risk Summary

Limb reduction anomalies have been reported with amitriptyline (1). However, analysis of 522,630 births, 86 with 1st trimester exposure to amitriptyline, did not confirm an association with this defect (2–9). Reported malformations other than limb reduction defects include (4, 8, 9):

> Micrognathia, anomalous right mandible, left pes equinovaruus (1 case)
> Swelling of hands and feet (1 case)
> Hypospadias (1 case)

Neonatal withdrawal following *in utero* exposure to other antidepressants (see Imipramine) has been reported but not with amitriptyline. However, the potential for this complication exists due to the close similarity among these compounds.

Urinary retention in the neonate has been associated with maternal use of nortriptyline, an amitriptyline metabolite (see Nortriptyline) (10).

Breast Feeding Summary

Amitriptyline and its metabolite, nortriptyline, are excreted into breast milk (11–13). Serum and milk concentrations of amitriptyline in one patient were 0.14 and 0.15 μg/ml, respectively, a milk:plasma ratio of 1.0 (11). No drug was detected in the infant's serum. In another patient, estimates indicated that the baby received about 1% of the mother's dose (13). No clinical signs of drug activity were observed in the infant.

Although levels of amitriptyline and its metabolite have not been detected in infant serum, the effects of exposure to small amounts in the milk are not known (11–14). The American Academy of Pediatrics considers amitriptyline compatible with breast-feeding (15).

References

1. McBride WG. Limb deformities associated with iminodibenzyl hydrochloride. Med J Aust 1972;1:492.
2. Australian Drug Evaluation Committee. Tricyclic antidepressants and limb reduction deformities. Med J Aust 1973;1:768–9.
3. Heinonen OP, Slone D, Shapiro S. *Birth Defects and Drugs in Pregnancy*. Littleton:Publishing Sciences Group, 1977:336–7.
4. Idanpaan-Heikkila J, Saxen L. Possible teratogenicity of imipramine/chloropyramine. Lancet 1973;2:282–3.
5. Rachelefsky GS, Glynt JW, Ebbin AJ, Wilson MG. Possible teratogenicity of tricyclic antidepressants. Lancet 1972;1:838.
6. Banister P, Dafoe C, Smith ESO, Miller J. Possible teratogenicity of tricyclic antidepressants. Lancet 1972;1:838–9.
7. Scanlon FJ. Use of antidepressant drugs during the first trimester. Med J Aust 1969;2:1077.
8. Crombie DL, Pinsent R, Fleming D. Imipramine in pregnancy. Br Med J 1972;1:745.
9. Kuenssberg EV, Knox JDE. Imipramine in pregnancy. Br Med J 1972;2:292.
10. Shearer WT, Schreiner RL, Marshall RE. Urinary retention in a neonate secondary to maternal ingestion of nortriptyline. J Pediatr 1972;81:570–2.
11. Bader TF, Newman K. Amitriptyline in human breast milk and the nursing infant's serum. Am J Psychiatry 1980;137;855–6.

12. Wilson JT, Brown D, Cherek DR, Dailey JW, Hilman B, Jobe PC, Manno BR, Manno JE, Redetzki HM, Stewart JJ. Drug excretion in human breast milk. Principles, pharmacokinetics and projected consequences. Clin Pharmacokinet 1980;5:1–66.
13. Brixen-Rasmussen L, Halgrener J, Jorgensen A. Amitriptyline and nortriptyline excretion in human breast milk. Psychopharmacology (Berlin) 1982;76:94–5.
14. Erickson SH, Smith GH, Heidrich F. Tricyclics and breast feeding. Am J Psychiartry 1979;136:1483.
15. Committee on Drugs, American Academy of Pediatrics. The transfer of drugs and other chemicals into human breast milk. Pediatrics 1983;72:375–83.

Name: **AMMONIUM CHLORIDE**

Class: **Expectorant/Urinary Acidifier**   Risk Factor: **B**

Fetal Risk Summary

The Collaborative Perinatal Project monitored 50,282 mother-child pairs, 365 of which had 1st trimester exposure to ammonium chloride as an expectorant in cough medications (1). For use anytime during pregnancy, 3,401 exposures were recorded (2). In neither case was evidence found to suggest a relationship to large categories of major or minor malformations. Three possible associations with individual malformations were found, but the statistical significance of these is unknown (3, 4). Independent confirmation is required to determine the actual risk:

Inguinal hernia (1st trimester only) (11 cases)
Cataract (6 cases)
Any benign tumor (17 cases)

When consumed in large quantities near term, ammonium chloride may cause acidosis in the mother and the fetus (5, 6). In some cases, the decreased pH and pCO_2, increased lactic acid, and reduced oxygen saturation were as severe as those seen with fatal apnea neonatorum. However, the newborns did not appear to be in distress.

Breast Feeding Summary

No data available.

References

1. Heinonen OP, Slone D, Shapiro S. *Birth Defects and Drugs in Pregnancy*. Littleton:Publishing Sciences Group, 1977:378–81.
2. *Ibid*, 442.
3. *Ibid*, 478.
4. *Ibid*, 496.
5. Goodlin RC, Kaiser IH. The effect of ammonium chloride induced maternal acidosis on the human fetus at term. I. pH, hemoglobin, blood gases. Am J Med Sci 1957;233:666–74.
6. Kaiser IH, Goodlin RC. The effect of ammonium chloride induced maternal acidosis on the human fetus at term. II. Electrolytes. Am J Med Sci 1958;235:549–54.

Name: **AMOBARBITAL**

Class: **Sedative/Hypnotic** Risk Factor: **D***

Fetal Risk Summary

Amobarbital is a member of the barbiturate class. The drug crosses the placenta, achieving levels in the cord serum similar to those in the maternal serum (1, 2). Single or continuous dosing of the mother near term does not induce amobarbital hydroxylation in the fetus as demonstrated by the prolonged elimination of the drug in the newborn (half-life 2.5 times maternal). An increase in the incidence of congenital defects in infants exposed *in utero* to amobarbital has been reported (3, 4). One survey of 1,369 patients exposed to multiple drugs found 273 who received amobarbital during the 1st trimester (3). Ninety-five of the exposed mothers delivered infants with major or minor abnormalities. Malformations associated with barbiturates, in general, were:

Anencephaly	Congenital dislocation of the hip
Congenital heart disease	Soft tissue deformity of the neck
Severe limb deformities	Hypospadias
Cleft lip and palate	Accessory auricle
Intersex	Polydactyly
Papilloma of the forehead	Nevus
Hydrocele	

The Collaborative Perinatal Project monitored 50,282 mother-child pairs, 298 of which had 1st trimester exposure to amobarbital (4). For use anytime during pregnancy, 867 exposures were recorded (5). A possible association was found between the use of the drug in the 1st trimester and the following:

Cardiovascular malformations (7 cases)
Polydactyly in blacks (2 cases in 29 blacks)
Genitourinary malformations other than hypospadias (3 cases)
Inguinal hernia (9 cases)
Clubfoot (4 cases)

In contrast to the above reports, a 1964 survey of 187 pregnant patients who had received various taken neuroleptics, including amobarbital, found a 3.1% incidence of malformations in the offspring (6). This is approximately the expected incidence of abnormalities in a nonexposed population. Arthrogryposis and multiple defects were reported in an infant exposed to amobarbital during the 1st trimester (7). The defects were attributed to immobilization of the limbs at the time of joint formation, multiple drug use, and active tetanus.

[* Risk Factor B according to manufacturer—Eli Lilly & Co, 1985.]

Breast Feeding Summary

No data available.

References

1. Kraver B, Draffan GH, Williams FM, Calre RA, Dollery CT, Hawkins DF. Elimination kinetics of amobarbital in mothers and newborn infants. Clin Pharmacol Ther 1973;14:442–7.

2. Draffan GH, Dollery CT, Davies DS, Krauer B, Williams FM, Clare RA, Trudinger BJ, Darling M, Sertel H, Hawkins DF. Maternal and neonatal elimination of amobarbital after treatment of the mother with barbiturates during late pregnancy. Clin Pharmacol Ther 1976;19:271–5.
3. Nelson MM, Forfar JO. Associations between drugs administered during pregnancy and congenital abnormalities of the fetus. Br Med J 1971;1:523–7.
4. Heinonen OP, Slone D, Shapiro S. Birth Defects and Drugs in Pregnancy. Littleton:Publishing Sciences Group, 1977:336, 344.
5. Ibid, 438.
6. Favre-Tissot M, Broussole P, Robert JM, Dumont L. An original clinical study of the pharmacologic-teratogenic relationship. Ann Med Psychol (Paris) 1967:389.
7. Jago RH. Arthrogryposis following treatment of maternal tetanus with muscle relaxants. Arch Dis Child 1970;45:277–9.

Name: **AMOXAPINE**

Class: **Antidepressant**   Risk Factor: **C_M**

Fetal Risk Summary

No reports linking the use of amoxapine with congenital defects have been located. Animal studies have demonstrated embryotoxicity and fetotoxicity but no teratogenic effects (1).

Breast Feeding Summary

No reports on the excretion of amoxapine into breast milk have been located. The American Academy of Pediatrics considers the drug compatible with breast-feeding (2).

References

1. Product information. Asendin. Lederle Laboratories, 1985.
2. Committee on Drugs, American Academy of Pediatrics. The transfer of drugs and other chemicals into human breast milk. Pediatrics 1983;72:375–83.

Name: **AMOXICILLIN**

Class: **Antibiotic**   Risk Factor: **B**

Fetal Risk Summary

Amoxicillin is a penicillin antibiotic similar to ampicillin (see also Ampicillin). No reports linking its use to congenital defects have been located. The Collaborative Perinatal Project monitored 50,282 mother-child pairs, 3,546 of which had 1st trimester exposure to penicillin derivatives (1). For use anytime during pregnancy, 7,171 exposures were recorded (2). In neither case was evidence found to suggest a relationship to large categories of major or minor malformations or to individual defects. Amoxicillin has been used as a single 3-g dose to treat bacteriuria in pregnancy without causing fetal harm (3).

Amoxicillin depresses both plasma-bound and urinary-excreted estriol (see also Ampicillin) (4). Urinary estriol was formerly used to assess the condition of the fetoplacental unit, but this is now done by measuring plasma unconjugated estriol which is not usually affected by amoxicillin.

Breast Feeding Summary

Amoxicillin is excreted into breast milk in low concentrations. Following a 1-g oral dose given to six mothers, peak milk levels occurred at 4–5 hours, averaging 0.9 μg/ml (range 0.68–1.3 μg/ml) (5). Mean milk:plasma ratios at 1, 2, and 3 hours were 0.014, 0.013, and 0.043, respectively. Although no adverse effects have been observed, three potential problems exist for the nursing infant: modification of bowel flora, direct effects on the infant (e.g., allergy/sensitization), and interference with the interpretation of culture results if a fever work-up is required.

References

1. Heinonen OP, Slone D, Shapiro S. *Birth Defects and Drugs in Pregnancy*. Littleton:Publishing Sciences Group, 1977:297–313.
2. *Ibid*, 435.
3. Masterton RG, Evans DC, Strike PW. Single-dose amoxycillin in the treatment of bacteriuria in pregnancy and the puerperium—a controlled clinical trial. Br J Obstet Gynaecol 1985;92:498–505.
4. Van Look PFA, Top-Huisman M, Gnodde HP. Effect of ampicillin or amoxycillin administration on plasma and urinary estrogen levels during normal pregnancy. Eur J Obstet Gynaecol Reprod Biol 1981;12:225–33.
5. Kafetzis D, Siafas C, Georgakopoulos P, Papadatos C. Passage of cephalosporins and amoxicillin into the breast milk. Acta Paediatr Scand 1981; 70:285–8.

Name: **AMPHOTERICIN B**

Class: **Antifungal Antibotic**   Risk Factor: **B**

Fetal Risk Summary

No reports linking the use of amphotericin B with congenital defects have been located. The Collaboratorive Perinatal Project monitored 50,282 mother-child pairs, 9 of which had 1st trimester exposure to amphotericin B (1). Numerous other reports have also described the use of amphotericin B during various stages of pregnancy, including the 1st trimester (2–17). No evidence of adverse fetal effects was found by these studies. Amphotericin B can be used during pregnancy in those patients who will clearly benefit from the drug.

Breast Feeding Summary

No data available.

References

1. Heinonen OP, Slone D, Shapiro S. *Birth Defects and Drugs in Pregnancy*. Littleton:Publishing Sciences Group, 1977:297.
2. Neiberg AD, Maruomatis F, Dyke J, Fayyad A. Blastomyces dermatitidis treated during pregnancy. Am J Obstet Gynecol 1977;128:911–2.
3. Philpot CR, Lo D. Cryptococcal meningitis in pregnancy. Med J Aust 1972;2:1005–7.
4. Aitken GWE, Symonds EM. Cryptococcal meningitis in pregnancy treated with amphotericin. Br J Obstet Gynaecol 1962;69:677–9.
5. Feldman R. Cryptococcosis of the CNS treated with amphotericin B during pregnancy. South Med J 1959;2:1415–7.
6. Kuo D. A case of torulosis of the central nervous system during pregnancy. Med J Aust 1962;1:558–60.
7. Crotty JM. Systemic mycotic infections in northern territory aborigines. Med J Aust 1965;1:184.
8. Littman ML. Cryptococcosis (torulosis). Current concepts and therapy. Am J Med 1959;27:976–8.
9. Mick R, Muller-Tyl E, Neufeld T. Comparison of the effectiveness of Nystatin and amphotericin B in the therapy of female genital mycoses. Wien Med Wochenschr 1975;125:131–5.

10. Silberfarb PM, Sarois GA, Tosh FE. Cryptococcosis and pregnancy. Am J Obstet Gynecol 1972;112:714–20.
11. McCoy MJ, Ellenberg JF, Killam AP. Coccidioidomycosis complicating pregnancy. Am J Obstet Gynecol 1980;137:739–40.
12. Curole DN. Cryptococcal meningitis in pregnancy. J Reprod Med 1981;26:317–9.
13. Sanford WG, Rasch JR, Stonehill RB. A therapeutic dilemma: the treatment of disseminated coccidioidomycosis with amphotericin B. Ann Intern Med 1962;56:553–63.
14. Harris RE. Coccidioidomycosis complicating pregnancy. Report of 3 cases and review of the literature. Obstet Gynecol 1966;28:401–5.
15. Smale LE, Waechter KG. Dissemination of coccidioidomycosis in pregnancy. Am J Obstet Gynecol 1970;107:356–9.
16. Hadsall FJ, Acquarelli MJ. Disseminated coccidioidomycosis presenting as facial granulomas in pregnancy: a report of two cases and a review of the literature. Laryngoscope 1973;83:51–8.
17. Ismail MA, Lerner SA. Disseminated blastomycosis in a pregnant woman. Review of amphotericin B usage during pregnancy. Am Rev Respir Dis 1982;126:350–3.

Name: **AMPICILLIN**

Class: **Antibiotic**   Risk Factor: **B**

Fetal Risk Summary

Ampicillin is a penicillin antibiotic (see also Penicillin G). The drug rapidly crosses the placenta into the fetal circulation and amniotic fluid (1–6). Fetal serum levels can be detected within 30 minutes and equilibrate with maternal serum in 1 hour. Amniotic fluid drug levels can be detected in 90 minutes, reaching 20% of the maternal serum peak in about 8 hours. The pharmacokinetics of ampicillin during pregnancy have been reported (7, 8).

Ampicillin depresses both plasma-bound and urinary-excreted estriol by inhibiting steroid conjugate hydrolysis in the gut (9–13). Urinary estriol was formerly used to assess the condition of the fetoplacental unit, depressed levels being associated with fetal distress. This assessment is now made by measuring plasma unconjugated estriol, which is not usually affected by ampicillin. An interaction between ampicillin and oral contraceptives resulting in pregnancy has been suspected (14, 15). Two studies, however, failed to confirm this interaction and concluded that alternate contraceptive methods were not necessary during ampicillin therapy (16, 17).

No reports linking the use of ampicillin with congenital defects have been located. The drug apparently does not exert a toxic effect on the developing fetus (16). The Collaborative Perinatal Project monitored 50,282 mother-child pairs, 3,546 of which had 1st trimester exposure to penicillin derivatives (18). For use anytime during pregnancy, 7,171 exposures were recorded (19). In neither case was evidence found to suggest a relationship to large categories of major or minor malformations or to individual defects. Based on these data, it is unlikely that ampicillin is teratogenic.

Breast Feeding Summary

Ampicillin is excreted into breast milk in low concentrations. Milk:plasma ratios have been reported up to 0.2 (20, 21). Candidiasis and diarrhea were observed in one infant whose mother was receiving ampicillin (22). Other reports of this effect have not been located. Although adverse effects are apparently rare, three potential problems exist for the nursing infant: modification of bowel flora, direct effects on the infant (e.g., allergic response/sensitization), and interference with the interpretation of culture results if a fever work-up is required.

References

1. Bray R, Boc R, Johnson W. Transfer of ampicillin into fetus and amniotic fluid from maternal plasma in late pregnancy. Am J Obstet Gynecol 1966;96:938–42.
2. MacAulay M, Abou-Sabe M, Charles D. Placental transfer of ampicillin. Am J Obstet Gynecol 1966;96:943–50.
3. Biro L, Ivan E, Elek E, Arr M. Data on the tissue concentration of antibiotics in man. Tissue concentrations of semi-synthetic penicillins in the fetus. Int Z Klin Pharmakol Ther Toxikol 1970;4:321–4.
4. Elek E, Ivan E, Arr M. Passage of penicillins from mother to foetus in humans. Int J Clin Pharmacol Ther Toxicol 1972;6:223–8.
5. Kraybill EN, Chaney NE, McCarthy LR. Transplacental ampicillin: inhibitory concentrations in neonatal serum. Am J Obstet Gynecol 1980;138:793–6.
6. Jordheim O, Hagen AG. Study of ampicillin levels in maternal serum, umbilical cord serum and amniotic fluid following administration of pivampicillin. Acta Obstet Gynecol Scand 1980;59:315–7.
7. Philipson A. Pharmacokinetics of ampicillin duing pregnancy. J Infect Dis 1977;136:370–6.
8. Noschel VH, Peiker G, Schroder S, Meinhold P, Muller B. Untersuchungren zur pharmakokinetik von antibiotika und sulfanilamiden in der schwangerschaft und unter der geburt. Zentralbl Gynaekol 1982;104:1514–8.
9. Willman K, Pulkkinen M. Reduced maternal plasma and urinary estriol during ampicillin treatment. Am J Obstet Gynecol 1971;109:893–6.
10. Boehn F, DiPietro D, Goss D. The effect of ampicillin administration on urinary estriol and serum estradiol in the normal pregnant patient. Am J Obstet Gynecol 1974;119:98–101.
11. Sybulski S, Maughan G. Effect of ampicillin administration on estradiol, estriol and cortisol levels in maternal plasma and on estriol levels in urine. Am J Obstet Gynecol 1976;124:379–81.
12. Aldercreutz H, Martin F, Lehtinen T, Tikkanen M, Pulkkinen M. Effect of ampicillin administration on plasma conjugated and unconjugated estrogen and progesterone levels in pregnancy. Am J Obstet Gynecol 1977;128:266–71.
13. Van Look PFA, Top-Huisman M, Gnodde HP. Effect of ampicillin or amoxycillin administration on plasma and urinary estrogen levels during normal pregnancy. Eur J Obstet Gynecol Reprod Biol 1981;12:225–33.
14. Dossetor J. Drug interactions with oral contraceptives. Br Med J 1975;4:467–8.
15. DeSano EA Jr, Hurley SC. Possible interactions of antihistamines and antibiotics with oral contraceptive effectiveness. Fertil Steril 1982;37:853–4.
16. Friedman CI, Huneke AL, Kim MH, Powell J. The effect of ampicillin on oral contraceptive effectiveness. Obstet Gynecol 1980;55:33–7.
17. Back DJ, Breckerridge AM, MacIver M, Orme M, Rowe PH, Staiger C, Thomas E, Tjia J. The effects of ampicillin on oral contraceptive steroids in women. Br J Clin Pharmacol 1982;14:43–8.
18. Heinonen OP, Slone D, Shapiro S. Birth Defects and Drugs in Pregnancy. Littleton:Publishing Sciences Group, 1977:297–313.
19. Ibid, 435.
20. Wilson J, Brown R, Cherek D, Dailey JW, Hilman B, Jobe PC, Manno BR, Manno JE, Redetzki HM, Stewart JJ. Drug excretion in human breast milk: principles, pharmacokinetics and projected consequences. Clin Pharmacol Ther 1980;5:1–66.
21. Knowles J. Excretion of drugs in milk—a review. J Pediatr 1965;66:1068–82.
22. Williams M. Excretion of drugs in milk. Pharm J 1976;217:219.

Name: **AMYL NITRITE**

Class: **Vasodilator**   Risk Factor: **C**

Fetal Risk Summary

Amyl nitrate is a rapid-acting, short-duration vasodilator used primarily for the treatment of angina pectoris. Due to the nature of its indication, experience in pregnancy is limited. The Collaborative Perinatal Project recorded seven 1st trimester exposures to amyl nitrite and nitroglycerin plus eight other patients exposed to other vasodilators (1). From this small group of 15 patients, four malformed children were produced, a statistically significant incidence ($p < 0.02$). It was not stated if amyl nitrite was taken by any of the mothers of the affected infants. Although the data serve as a warning, the number of patients is so small that conclusions as to the relative safety of amyl nitrite in pregnancy cannot be made.

Breast Feeding Summary

No data available.

References

1. Heinonen OP, Slone D, Shapiro S. *Birth Defects and Drugs in Pregnancy.* Littleton:Publishing Sciences Group, 1977:371–3.

Name: **ANILERIDINE**

Class: **Narcotic Analgesic**   Risk Factor: **B***

Fetal Risk Summary

No reports linking the use of anileridine with congenital defects have been located. Usage in pregnancy is primarily confined to labor. Withdrawal may occur in infants exposed *in utero* to prolonged maternal treatment with anileridine. Respiratory depression in the neonate similar to that produced by meperidine or morphine should be expected (1).

[* Risk Factor D if used for prolonged periods or in high doses at term.]

Breast Feeding Summary

No data available.

References

1. Bonica J. *Principles and Practice of Obstetric Analgesia and Anesthesia.* Philadelphia:FA Davis Company, 1967:250.

Name: **ANISINDIONE**

Class: **Anticoagulant**   Risk Factor: **D**

Fetal Risk Summary

See Coumarin Derivatives.

Breast Feeding Summary

See Coumarin Derivatives.

Name: **ANISOTROPINE**

Class: **Parasympatholytic**   Risk Factor: **C**

Fetal Risk Summary

Anisotropine is an anticholinergic quaternary ammonium methylbromide. In a large prospective study, 2,323 patients were exposed to this class of drugs during the 1st trimester, two of whom took anisotropine (1). A possible association was found between the total group and minor malformations.

Breast Feeding Summary

No data available (see also Atropine).

References

1. Heinonen OP, Slone D, Shapiro S. *Birth Defects and Drugs in Pregnancy*. Littleton:Publishing Sciences Group, 1977:346–53.

Name: **ANTAZOLINE**

Class: **Antihistamine**   Risk Factor: **C**

Fetal Risk Summary

No data available. See Diphenhydramine for representative agent in this class.

Breast Feeding Summary

No data available.

Name: **APROBARBITAL**

Class: **Sedative/Hypnotic**   Risk Factor: **C**

Fetal Risk Summary

No data available.

Breast Feeding Summary

No data available.

Name: **APROTININ**

Class: **Hemostatic**   Risk Factor: **C**

Fetal Risk Summary

No reports linking the use of aprotinin and congenital defects have been located. The drug crosses the placenta and decreases fibrinolytic activity in the newborn (1). The drug has been used safely in severe accidental hemorrhage with coagulation where labor was not established (2).

Breast Feeding Summary

No data available.

References

1. Hoffhauer H, Dobbeck P. Untersuchungen uber die plactapassage des kallikrein-inhibitors. Klin Wochenschr 1970;48:183–4.
2. Sher G. Trasylol in cases of accidental hemorrhage with coagulation disorder and associated uterine inertia. S Afr Med J 1974;48:1452–5.

Name: **ASPIRIN**

Class: **Analgesic/Antipyretic**   Risk Factor: **C***

Fetal Risk Summary

Aspirin is the most frequently ingested drug in pregnancy, either as a single agent or in combination with other drugs (1). (The terms "aspirin" and "salicylate" are used interchangeably in this monograph unless specifically separated.)

In eight surveys totaling over 54,000 patients, aspirin was consumed sometime during gestation by slightly over 33,000 (61%) (2–9). The true incidence is probably much higher than this since many patients either do not remember taking aspirin or consume drug products without realizing they contain large amounts of salicylates (2, 4, 8). Evaluation of the effects of aspirin on the fetus is thus difficult due to this common, and often hidden, exposure. However, some toxic effects on the mother and fetus from large doses of salicylates have been known since 1893 (10).

Aspirin consumption during pregnancy may produce adverse effects in the mother: anemia, antepartum and/or postpartum hemorrhage, prolonged gestation, and prolonged labor (5, 11–14). The increased length of labor and frequency of postmaturity result from the inhibition of prostaglandin synthetase by aspirin. Aspirin has been shown to significantly delay the induced abortion time in nulliparous, but not multiparous, patients, by this same mechanism (15). In an Australian study, regular aspirin ingestion was also found to increase the number of complicated deliveries (cesarean sections, breech, and forceps (5). Small doses of aspirin may decrease urinary estriol excretion (16).

Aspirin, either alone or in combination with β-mimetics, has been used to treat premature labor (17–19). While adverse effects in the newborn were infrequent, maternal complications in one study included non-dose-related prolonged bleeding times and dose-related vertigo, tinnitus, headache, and hyperventilation (19).

Failure of intrauterine devices to prevent conception has been described in two patients consuming frequent doses of aspirin (20). The anti-inflammatory action of aspirin was proposed as the mechanism of the failure.

Low-dose aspirin (about 85 mg/day) was used to treat maternal thrombocytopenia (platelet counts <60,000/mm^3) in 19 patients with either intrauterine growth retardation or toxemia (21). In five women who had a definite response to the aspirin, no improvement in plasma volume or fetal welfare was demonstrated.

Fetal and newborn effects, other than congenital defects, from aspirin exposure *in utero* may include increased perinatal mortality, intrauterine growth retardation, congenital salicylate intoxication, and depressed albumin-binding capacity (2, 5, 12, 22–24). For the latter effect, no increase in the incidence of jaundice was observed (2). Perinatal mortality in the Australian study was usually a result of stillbirths more than neonatal deaths (5, 22). Some of the stillbirths were associated with antepartum hemorrhage while others may have been due to closure of the ductus arteriosus *in utero* (25). Closure of the ductus has been shown in animals to be due to aspirin inhibition of prostaglandin synthetase. However, a large prospective American study involving 41,337 patients, 64% of whom used aspirin sometime during gestation, failed to show that aspirin was a cause of stillbirths, neonatal deaths, or reduced birth weight (26). The difference between these findings probably relates to the chronic or intermittent use of higher doses by the patients in the Australian study (25). Excessive use of aspirin was blamed for the stillbirth of a fetus in whom salicylate levels in the blood and liver were 25–30 and 12 mg/100 ml, respectively (27). Congenital salicylate intoxication was found in two newborns exposed to high aspirin doses prior to delivery (23, 24). Although both infants survived, one infant exhibited withdrawal symptoms, consisting of hypertonia, agitation, a shrill piercing cry, and increased reflex irritability, beginning on the 2nd neonatal day (24). Serum salicylate level was 31 mg/100 ml. Most of the symptoms gradually subsided over 6 weeks, but some mild hypertonia may have persisted.

Aspirin given in low doses during the week prior to delivery may affect the clotting ability of the newborn (28–34). In the initial studies by Bleyer and Breckenridge (28), 3 of 14 newborns exposed to aspirin within 1 week of delivery had minor hemorrhagic phenomena vs only 1 of 17 nonexposed controls. Collagen-induced platelet aggregation was absent in the aspirin group, and, although of less clinical significance, Factor XII activity was markedly depressed. A direct correlation was found between Factor XII activity and the interval between the last dose of aspirin and birth. Neonatal purpuric rash with depressed platelet function has also been observed after maternal use of aspirin close to term (34). The use of salicylates other than aspirin may not be a problem since the acetyl moiety is apparently required to depress platelet function (35–37). In a 1982 study, 10 mothers consuming less than 1 g of aspirin within 5 days of delivery had excessive intrapartum or postpartum blood loss, resulting in markedly lower hemoglobulin levels than controls (13, 14). One mother required a transfusion. Bleeding complications seen in 9 of the 10 infants included numerous petechiae over the presenting part, hematuria, a cephalohematoma, subconjunctival hemorrhage, and bleeding from a circumcision. No life-threatening hemorrhage, effect on Apgar scores, or increased hospital stay was found, nor was bleeding observed in seven mother-infant pairs when aspirin consumption occurred 6–10 days before delivery (13, 14).

An increased incidence of intracranial hemorrhage (ICH) in premature or low-birth-weight infants may occur after maternal aspirin use near birth (38). Computed tomographic screening for ICH was conducted on 108 infants 3–7 days after delivery. All of the infants were either 34 weeks or less in gestation or 1,500 g or less in birth weight. A total of 53 (49%) developed ICH, including 12 (71%) of the 17 aspirin-exposed newborns. This incidence was statistically significant ($p < 0.05$) when compared to the 41 (45%) non-aspirin-exposed infants who developed ICH. The conclusions of this study have been challenged and defended (39, 40). In view of the potentially serious outcome, however, aspirin should be used with extreme caution by patients in danger of premature delivery.

Aspirin readily crosses the placenta (10). When given near term, higher concentrations are found in the neonate than in the mother (41). The kinetics of salicylate elimination in the newborn have been studied (41–43).

The relationship between aspirin and congenital defects is controversial. Several studies have examined this question with findings either supporting or denying a relationship. In two large retrospective studies, mothers of 1,291 malformed infants were found to have consumed aspirin during pregnancy more frequently than mothers of normal infants (44, 45). In a retrospective survey of 599 children with oral clefts, use of salicylates in the 1st trimester was almost three times more frequent in the mothers of children with this defect (46). Reviewing these studies, Collins (26) noted several biases, including the fact that they were retrospective, that could account for the results. Three other reports of aspirin teratogenicity involving a total of 10 infants have been located (47–49). In each of these cases, other drugs and factors were present. A 1985 study found a possible association between the use of aspirin in early pregnancy and congenital heart disease (50). The risk for defects in septation of the truncus arteriosus was increased about 2-fold over that in nonexposed controls.

The Collaborative Perinatal Project monitored 50,282 mother-child pairs, 14,864 of which used aspirin during the 1st trimester (6). For use anytime during pregnancy, 32,164 (64%) exposures were recorded. This prospective study did not find evidence of a teratogenic effect with aspirin. However, the data did not exclude the possibility that grossly excessive doses of aspirin may be teratogenic. An Australian study of 144 infants of mothers who took aspirin regularly in pregnancy also failed to find an association between salicylates and malformations (22). Based on these studies and the fact that aspirin usage in pregnancy is so common, it is not possible to determine the teratogenic risk of salicylates, if indeed it exists.

In summary, the use of aspirin during pregnancy, especially of chronic or intermittent high doses, should be avoided. The drug may affect maternal and newborn hemostasis mechanisms, leading to an increased risk of hemorrhage. High doses may be related to increased perinatal mortality, intrauterine growth retardation, and teratogenic effects. Low doses do not seem to carry these risks. Near term, aspirin may prolong gestation and labor even in very low doses. Although aspirin has been used as a tocolytic agent, serious bleeding complications may occur in the newborn and the benefit:risk ratio has not been adequately studied. If an analgesic or antipyretic drug is needed, acetaminophen should be considered.

[* Risk Factor D if used in the 3rd trimester.]

Breast Feeding Summary

Aspirin and other salicylates are excreted into breast milk in low concentrations. Sodium salicylate was first demonstrated in human milk in 1935 (51). In one study of a mother taking 4 g daily, no detectable salicylate in her milk or in her infant's serum was found, but the test sensitivity was only 50 µg/ml (52). Reported milk concentrations are much lower than this level. Following single or repeated oral doses, peak milk levels occurred at around 3 hours and ranged from 1.1 to 10 µg/ml (53, 54). This represented a milk:plasma ratio of 0.03–0.08 at 3 hours. Since salicylates are eliminated more slowly from milk than from plasma, the ratio increased to 0.34 at 12 hours (54). Peak levels have also been reported to occur at 9 hours (55). Only one report has attributed infant toxicity to salicylates obtained in mother's milk (56). A 16-day-old female infant developed severe salicylate intoxication with a serum salicylate level of 24 mg/100 ml on the 3rd hospital day. Milk and maternal serum levels were not obtained. Although the parents denied giving the baby aspirin or other salicylates, it is unlikely, based on the above reports, that she could have received the drug from the mother's milk in the quantities found. Adverse effects on platelet function in the nursing infant exposed to aspirin via the mother's milk have not been reported but are a potential risk.

References

 1. Corby DG. Aspirin in pregnancy: maternal and fetal effects. Pediatrics 1978;62(Suppl):930–7.
 2. Palmisano PA, Cassady G. Salicylate exposure in the perinate. JAMA 1969;209:556–8.
 3. Forfar JO, Nelson MM. Epidemiology of drugs taken by pregnant women: drugs that may affect the fetus adversely. Clin Pharmacol Ther 1973;14:632–42.
 4. Finnigan D, Burry AF, Smith IDB. Analgesic consumption in an antenatal clinic survey. Med J Aust 1974;1:761–2.
 5. Collins E, Turner G. Maternal effects of regular salicylate ingestion in pregnancy. Lancet 1975;2:335–7.
 6. Slone D, Heinonen OP, Kaufman DW, Siskind V, Monson RR, Shapiro S. Aspirin and congenital malformations. Lancet 1976;1:1373–5.
 7. Hill RM, Craig JP, Chaney MD, Tennyson LM, McCulley LB. Utilization of over-the-counter drugs during pregnancy. Clin Obstet Gynecol 1977;20:381–94.
 8. Harrison K, Thomas I, Smith I. Analgesic use during pregnancy. Med J Aust 1978;2:161.
 9. Bodendorfer TW, Briggs GG, Gunning JE. Obtaining drug exposure histories during pregnancy. Am J Obstet Gynecol 1979;135:490–4.
10. Jackson AV. Toxic effects of salicylate on the foetus and mother. J Pathol Bacteriol 1948;60:587–93.
11. Lewis RN, Schulman JD. Influence of acetylsalicylic acid, an inhibitor of prostaglandin synthesis, on the duration of human gestation and labour. Lancet 1973;2:1159–61.
12. Rudolph AM. Effects of aspirin and acetaminophen in pregnancy and in the newborn. Arch Intern Med 1981;141:358–63.
13. Stuart MJ, Gross SJ, Elrad H, Graeber JE. Effects of acetylsalicylic-acid ingestion on maternal and neonatal hemostasis. N Engl J Med 1982;307:909–12.
14. Stuart MJ. Aspirin and maternal or neonatal hemostasis. N Engl J Med 1983;308:281.
15. Niebyl JR, Blake DA, Burnett LS, King TM. The influence of aspirin on the course of induced midtrimester abortion. Am J Obstet Gynecol 1976;124:607–10.
16. Castellanos JM, Aranda M, Cararach J, Cararach V. Effect of aspirin on oestriol excretion in pregnancy. Lancet 1975;1:859.
17. Babenerd VJ, Kyriakidis K. Acetylsalicylic acid in the prevention of premature delivery. Fortschr Med 1979;97:463–6.
18. Wolff F, Bolte A, Berg R. Does an additional administration of acetylsalicylic acid reduce the requirement of betamimetics in tocolytic treatment? Geburtshilfe Frauenheilkd 1981;41:293–6.
19. Wolff F, Berg R, Bolte A. Clinical study of the labour inhibiting effects and side effects of acetylsalicylic acid (ASA). Geburtshilfe Frauenheilkd 1981;41:96–100.
20. Buhler M, Papiernik E. Successive pregnancies in women fitted with intrauterine devices who take antiinflammatory drugs. Lancet 1983;1:483.
21. Goodlin RC. Correction of pregnancy-related thrombocytopenia with aspirin without improvement in fetal outcome. Am J Obstet Gynecol 1983;146:862–4.

22. Turner G, Collins E. Fetal effects of regular salicylate ingestion in pregnancy. Lancet 1975;2:338–9.

23. Earle R Jr. Congenital salicylate intoxication—report of a case. N Engl J Med 1961;265:1003–4.

24. Lynd PA, Andreasen AC, Wyatt RJ. Intrauterine salicylate intoxication in a newborn. A case report. Clin Pediatr (Phila) 1976;15:912–3.

25. Shapiro S, Monson RR, Kaufman DW, Siskind V, Heinonen OP, Slone D. Perinatal mortality and birth-weight in relation to aspirin taken during pregnancy. Lancet 1976;1:1375–6.

26. Collins E. Maternal and fetal effects of acetaminophen and salicylates in pregnancy. Obstet Gynecol 1981;58(Suppl):57S–62S.

27. Aterman K, Holzbecker M, Ellenberger HA. Salicylate levels in a stillborn infant born to a drug-addicted mother, with comments on pathology and analytical methodology. Clin Toxicol 1980;16:263–8.

28. Bleyer WA, Breckenridge RJ. Studies on the detection of adverse drug reactions in the newborn. II. The effects of prenatal aspirin on newborn hemostasis. JAMA 1970;213:2049–53.

29. Corby DG, Schulman I. The effects of antenatal drug administration on aggregation of platelets of newborn infants. J Pediatr 1971;79:307–13.

30. Casteels-Van Daele M, Eggermont E, de Gaetano G, Vermijlen J. More on the effects of antenatally administered aspirin on aggregation of platelets of neonates. J Pediatr 1972;80:685–6.

31. Haslam RR, Ekert H, Gillam GL. Hemorrhage in a neonate possible due to maternal ingestion of salicylate. J Pediatr 1974;84:556–7.

32. Ekert H, Haslam RR. Maternal ingested salicylate as a cause of neonatal hemorrhage. Reply. J Pediatr 1974;85:738.

33. Pearson H. Comparative effects of aspirin and acetaminophen on hemostasis. Pediatrics 1978;62(Suppl):926–9.

34. Haslam RR. Neonatal purpura secondary to maternal salicylism. J Pediatr 1975;86:653.

35. O'Brien JR. Effects of salicylates on human platelets. Lancet 1968;1:779–83.

36. Weiss HJ, Aledort ML, Shaul I. The effect of salicylates on the haemostatic properties of platelets in man. J Clin Invest 1968;47:2169–80.

37. Bleyer WA. Maternal ingested salicylates as a cause of neonatal hemorrhage. J Pediatr 1974;85:736–7.

38. Rumack CM, Guggenheim MA, Rumack BH, Peterson RG, Johnson ML, Braithwaite WR. Neonatal intracranial hemorrhage and maternal use of aspirin. Obstet Gynecol 1981;58(Suppl):52S–6S.

39. Soller RW, Stander H. Maternal drug exposure and perinatal intracranial hemorrhage. Obstet Gynecol 1981;58:735–7.

40. Corby DG. Editorial comment. Obstet Gynecol 1981;58:737–40.

41. Levy G, Procknal JA, Garrettson LK. Distribution of salicylate between neonatal and maternal serum at diffusion equilibrium. Clin Pharmacol Ther 1975;18:210–4.

42. Levy G, Garrettson LK. Kinetics of salicylate elimination by newborn infants of mothers who ingested aspirin before delivery. Pediatrics 1974;53:201–10.

43. Garrettson LK, Procknal JA, Levy G. Fetal acquisition and neonatal elimination of a large amount of salicylate. Study of a neonate whose mother regularly took therapeutic doses of aspirin during pregnancy. Clin Pharmacol Ther 1975;17:98–103.

44. Richards ID. Congenital malformations and environmental influences in pregnancy. Br J Prev Soc Med 1969;23:218–25.

45. Nelson MM, Forfar JO. Associations between drugs administered during pregnancy and congenital abnormalities of the fetus. Br Med J 1971;1:523–7.

46. Saxen I. Associations between oral clefts and drugs during pregnancy. Int J Epidemiol 1975;4:37–44.

47. Benawra R, Mangurten HH, Duffell DR. Cyclopia and other anomalies following maternal ingestion of salicylates. J Pediatr 1980;96:1069–71.

48. McNiel JR. The possible effect of salicylates on the developing fetus. Brief summaries of eight suggestive cases. Clin Pediatr (Phila) 1973;12:347–50.

49. Sayli BS, Asmaz A, Yemisci B. Consanguinity, aspirin, and phocomelia. Lancet 1966;1:876.

50. Zierler S, Rothman KJ. Congenital heart disease in relation to maternal use of Bendectin and other drugs in early pregnancy. N Engl J Med 1985;313:347–52.

51. Kwit NT, Hatcher RA. Excretion of drugs in milk. Am J Dis Child 1935;49:900–4.

52. Erickson SH, Oppenheim GL. Aspirin in breast milk. J Fam Pract 1979;8:189–90.

53. Weibert RT, Bailey DN. Salicylate excretion in human breast milk. Presented at the 1979 Seminar

of the California Society of Hospital Pharmacists, Los Angeles, October 13, 1979, Abstr. 7.

54. Findlay JWA, DeAngelis RL, Kearney MF, Welch RM, Findley JM. Analgesic drugs in breast milk and plasma. Clin Pharmacol Ther 1981;29:625–33.

55. Anderson PO. Drugs and breast feeding—a review. Drug Intell Clin Pharm 1977;11:208–23.

56. Clark JH, Wilson WG. A 16-day-old breast-fed infant with metabolic acidosis caused by salicylate. Clin Pediatr (Phila) 1981;20:53–4.

Name: **ATENOLOL**

Class: **Sympatholytic (β-Adrenergic Blocker)**   Risk Factor: **C$_M$**

Fetal Risk Summary

Atenolol is a cardioselective β-adrenergic blocking agent used for the treatment of hypertension. The drug readily crosses the placenta to the fetus, producing steady state fetal levels that are approximately equal to those in the maternal serum (1–6). In 11 pregnant patients treated with 100 mg/day, the serum half-life (8.1 hours) and the 24-hour urinary excretion (52 mg) were similar to those in nonpregnant women (6).

Safe use of atenolol for the treatment of hypertension in the pregnant woman has been documented by several investigators (5, 7–12). No fetal malformations attributable to atenolol have been reported, but experience with the drug during the 1st trimester is lacking. Reduced birth weight and persistent β-blockade in the newborn have been observed after atenolol exposure.

In a nonrandomized study comparing atenolol with two other β-blockers for the treatment of hypertension during pregnancy, the mean birth weights of atenolol-exposed babies were markedly lower than those of infants exposed *in utero* to either acebutolol or pindolol (2,745 g vs 3,160 g vs 3,375 g) (12, 13). A similar study comparing atenolol with labetalol found a significant difference in the birth weights of the two groups, 2,750 g vs 3,280 g ($p < 0.001$) (4). No difference was found in the birth weights of atenolol- vs placebo-exposed infants (2,961 g vs 3,017 g) in a randomized, double-blind investigation of 120 pregnant women with mild to moderate hypertension (10). The differences observed in the above studies may be related to the severity of the maternal hypertension combined with the more pronounced maternal bradycardia noted in atenolol-treated women, resulting in placental insufficiency. Intrauterine fetal deaths have been observed in women with severe hypertension treated with atenolol, but this has also occurred with other β-blockers and in hypertensive women not treated with drugs (4, 10, 14).

In eight mothers treated with atenolol or pindolol, a decrease in the basal fetal heart rate was noted only in atenolol-exposed fetuses (15). Before and during treatment fetal heart rates in the atenolol patients were 136 and 120 beats/min while the rates for the pindolol group were 128 and 132 beats/min. In 60 patients treated with atenolol for pregnancy-induced hypertension, no effect was observed on fetal heart rate pattern in response to uterine contractions (16). Accelerations, variables, and late decelerations were all easily distinguishable (16).

Persistent β-blockade was observed in a newborn whose mother was treated with atenolol, 100 mg/day, for hypertension (2). At 15 hours of age, the otherwise normal infant developed bradycardia at rest and when crying, and hypotension.

Serum atenolol level was 0.24 μg/ml. Urinary excretion of the drug during the first 7 days ranged from 0.85 to 0.196 μg/ml. In another study, 39% (18 of 46) of the newborns exposed to atenolol developed bradycardia compared to only 10% (4 of 39) of placebo-exposed newborns ($p < 0.01$) (10). None of the infants required treatment for the lowered heart rate.

Exposure to atenolol *in utero* apparently has no effect on infant growth or behavior. No differences were noted in the development at 1 year of age of offspring from mothers treated during the 3rd trimester for mild to moderate pregnancy-induced hypertension with either bed rest alone or rest combined with atenolol (17). The mean duration of therapy in the atenolol-treated patients was 5 weeks.

Newborns exposed to atenolol near delivery should be closely observed during the first 24–48 hours for signs and symptoms of β-blockade. Long-term effects of *in utero* exposure to this class of drugs have not been studied but warrant evaluation.

Breast Feeding Summary

Atenolol is excreted into breast milk (3, 6, 18–21). The drug is a weak base, and accumulation in the milk occurs with concentrations significantly greater than corresponding plasma levels (3, 18–21). Peak milk concentrations after single (50 mg) and continuous dosing (25–100 mg/day) regimens were 3.6 and 2.9 times greater than simultaneous plasma levels (20). Atenolol has been found in the serum and urine of breast-fed infants in some studies (3, 6, 18). Other studies have been unable to detect the drug in the infant serum (test limit 10 ng/ml) (19, 20). Although no adverse reactions have been observed, nursing infants should be closely monitored for bradycardia and other signs and symptoms of β-blockade. Long-term effects on infants exposed to β-blockers from breast milk have not been studied but warrant evaluation. The American Academy of Pediatrics considers atenolol compatible with breast-feeding (22).

References

1. Melander A, Niklasson B, Ingemarsson I, Liedholm H, Schersten B, Sjoberg NO. Transplacental passage of atenolol in man. Eur J Clin Pharmacol 1978;14:93–4.
2. Woods DL, Morrell DF. Atenolol: side effects in a newborn infant. Br Med J 1982;285:691–2.
3. Liedholm H. Transplacental passage and breast milk accumulation of atenolol in humans. Drugs 1983;25(Suppl 2):217–8.
4. Lardoux H, Gerard J, Blazquez G, Chouty F, Flouvat B. Hypertension in pregnancy: evaluation of two beta blockers atenolol and labetalol. Eur Heart J 1983;4(Suppl G):35–40.
5. Liedholm H. Atenolol in the treatment of hypertension of pregnancy. Drugs 1983;25(Suppl 2):206–11.
6. Thorley KJ. Pharmacokinetics of atenolol in pregnancy and lactation. Drugs 1983;25(Suppl 2):216–7.
7. Dubois D, Petitcolas J, Temperville B, Klepper A. Beta blockers and high-risk pregnancies. Int J Biol Res Pregnancy 1980;1:141–5.
8. Thorley KJ, McAinsh J, Cruickshank JM. Atenolol in the treatment of pregnancy-induced hypertension. Br J Clin Pharmacol 1981;12:725–30.
9. Rubin PC, Butters L, Low RA, Reid JL. Atenolol in the treatment of essential hypertension during pregnancy. Br J Clin Pharmacol 1982;14:279–81.
10. Rubin PC, Butters L, Clark DM, Reynolds B, Sumner DJ, Steedman D, Low RA, Reid JL. Placebo-controlled trial of atenolol in treatment of pregnancy-associated hypertension. Lancet 1983;1:431–4.
11. Rubin PC, Butters L, Low RA, Clark DC, Reid JL. Atenolol in the management of hypertension during pregnancy. Drugs 1983;25(Suppl 2):212–4.

12. Dubois D, Peticolas J, Temperville B, Klepper A. Treatment with atenolol of hypertension in pregnancy. Drugs 1983;25(Suppl 2):215–8.
13. Dubois D, Petitcolas J, Temperville B, Klepper A, Catherine CH. Treatment of hypertension in pregnancy with β-adrenoceptor antagonists. Br J Clin Pharmacol 1982;13(Suppl):375S–8S.
14. Lubbe WF. More on beta-blockers in pregnancy. N Engl J Med 1982;307:753.
15. Ingemarsson I, Liedholm H, Montan S, Westgren M, Melander A. Fetal heart rate during treatment of maternal hypertension with beta-adrenergic antagonists. Acta Obstet Gynecol Scand 1984;118(Suppl):95–7.
16. Rubin PC, Butters L, Clark D, Sumner D, Belfield A, Pledger D, Low RAL, Reid JL. Obstetric aspects of the use in pregnancy-associated hypertension of the β-adrenoceptor antagonist atenolol. Am J Obstet Gynecol 1984;150:389–92.
17. Reynolds B, Butters L, Evans J, Adams T, Rubin PC. First year of life after the use of atenolol in pregnancy associated hypertension. Arch Dis Child 1984;59:1061–3.
18. Liedholm H, Melander A, Bitzen PO, Helm G, Lonnerholm G, Mattiasson I, Nilsson B, Wahlin-Boll E. Accumulation of atenolol and metoprolol in human breast milk. Eur J Clin Pharmacol 1981;20:229–31.
19. Kulas J, Lunell NO, Rosing U, Steen B, Rane A. Atenolol and metoprolol. A comparison of their excretion into human breast milk. Acta Obstet Gynecol Scand 1984;118(Suppl):65–9.
20. White WB, Andreoli JW, Wong SH, Cohn RD. Atenolol in human plasma and breast milk. Obstet Gynecol 1984;63:42S–4S.
21. White WB. Management of hypertension during lactation. Hypertension 1984;6:297–300.
22. Committee on Drugs, American Academy of Pediatrics. The transfer of drugs and other chemicals into human breast milk. Pediatrics 1983;72:375–83.

Name: ATROPINE

Class: **Parasympatholytic**   Risk Factor: **C**

Fetal Risk Summary

Atropine, an anticholinergic, rapidly crosses the placenta (1–3). The drug has been used to test placental function in high-risk obstetrical patients by producing fetal vagal blockade and subsequent tachycardia (4). The Collaborative Perinatal Project monitored 50,282 mother-child pairs, 401 of which used atropine in the 1st trimester (5). For use anytime during pregnancy, 1,198 exposures were recorded (6). In neither case was evidence found for an association with malformations. However, when the group of parasympatholytics was taken as a whole (2,323 exposures), a possible association with minor malformations was found (5). Atropine has been used to reduce gastric secretions prior to cesarean section without producing fetal or neonatal effects (7, 8). In a study comparing atropine and glycopyrrolate, 10 women in labor received 0.01 mg/kg of atropine intravenously (9). No statistically significant changes were noted in fetal heart rate or variability nor was there any effect on uterine activity.

Breast Feeding Summary

The passage of atropine into breast milk is controversial (10). It has not been adequately documented if measurable amounts are excreted or, if excretion does occur, whether this may affect the nursing infant. Although neonates are particularly sensitive to anticholinergic agents, no adverse effects have been reported in nursing infants whose mothers were taking atropine (11).

References

1. Nishimura H, Tanimura T. *Clinical Aspects of the Teratogenicity of Drugs.* New York: American Elsevier, 1976:63.
2. Kivalo I, Saarikoski S. Placental transmission of atropine at full-term pregnancy. Br J Anaesth 1977;49:1017–21.
3. Kanto J, Virtanen R, Iisalo E, Maenpaa K, Liukko P. Placental transfer and pharmacokinetics of atropine after a single maternal intravenous and intramuscular administration. Acta Anaesth Scand 1981;25:85–8.
4. Hellman LM, Fillisti LP. Analysis of the atropine test for placental transfer in gravidas with toxemia and diabetes. Am J Obstet Gynecol 1965;91:797–805.
5. Heinonen OP, Slone D, Shapiro S. *Birth Defects and Drugs in Pregnancy.* Littleton:Publishing Sciences Group, 1977:346–53.
6. *Ibid*, 439.
7. Diaz DM, Diaz SF, Marx GF. Cardiovascular effects of glycopyrrolate and belladonna derivatives in obstetric patients. Bull NY Acad Med 1980;56:245–8.
8. Roper RE, Salem MG. Effects of glycopyrrolate and atropine combined with antacid on gastric acidity. Br J Anaesth 1981;53:1277–80.
9. Abboud T, Raya J, Sadri S, Grobler N, Stine L, Miller F. Fetal and maternal cardiovascular effects of atropine and glycopyrrolate. Anesth Analg 1983;62:426–30.
10. Stewart JJ. Gastrointestinal drugs. In Wilson JT, ed. *Drugs in Breast Milk.* Balgowlah, Australia: ADIS Press, 1981:65–71.
11. Committee on Drugs, American Academy of Pediatrics. The transfer of drugs and other chemicals into human breast milk. Pediatrics 1983;72:375–83.

Name: **AUROTHIOGLUCOSE**

Class: **Gold Compound**   Risk Factor: **C**

Fetal Risk Summary

See Gold Sodium Thiomalate

Breast Feeding Summary

See Gold Sodium Thiomalate

Name: **AZATADINE**

Class: **Antihistamine**   Risk Factor: **B$_M$**

Fetal Risk Summary

No data available. See Diphenhydramine for representative agent in this class.

Breast Feeding Summary

No data available.

Name: **AZATHIOPRINE**

Class: **Antineoplastic/Immunosuppressant**   Risk Factor: **D**

Fetal Risk Summary

Azathioprine is used primarily in patients with renal or liver transplants or in those with inflammatory bowel disease. Prednisone is commonly combined with azathioprine in these patients. The drug crosses the placenta and trace amounts of its active metabolite, mercaptopurine, have been found in fetal blood (see also Mercaptopurine) (1). Experience in pregnancy is limited, but most investigators have found azathioprine to be relatively safe (2–16). However, transient chromosomal aberrations were found in one infant after *in utero* exposure (17). Congenital defects have been observed in two exposed infants: pulmonary valvular stenosis and preaxial polydactyly (type 1) (18, 19). In a third case, a mother received a renal transplant at the 12th–14th week of gestation and was then treated with azathioprine and prednisone (20). The infant, delivered prematurely at 34–35 weeks, had hypothyroidism and an atrial septal defect. The child was small for her age at 2.5 years.

Immunosuppression of the newborn was observed in one infant whose mother received 150 mg of azathioprine and 30 mg of prednisone daily throughout pregnancy (8). The suppression was characterized by lymphopenia, decreased survival of lymphocytes in culture, absence of IgM, and reduced levels of IgG. Recovery occurred at about 15 weeks of age. An infant exposed to 125 mg of azathioprine plus 12.5 mg of prednisone daily during pregnancy was born with pancytopenia and severe combined immune deficiency (21). The infant died at 28 days from complications brought on by irreversible bone marrow and lymphoid hypoplasia. To avoid neonatal leukopenia and thrombocytopenia, maternal doses of azathioprine were reduced during the 3rd trimester in a 1985 study (22). The authors of this research found a significant correlation between maternal leukocyte counts at 32 weeks gestation and at delivery and cord blood leukocyte count. If the mother's count was at or below 1 standard deviation for normal pregnancy, her dose of azathioprine was halved. Before this technique was used, several newborns had leukopenia and thrombocytopenia, but no low levels were measured after institution of the new procedure.

Azathioprine has been reported to interfere with the effectiveness of an intrauterine contraceptive device (IUD) (23). Two renal transplant patients, maintained on azathioprine and prednisone, each received a copper IUD (Cu7). Both became pregnant with the IUD in place. No defects were noted in either newborn, although one was delivered prematurely. The authors recommend other means of contraception in sexually active women receiving azathioprine/prednisone.

Breast Feeding Summary

No data available.

References

1. Sarrikoski S, Seppala M. Immunosuppression during pregnancy. Transmission of azathioprine and its metabolites from the mother to the fetus. Am J Obstet Gynecol 1973;115:1100–6.
2. Gillibrand PN. Systemic lupus erythematosus in pregnancy treated with azathioprine. Proc R Soc Med 1966;59:834.

3. Board JA, Lee HM, Draper DA, Hume DM. Pregnancy following kidney homotransplantation from a non-twin: report of a case with concurrent administration of azathioprine and prednisone. Obstet Gynecol 1967;29:318–23.

4. Kaufmann JJ, Dignam W, Goodwin WE, Martin DC, Goldman R, Maxwell MH. Successful, normal childbirth after kidney homotransplantation. JAMA 1967;200:338–41.

5. Anonymous. Eleventh annual report of human renal transplant registry. JAMA 1973;216:1197.

6. Nolan GH, Sweet RL, Laros RK, Roure CA. Renal cadaver transplantation followed by successful pregnancies. Obstet Gynecol 1974;43:732–8.

7. Sharon E, Jones J, Diamond H, Kaplan D. Pregnancy and azathioprine in systemic lupus erythematosus. Am J Obstet Gynecol 1974;118:25–7.

8. Cote CJ, Meuwissen HJ, Pickering RJ. Effects on the neonate of prednisone and azathioprine administered to the mother during pregnancy. J Pediatr 1974;85:324–8.

9. Erkman J, Blythe JG. Azathioprine therapy complicated by pregnancy. Obstet Gynecol 1972;40:708–9.

10. Price HV, Salaman JR, Laurence KM, Langmaid H. Immunosuppressive drugs and the foetus. Transplantation 1976;21:294–8.

11. The Registration Committee of the European Dialysis and Transplant Association. Successful pregnancies in women treated by dialysis and kidney transplantation. Br J Obstet Gynaecol 1980;87:839–45.

12. Golby M. Fertility after renal transplantation. Transplantation 1970;10:201–7.

13. Rabau-Friedman E, Mashiach S, Cantor E, Jacob ET. Association of hypoparathyroidism and successful pregnancy in kidney transplant recipient. Obstet Gynecol 1982;59:126–8.

14. Myers RL, Schmid R, Newton JJ. Childbirth after liver transplantation. Transplantation 1980;29:432.

15. Williams PF, Johnstone M. Normal pregnancy in renal transplant recipient with history of eclampsia and intrauterine death. Br Med J 1982;285:1535.

16. Westney LS, Callender CO, Stevens J, Bhagwanani SG, George JPA, Mims OL. Successful pregnancy with sickle cell disease and renal transplantation. Obstet Gynecol 1984;63:752–5.

17. Leb DE, Weisskopf B, Kanovitz BS. Chromosome aberrations in the child of a kidney transplant recipient. Arch Intern Med 1971;128:441–4.

18. Nishimura H, Tanimura T. *Clinical Aspects of the Teratogenicity of Drugs*. New York:American Elsevier, 1976:106–7.

19. Williamson RA, Karp LE. Azathioprine teratogenicity: review of the literature and case report. Obstet Gynecol 1981;58:247–50.

20. Burleson RL, Sunderji SG, Aubry RH, Clark DA, Marbarger P, Cohen RS, Scruggs BF, Lagraff S. Renal allotransplantation during pregnancy. Successful outcome for mother, child, and kidney. Transplantation 1983;36:334.

21. DeWitte DB, Buick MK, Cyran SE, Maisels MJ. Neonatal pancytopenia and severe combined immunodeficiency associated with antenatal administration of azathioprine and prednisone. J Pediatr 1984;105:625–8.

22. Davison JM, Dellagrammatikas H, Parkin JM. Maternal azathioprine therapy and depressed haemopoiesis in the babies of renal allograft patients. Br J Obstet Gynaecol 1985;92:233–9.

23. Zerner J, Doil KL, Drewry J, Leeber DA. Intrauterine contraceptive device failures in renal transplant patients. J Reprod Med 1981;26:99–102.

Name: **BACAMPICILLIN**

Class: **Antibiotic**   Risk Factor: **B_M**

Fetal Risk Summary

Bacampicillin, a penicillin antibiotic, is converted to ampicillin during absorption from the gastrointestinal tract (see Ampicillin).

Breast Feeding Summary

See Ampicillin.

Name: **BACITRACIN**

Class: **Antibiotic**   Risk Factor: **C**

Fetal Risk Summary

No reports linking the use of bacitracin with congenital defects have been located. The drug is primarily used topically, although the injectable form is available. One study listed 18 patients exposed to the drug in the 1st trimester (1). The route of administration was not specified. No association with malformations was found.

Breast Feeding Summary

No data available.

References

1. Heinonen OP, Slone D, Shapiro S. *Birth Defects and Drugs in Pregnancy*. Littleton:Publishing Sciences Group, 1977:297, 301.

Name: **BELLADONNA**

Class: **Parasympatholytic**   Risk Factor: **C**

Fetal Risk Summary

Belladonna is an anticholinergic agent. The Collaborative Perinatal Project monitored 50,282 mother-child pairs, 554 of which used belladonna in the 1st trimester (1). Belladonna was found to be associated with malformations in general and with minor malformations. For use anytime during pregnancy, 1,355 exposures were recorded (2). No association was found in this case.

Breast Feeding Summary

See Atropine.

References

1. Heinonen OP, Slone D, Shapiro S. *Birth Defects and Drugs in Pregnancy*. Littleton:Publishing Sciences Group, 1977:346–53.
2. *Ibid*, 439.

Name: **BENDROFLUMETHIAZIDE**

Class: **Diuretic**   Risk Factor: **D***

Fetal Risk Summary

See Chlorothiazide.

[* Risk Factor C according to manufacturer—E. R. Squibb & Sons, 1985.]

Breast Feeding Summary

Bendroflumethiazide has been used to suppress lactation (see Chlorothiazide).

Name: **BENZTHIAZIDE**

Class: **Diuretic**   Risk Factor: **D**

Fetal Risk Summary

See Chlorothiazide.

Breast Feeding Summary

See Chlorothiazide.

Name: **BENZTROPINE**

Class: **Parasympatholytic**   Risk Factor: **C**

Fetal Risk Summary

Benztropine is an anticholinergic agent structurally related to atropine (see also Atropine). It also has antihistaminic activity. In a large prospective study, 2,323 patients were exposed to this class of drugs during the 1st trimester, 4 of whom took benztropine (1). A possible association was found between the total group and minor malformations. Paralytic ileus has been observed in two newborns exposed to chlorpromazine and benztropine at term (2). In one of these infants, other anticholinergic drugs may have contributed to the effect (see Doxepin). The small left colon syndrome was characterized by decreased intestinal motility, abdominal distention, vomiting, and failure to pass meconium. The condition cleared rapidly in both infants following a Gastrografin enema.

Breast Feeding Summary

No data available (see Atropine).

References

1. Heinonen OP, Slone D, Shapiro S. *Birth Defects and Drugs in Pregnancy*. Littleton:Publishing Sciences Group, 1977:346–53.
2. Falterman CG, Richardson CJ. Small left colon syndrome associated with maternal ingestion of psychotropic drugs. J Pediatr 1980;97:308–10.

Name: β-**CAROTENE**

Class: **Vitamin** Risk Factor: **C**

Fetal Risk Summary

β-Carotene, a natural precursor to vitamin A found in green and yellow vegetables as well as commercially available, is partially converted in the small intestine to vitamin A (1). Even with therapeutic doses of the drug, serum levels of vitamin A do not rise above normal. No reports of the therapeutic use of this vitamin in human pregnancy have been located. Studies in animals have failed to show a teratogenic effect (see also Vitamin A) (2).

Breast Feeding Summary

No data available.

References

1. American Hospital Formulary Service. *Drug Information 1985*. Bethesda: American Society of Hospital Pharmacists, 1985:1680–1.
2. Nishimura H, Tanimura T. *Clinical Aspects of The Teratogenicity of Drugs*. New York:American Elsevier, 1978:252.

Name: **BETAMETHASONE**

Class: **Corticosteroid** Risk Factor: **C**

Fetal Risk Summary

No reports linking the use of betamethasone with congenital defects have been located. Betamethasone is often used in patients with premature labor at about 26–34 weeks gestation to stimulate fetal lung maturation (1–14). The benefits of this therapy are:

Reduction in incidence of respiratory distress syndrome (RDS)
Decreased severity of RDS if it occurs
Decreased incidence of, and mortality from, intracranial hemorrhage
Increased survival of premature infants

Betamethasone crosses the placenta to the fetus (15). The drug is partially metabolized (47%) by the perfused placenta to its inactive 11-ketosteroid derivative but less so than other corticosteroids, although the differences are not statistically significant (16).

In patients with premature rupture of the membranes (PROM), administration of betamethasone to the mother does not always reduce the frequency of RDS or perinatal mortality (17–21). An increased risk of maternal infection has also been observed in patients with PROM treated with corticosteroids (18, 19). In a study comparing betamethasone therapy with nonsteroid management of women with PROM, neonatal sepsis was observed in 23% (5 of 22) of steroid-exposed newborns vs only 2% (1 of 46) of the nonsteroid-exposed group (20). A 1985 study also found increased neonatal sepsis in exposed newborns who were delivered more than 48 hours after PROM, 18.6% (14 of 75) vs 7.4% (4 of 54) nonexposed controls (21). In addition, moderate to severe respiratory morbidity was increased over controls, 21.3% vs 11.1%, as well as overall mortality, 8% vs 1.8% (21). Other reports, however, have noted beneficial effects of betamethasone administration to patients with PROM with no increase in infectious morbidity (22, 23).

Betamethasone therapy is less effective in decreasing the incidence of RDS in male infants than in female infants (22, 24). The reasons for this difference have not been discovered. Slower lung maturation in male fetuses has been cited as a major contributing factor to the sex differential noted in neonatal mortality (25).

An increased incidence of hypoglycemia in newborns exposed *in utero* to betamethasone has been reported (26). Other reports have not observed this effect.

In the initial study examining the effect of betamethasone on RDS, Liggins and Howie (1) reported an increased risk of fetal death in patients with severe preeclampsia. They proposed that the corticosteroid had an adverse effect on placentas already damaged by vascular disease. A second study did not confirm these findings (7).

Leukocytosis was observed in a 880-g, 30 weeks gestation female infant whose mother received 12 mg of betamethasone 4 hours prior to delivery (27). The WBC count returned to normal in about 1 week. A 1984 study examined the effect of betamethasone on leukocyte counts in mothers with PROM or premature labor (28). No effect, as compared to untreated controls, was found in either group.

Respiratory crisis secondary to acute exacerbation of muscular weakness was described in a woman with myasthenia gravis treated with betamethasone and ritodrine for premature labor (29). Adrenocorticosteroids are known to aggravate myasthenia gravis so the condition was thought to be due to betamethasone. Hypertensive crisis associated with the use of ritodrine and betamethasone has been reported (30). Systolic blood pressure was above 300 mm Hg with a diastolic pressure of 120 mm Hg. Although the hypertension was probably caused by ritodrine, it is not known if the corticosteroid was a contributing factor.

The effect of betamethasone administration on patent ductus arteriosus (PDA) was investigated in premature infants with birth weights less than 2,000 g (31). Infants of nontreated mothers had a PDA incidence of 44% vs 6.5% for infants of treated mothers ($p < 0.01$).

A 1984 article has discussed the potential benefits of combining thyroid hormones with corticosteroids to produce an additive or synergistic effect on fetal lung phosphatidylcholine synthesis (32). The therapy, according to Ballard, would offer advantages over corticosteroid therapy alone, but is presently not possible due to the lack of commercially available thyroid stimulators that cross the placenta. The thyroid hormones, T_4 and T_3, are poorly transported across the placenta and thus would not be effective.

Although human studies have usually shown a benefit, the use of corticosteroids in animals has been associated with several toxic effects (33, 34):

Reduced fetal head circumference
Reduced fetal adrenal weight
Increased fetal liver weight
Reduced fetal thymus weight
Reduced placental weight

Fortunately, none of these effects has been observed in human investigations. In children born of mothers treated with betamethasone for premature labor, studies conducted at ages 4 and 6 years have found no differences with controls in cognitive and psychosocial development (35, 36).

Breast Feeding Summary

No data available.

References

1. Liggins GC, Howie RN. A controlled trial of antepartum glucocorticoid treatment for prevention of the respiratory distress syndrome in premature infants. Pediatrics 1972;50:515–25.
2. Gluck L. Administration of corticosteroids to induce maturation of fetal lung. Am J Dis Child 1976; 130:976–8.
3. Ballard RA, Ballard PL. Use of prenatal glucocorticoid therapy to prevent respiratory distress syndrome: a supporting view. Am J Dis Child 1976;130:982–7.
4. Mead PB, Clapp JF III. The use of betamethasone and timed delivery in management of premature rupture of the membranes in the preterm pregnancy. J Reprod Med 1977;19:3–7.
5. Block MF, Kling OR, Crosby WM. Antenatal glucocorticoid therapy for the prevention of respiratory distress syndrome in the premature infant. Obstet Gynecol 1977;50:186–90.
6. Ballard RA, Ballard PL, Granberg JP, Sniderman S. Prenatal administration of betamethasone for prevention of respiratory distress syndrome. J Pediatr 1979;94:97–101.
7. Nochimson DJ, Petrie RH. Glucocorticoid therapy for the induction of pulmonary maturity in severely hypertensive gravid women. Am J Obstet Gynecol 1979;133:449–51.
8. Eggers TR, Doyle LW, Pepperell RJ. Premature labour. Med J Aust 1979;1:213–6.
9. Doran TA, Swyer P, MacMurray B, et al. Results of a double-blind controlled study on the use of betamethasone in the prevention of respiratory distress syndrome. Am J Obstet Gynecol 1980;136:313–20.
10. Schutte MF, Treffers PE, Koppe JG, Breur W. The influence of betamethasone and orciprenaline on the incidence of respiratory distress syndrome in the newborn after preterm labour. Br J Obstet Gynaecol 1980;87:127–31.
11. Dillon WP, Egan EA. Aggressive obstetric management in late second-trimester deliveries. Obstet Gynecol 1981;58:685–90.

12. Johnson DE, Munson DP, Thompson TR. Effect of antenatal administration of betamethasone on hospital costs and survival of premature infants. Pediatrics 1981;68:633–7.
13. Bishop EH. Acceleration of fetal pulmonary maturity. Obstet Gynecol 1981;58(Suppl):48S–51S.
14. Ballard PL, Ballard RA. Corticosteroids and respiratory distress syndrome: status 1979. Pediatrics 1979;63:163–5.
15. Ballard PL, Granberg P, Ballard RA. Glucocorticoid levels in maternal and cord serum after prenatal betamethasone therapy to prevent respiratory distress syndrome. J Clin Invest 1975;56:1548–54.
16. Levitz M, Jansen V, Dancis J. The transfer and metabolism of corticosteroids in the perfused human placenta. Am J Obstet Gynecol 1978;132:363–6.
17. Eggers TR, Doyle LW, Pepperell RJ. Premature rupture of the membranes. Med J Aust 1979;1:209–13.
18. Garite TJ, Freeman RK, Linzey EM, Braly PS, Dorchester WL. Prospective randomized study of corticosteroids in the management of premature rupture of the membranes and the premature gestation. Am J Obstet Gynecol 1981;141:508–15.
19. Garite TJ. Premature rupture of the membranes: the enigma of the obstetrician. Am J Obstet Gynecol 1985;151:1001–5.
20. Nelson LH, Meis PJ, Hatjis CG, Ernest JM, Dillard R, Schey HM. Premature rupture of membranes: a prospective, randomized evaluation of steroids, latent phase, and expectant management. Obstet Gynecol 1985;66:55–8.
21. Simpson GF, Harbert GM Jr. Use of β-methasone in management of preterm gestation with premature rupture of membranes. Obstet Gynecol 1985;66:168–75.
22. Kuhn RJP, Speirs AL, Pepperell RJ, Eggers TR, Doyle LW, Hutchison A. Betamethasone, albuterol, and threatened premature delivery: benefits and risks. Obstet Gynecol 1982;60:403–8.
23. Schmidt PL, Sims ME, Strassner HT, Paul RH, Mueller E, McCart D. Effect of antepartum glucocorticoid administration upon neonatal respiratory distress syndrome and perinatal infection. Am J Obstet Gynecol 1984;148:178–86.
24. Ballard PL, Ballard RA, Granberg JP, et al. Fetal sex and prenatal betamethasone therapy. J Pediatr 1980;97:451–4.
25. Khoury MJ, Marks JS, McCarthy BJ, Zaro SM. Factors affecting the sex differential in neonatal mortality: the role of respiratory distress syndrome. Am J Obstet Gynecol 1985;151:777–82.
26. Papageorgiou AN, Desgranges MF, Masson M, Colle E, Shatz R, Gelfand MM. The antenatal use of betamethasone in the prevention of respiratory distress syndrome: a controlled double-blind study. Pediatrics 1979;63:73–9.
27. Bielawski D, Hiatt IM, Hegyi T. Betamethasone-induced leukaemoid reaction in pre-term infant. Lancet 1978;1:218–9.
28. Ferguson JE, Hensleigh PA, Gill P. Effects of betamethasone on white blood cells in patients with premature rupture of the membranes and preterm labor. Am J Obstet Gynecol 1984;150:439–41.
29. Catanzarite VA, McHargue AM, Sandberg EC, Dyson DC. Respiratory arrest during therapy for premature labor in a patient with myasthenia gravis. Obstet Gynecol 1984;64:819–22.
30. Gonen R, Samberg I, Sharf M. Hypertensive crisis associated with ritodrine infusion and betamethasone administration in premature labor. Eur J Obstet Gynecol Reprod Biol 1982;13:129–32.
31. Waffarn F, Siassi B, Cabal LA, Schmidt PL. Effect of antenatal glucocorticoids on clinical closure of the ductus arteriosus. Am J Dis Child 1983;137:336–8.
32. Ballard PL. Combined hormonal treatment and lung maturation. Semin Perinatol 1984;8:283–92.
33. Taeusch HW Jr. Glucocorticoid prophylaxis for respiratory distress syndrome: a review of potential toxicity. J Pediatr 1975;87:617–23.
34. Johnson JWC, Mitzner W, London WT, Palmer AE, Scott R. Betamethasone and the rhesus fetus: multisystemic effects. Am J Obstet Gynecol 1979;133:677–84.
35. MacArthur BA, Howie RN, Dezoete JA, Elkins J. Cognitive and psychosocial development of 4-year-old children whose mothers were treated antenatally with betamethasone. Pediatrics 1981;68:638–43.
36. MacArthur BA, Howie RN, Dezoete JA, Elkins J. School progress and cognitive development of 6-year-old children whose mothers were treated antenatally with betamethasone. Pediatrics 1982;70:99–105.

Name: **BETHANECHOL**

Class: **Parasympathomimetic (Cholinergic)**   Risk Factor: **C$_M$**

Fetal Risk Summary

The use of bethanechol in pregnancy has been reported, but too few data are available to analyze (1).

Breast Feeding Summary

Although specific data on the excretion of bethanechol into breast milk are lacking, one author cautioned that mothers receiving regular therapy with this drug should not breast-feed (2). Abdominal pain and diarrhea have been reported in a nursing infant exposed to bethanechol in milk (3).

References

1. Heinonen OP, Slone D, Shapiro S. *Birth Defects and Drugs in Pregnancy*. Littleton:Publishing Sciences Group, 1977:345–56.
2. Platzker ACD, Lew CD, Stewart D. Drug "administration" via breast milk. Hosp Pract 1980;15:111–122.
3. Shore MF. Drugs can be dangerous during pregnancy and lactations. Can Pharm J 1970;103:358. As cited in: Committee on Drugs, American Academy of Pediatrics. The transfer of drugs and other chemicals into human breast milk. Pediatrics 1983;72:375–83.

Name: **BIPERIDEN**

Class: **Parasympatholytic**   Risk Factor: **C$_M$**

Fetal Risk Summary

Biperiden is an anticholinergic agent used in the treatment of parkinsonism. No reports of its use in pregnancy have been located (see also Atropine).

Breast Feeding Summary

No data available (see also Atropine).

Name: **BLEOMYCIN**

Class: **Antineoplastic**   Risk Factor: **D**

Fetal Risk Summary

No reports linking the use of bleomycin with congenital defects have been located. Chromosomal aberrations in human marrow cells have been reported but the significance to the fetus is not known (1). Two separate cases of non-Hodgkin's lymphoma in pregnancy were treated during the 2nd and 3rd trimesters with bleomycin and other antineoplastic agents (2, 3). Normal infants without anomalies or chromosome changes were delivered.

Combination chemotherapy with bleomycin was used for teratoma of the testis in two men (4). In both cases, recovery of spermatogenesis with apparently successful fertilization occurred but the possibility of alternate paternity could not be excluded.

Breast Feeding Summary

No data available.

References

1. Bornstein RS, Hungerford DA, Haller G, Engstrom PF, Yarbro JW. Cytogenic effects of bleomycin therapy in man. Cancer Res 1971;31:2004–7.
2. Ortega J. Multiple agent chemotherapy including bleomycin of non-Hodgkin's lymphoma during pregnancy. Cancer 1977;40:2829–35.
3. Falkson HC, Simson IW, Falkson G. Non-Hodgkin's lymphoma in pregnancy. Cancer 1980;45:1679–82.
4. Rubery ED. Return of fertility after curative chemotherapy for disseminated teratoma of testis. Lancet 1983;1:186.

Name: **BRETYLIUM**

Class: **Antiarrhythmic**   Risk Factor: **C**

Fetal Risk Summary

Bretylium, a quaternary ammonium compound, is an adrenergic blocker used as an antiarrhythmic agent. No information on its use in pregnancy has been located. Hypotension has been observed in 50% of patients after bretylium (1). Although reports are lacking, reduced uterine blood flow with fetal hypoxia (bradycardia) is a potential risk. The manufacturer states that bretylium may be used in life-threatening situations if the expected benefits outweigh the unknown potential risks to the fetus (1).

Breast Feeding Summary

No data available.

References

1. Product information. Bretylol. American Critical Care, 1985.

Name: **BROMIDES**

Class: **Anticonvulsant/Sedative**   Risk Factor: **D**

Fetal Risk Summary

The Collaborative Perinatal Project monitored 50,282 mother-child pairs, 986 of which had 1st trimester exposure to bromides (1). For use anytime during pregnancy, 2,610 exposures were recorded (2). In neither case was evidence found to suggest a relationship to large categories of major or minor malformations. Four possible associations with individual malformations were found but the statistical significance of these are unknown and independent confirmation is required:

Polydactyly (14 cases)
Gastrointestinal malformations (10 cases)
Clubfoot (7 cases)
Congenital dislocation of hip (anytime use) (92 cases)

There have been two case reports of intrauterine growth retardation and subsequent failure to thrive (3 ,4). One of these affected infants also had congenital heart disease. More study is needed to establish a relationship between the use of bromides and congenital defects. Neonatal bromide intoxication from transplacental accumulation has been described (5, 6). Symptoms of neonatal bromism are generally nonspecific and include poor suck response, diminished Moro reflex, and hypotonia. Monitoring of serum bromide concentrations is recommended in neonates with *in utero* exposure.

Breast Feeding Summary

Bromide appears in breast milk. Kwit and Hatcher (7) reported breast milk concentrations of 1,666 μg/ml in two patients given 5 g daily for 1 month. A case of drowsiness and rash in a breast-fed infant appeared in 1921 (8). Breast-feeding is not recommended in patients receiving bromide-containing medications.

References

1. Heinonen OP, Slone D, Shapiro S. *Birth Defects and Drugs in Pregnancy*. Littleton:Publishing Sciences Group, 1977;402–6.
2. *Ibid*, 444.
3. Rossiter EJR, Rendel-Short TJ. Congenital effects of bromism? Lancet 1972; 2:705.
4. Opitz JM, Grosse RF, Haneberg B. Congenital effects of bromism? Lancet 1972;1:91.
5. Pleasure JR, Blackburn MG. Neonatal bromide intoxication: prenatal ingestion of a large quantity of bromides with transplacental accumulation in the fetus. Pediatrics 1975;55:503–6.
6. Mangurten HH, Ban R. Neonatal hypotonia secondary to transplacental bromism. J Pediatr 1974;85:426–8.
7. Kwit NT, Hatcher RA. Excretion of drugs in milk. Am J Dis Child 1935;49:900– 4.
8. Van der Bogert F. Bromin poisoning through mother's milk. Am J Dis Child 1921;21:167.

Name: **BROMOCRIPTINE**

Class: **Miscellaneous** Risk Factor: **C$_M$**

Fetal Risk Summary

Bromocriptine has been used during all stages of pregnancy. In 1982, Turkalj and co-workers (1) reviewed the results of 1,410 pregnancies in 1,335 women exposed to bromocriptine during gestation. The drug, used for the treatment of infertility due to hyperprolactinemia or pituitary tumors including acromegaly, was usually discontinued as soon as pregnancy was confirmed. The mean duration of exposure after conception was 21 days. The review included all reported cases from 1973, the year bromocriptine was introduced, through 1980. Since then, 11 other studies have reported the results of treatment in 121 women with 145 pregnancies (2–12). The results of the pregnancies in the combined studies are:

Total patients/Pregnancies	1456/1555
Liveborn infants	1369 (88%)
Stillborn infants	5 (0.3%)
Multiple pregnancies (30 twins/3 triplets)	33*(2.1%)
Spontaneous abortions	166 (10.7%)
Elective abortions	26 (1.7%)
Extrauterine pregnancies	12 (0.8%)
Hydatidiform moles (2 patients)	3 (0.2%)
Pregnant at time of report-outcome unknown	10

   * 2 women with twins were also treated with clomiphene or gonadotropin

A total of 48 (3.5%) of the 1374 liveborn/stillborn infants had detectable anomalies at birth (1, 2). This incidence is similar to the expected rate of congenital defects found in the general population. In the review of Turkalj et al., the mean duration of fetal exposure to bromocriptine was similar between children with congenital abnormalities and normal children. No distinguishable pattern of anomalies was found. Malformations detected at birth were:

Major	No.	Minor	No.
Down's syndrome	2	Bat ear/plagiocephalus	1
Hydrocephalus/multiple atresia of esophagus and intestine	1	Cleft palate	1
		Ear lobe deformity	1
Microcephalus/encephalopathy	1	Head posture constrained	1
Omphalocele/talipes	1	Hip dislocation (aplasia of cup)	9
Pulmonary artery atresia	1	Hydrocele	3
Reduction deformities	4	Hydrocele/omphalocele	1
Renal agenesis	1	Hydrospadius	1
Pierre Robin syndrome	1	Inguinal hernia	2
		Skull soft/open fontanelle	1
		Single palmar crease	1
		Single umbilical artery	1
		Syndactyly	2
		Talipes	5
		Umbilical hernia	1
		Cutaneous hemangioma	4
		Testicular ectopia (spontaneous correction at age 7 months)	1
Total	12	Total	36

Long-term studies on 213 children followed up to 6 years of age have shown normal mental and physical development (1, 2).

In summary, bromocriptine apparently does not pose a significant risk to the fetus. The pattern and incidence of anomalies are similar to those expected in a nonexposed population.

Breast Feeding Summary

Since bromocriptine is indicated for the prevention of physiologic lactation, breast-feeding is not possible during therapy (13, 14). However, in one report, a mother taking 5 mg/day for a pituitary tumor was able to successfully breast-feed her infant (3). No effects on the infant were mentioned. Because bromocriptine suppresses lactation, the American Academy of Pediatrics considers the drug contraindicated during breast-feeding (15).

References

1. Turkalj I, Braun P, Krupp P. Surveillance of bromocriptine in pregnancy. JAMA 1982;247:1589–91.
2. Konopka P, Raymond JP, Merceron RE, Seneze J. Continuous administration of bromocriptine in the prevention of neurological complications in pregnant women with prolactinomas. Am J Obstet Gynecol 1983;146:935–8.
3. Canales ES, Garcia IC, Ruiz JE, Zarate A. Bromocriptine as prophylactic therapy in prolactinoma during pregnancy. Fertil Steril 1981;36:524–6.
4. Bergh T, Nillius SJ, Larsson SG, Wide L. Effects of bromocriptine-induced pregnancy on prolactin-secreting pituitary tumors. Acta Endocrinol (Copenh) 1981;98:333.
5. Yuen BH, Cannon W, Sy L, Booth J, Burch P. Regression of pituitary microadenoma during and following bromocriptine therapy: persistent defect in prolactin regulation before and throughout pregnancy. Am J Obstet Gynecol 1982;142:634–9.
6. Maeda T, Ushiroyama T, Okuda K, Fujimoto A, Ueki M, Sugimoto O. Effective bromocriptine treatment of a pituitary macroadenoma during pregnancy. Obstet Gynecol 1983;61:117–21.
7. Hammond CB, Haney AF, Land MR, van der Merwe JV, Ory SJ, Wiebe RH. The outcome of pregnancy in patients with treated and untreated prolactin-secreting pituitary tumors. Am J Obstet Gynecol 1983;147: 148–57.
8. Cundy T, Grundy EN, Melville H, Sheldon J. Bromocriptine treatment of acromegaly following spontaneous conception. Fertil Steril 1984;42:134–6.
9. Randall S, Laing I, Chapman AJ, Shalet SM, Beardwell CG, Kelly WF, Davies D. Pregnancies in women with hyperprolactinaemia: obstetric and enocrinological management of 50 pregnancies in 37 women. Br J Obstet Gynaecol 1982;89:20–33.
10. Andersen AN, Starup J, Tabor A, Jensen HK, Westergaard JG. The possible prognostic value of serum prolactin increment during pregnancy in hyperprolactinaemic patients. Acta Endocrinol (Copenh) 1983;102:1–5.
11. van Roon E, van der Vijver JCM, Gerretsen G, Hekster REM, Wattendorff RA. Rapid regression of a suprasellar extending prolactinoma after bromocriptine treatment during pregnancy. Fertil Steril 1981;36:173–77.
12. Crosignani P, Ferrari C, Mattei AM. Visual field defects and reduced visual acuity during pregnancy in two patients with prolactinoma: rapid regression of symptoms under bromocriptine. Case reports. Br J Obstet Gynaecol 1984;91:821–3.
13. Product information. Parlodel. Sandoz Pharmaceuticals, 1985.
14. Thorbert G, Akerlund M. Inhibition of lactation by cyclofenil and bromocriptine. Br J Obstet Gynaecol 1983;90:739–42.
15. Committee on Drugs, American Academy of Pediatrics. The transfer of drugs and other chemicals into human breast milk. Pediatrics 1983;72:375–83.

Name: **BROMODIPHENHYDRAMINE**

Class: **Antihistamine** Risk Factor: **C**

Fetal Risk Summary

Bromodiphenhydramine is a derivative of diphenhydramine (see Diphenhydramine).

Breast Feeding Summary

No data available.

Name: **BROMPHENIRAMINE**

Class: **Antihistamine**   Risk Factor: C_M

Fetal Risk Summary

The Collaborative Perinatal Project monitored 50,282 mother-child pairs, 65 of which had 1st trimester exposure to brompheniramine (1). Based on 10 malformed infants, a statistically significant association ($p < 0.01$) was found between this drug and congenital defects. This relationship was not found with other antihistamines. For use anytime during pregnancy, 412 exposures were recorded (2). In this case, no evidence was found for an association with malformations.

Breast Feeding Summary

A single case report has been located describing adverse effects in a 3-month-old nursing infant of a mother consuming a long-acting preparation containing 6 mg of dexbrompheniramine and 120 mg of d-isoephedrine (3). The mother had begun taking the preparation on a twice daily schedule about 1 or 2 days prior to the onset of symptoms in the infant. Symptoms consisted of irritability, excessive crying, and disturbed sleeping patterns which resolved spontaneously within 12 hours when breast-feeding was stopped. One manufacturer considers the drug contraindicated for nursing mothers (4).

References

1. Heinonen OP, Slone D, Shapiro S. *Birth Defects and Drugs in Pregnancy*. Littleton:Publishing Sciences Group, 1977:322–5.
2. *Ibid*, 437.
3. Mortimer EA Jr. Drug toxicity from breast milk? Pediatrics 1977;60:780–1.
4. Product information. Dimetane. AH Robins Company, 1985.

Name: **BUCLIZINE**

Class: **Antihistamine/Antiemetic**   Risk Factor: **C**

Fetal Risk Summary

Buclizine is a piperazine antihistamine which is used as an antiemetic (see also Cyclizine and Meclizine for closely related drugs). The drug is teratogenic in animals, but its effects on the human fetus have not been thoroughly studied.

The Collaborative Perinatal Project monitored 50,282 mother-child pairs, 44 of which had 1st trimester exposure to buclizine (1). No evidence was found to suggest a relationship to large categories of major or minor malformations. For use anytime during pregnancy, 62 exposures were recorded (2). A possible association with congenital defects, based on the report of three malformed children, was found from this exposure.

The manufacturer considers the drug to be contraindicated in early pregnancy (3).

Breast Feeding Summary

No data available.

References

1. Heinonen OP, Slone D, Shapiro S. *Birth Defects and Drugs in Pregnancy*. Littleton:Publishing Sciences Group, 1977:323–4.
2. *Ibid*, 437.
3. Product information. Bucladin. Stuart Pharmaceuticals, 1985.

Name: **BUSULFAN**

Class: **Antineoplastic** Risk Factor: **D**

Fetal Risk Summary

Busulfan is an alkylating antineoplastic agent. The use of this drug has been reported in 33 pregnancies, 22 in the 1st trimester (1). Six malformed infants have been observed (1–4):

Unspecified malformations, aborted
   at 20 weeks (1 case)
Anomalous deviation left lobe liver,
   bilobar spleen, pulmonary atelectasis (1 case)
Pyloric stenosis (1 case)
Cleft palate, microphthalmia, cytomegaly, hypoplasia
   of ovaries and thyroid gland, corneal opacity,
   intrauterine growth retardation (IUGR) (1 case)
Myeloschisis, aborted at 6 weeks (1 case)
IUGR, left hydronephrosis and hydroureter, absent
   right kidney and ureter, hepatic subcapsular
   calcifications (1 case)

Data from one review indicated that 40% of the infants exposed to anticancer drugs were of low birth weight (1). This finding was not related to the timing of the exposure. Long-term studies of growth and mental development in offspring exposed to busulfan during the 2nd trimester, the period of neuroblast multiplication, have not been conducted (5). Chromosomal damage has been associated with busulfan therapy, but the potential for future teratogenicity is unknown (6). Irregular menses and amenorrhea, the latter at times permanent, have been reported in women receiving busulfan (7, 8).

Breast Feeding Summary

No data available.

References

1. Nicholson HO. Cytotoxic drugs in pregnancy: review of reported cases. J Obstet Gynaecol Br Commonw 1968;75:307–12.

2. Diamond I, Anderson MM, McCreadie SR. Transplacental transmission of busulfan (Myleran) in a mother with leukemia: production of fetal malformation and cytomegaly. Pediatrics 1960;25:85–90.
3. Abramovici A, Shaklai M, Pinkhas J. Myeloschisis in a six weeks embryo of a leukemic woman treated by busulfan. Teratology 1978;18:241–6.
4. Gililland J, Weinstein L. The effects of cancer chemotherapeutic agents on the developing fetus. Obstet Gynecol Survey 1983;38:6–13.
5. Dobbing J. Pregnancy and leukaemia. Lancet 1977;1:1155.
6. Gebhart E, Schwanitz G, Hartwich G. Chromosomal aberrations during busulphan therapy. Dtsch Med Wochenschr 1974;99:52–6.
7. Galton DAG, Till M, Wiltshaw E. Busulfan: summary of clinical results. Ann NY Acad Sci 1958;68:967–73.
8. Schilsky RL, Lewis BJ, Sherins RJ, Young RC. Gonadal dysfunction in patients receiving chemotherapy for cancer. Ann Intern Med 1980;93:109–14.

Name: **BUTALBITAL**

Class: **Sedative**   Risk Factor: **C***

Fetal Risk Summary

Butalbital is a short-acting barbiturate that is contained in a number of analgesic mixtures. In a large prospective study, 112 patients were exposed to this drug during the 1st trimester (1). No association with malformations was found. Severe neonatal withdrawal was described in a male infant whose mother took 150 mg of butalbital daily during the last 2 months of pregnancy in the form of a proprietary headache mixture (Esgic—butalbital 50 mg, caffeine 40 mg, and acetaminophen 325 mg per dose) (2). The infant was also exposed to oxycodone, pentazocine, and acetaminophen during the 1st trimester, but apparently these had been discontinued prior to the start of the butalbital product. Onset of withdrawal occurred within 2 days of birth.

[* Risk Factor D if used for prolonged periods or in high doses at term.]

Breast Feeding Summary

No data available (see also Pentobarbital).

References

1. Heinonen OP, Slone D, Shapiro S. *Birth Defects and Drugs in Pregnancy*. Littleton:Publishing Sciences Group, 1977:336–7.
2. Ostrea EM. Neonatal withdrawal from intrauterine exposure to butalbital. Am J Obstet Gynecol 1982;143:597–9.

Name: **BUTAPERAZINE**

Class: **Tranquilizer**   Risk Factor: **C**

Fetal Risk Summary

Butaperazine is a piperazine phenothiazine in the same group as prochlorperazine (see Prochlorperazine). The phenothiazines readily cross the placenta (1). No specific information on the use of butaperazine in pregnancy has been located.

Although occasional reports have attempted to link various phenothiazine compounds with congenital malformations, the bulk of the evidence indicates that these drugs are safe for the mother and fetus (see also Chlorpromazine).

Breast Feeding Summary

No data available.

References

1. Moya F, Thorndike V. Passage of drugs across the placenta. Am J Obstet Gynecol 1962;84:1778–98.

Name: **BUTORPHANOL**

Class: **Analgesic**   Risk Factor: **B***

Fetal Risk Summary

No reports linking the use of butorphanol with congenital defects have been located. Since it has both narcotic agonist and antagonist properties, prolonged use during gestation may result in fetal addiction with subsequent withdrawal in the newborn (see also Pentazocine).

At term, butophanol rapidly crosses the placenta, producing cord serum levels averaging 84% of maternal concentrations (1, 2). Depressant effects on the newborn from *in utero* exposure during labor are similar to those seen with meperidine (1–3).

The use of 1 mg of butorphanol combined with 25 mg of promethazine administered intravenously to a woman in active labor was associated with a sinusoidal fetal heart rate pattern (4). Onset of the pattern occurred 6 minutes after drug injection and persisted for approximately 58 minutes. The newborn infant showed no effects from the abnormal heart pattern.

A study comparing neonatal neurobehavior was conducted in 135 patients during their first day of life (5). Maternal analgesia consisted of 1 mg of butorphanol (68 patients) or 40 mg of meperidine (67 patients). No difference between the drugs was observed.

[* Risk Factor D if used for prolonged periods or in high doses at term.]

Breast Feeding Summary

Butorphanol passes into breast milk in concentrations paralleling levels in maternal serum (2). Milk:plasma ratios after intramuscular (12 mg) or oral (8 mg) doses were 0.7 and 1.9, respectively. Using 2 mg intramuscularly or 8 mg orally four times a day would result in 4 μg excreted in the full daily milk output (1000 ml). Although it has not been studied, this amount is probably insignificant. The American Academy of Pediatrics considers butorphanol compatible with breast-feeding (6).

References

1. Maduska AL, Hajghassemali M. A double-blind comparison of butorphanol and merperidine in labour: maternal pain relief and effect on the newborn. Can Anaesth Soc J 1978;25:398–404.

2. Pittman KA, Smyth RD, Losada M, Zighelboim I, Maduska AL, Sunshine A. Human perinatal distribution of butorphanol. Am J Obstet Gynecol 1980;138:797–800.
3. Quilligan EJ, Keegan KA, Donahue MJ. Double-blind comparison of intravenously injected butorphanol and meperidine in parturients. Int J Gynaecol Obstet 1980;18:363–7.
4. Angel JL, Knuppel RA, Lake M. Sinusoidal fetal heart rate pattern associated with intravenous butorphanol administration: a case report. Am J Obstet Gynecol 1984;149:465–7.
5. Hodgkinson R, Huff RW, Hayashi RH, Husain FJ. Double-blind comparison of maternal analgesia and neonatal neurobehaviour following intravenous butorphanol and meperidine. J Int Med Res 1979;7:224–30.
6. Committee on Drugs, American Academy of Pediatrics. The transfer of drugs and other chemicals into human breast milk. Pediatrics 1983;72:375–83.

Name: **BUTRIPTYLINE**

Class: **Antidepressant**   Risk Factor: **D**

Fetal Risk Summary

No data available (see Imipramine).

Breast Feeding Summary

No data available (see Imipramine).

C

Name: **CAFFEINE**

Class: **Central Stimulant**   Risk Factor: **B**

Fetal Risk Summary

Caffeine is one of the most popular drugs in North America and many other parts of the world. It is frequently used in combination products containing aspirin, phenacetin, and codeine and is present in a number of commonly consumed beverages, such as coffee, teas, and colas. The Food and Drug Administration has removed caffeine from the list of drugs "generally regarded as safe" and has issued a warning regarding the consumption of caffeine during pregnancy (1, 2).

Caffeine crosses the placenta, and fetal blood and tissue levels similar to maternal concentrations are achieved (3–5). Cord blood levels of 1–1.6 μg/ml have been measured (3). Caffeine has also been found in newborns exposed to theophylline *in utero* (6).

The mutagenicity and carcinogenicity of caffeine have been evaluated in over 50 studies involving laboratory animals, human and animal cell tissue cultures, and human lymphocytes *in vivo* (3). The significance of mutagenic and carcinogenic effects found in nonmammalian systems has not been established in man.

The Collaborative Perinatal Project monitored 50,282 mother-child pairs, 5,378 of which had 1st trimester exposure to caffeine (7). No evidence of a relationship to congenital defects was found. For use anytime during pregnancy, 12,696 exposures were recorded (8). In this case, slightly increased relative risks were found for musculoskeletal defects, hydronephrosis, adrenal anomalies, and hemangiomas/granulomas, but the results are uninterpretable without independent confirmation (8). A follow-up analysis by the Collaborative Perinatal Project on 2,030 malformed infants and maternal use of caffeine-containing beverages does not support caffeine as a teratogen (9). Other reports have also found no association between the use of caffeine during pregnancy and congenital malformations (10–12).

Several authors have associated high caffeine consumption (6–8 cups of coffee per day) with decreased fertility, increased incidence of spontaneous abortion, and low birth weights (3, 13–17). Unfortunately, few of these studies have isolated the effects of caffeine from cigarette or alcohol use, both of which are positively associated with caffeine consumption (3). One German study has observed that high coffee use alone is associated with low birth weights (18). The Delivery Interview Program at the Boston Hospital for Women assessed the effects of coffee consumption in more than 12.400 women. Low birth weights and short gestation occurred more often among offspring of women who drank 4 or more cups of coffee per day and who also smoked (19). No relationship between low birth weights/short gestation and caffeine was found after controlling for smoking, alcohol intake, and demographic characteristics.

The altering of catecholamine levels by the presence of caffeine is of concern (20). However, the significance of this pharmacological effect on normal human development is not understood.

In summary, caffeine consumption in pregnancy in moderate amounts does not seem to pose a risk to the fetus. Use of high doses (>6–8 cups of coffee per day) may be associated with complications, including infertility, but other factors may be involved.

Breast Feeding Summary

Caffeine is excreted into breast milk (21–26). Milk:plasma ratios of 0.5 and 0.76 have been reported (22, 23). Following ingestion of coffee or tea containing known amounts of caffeine (36–335 mg), peak milk levels of 2.09–7.17 μg/ml occurred within 1 hour (24). An infant consuming 90 ml of milk every 3 hours would ingest 0.01–1.64 mg of caffeine over 24 hours after the mother drank a single cup of caffeinated beverage (24).

In another study, peak milk levels after a 100-mg dose were 3.0 μg/ml at 1 hour (23). In this and an earlier study, the authors estimated a nursing infant would receive 1.5–3.1 mg of caffeine after the mother drank a single cup of coffee (22, 23).

The amounts described above are probably too low to be clinically significant. However, accumulation may occur in infants when mothers use moderate to heavy amounts of caffeinated beverages. The elimination half-life of caffeine is approximately 80 hours in term newborns and 97.5 hours in premature babies (25). Irritability and poor sleeping patterns have been observed in nursing infants during periods of heavy maternal use of caffeine (26).

References

1. Morris MB, Weinstein L. Caffeine and the fetus: is trouble brewing? Am J Obstet Gynecol 1981;140:607–10.
2. Goyan JE. Statement by the Commissioner of Food and Drugs, FDA press release. Washington, DC, September 4, 1980(P80-36):3.
3. Soyka LF. Caffeine ingestion during pregnancy: in utero exposure and possible effects. Semin Perinatol 1981;5:305–9.
4. Goldstein A, Warren R. Passage of caffeine into human gonadal and fetal tissue. Biochem Pharmacol 1962;17:166–8.
5. Parsons WD, Aranda JV, Neims AH. Elimination of transplacentally acquired caffeine in fullterm neonates. Pediatr Res 1976;10:333.
6. Brazier JL, Salle B. Conversion of theophylline to caffeine by the human fetus. Semin Perinatol 1981;5:315–20.
7. Heinonen OP, Slone D, Shapiro S. Birth Defects and Drugs in Pregnancy. Littleton:Publishing Sciences Group, 1977:366–70.
8. Ibid, 493–4.
9. Rosenberg L, Mitchell AA, Shapiro S, Slone D. Selected birth defects in relation to caffeine-containing beverages. JAMA 1982;247:1429–32.
10. Van't Hoff W. Caffeine in pregnancy. Lancet 1982;1:1020.
11. Kurppa K, Holmberg PC, Kuosma E, Saxen L. Coffee consumption during pregnancy. N Engl J Med 1982;306:1548–9.
12. Curatolo PW, Robertson D. The health consequences of caffeine. Ann Intern Med 1983;98(Part 1):641–53.
13. Weathersbee PS, Olsen LK, Lodge JR. Caffeine and pregnancy. Postgrad Med 1977;62:64–9.
14. Anonymous. Caffeine and birth defects—another negative study. Pediatr Alert 1982;7:23–4.

15. Hogue CJ. Coffee in pregnancy. Lancet 1981;2:554.
16. Weathersbee PS, Lodge JR, Caffeine: its direct and indirect influence on reproduction. J Reprod Med 1977;19:55–63.
17. Lechat MF, Borlee I, Bouckaert A, Misson C. Caffeine study. Science 1980;207:1296–7.
18. Mau G, Netter P. Kaffee- und alkoholkonsum-riskofaktoren in der schwangerschaft? Geburtshilfe Frauenheilkd 1974;34:1018–22.
19. Linn S, Schoenbaum SC, Monson RR, Rosner B, Stubblefield PG, Ryan KJ. No association between coffee consumption and adverse outcomes of pregnancy. N Engl J Med 1982;306:141–5.
20. Bellet S, Roman L, DeCastro O, et al. Effect of coffee ingestion on catecholamine release. Metabolism 1969;18:288–91.
21. Jobe PC. Psychoactive substances and antiepileptic drugs. In Wilson JT, ed. Drugs in Breast Milk. Balgowlah, Australia: ADIS Press, 1981:40.
22. Tyrala EE, Dodson WE. Caffeine secretion into breast milk. Arch Dis Child 1979;54:787–800.
23. Sargraves R, Bradley JM, Delgado MJM, Wagner D, Sharpe GL, Stavchansky S. Pharmacokinetics of caffeine in human breast milk after a single oral dose of caffeine. Drug Intell Clin Pharm 1984;18:507 (Abstr).
24. Berlin CM Jr, Denson HM, Daniel CH, Ward RM. Disposition of dietary caffeine in milk, saliva, and plasma of lactating women. Pediatrics 1984;73:59–63.
25. Berlin CM Jr. Excretion of the methylxanthines in human milk. Semin Perinatol 1981;5:389–94.
26. Hill RM, Craig JP, Chaney MD, Tennyson LM, McCulley LB. Utilization of over-the-counter drugs during pregnancy. Clin Obstet Gynecol 1977;20:381–94.

Name: CALCIFEDIOL
Class: **Vitamin**   Risk Factor: **A***

Fetal Risk Summary

Calcifediol is converted in the kidneys to calcitriol, one of the active forms of vitamin D. See Vitamin D.

[* Risk Factor D if used in doses above the RDA.]

Breast Feeding Summary

See Vitamin D.

Name: CALCITONIN
Class: **Calcium Regulation Hormone**   Risk Factor: **B**

Fetal Risk Summary

No reports linking the use of calcitonin with congenital defects have been located. Marked increases of calcitonin concentrations in fetal serum over maternal levels has been demonstrated at term (1). The significance of this finding is unknown. The hormone does not cross the placenta (2).

Breast Feeding Summary

No data available. Calcitonin has been shown to inhibit lactation in animals. Mothers wishing to breast-feed should be informed of this potential complication (2).

References

1. Kovarik J, Woloszczuk W, Linkesch W, Pavelka R. Calcitonin in pregnancy. Lancet 1980;1:199–200.
2. Product information. Calcimar. Armour Pharmaceutical Company, 1985.

Name: **CALCITRIOL**

Class: **Vitamin**   Risk Factor: **A***

Fetal Risk Summary

Calcitriol is one of three physiologically active forms of vitamin D. See Vitamin D.

[* Risk Factor D if used in doses above RDA.]

Breast Feeding Summary

See Vitamin D.

Name: **CAMPHOR**

Class: **Antipruritic/Local Anesthetic**   Risk Factor: **C**

Fetal Risk Summary

No reports linking the use of topically applied camphor with congenital defects have been located. Camphor is toxic and potentially a fatal poison if taken orally in sufficient quantities. Four cases of fetal exposure after accidental ingestion, including a case of fetal death and neonatal respiratory failure, have been reported (1–4). The drug crosses the placenta (2).

Breast Feeding Summary

No data available.

References

1. Figgs J, Hamilton R, Homel S, McCabe J. Camphorated oil intoxication in pregnancy. Report of a case. Obstet Gynecol 1965;25:255–8.
2. Weiss J, Catalano P. Camphorated oil intoxication during pregnancy. Pediatrics 1973;52:713–4.
3. Blackman WB, Curry HB. Camphor poisoning: report of case occurring during pregnancy. J Fla Med Assoc 1957;43:99.
4. Jacobziner H, Raybin HW. Camphor poisoning. Arch Pediatr 1962;79:28.

Name: **CAPTOPRIL**

Class: **Antihypertensive**   Risk Factor: **C$_M$**

Fetal Risk Summary

A malformed fetus was apparently discovered following voluntary abortion in a patient with renovascular hypertension (1). The patient had been treated during the 1st trimester with captopril, propranolol, and amiloride. The left leg ended at mid-thigh without distal development, and no obvious skull formation was noted above the brain tissue. However, because of the very small size of the fetus (1.5 cm), the pathologist could not be certain that the defects were not a result of the abortion (2). In a second case, a pregnant woman with nephrotic syndrome and arterial hypertension was treated throughout pregnancy with captopril and acebutolol (3). Intrauterine growth retardation, due either to the drug therapy or to severe maternal disease, was identified early in the 2nd trimester and became progressively worse. The growth-retarded male infant was delivered prematurely at 34 weeks by cesarean section. Captopril was found in the cord blood with levels in the mother and fetus less than 100 ng/ml 4 hours after the last dose. Angiotensin-converting enzyme activity was below normal limits in both the mother and the newborn. Neonatal respiratory arrest occurred 15 minutes after delivery, with varying degrees of hypotension persisting over the first 10 days. A patent ductus arteriosus was also present.

Captopril is embryocidal in animals and has been shown to cause an increase in stillbirths in some species (4). Because of this toxicity, a committee of the National Institutes of Health recommends that captopril be avoided during pregnancy (5).

Breast Feeding Summary

Captopril is excreted into breast milk in low concentrations. In 12 mothers given 100 mg three times a day, average peak milk levels of 4.7 ng/ml at 3.8 hours after their last dose were produced (6, 7). This represented an average milk:plasma ratio of 0.012. No differences were found in captopril levels in pre- and postdrug milk samples. No effects on the nursing infants were observed. The American Academy of Pediatrics considers captopril compatible with breast-feeding (8).

References

1. Duminy PC, Burger PT. Fetal abnormality associated with the use of captopril during pregnancy. S Afr Med J 1981;60:805.
2. Broude AM. Fetal abnormality associated with captropril during pregnancy. S Afr Med J 1982;61:68.
3. Boutroy MJ, Vert P, Hurault de Ligny B, Miton A. Captopril administration in pregnancy impairs fetal angiotensin converting enzyme activity and neonatal adaptation. Lancet 1984;2:935–6.
4. Pipkin FB, Turner SR, Symonds EM. Possible risk with captopril in pregnancy: some animal data. Lancet 1980;1:1256.
5. Anonymous. The 1984 report of the Joint National Committee on Detection, Evaluation, and Treatment of High Blood Pressure. Arch Intern Med 1984;144:1045–6.
6. Devlin RG, Fleiss PM. Selective resistance to the passage of captopril into human milk. Clin Pharmacol Ther 1980;27:250.
7. Devlin RG, Fleiss PM. Captopril in human blood and breast milk. J Clin Pharmacol 1981;21:110–3.
8. Committee on Drugs, American Academy of Pediatrics. The transfer of drugs and other chemicals into human breast milk. Pediatrics 1983;72:375–83.

Name: CARBACHOL

Class: Parasympathomimetic (Cholinergic)   Risk Factor: C

Fetal Risk Summary

Carbachol is used in the eye. No reports of its use in pregnancy have been located. As a quaternary ammonium compound, it is ionized at physiologic pH, and transplacental passage in significant amounts would not be expected.

Breast Feeding Summary

No data available.

Name: **CARBAMAZEPINE**

Class: **Anticonvulsant**   Risk Factor: **C$_M$**

Fetal Risk Summary

Carbamazepine, a tricyclic anticonvulsant, has been in clinical use since 1962. The drug crosses the placenta with highest concentrations found in fetal liver and kidneys (1–3). Fetal levels are approximately 50–80% of those of maternal serum (3).

Use of carbamazepine during the 1st trimester has been reported in over 500 pregnancies (4–15). Multiple anomalies were found in one stillborn infant where carbamazepine was the only anticonvulsant used by the mother (11). These included closely set eyes, flat nose with single nasopharynx, polydactyly, atrial septal defect, patent ductus arteriosus, absent gallbladder and thyroid gland, and collapsed fontanel. Individual defects observed in this and other cases include talipes, meningomylocele, anal atresia, ambiguous genitalia, congenital heart disease, hypertelorism, hypoplasia of the nose, cleft lip, congenital hip dislocation, inguinal hernia, hypoplasia of the nails, and torticollis (4–13). Decreased head circumference, 7 mm less than controls, has been observed in infants exposed only to carbamazepine during gestation (15). The head size was still small by 18 months of age with no catch-up growth evident. In a 1982 review, Janz (16) stated that nearly all possible malformations had been observed in epileptic patients. Minor malformations, such as those seen in the fetal hydantoin syndrome (see Phenytoin), have also been observed with carbamazepine monotherapy, causing Janz to conclude that the term "fetal hydantoin syndrome" was misleading (16).

Whether or not carbamazepine is teratogenic is still open to question. Drug therapy, the disease itself, genetic factors, or a combination of these may be related to the defects observed in the offspring of epileptic mothers. Of interest in this regard, Nakane and co-workers (8) found no statistical relationship between carbamazepine and malformations. Carbamazepine has been recommended as the drug of choice in women at risk of pregnancy who require anticonvulsant therapy for the first time (17).

Placental function in women taking carbamazepine has been evaluated (14). No effect was detected from carbamazepine as measured by serum human placental lactogen, 24-hour urinary total estriol excretion, placental weight, and birth weight.

The effect of carbamazepine on maternal and fetal vitamin D metabolism was examined in a 1984 study (18). In comparison to normal controls, several significant differences were found in the level of various vitamin D compounds and in serum calcium, but the values were still within normal limits. No alterations were found in alkaline phosphatase and phosphate concentrations. The authors doubted if the observed differences were of major clinical significance.

Breast Feeding Summary

Carbamazepine is excreted into breast milk producing milk:plasma ratios of 0.24–0.69 (1, 3, 6, 11, 19). The amount of carbamazepine measured in infant serum is low with typical levels around 0.4 μg/ml, but may be as high as 0.5–1.8 μg/ml (1). Accumulation does not seem to occur. The American Academy of Pediatrics considers the drug compatible with breast-feeding (20).

References

1. Pynnonen S, Knato J, Stilanpaa M, Erkkola R. Carbamazepine: placental transport, tissue concentrations in the foetus and newborns, and level milk. Acta Pharmacol Toxicol 1977;41:244–53.
2. Rane A, Bertilsson L, Palmer L. Disposition of placentally transferred carbamazepine (Tegretol) in the newborn. Eur J Clin Pharmacol 1975;8:283–4.
3. Nau H, Kuhnz W, Egger HJ, Rating D, Helge H. Anticonvulsants during pregnancy and lactation: transplacental, maternal and neonatal pharmacokinetics. Clin Pharmacokinet 1982;7:508–43.
4. Geigy Pharmaceuticals. Tegretol in epilepsy. In *Monograph 319-80950*. Ardsley:Ciba-Geigy, 1978:18–19.
5. McMullin GP. Teratogenic effects of anticonvulsants. Br Med J 1971;4:430.
6. Pynnonen S, Sillanpaa M. Carbamazepine and mother's milk. Lancet 1975;2:563.
7. Lander CM, Edwards VE, Endie MJ, Tyrer JH. Plasma anticonvulsant concentrations during pregnancy. Neurology 1977;27:128–31.
8. Nakane Y, Okuma T, Takahashi R, et al. Multi-institutional study on the teratogenicity and fetal toxicity to antiepileptic drugs: a report of a collaborative study group in Japan. Epilepsia 1980;21:633–80.
9. Janz D. The teratogenic risk of antiepileptic drugs. Epilepsia 1975;16:159–69.
10. Meyer JG. Teratogenic risk of anticonvulsants and the effects on pregnancy and birth. Eur Neurol 1979;10:179–90.
11. Niebly JR, Blake DA, Freeman JM, Luff RD. Carbamazepine levels in pregnancy and lactation. Obstet Gynecol 1979;53:130–40.
12. Hicks EP. Carbamazepine in two pregnancies. Clin Exp Neurol 1979;16:269–75.
13. Thomas D, Buchanan N. Teratogenic effects of anticonvulsants. J Pediatr 1981;99:163.
14. Hiilesmaa VK. Evaluation of placental function in women on antiepileptic drugs. J Perinat Med 1983;11:187–92.
15. Hiilesmaa VK, Teramo K, Granstrom ML, Bardy AH. Fetal head growth retardation associated with maternal antiepileptic drugs. Lancet 1981;2:165–7.
16. Janz D. Antiepileptic drugs and pregnancy: altered utilization patterns and teratogenesis. Epilepsia 1982;23(Suppl 1):S53–S63.
17. Paulson GW, Paulson RB. Teratogenic effects of anticonvulsants. Arch Neurol 1981;38:140–3.
18. Markestad T, Ulstein M, Strandjord RE, Aksnes L, Aarskog D. Anticonvulsant drug therapy in human pregnancy: effects on serum concentrations of vitamin D metabolites in maternal and cord blood. Am J Obstet Gynecol 1984;150:254–8.
19. Kok THHG, Taitz LS, Bennett MJ, Holt DW. Drowsiness due to clemastine transmitted in breast milk. Lancet 1982;1:914–5.
20. Committee on Drugs, American Academy of Pediatrics. The transfer of drugs and other chemicals into human breast milk. Pediatrics 1983;72:375–83.

Name: **CARBARSONE**

Class: **Amebicide**   Risk Factor: **D**

Fetal Risk Summary

No reports linking the use of carbarsone with congenital defects have been located. However, carbarsone contains approximately 29% arsenic, which has been associated with lesions of the central nervous system (1). In view of potential tissue accumulation and reported fetal fatalities secondary to arsenic poisonings, carbarsone is not recommended during pregnancy (1, 2).

Breast Feeding Summary

No data available.

References

1. Arnold W. Morphologic und pathogenese der Salvarsan-schadigungen des zentralnervensystems. Virchows Arch (Pathol Anat) 1944;311:1.
2. Lugo G, Cassady G, Palmisano P. Acute maternal arsenic intoxication with neonatal death. Am J Dis Child 1969;117:328.

Name: **CARBENICILLIN**

Class: **Antibiotic**   Risk Factor: **B**

Fetal Risk Summary

Carbenicillin is a penicillin antibiotic (see also Penicillin G). The drug crosses the placenta and distributes to most fetal tissues (1, 2). Following a 4-g intramuscular dose, mean peak concentrations in cord and maternal serums at 2 hours were similar. Amniotic fluid levels averaged 7–11% of maternal peak concentrations.

No reports linking the use of carbenicillin with congenital defects have been located. The Collaborative Perinatal Project monitored 50,282 mother-child pairs, 3,546 of which had documented 1st trimester exposure to penicillin derivatives (3). For use anytime during pregnancy, 7,171 exposures were recorded (4). In neither case was evidence found to suggest a relationship to large categories of major or minor malformations or to individual defects.

Breast Feeding Summary

No data available (see Penicillin G).

References

1. Biro L, Ivan E, Elek E, Arr M. Data on the tissue concentration of antibiotics in man. Tissue concentrations of semi-synthetic penicillins in the fetus. Int Z Pharmakol Ther Toxikol 1970;4:321–4.
2. Elek E, Ivan E, Arr M. Passage of penicillins from mother to foetus in humans. Int J Clin Pharmacol Ther Toxicol 1972;6:223–8.
3. Heinonen OP, Slone D, Shapiro S. *Birth Defects and Drugs in Pregnancy.* Littleton:Publishing Sciences Group, 1977:297–313.
4. *Ibid*, 435.

Name: **CARBIMAZOLE**

Class: **Antithyroid**   Risk Factor: **D**

Fetal Risk Summary

Carbimazole is converted in vivo to methimazole (1). See Methimazole.

Breast Feeding Summary

See Methimazole.

References

1. Haynes RC Jr, Murad F. Thyroid and antithyroid drugs. In Gilman AG, Goodman LS, Gilman A, eds. *The Pharmacological Basis of Therapeutics*, ed. 5. New York:Macmillan Publishing Co, 1980:1411.

Name: **CARBINOXAMINE**

Class: **Antihistamine**   Risk Factor: **C**

Fetal Risk Summary

No data available. See Diphenhydramine for representative agent in this class.

Breast Feeding Summary

No data available.

Name: **CARPHENAZINE**

Class: **Tranquilizer**   Risk Factor: **C**

Fetal Risk Summary

Carphenazine is a piperazine phenothiazine in the same group as prochlorperazine (see Prochlorperazine). Phenothiazines readily cross the placenta (1). No specific information on the use of carphenazine in pregnancy has been located. Although occasional reports have attempted to link various phenothiazine compounds with congenital malformations, the bulk of the evidence indicates these drugs are safe for the mother and fetus (see also Chlorpromazine).

Breast Feeding Summary

No data available.

References

1. Moya F, Thorndike V. Passage of drugs across the placenta. Am J Obstet Gynecol 1962;84:1778–98.

Name: **CASANTHRANOL**

Class: **Purgative**   Risk Factor: **C**

Fetal Risk Summary

Casanthranol is an anthraquinone purgative. In a large prospective study, 109 patients were exposed to this agent during pregnancy, 21 in the 1st trimester (1). No evidence of an increased risk for malformations was found (see also Cascara Sagrada).

Breast Feeding Summary

See Cascara Sagrada.

References

1. Heinonen OP. Slone D, Shapiro S. *Birth Defects and Drugs in Pregnancy*. Littleton:Publishing Sciences Group, 1977:384–7, 442.

Name: **CASCARA SAGRADA**

Class: **Purgative**   Risk Factor: **C**

Fetal Risk Summary

Cascara sagrada is an anthraquinone purgative. In a large prospective study, 53 mother-child pairs were exposed to cascara sagrada during the 1st trimester (1). Although the numbers are small, no evidence for an increased risk of malformations was found. For use anytime during pregnancy, 188 exposures were recorded (2). The relative risk for anomalies was higher than expected in this group for benign tumors, but the statistical significance is unknown and independent confirmation is required (2).

Breast Feeding Summary

Most reviewers acknowledge the presence of anthraquinones in breast milk and warn of the consequences for the nursing infant (3-5). A comprehensive review that describes the excretion of laxatives into human milk has been published (6). The authors state that little is actually known about the presence of these agents in breast milk. Two reports suggest an increased incidence of diarrhea in infants when nursing mothers are given cascara sagrada or senna for postpartum constipation (7, 8).

References

1. Heinonen OP, Slone D, Shapiro S. *Birth Defects and Drugs in Pregnancy*. Littleton:Publishing Sciences Group, 1977:384–7.
2. *Ibid*, 438, 442, 497.
3. Knowles JA. Breast milk: a source of more than nutrition for the neonate. Clin Toxicol 1974;7:69–82.
4. O'Brien TE. Excretion of drugs in human milk. Am J Hosp Pharm 1974;31:844–54.
5. Edwards A. Drugs in breast milk—a review of the recent literature. Aust J Hosp Pharm 1981;11:27–39.
6. Stewart JJ. Gastrointestinal drugs. In Wilson JT, ed. *Drugs in Breast Milk*. Balgowlah, Australia: ADIS Press, 1981:65–71.
7. Tyson RM, Shrader EA, Perlman HH. Drugs transmitted through breast milk. Part I. Laxatives. J Pediatr 1937;11:824–32.
8. Greenleaf JO, Leonard HSD. Laxatives in the treatment of constipation in pregnant and breast-feeding mothers. Practitioner 1973;210:259–63.

Name: **CEFACLOR**

Class: **Antibiotic**   Risk Factor: **B$_M$**

Fetal Risk Summary

Cefaclor is a cephalosporin antibiotic. No reports on its use in pregnancy have been located.

Breast Feeding Summary

Cefaclor is excreted into breast milk in low concentrations. Following a single 500-mg oral dose, average milk levels ranged from 0.16–0.21 μg/ml over a 5-hour period (1). Only trace amounts of the antibiotic could be measured at 1 and 6 hours. Although these levels are low, three potential problems exist for the nursing infant: modification of bowel flora, direct effects on the infant, and interference with the interpretation of culture results if a fever work-up is required.

References

1. Takase Z. Clinical and laboratory studies of cefaclor in the field of obstetrics and gynecology. Chemotherapy (Tokyo) 1979;27(Suppl):668.

Name: **CEFADROXIL**

Class: **Antibiotic**   Risk Factor: **B$_M$**

Fetal Risk Summary

Cefadroxil is a cephalosporin antibiotic. No controlled studies on its use in pregnancy have been located. At term, a 500-mg oral dose produced an average peak cord serum level of 4.6 μg/ml at 2.5 hours (about 40% of maternal serum) (1). Amniotic fluid levels achieved a peak of 4.4 μg/ml at 10 hours. No infant data were given.

Breast Feeding Summary

Cefadroxil is excreted into breast milk in low concentrations. Following a single 500-mg oral dose, peak milk levels of about 0.6–0.7 μg/ml occurred at 5–6 hours (1). A 1-g oral dose given to six mothers produced peak milk levels averaging 1.83 μg/ml (range 1.2–2.4 μg/ml) at 6–7 hours (2). In this latter group, milk:plasma ratios at 1, 2, and 3 hours were 0.009, 0.011, and 0.019, respectively. Although these levels are low, three potential problems exist for the nursing infant: modification of bowel flora, direct effects on the infant, and interference with the interpretation of culture results if a fever work-up is required. The American Academy of Pediatrics considers cefadroxil compatible with breast-feeding (3).

References

1. Takase Z, Shirafuji H, Uchida M. Experimental and clinical studies of cefadroxil in the treatment of infections in the field of obstetrics and gynecology. Chemotherapy (Tokyo) 1980;28(Suppl 2):424–31.

2. Kafetzi D, Siafas C, Georgakopoulos P, Papdatos C. Passage of cephalosporins and amoxicillin into the breast milk. Acta Paediatr Scand 1981;70:285–8.
3. Committee on Drugs, American Academy of Pediatrics. The transfer of drugs and other chemicals into human breast milk. Pediatrics 1983;72:375–83.

Name: **CEFAMANDOLE**

Class: **Antibiotic**   Risk Factor: **B$_M$**

Fetal Risk Summary

Cefamandole is a cephalosporin antibiotic. No controlled studies on its use in pregnancy have been located. Although pregnant patients were excluded from clinical trials of cefamandole, one patient did receive the drug in the 1st trimester (1). No apparent adverse effects were noted in the newborn.

Breast Feeding Summary

Cefamandole is excreted into breast milk in low concentrations. Following a 1-g intravenous dose, average milk levels in four patients ranged from 0.46 (1 hour) to 0.19 μg/ml (6 hours) (1). The milk:plasma ratio at 1 hour was 0.02. No neonate information was given. Although these levels are low, three potential problems exist for the nursing infant: modification of bowel flora, direct effects on the infant and interference with the interpretation of culture results if a fever work-up is required.

References

1. Anderson JT, Medical Research–Marketed Products, Clinical Investigation Division, Lilly Research Laboratories, May 12, 1981. Personal communication.

Name: **CEFATRIZINE**

Class: **Antibiotic**   Risk Factor: **B$_M$**

Fetal Risk Summary

Cefatrizine is a cephalosporin antibiotic. No controlled studies on its use in pregnancy have been located. Transplacental passage of cefatrizine has been demonstrated in women undergoing elective therapeutic surgical abortion in the 1st and 2nd trimesters (1). None of the fetuses from prostaglandin F$_{2a}$ abortions revealed evidence of cefatrizine.

Breast Feeding Summary

Most cephalosporins are excreted into breast milk in low concentrations, but data for cefatrizine are lacking. For potential problems during breast feeding, see Cephalothin.

References

1. Bernard B, Thielen P, Garcia-Cazares SJ, Ballard CA. Maternal-fetal pharmacology of cefatrizine in the first 20 weeks of pregnancy. Antimicrob Agents Chemother 1977;12:231–6.

Name: **CEFAZOLIN**

Class: **Antibiotic** Risk Factor: **B_M**

Fetal Risk Summary

Cefazolin is a cephalosporin antibiotic. No controlled studies on its use in pregnancy have been located. Cefazolin crosses the placenta into the cord serum and amniotic fluid (1–4). In early pregnancy, distribution is limited to the body fluids, and these concentrations are considerably lower than those found in the 2nd and 3rd trimesters (2). At term, 15–70 minutes after a 500-mg dose, cord serum levels ranged from 35 to 69% of maternal serum (3). The maximum concentration in amniotic fluid after 500 mg was 8 μg/ml at 2.5 hours (4). No data on the newborns were given.

Breast Feeding Summary

Cefazolin is excreted into breast milk in low concentrations. Following a 2-g intravenous dose, average milk levels ranged from 1.2 to 1.5 μg/ml over 4 hours (milk:plasma ratio 0.02) (5). When cefazolin was given as a 500-mg intramuscular dose, one to three times daily, the drug was not detectable (4). Although these levels are low, three potential problems exist for the nursing infant: modification of bowel flora, direct effects on the infant, and interference with the interpretation of culture results if a fever work-up is required. The American Academy of Pediatrics considers cefazolin compatible with breast-feeding (6).

References

1. Dekel A, Elian I, Gibor Y, Goldman JA. Transplacental passage of cefazolin in the first trimester of pregnancy. Eur J Obstet Gynecol Reprod Biol 1980;10:303–7.
2. Bernard B, Barton L, Abate M, Ballard CA. Maternal-fetal transfer of cefazolin in the first twenty weeks of pregnancy. J Infect Dis 1977;136:377–82.
3. Cho N, Ito T, Saito T, et al. Clinical studies on cefazolin in the field of obstetrics and gynecology. Chemotherapy (Tokyo) 1970;18:770–7.
4. von Kobyletzki D, Reither K, Gellen J, Kanyo A, Glocke M. Pharmacokinetic studies with cefazolin in obstetrics and gynecology. Infection 1974;2(Suppl):60–7.
5. Yoshioka H, Cho K, Takimato M, Maruyama S, Shimizu T. Transfer of cefazolin into human milk. J Pediatr 1979;94:151–2.
6. Committee on Drugs, American Academy of Pediatrics. The transfer of drugs and other chemicals into human breast milk. Pediatrics 1983;72:375–83.

Name: **CEFONICID**

Class: **Antibiotic** Risk Factor: **B_M**

Fetal Risk Summary

Cefonicid is a cephalosporin antibiotic. No studies on its use in pregnancy are available (1).

Breast Feeding Summary

Cefonicid is excreted into breast milk in low concentrations. Milk levels 1 hour after a 1-g intramuscular dose were equal to or less than 0.3 μg/ml, averaging 0.16 μg/ml (2). Although these concentrations are low, three potential problems exist for the nursing infant: modification of bowel flora, direct effects on the infant, and interference with the interpretation of culture results if a fever work-up is required.

References

1. Evrard HM, Smith Kline & French Laboratories, 1985. Personal communication.
2. Lou MA Sr, Wu YH, Jacob LS, Pitkin DH. Penetration of cefonicid into human breast milk and various body fluids and tissues. Rev Infect Dis 1984;6(Suppl 4):S816–20.

Name: **CEFOPERAZONE**

Class: **Antibiotic**   Risk Factor: B_M

Fetal Risk Summary

Cefoperazone is a cephalosporin antibiotic. Following a 1-g intravenous (IV) or intramuscular dose, cord blood levels averaged 34.4 and 33.2%, respectively, of the maternal serum (1). Peak concentrations occurred at about 1 hour after both IV and intramuscular doses. Amniotic fluid levels were 3–4 μg/ml within 6 hours of administration. Continuous IV dosing (1 g given two to four times every 12 hours) produced higher levels with cord blood averaging 40–48% of maternal serum and amniotic fluid levels increasing to 3.8–8.8 μg/ml. In a second study, 1 g IV produced peak cord blood concentrations averaging about 45% of maternal serum (25 μg/ml vs 56.1 μg/ml) at 70 minutes with amniotic fluid concentrations varying between 2.8 and 4.8 μg/ml at 180 minutes (2). No effects on the newborns were reported in either study.

Breast Feeding Summary

Cefoperazone is excreted into breast milk in low concentrations. An IV dose of 1 g produced milk levels ranging from 0.4 to 0.9 μg/ml (3). Although these concentrations are low, three potential problems exist for the nursing infant: modification of bowel flora, direct effects on the infant, and interference with the interpretation of culture results if a fever work-up is required.

References

1. Matsuda S, Tanno M, Kashiwagura T, Furuya H. Placental transfer of cefoperazone (T-1551) and a clinical study of its use in obstetrics and gynecological infections. Curr Chemother Infect Dis 1979;2:167–8.
2. Shimizu K. Cefoperazone: absorption, excretion, distribution, and metabolism. Clin Ther 1980;3(Special Issue):60–79.
3. Jacobson CE, Roerig, 1985. Data on file.

Name: **CEFORANIDE**

Class: **Antibiotic**   Risk Factor: B_M

Ceforanide is a cephalosporin antibiotic. No data on its use in pregnancy have been located.

Breast Feeding Summary

No studies on the excretion of ceforanide into breast milk have been located. Like other cephalosporins, however, excretion should be expected resulting in three potential problems for the nursing infant: modification of bowel flora, direct effects on the infant, and interference with the interpretation of culture results if a fever work-up is required.

Name: **CEFOTAXIME**

Class: **Antibiotic**   Risk Factor: **B$_M$**

Fetal Risk Summary

Cefotaxime is a cephalosporin antibiotic. No controlled studies on its use in pregnancy have been located. During the 2nd trimester, the drug readily crosses the placenta (1). The half-lives of cefotaxime in fetal serum and in amniotic fluid were 2.3 and 2.8 hours, respectively.

Breast Feeding Summary

Cefotaxime is excreted into breast milk in low concentrations. Following a 1-g intravenous dose, mean peak milk levels of 0.33 μg/ml were measured at 2–3 hours (1, 2). The half-life in milk ranged from 2.36 to 3.89 hours (mean 2.93). The milk:plasma ratio at 1, 2, and 3 hours were 0.027, 0.09, and 0.16, respectively. Although these levels are low, three potential problems exist for the nursing infant: modification of bowel flora, direct effects on the infant, and interference with the interpretation of culture results if a fever work-up is required. The American Academy of Pediatrics considers cefotaxime compatible with breast-feeding (3).

References

1. Kafetzis DA, Lazarides CV, Siafas CA, Georgakopoulos PA, Papadatos CJ. Transfer of cefotaxime in human milk and from mother to foetus. J Antimicrob Chemother 1980;6(Suppl A):135–41.
2. Kafetzis DA, Siafas CA, Georgakopoulos PA, Papadatos CJ. Passage of cephalosporins and amoxicillin into the breast milk. Acta Paediatr Scand 1981;70:285–8.
3. Committee on Drugs, American Academy of Pediatrics. The transfer of drugs and other chemicals into human breast milk. Pediatrics 1983;72:375–83.

Name: **CEFOXITIN**

Class: **Antibiotic**   Risk Factor: **B**

Fetal Risk Summary

Cefoxitin is a cephalosporin antibiotic. No controlled studies of its use in pregnancy have been located but multiple reports have described its transplacental passage (1–13). Two patients were given 1 g intravenously just prior to therapeutic abortion at 9 and 10 weeks gestation (9). At 55 minutes, the serum level in one woman was

10.5 μg/ml, whereas no drug was found in the fetal tissues. At 4.25 hours in the second patient, the maternal serum level was nil, whereas the fetal tissue level was 35.7 μg/ml.

At term, following intramuscular or rapid intravenous doses of 1 or 2 g, cord serum levels up to 22 μg/ml (11–90%) of maternal levels have been measured (6–9). Amniotic fluid concentrations peaked at 2–3 hours in the 3–15 μg/ml range (6, 7, 9, 10, 13). No apparent adverse effects were noted in any of the newborns.

Breast Feeding Summary

Cefoxitin is excreted into breast milk in low concentrations (5, 9, 11, 12). Up to 2 μg/ml have been detected in the milk of women receiving therapeutic doses (14). No data on the infants were given. Although these levels are low, three potential problems exist for the nursing infant: modification of bowel flora, direct effects on the infant, and interference with the interpretation of culture results if a fever work-up is required.

References

1. Bergone-Berezin B, Kafe H, Berthelot G, Morel O, Benard Y. Pharmacokinetic study of cefoxitin in bronchial secretions. In *Current Chemotherapy: Proceedings of the 10th International Congress of Chemotherapy*, Zurich, Switzerland, September 18–23, 1977; Washington, DC: American Society for Microbiology, 1978.
2. Aokawa H, Minagawa M, Yamamiohi K, Sugiyama A. Studies on cefoxitin. Chemotherapy (Tokyo) 1977;(Suppl):394.
3. Matsuda S, Tanno M, Kashiwakura S, Furuya H. Basic and clinical studies on cefoxitin. Chemotherapy (Tokyo) 1977;(Suppl):396.
4. Berthelot G, Bergogne-Berezin B, Morel O, Kafe H, Benard Y. Cefoxitin: pharmacokinetic study in bronchial secretions-transplacental diffusion. In *Current Chemotherapy: Proceedings of the 10th International Congress of Chemotherapy*, Zurich, Switzerland, September 18–23, 1977; Washington, DC: American Society for Microbiology, 1978.
5. Mashimo K, Mihashi S, Fukaya I, Okubo B, Ohgob M, Saito A. New drug symposium. IV. Cefoxitin. Chemotherapy (Tokyo) 1978;26:114–9.
6. Matsuda S, Tanno M, Kashiwakura T, Furuya H. Laboratory and clinical studies on cefoxitin in the field of obstetrics and gynecology. Chemotherapy (Tokyo) 1978;26(Suppl 1):460–7.
7. Cho N, Ubhara K, Suigizaki K, et al. Clinical studies of cefoxitin in the field of obstetrics and gynecology. Chemotherapy (Tokyo) 1978;26(Suppl 1):468–75.
8. Seiga K, Minagawa M, Yamaji K, Sugiyama Y. Study on cefoxitin. Chemotherapy (Tokyo) 1978;26(Suppl 1):491–501.
9. Takase Z, Shirafuji H, Uchida M. Clinical and laboratory studies on cefoxitin in the field of obstetrics and gynecology. Chemotherapy (Tokyo) 1978;26(Suppl 1):502–5.
10. Bergogne-Berezin B, Lambert-Zeohovsky N, Rouvillois JL. Placental transfer of cefoxitin. Paper presented at the 18th Interscience Conference on Antimicrobial Agents and Chemotherapy, Atlanta, GA, October 1–4, 1978, Program Abstract No. 314.
11. Brogden RN, Heel RC, Speight TM, Avery GS. Cefoxitin: A review of its antibacterial activity, pharmacological properties and therapeutic use. Drugs 1979;17:1–37.
12. Dubois M, Delapierre D, Demonty J, Lambotte R, Dresse A. Transplacental and mammary transfer of cefoxitin. Paper presented at 11th International Congress of Chemotherapy and 19th Interscience Conference on Antimicrobial Agents and Chemotherapy, Boston, MA, October 1–5, 1979, Program Abstract No. 118.
13. Bergogne-Berezin B, Morel O, Kafe H, et al. Pharmacokinetic study of cefoxitin in man: diffusion into the bronchi and transfer across the placenta. Therapie 1979;34:345–54.
14. Whalen JJ, Merck Sharp and Dohme, May 13, 1981. Personal communication.

Name: **CEFTIZOXIME**

Class: **Antibiotic**   Risk Factor: **B$_M$**

Fetal Risk Summary

Ceftizoxime is a cephalosporin antibiotic. Following 1- or 2-g intravenous doses administered to women at term, peak cord blood levels occurred at 1–2 hours with concentrations ranging between 12 and 30 μg/ml (1–5). Amniotic fluid concentrations were lower with peak levels of 10–20 μg/ml at 2–3 hours. The mean fetal:maternal ratio reported in one group of patients after a 2-g intravenous dose was 0.28 (5). No adverse fetal or newborn effects were noted in any of the trials.

Breast Feeding Summary

Ceftizoxime is excreted into breast milk in low concentrations (5, 6). Mean levels following single doses of 1 and 2 g were less than 0.5 μg/ml. Although these levels are low, three potential problems exist for the nursing infant: modification of bowel flora, direct effects on the infant and interference with the interpretation of culture results if a fever work-up is required.

References

1. Cho N, Fukunaga K, Kunii K. Studies on ceftizoxime (CZX) in the field of obstetrics and gynecology. Chemotherapy (Tokyo) 1980;28(Suppl 5):821–30.
2. Matsuda S, Seida A. Clinical use of ceftizoxime in obstetrics and gynecology. Chemotherapy (Tokyo) 1980;28(Suppl 5):812–20.
3. Okada E, Kawada A, Shirakawa N. Clinical studies on transplacental diffusion of ceftizoxime into fetal blood and treatment of infections in obstetrics and gynecology. Chemotherapy (Tokyo) 1980;28(Suppl 5):874–87.
4. Seiga K, Minagawa M, Egawa J, Yamaji K, Sugiyama Y. Clinical and laboratory studies on ceftizoxime (CZX) in the field of obstetrics and gynecology. Chemotherapy (Tokyo) 1980;28(Suppl 5):845–62.
5. Motomura R, Kohno M, Mori H, Yamabe T. Basic and clinical studies of ceftizoxime in obstetrics and gynecology. Chemotherapy (Tokyo) 1980;28(Suppl 5):888–99.
6. Gerding DN, Peterson LR. Comparative tissue and extravascular fluid concentrations of ceftizoxime. J Antimicrob Chemother 1982;10(Suppl C):105–16.

Name: **CEFTRIAXONE**

Class: **Antibiotic**   Risk Factor: **B$_M$**

Fetal Risk Summary

Ceftriaxone is a cephalosporin antibiotic. Peak levels in cord blood following 1- or 2-g intravenous doses occurred at 4 hours with concentrations varying between 19.6–40.6 μg/ml (1–8 hours) (1–3). Amniotic fluid levels over 24 hours ranged from 2.2–23.4 μg/ml with peak levels occurring at 6 hours (1–3). Ceftriaxone concentrations in the first voided newborn urine were highly variable, ranging from 6 to 92 μg/ml. Elimination half-lives from cord blood (7 hours), amniotic fluid (6.8 hours), and placenta (5.4 hours) were nearly identical to those of maternal serum (1, 2, 4). No adverse effects in the newborns were mentioned.

Breast Feeding Summary

Ceftriaxone is excreted into breast milk in low concentrations. Following either 1- or 2-g intravenous or intramuscular doses, peak levels of 0.5–0.7 μg/ml occurred at 5 hours, approximately 3–4% of maternal serum (1, 2). High protein binding in maternal serum probably limited transfer to the milk (1, 2). The antibiotic was still detectable in milk at 24 hours (1). Elimination half-lives after intravenous and intramuscular doses were 12.8 and 17.3 hours, respectively (1). Chronic dosing would eventually produce calculated steady-state levels in 1.5–3 days in the 3–4 μg/ml range (2). Although these levels are low, three potential problems exist for the nursing infant: modification of bowel flora, direct effects on the infant, and interference with the interpretation of culture results if a fever work-up is required.

References

1. Kafetzis DA, Brater DC, Fanoursakis JE, Voyatzis J, Georgakopoulos P. Placental and breast-milk transfer of ceftriaxone (C). In *Proceedings of the 22nd Interscience Conference on Antimicrobial Agents and Chemotherapy*, Miami, FL, October 4–6, 1982:155; New York:Academic Press, 1983.
2. Kafetzis DA, Brater DC, Fanourgakis JE, Voyatzis J, Georgakopoulos P. Ceftriaxone distribution between maternal blood and fetal blood and tissues at parturition and between blood and milk postpartum. Antimicrob Agents Chemother 1983;23:870–3.
3. Cho N, Kunii K, Fukunago K, Komoriyama Y. Antimicrobial activity, pharmacokinetics and clinical studies of ceftriaxone in obstetrics and gynecology. In *Proceedings of the 13th International Congress on Chemotherapy*, Vienna, Austria, August 28–September 2, 1983:100/64–66; Princeton:Excerpta Medica, 1984.
4. Graber H, Magyar T. Pharmacokinetics of ceftriaxone in pregnancy. Am J Med 1984;77:117–8.

Name: **CEFUROXIME**

Class: **Antibiotic**   Risk Factor: **B$_M$**

Fetal Risk Summary

Cefuroxime is a cephalosporin antibiotic. No controlled studies on its use in pregnancy have been located. Cefuroxime readily crosses the placenta in late pregnancy and labor achieving therapeutic concentrations in fetal serum and amniotic fluid (1–5). Therapeutic antibiotic levels in infants can be demonstrated up to 6 hours after birth with measurable concentrations persisting for 26 hours. The pharmacokinetics of cefuroxime in pregnancy have been reported (7). The antibiotic has been used for the treatment of pyelonephritis in pregnancy (8). Adverse effects in the newborn after *in utero* exposure have not been observed.

Breast Feeding Summary

Most cephalosporins are excreted into breast milk in low concentrations, but data for cefuroxime are lacking. For potential problems during breast feeding, see Cephalothin.

References

1. Craft I, Mullinger BM, Kennedy MRK. Placental transfer of cefuroxime. Br J Obstet Gynaecol 1981;88:141–5.
2. Bousfield P, Browning AK, Mullinger BM, Elstein M. Cefuroxime: potential use in pregnant women at term. Br J Obstet Gynaecol 1981;88:146–9.

3. Bergogne–Berezin E, Pierre J, Even P, Rouvillois JL, Dumez Y. Study of penetration of cefuroxime into bronchial secretions and of its placental transfer. Therapie 1980;35:677–84.
4. Tzingounis V, Makris N, Zolotas J, Michalas S, Aravantinos D. Cefuroxime prophylaxis in caesarean section. Pharmatherapeutica 1982;3:140–2.
5. Coppi G, Berti MA, Chehade A, Franchi I, Magro B. A study of the transplacental transfer of cefuroxime in humans. Curr Ther Res 1982;32:712–6.
6. Bousefield PF. Use of cefuroxime in pregnant women at term. Res Clin Forums 1984;6:53–8.
7. Philipson A, Stiernstedt G. Pharmacokinetics of cefuroxime in pregnancy. Am J Obstet Gynecol 1982;142:823–8.
8. Faro S, Pastorek JG II, Plauche WC, Korndorffer FA, Aldridge KE. Short-course parenteral antibiotic therapy for pyelonephritis in pregnancy. South Med J 1984;77:455–7.

Name: **CEPHALEXIN**

Class: **Antibiotic**   Risk Factor: **B**$_M$

Fetal Risk Summary

Cephalexin is a cephalosporin antibiotic. Several reports have described the administration of cephalexin to pregnant patients in various stages of gestation (1–8). None of these has linked the use of cephalexin with congenital defects or toxicity in the newborn.

Transplacental passage of cephalexin has been demonstrated only near term (1, 2). Following a 1-g oral dose, peak concentrations (μg/ml) for maternal serum, cord serum, and amniotic fluid were about 34 (1 hour), 11 (4 hours), and 13 (6 hours), respectively (2). Patients in whom labor was induced were observed to have falling concentrations of cephalexin in all samples when labor was prolonged beyond 18 hours (3). In one report, all fetal blood samples gave a negative Coombs' reaction (1).

The manufacturer has unpublished information on 46 patients treated with cephalexin during pregnancy (9). Two of these patients received the drug from 1–2 months prior to conception to term. No effects on the fetus attributable to the antibiotic were observed. Results of follow-up examination on one infant at 2 months were normal.

Breast Feeding Summary

Cephalexin is excreted into breast milk in low concentrations. A 1-g oral dose given to six mothers produced peak milk levels at 4–5 hours averaging 0.51 μg/ml (range 0.24–0.85 μg/ml) (10). Mean milk:plasma ratios at 1, 2, and 3 hours were 0.008, 0.021, and 0.14, respectively. Although these levels are low, three potential problems exist for the nursing infant: modification of bowel flora, direct effects on the infant, and interference with the interpretation of culture results if a fever work-up is required.

References

1. Paterson ML, Henderson A, Lunan CB, McGurk S. Transplacental transfer of cephalexin. Clin Med 1972;79:22–4.
2. Creatsas G, Pavlatos M, Lolis D, Kaskarelis D. A study of the kinetics of cephapirin and cephalexin in pregnancy. Curr Med Res Opin 1980;7:43–6.

3. Hirsch HA. Behandlung von harnwegsinfektionen in gynakologic und geburtshilfe mit cephalexin. Int J Clin Pharmacol 1969;2(Suppl):121–3.
4. Brumfitt W, Pursell R. Double-blind trial to compare ampicillin, cephalexin, co-trimoxazole, and trimethoprim in treatment of urinary infection. Br Med J 1972;2:673–6.
5. Mizuno S, Metsuda S, Mori S. *Clinical Evaluation of Cephalexin in Obstetrics and Gynaecology: Proceedings of a Symposium on the Clinical Evaluation of Cephalexin*. Royal Society of Medicine, London, June 2 and 3, 1969.
6. Guttman D. *Cephalexin in Urinary Tract Infections—Preliminary Results, Proceedings of a Symposium on the Clinical Evaluation of Cephalexin*. Royal Society of Medicine, London, June 2 and 3, 1969.
7. Soto RF, Fesbre F, Cordido A, et al. Ensayo con cefalexina en el tratamiento de infecciones urinarias en pacientes embarazadas. Rev Obstet Ginecol Venez 1972;32:637–41.
8. Campbell-Brown M, McFadyen IR. Bacteriuria in pregnancy treated with a single dose of cephalexin. Br J Obstet Gynaecol 1983;90:1054–9.
9. Lynch CL, Medical Research—Marketed Products, Clinical Investigation Division, Dista Products, 1981. Personal communication.
10. Kafetzis D, Siafas C, Georgakopoulos P, Papadatos CJ. Passage of cephalosporins and amoxicillin into the breast milk. Acta Paediatr Scand 1981;70:285–8.

Name: **CEPHALOTHIN**

Class: **Antibiotic**   Risk Factor: B_M

Fetal Risk Summary

Cephalothin, a cephalosporin antibiotic, has been used during all stages of gestation (1–3). No reports linking this use with congenital defects or toxicity in the newborn have been located. The drug crosses the placenta and distributes in fetal tissues (4–10). Following a 1-g dose, average peak cord serum levels were found at 1–2 hours for the intramuscular route (2.8 μg/ml; 16% of maternal peak), and at 10 minutes for intravenous administration (12.5 μg/ml; 41% of maternal) (4–6). In amniotic fluid, cephalothin was slowly concentrated reaching an average level of 21 μg/ml at 4–5 hours (5).

Breast Feeding Summary

Cephalothin is excreted into breast milk in low concentrations. A 1-g intravenous bolus dose given to six mothers produced peak milk levels at 1–2 hours averaging 0.51 μg/ml (range 0.36–0.62 μg/ml) (11). Mean milk:plasma ratios at 1, 2, and 3 hours were 0.073, 0.26, and 0.50, respectively. Although these levels are low, three potential problems exist for the nursing infant: modification of bowel flora, direct effects on the infant, and interference with the interpretation of culture results if a fever work-up is required.

References

1. Cunningham FG, Morris GB, Mickal A. Acute pyelonephritis of pregnancy: a clinical review. Obstet Gynecol 1973;42:112–7.
2. Harris RE, Gilstrap LC. Prevention of recurrent pyelonephritis during pregnancy. Obstet Gynecol 1974;44:637–41.
3. Moro M, Andrews M. Prophylactic antibiotics in cesarean section. Obstet Gynecol 1974;44:688–92.

4. MacAulay MA, Charles D. Placental transfer of cephalothin. Am J Obstet Gynecol 1968;100:940–5.
5. Sheng KT, Huang NN, Promadhattavedi V. Serum concentrations of cephalothin in infants and children and placental transmission of the antibiotic. Antimicrob Agents Chemother 1964:200–6.
6. Fukada M. Studies on chemotherapy during the perinatal period with special reference to such derivatives of cephalosporin C as cefazolin, cephaloridine and cephalothin. Jpn J Antibiot 1973;26:197–212.
7. Paterson L, Henderson A, Lunan CB, McGurk S. Transfer of cephalothin sodium to the fetus. J Obstet Gynaecol Br Commonw 1970;77:565–6.
8. Morrow S, Palmisano P, Cassady G. The placental transfer of cephalothin. J Pediatr 1968;73:262–4.
9. Stewart KS, Shafi M, Andrews J, Williams JD. Distribution of parenteral ampicillin and cephalosporins in late pregnancy. J Obstet Gynaecol Br Commonw 1973;80:902–8.
10. Corson SL, Bolognese RJ. The behavior of cephalothin in amniotic fluid. J Reprod Med 1970;4:105–8.
11. Kafetzis D, Siafas C, Georgakopoulos P, Papadatos CJ. Passage of cephalosporins and amoxicillin into the breast milk. Acta Paediatr Scand 1981;70:285–8.

Name: **CEPHAPIRIN**

Class: **Antibiotic** Risk Factor: **B$_M$**

Fetal Risk Summary

Cephapirin is a cephalosporin antibiotic. At term, following a 1-g intramuscular dose, peak concentrations (μg/ml) for maternal serum, cord serum and amniotic fluid were about 17 (0.5 hours), 10 (4 hours) and 13 (6 hours), respectively (1). No data on the newborns were given.

Breast Feeding Summary

Cephapirin is excreted into breast milk in low concentrations. A 1-g intravenous bolus dose given to six mothers produced peak milk levels at 1–2 hours averaging 0.49 μg/ml (range 0.30–0.64 μg/ml) (2). Mean milk:plasma ratios at 1, 2, and 3 hours were 0.068, 0.250, and 0.480, respectively. Although these levels were low, three potential problems exist for the nursing infant: modification of bowel flora, direct effects on the infant, and interference with the interpretation of culture results if a fever work-up is required.

References

1. Creatsas G, Pavlatos M, Lolis D, Kasharelis D. A study of the kinetics of cephapirin and cefalexin in pregnancy. Curr Med Res Opin 1980;7:43–6.
2. Kafetzis D, Siafas C, Georgakopoulos P, Papadatos CJ. Passage of cephalosporins and amoxicillin into the breast milk. Acta Paediatr Scand 1981;70:285–8.

Name: **CEPHRADINE**

Class: **Antibiotic** Risk Factor: **B$_M$**

Fetal Risk Summary

Cephradine is a cephalosporin antibiotic The drug rapidly crosses the placenta throughout gestation (1–4). In the 1st and 2nd trimesters, intravenous (IV) or oral doses produce amniotic fluid levels in the 1 μg/ml range or less. Between 15 and

30 weeks of gestation, a 1-g IV dose produces therapeutjc fetal levels peaking in 40–50 minutes (1). At term, oral doses of 2 g/day for 2 days or more allowed cephradine to concentrate in the amniotic fluid, producing levels in the range of 3 to 15 μg/ml (2,3). A 2-g IV dose 17 minutes prior to delivery produced high cord serum levels (29 μg/ml) but low amniotic fluid concentrations (1.1 μg/ml) (4). Serum samples taken from two of the newborns within 20 hours of birth indicated that cephradine is excreted by the neonate (4). No other infant data were given in any of the studies.

Breast Feeding Summary

Cephradine is excreted into breast milk in low concentrations. After 500 mg orally every 6 hours for 48 hours, constant milk concentrations of 0.6 μg/ml were measured over 6 hours, a milk:plasma ratio of about 0.2 (2, 3). Although these levels are low, three potential problems exist for the nursing infant: modification of bowel flora, direct effects on the infant, and interference with the interpretation of culture results if a fever work-up is required.

References

1. Lange IR, Rodeck C, Cosgrove R. The transfer of cephradine across the placenta. Br J Obstet Gynaecol 1984;91:551–4.
2. Mischler TW, Corson SL, Bolognese RJ, Letocha MJ, Neiss ES. Presence of cephradine in body fluids of lactating and pregnant women. Clin Pharmacol Ther 1974;15:214.
3. Mischler TW, Corson SL, Larranaga A, Bolognese RJ, Neiss ES, Vukovich RA. Cephradine and epicillin in body fluids of lactating and pregnant women. J Reprod Med 1978;21:130–6.
4. Craft I, Forster TC. Materno-fetal cephradine transfer in pregnancy. Antimicrob Agents Chemother 1978;14:924–6.

Name: **CHLORAL HYDRATE**

Class: **Sedative/Hypnotic**   Risk Factor: **C$_M$**

Fetal Risk Summary

No reports linking the use of chloral hydrate with congenital defects have been located. The drug has been given in labor and demonstrated in cord blood at concentrations similar to maternal levels (1). Sedative effects on the neonate have not been studied.

Breast Feeding Summary

Chloral hydrate and its active metabolite are excreted into breast milk. Peak concentrations of about 8 μg/ml were obtained about 45 minutes after a 1.3-g rectal dose (2). Only trace amounts are detectable after 10 hours.

Mild drowsiness was observed in the nursing infant of a mother taking 1,300 mg of dichloralphenazone every evening (3). The mother was also consuming chlorpromazine, 100 mg three times daily. Dichloralphenazone is metabolized to trichloroethanol, the same active metabolite of chloral hydrate. Milk levels of trichloroethanol were 60–80% of the maternal serum. The highest milk concentration measured was 0.27 mg/100 ml. Infant growth and development remained normal during the exposure and at follow-up 3 months after the drug was stopped.

References

1. Bernstine JB, Meyer AE, Hayman HB. Maternal and fetal blood estimation following the administration of chloral hydrate during labor. J Obstet Gynaecol Br Emp 1954;61:683–5.
2. Berstine JB, Meyer AE, Berstine RL. Maternal blood and breast milk estimation following the administration of chloral hydrate during the puerperium. J Obstet Gynaecol Br Emp 1956;63:228–31.
3. Lacey JH. Dichloralphenazone and breast milk. Br Med J 1971;4:684.

Name: **CHLORAMBUCIL**

Class: **Antineoplastic** Risk Factor: D_M

Fetal Risk Summary

Chlorambucil has been used during pregnancy without causing congenital malformations (1, 2). However, there are two reports of unilateral agenesis of the left kidney and ureter in male fetuses following 1st trimester exposure to chlorambucil (3, 4). Similar defects have been found in animals exposed to the drug (5). In a third case, a pregnant patient was treated with chlorambucil at the 10th week of gestation (6). A full term infant was delivered but died 3 days later of multiple cardiovascular anomalies.

Chlorambucil is mutagenic as well as carcinogenic (7–11). These effects have not been reported in newborns following *in utero* exposure. Data from one review indicated that 40% of the infants exposed to anticancer drugs were of low birth weight (12). Long-term studies of growth and mental development in offspring exposed to chlorambucil during the 2nd trimester, the period of neuroblast multiplication, have not been conducted (13). Amenorrhea and reversible azoospermia with high doses have been reported (14–17).

Breast Feeding Summary

No data available.

References

1. Sokal JE, Lessmann EM. Effects of cancer chemotherapeutic agents on the human fetus. JAMA 1960;172:1765–71.
2. Jacobs C, Donaldson SS, Rosenberg SA, Kaplan HS. Management of the pregnant patient with Hodgkin's disease. Ann Intern Med 1981;95:669–75.
3. Shotton D, Monie IW. Possible teratogenic effect of chlorambucil on a human fetus. JAMA 1963;186:74–5.
4. Steege JF, Caldwell DS. Renal agenesis after first trimester exposure to chlorambucil. South Med J 1980;73:1414–5.
5. Monie IW. Chlorambucil-induced abnormalities of urogenital system of rat fetuses. Anat Rec 1961;139:145.
6. Thompson J, Conklin KA. Anesthetic management of a pregnant patient with scleroderma. Anesthesiology 1983;59:69–71.
7. Lawler SD, Lele KP. Chromosomal damage induced by chlorambucil and chronic lymphocytic leukemia. Scand J Haematol 1972;9:603–12.
8. Westin J. Chromosome abnormalities after chlorambucil therapy of polycythemia vera. Scand J Haematol 1976;17:197–204.
9. Catovsky D, Galton DAG. Myelomonocytic leukaemia supervening on chronic lymphocytic leukaemia. Lancet 1971;1:478–9.

10. Rosner R. Acute leukemia as a delayed consequence of cancer chemotherapy. Cancer 1976;37:1033–6.
11. Reimer RR, Hover R, Fraumeni JF, Young RC. Acute leukemia after alkylating-agent therapy of ovarian cancer. N Engl J Med 1977;297:177–81.
12. Nicholson HO. Cytotoxic drugs in pregnancy: review of reported cases. J Obstet Gynaecol Br Commonw 1968;75:307–12.
13. Dobbing J. Pregnancy and leukaemia. Lancet 1977;1:1155.
14. Freckman HA, Fry HL, Mendex FL, Maurer ER. Chlorambucil-prednisolone therapy for disseminated breast carcinoma. JAMA 1964;189:111–4.
15. Richter P, Calamera JC, Morganfeld MC, Kierszenbaum AL, Lavieri JC, Mancinni RE. Effect of chlorambucil on spermatogenesis in the human malignant lymphoma. Cancer 1970;25:1026–30.
16. Morgenfeld MC, Goldberg V, Parisier H, Bugnard SC, Bur GE. Ovarian lesions due to cytostatic agents during the treatment of Hodgkin's disease. Surg Gynecol Obstet 1972;134:826–8.
17. Schilsky RL, Lewis BJ, Sherins RJ, Young RC. Gonadal dysfunction in patients receiving chemotherapy for cancer. Ann Intern Med 1980;93:109–14.

Name: **CHLORAMPHENICOL**

Class: **Antibiotic**   Risk Factor: **C**

Fetal Risk Summary

No reports linking the use of chloramphenicol with congenital defects have been located. The drug crosses the placenta at term, producing cord serum concentrations 30–106% of maternal levels (1, 2).

The Collaborative Perinatal Project monitored 50,282 mother-child pairs, 98 of which had 1st trimester exposure to chloramphenicol (3). For use anytime during pregnancy, 348 exposures were recorded (4). In neither case was evidence found to suggest a relationship to large categories of major or minor malformations or to individual defects. A 1977 case report described a 14-day course of intravenous chloramphenicol, 2 g daily, given to a patient with typhoid fever in the 2nd trimester (5). A normal infant was delivered at term. Twenty-two patients, in various stages of gestation, were treated with chloramphenicol for acute pyelonephritis (6). No difficulties in the newborn could be associated with the antibiotic. In a controlled study, 110 patients received one to three antibiotics during the 1st trimester for a total of 589 weeks (7). Chloramphenicol was given for a total of 205 weeks. The incidence of birth defects was similar to that incontrols.

Although apparently nontoxic to the fetus, the use of chloramphenicol should be used with caution at term. Although specific details were not provided, one report claimed that cardiovascular collapse (gray syndrome) developed in babies delivered from mothers treated with chloramphenicol during the final stage of pregnancy (8). Additional reports of this severe adverse effect have not been located, although it is well known that newborns exposed directly to high doses of chloramphenicol may develop the gray syndrome (9–11). Because of this risk, some authors consider the drug to be contraindicated during pregnancy (12).

Breast Feeding Summary

Chloramphenicol is excreted into human breast milk. Levels of two milk samples, separated by 24 hours, from the same patient were reported as 16 and 25 µg/ml, representing milk:plasma ratios of 0.51 and 0.61, respectively (13). Both active drug and inactive metabolite were measured. No effect on the infant was mentioned. No infant toxicity was mentioned in a 1964 report that found peak levels occurring in milk 1–3 hours after a single 1-g oral dose (14). In a similar study, continuous excretion of chloramphenicol into breast milk was established after the 1st day of therapy (15). Minimum and maximum milk concentrations were determined for five patients receiving 250 mg orally every 6 hours (0.54 and 2.84 μg/ml) and for five patients receiving 500 mg orally every 6 hours (1.75 and 6.10 μg/ml). No infant data were given.

The safety of maternal chloramphenicol consumption and breast-feeding is controversial. The American Academy of Pediatrics considers the antibiotic compatible with breast-feeding (16). However, another publication recommends chloramphenicol not be used in the lactating patient (17). Milk levels of this antibiotic are too low to precipitate the gray syndrome, but a theoretical risk exists for bone marrow depression. Two other potential problems exist for the nursing infant: modification of bowel flora and interference with the interpretation of culture results if a fever work-up is required. Several adverse effects, reported in 50 breast-fed infants whose mothers were being treated with chloramphenicol, were refusal of the breast, falling asleep during feeding, intestinal gas, and heavy vomiting after feeding (18).

References

1. Scott WC, Warner RF. Placental transfer of chloramphenicol (Chloromycetin). JAMA 1950;142:1331–2.
2. Ross S, Burke RG, Sites J, Rice EC, Washington JA. Placental transmission of chloramphenicol (Chloromycetin). JAMA 1950;142:1361.
3. Heinonen OP, Slone D, Shapiro S. Birth Defects and Drugs in Pregnancy. Littleton:Publishing Sciences Group, 1977:297–301.
4. Ibid, 435.
5. Schiffman P, Samet CM, Fox L, Neimand KM, Rosenberg ST. Typhoid fever in pregnancy—with probable typhoid hepatitis. NY State J Med 1977;77:1778–9.
6. Cunningham FG, Morris GB, Mickal A. Acute pyelonephritis of pregnancy: a clinical review. Obstet Gynecol 1973;42:112–7.
7. Ravid R, Roaff R. On the possible teratogenicity of antibiotic drugs administered during pregnancy. In Klingberg MA, Abramovici H, Chemke J, eds. Drugs and Fetal Development. New York:Plenum Press, 1972:505–10.
8. Oberheuser F. Praktische erfahrungen mit medikamenten in der schwangerschaft. Therapiewoche 1971;31:2200. As reported in Manten A. Antibiotic drugs. In Dukes MNG, ed. Meyler's Side Effects of Drugs, Vol VIII. New York:American Elsevier, 1975:604.
9. Sutherland JM. Fatal cardiovascular collapse of infants receiving large amounts of chloramphenicol. J Dis Child 1959;97:761–7.
10. Weiss CV, Glazko AJ, Weston JK. Chloramphenicol in the newborn infant. A physiologic explanation of its toxicity when given in excessive doses. N Engl J Med 1960;262:787–94.
11. Oberheuser F. Praktische erfahrungen mit medikamenten in der schwangerschaft. Therapiewoche 1971;31:2200.
12. Schwarz RH, Crombleholme WR. Antibiotics in pregnancy. South Med J 1979;72:1315–8.
13. Smadel JE, Woodward TE, Ley HL Jr, Lewthwaite R. Chloramphenicol (Chloromycetin) in the treatment of tsutsugamushi disease (scrub typhus). J Clin Invest 1949;28:1196–215.
14. Prochazka J, Havelka J, Hejzlar M. Excretion of chloramphenicol by human milk. Cas Lek Cesk 1964;103:378–80.
15. Prochazka J, Hejzlar M, Popov V, Viktorinova D, Prochazka J. Excretion of chloramphenicol in human milk. Chemotherapy 1968;13:204–11.
16. Committee on Drugs, American Academy of Pediatrics. The transfer of drugs and other chemicals into human breast milk. Pediatrics 1983;72:375–83.

17. Anonymous. Update: drugs in breast milk. Med Lett Drugs Ther 1979;21:21–4.

18. Havelka J, Frankova A. Contribution to the question of side effects of chloramphenicol therapy in newborns. Cesk Pediatr 1972;21:31–3.

Name: **CHLORCYCLIZINE**

Class: **Antihistamine**   Risk Factor: **C**

Fetal Risk Summary

No data available. See Meclizine for representative agent in this class.

Breast Feeding Summary

No data available.

Name: **CHLORDIAZEPOXIDE**

Class: **Sedative**   Risk Factor: **D**

Fetal Risk Summary

Chlordiazepoxide is a benzodiazepine (see also Diazepam). In a study evaluating 19,044 live births, the use of chlordiazepoxide was associated with a greater than 4-fold increase in severe congenital anomalies (1). In 172 patients exposed to the drug during the first 42 days of gestation, the following defects were observed: mental deficiency; spastic diplegia and deafness; microcephaly and retardation; duodenal atresia; and Meckel's diverticulum (1). Although not statistically significant, an increased fetal death rate was also found with maternal chlordiazepoxide ingestion (1). A survey of 390 infants with congenital heart disease matched with 1,254 normal infants found a higher rate of exposure to several drugs, including chlordiazepoxide, in the offspring with defects (2). Other studies have not confirmed a relationship with increased defects or mortality (3–6).

The Collaborative Perinatal Project monitored 50,282 mother-child pairs, 257 of which were exposed in the 1st trimester to chlordiazepoxide (4, 7). No association with large classes of malformations or to individual defects was found.

Neonatal withdrawal consisting of severe tremulousness and irritability has been attributed to maternal use of chlordiazepoxide (8). The onset of withdrawal symptoms occurred on the 26th day of life. Chlordiazepoxide readily crosses the placenta at term in an approximate 1:1 ratio (9–11). The drug has been used to reduce pain during labor, but the maternal benefit was not significant (12, 13). Marked depression was observed in three infants whose mothers received chlordiazepoxide within a few hours of delivery (11). The infants were unresponsive, hypotonic, hypothermic, and fed poorly. Hypotonicity persisted for up to a week. In other studies depression has not been seen (9, 10).

Breast Feeding Summary

No data available (see Diazepam).

References

1. Milkovich L, van den Berg BJ. Effects of prenatal meprobamate and chlordiazepoxide hydrochloride on human embryonic and fetal development. N Engl J Med 1974;291:1268–71.
2. Rothman KJ, Fyler DC, Golblatt A, Kreidberg MB. Exogenous hormones and other drug exposures of children with congenital heart disease. Am J Epidemiol 1979;109:433–9.
3. Crombie DL, Pinsent RJ, Fleming DM, Rumeau-Rouguette C, Goujard J, Huel G. Fetal effects of tranquilizers in pregnancy. N Engl J Med 1975;293:198–9.
4. Hartz SC, Heinonen OP, Shapiro S, Siskind V, Slone D. Antenatal exposure to meprobamate and chlordiazepoxide in relation to malformations, mental development, and childhood mortality. N Engl J Med 1975;292:726–8.
5. Bracken MB, Holford TR. Exposure to prescribed drugs in pregnancy and association with congenital malformations. Obstet Gynecol 1981;58:336–44.
6. Committee on Drugs, American Academy of Pediatrics. Psychotropic drugs in pregnancy and lactation. Pediatrics 1982;69:241–4.
7. Heinonen OP, Slone D, Shapiro S. *Birth Defects and Drugs in Pregnancy*. Littleton:Publishing Sciences Group, 1977:336–7.
8. Athinarayanan P, Pierog SH, Nigam SK, Glass L. Chlordiazepoxide withdrawal in the neonate. Am J Obstet Gynecol 1976;124:212–3.
9. Decancq HG Jr, Bosco JR, Townsend EH Jr. Chlordiazepoxide in labour: its effect on the newborn infant. J Pediatr 1965;67:836–40.
10. Mark PM, Hamel J. Librium for patients in labor. Obstet Gynecol 1968;32:188–94.
11. Stirrat GM, Edington PT, Berry DJ. Transplacental passage of chlordiazepoxide. Br Med J 1974;2:729.
12. Duckman S, Spina T, Attardi M, Meyer A. Double-blind study of chlordiazepoxide in obstetrics. Obstet Gynecol 1964;24:601–5.
13. Kanto JH. Use of benzodiazepines during pregnancy, labour and lactation, with particular reference to pharmacokinetic considerations. Drugs 1982;23:354–80.

Name: **CHLOROQUINE**

Class: **Antimalarial**   Risk Factor: **C**

Fetal Risk Summary

Chloroquine is the drug of choice for the prophylaxis and treatment of sensitive malaria species during pregnancy (1–4). The drug is generally considered safe for this purpose by most authorities (1–6). Defects have been reported in three infants delivered from one mother who took 250–500 mg of chloroquine per day during pregnancy (7). In addition, this woman also had two normal infants, who had not been exposed to chloroquine during gestation and one normal infant who had been exposed. Anomalies in the three infants were:

Wilms' tumor at age 4 years, left-sided
   hemihypertrophy (1 infant)
Cochleovestibular paresis (2 infants)

A 1985 report summarized the results of 169 infants exposed *in utero* to 300 mg of chloroquine base once weekly throughout pregnancy (8). The control group consisted of 454 nonexposed infants. Two infants (1.2%) in the study group had anomalies (tetralogy of Fallot and congenital hypothyroidism) compared to four control infants who had defects (0.9%). Based on these data, the authors concluded that chloroquine does not have a strong teratogenic effect, but a small increase in birth defects could not be excluded (8).

Breast Feeding Summary

Chloroquine does not appear to be excreted in measurable amounts in the breast milk (9). The American Academy of Pediatrics considers the drug compatible with breast-feeding (10).

References

1. Gilles HM, Lawson JB, Sibelas M, Voller A, Allan N. Malaria, anaemia and pregnancy. Ann Trop Med Parasitol 1969;63:245–63.
2. Diro M, Beydoun SN. Malaria in pregnancy. South Med J 1982;75:959–62.
3. Anonymous. Malaria in pregnancy. Lancet 1983;2:84–5.
4. Strang A, Lachman E, Pitsoe SB, Marszalek A, Philpott RH. Malaria in pregnancy with fatal complications: case report. Br J Obstet Gynaecol 1984;91:399–403.
5. Ross JB, Garatsos S. Absence of chloroquine induced ototoxicity in a fetus. Arch Dermatol 1974;109:573.
6. Lewis R, Lauresen NJ, Birnbaum S. Malaria associated with pregnancy. Obstet Gynecol 1973;42:698–700.
7. Hart CW, Naunton RF. The ototoxicity of chloroquine phosphate. Arch Otolaryngol 1964;80:407–12.
8. Wolfe MS, Cordero JF. Safety of chloroquine in chemosuppression of malaria during pregnancy. Br Med J 1985;290:1466–7.
9. Anderson PO. Drugs and breast feeding. Drug Intell Clin Pharm 1977;11:210–1.
10. Committee on Drugs, American Academy of Pediatrics. The transfer of drugs and other chemicals into human breast milk. Pediatrics 1983;72:375–83.

Name: **CHLOROTHIAZIDE**

Class: **Diuretic**   Risk Factor: **D**

Fetal Risk Summary

Chlorothiazide is a member of the thiazide group of diuretics. The information in this monograph applies to all members of the group, including the structurally related diuretics, chlorthalidone, metolazone, and quinethazone. Thiazide and related diuretics are rarely administered during the 1st trimester. In the past, when these drugs were routinely given to prevent or treat toxemia, therapy was usually begun in the 2nd or 3rd trimesters and adverse effects in the fetus were rare (1–10). No increases in the incidence of congenital defects were discovered and thiazides were considered nonteratogenic (11–14). In contrast, the Collaborative Perinatal Project monitored 50,282 mother-child pairs, 233 of which were exposed in the 1st trimester to thiazide or related diuretics (15). All of the mothers had cardiovascular disorders, which makes interpretation of the data difficult. However, an increased risk for malformations was found for chlorthalidone (20 patients) and miscellaneous thiazide diuretics (35 patients, excluding chlorothiazide and hydrochlorothiazide). For use anytime during pregnancy, 17,492 exposures were recorded and only polythiazide showed a slight increase in risk (16).

Many investigators consider diuretics contraindicated in pregnancy, except for patients with heart disease, since they do not prevent or alter the course of toxemia, and they may decrease placental perfusion (7, 17–21). A 1984 study determined that the use of diuretics for hypertension in pregnancy prevented normal plasma volume expansion and did not change perinatal outcome (22). In 4,035 patients treated for edema in the last half of the 3rd trimester (hypertensive patients were excluded), higher rates were found for induction of labor, stimulation of labor, uterine inertia, meconium staining, and perinatal mortality (20). All except perinatal mortality showed a statistically significant difference from 13,103 controls. Shoemaker and co-workers (23) found a decrease in endocrine function of the placenta as measured by placental clearance of estradiol in three patients treated with hydrochlorothiazide.

Chlorothiazide readily crosses the placenta at term and fetal serum levels may equal those of the mother (24). Chlorthalidone also crosses the placenta and at term, fetal serum levels may equal those of the mother (25). Other diuretics probably cross to the fetus in similar amounts, although specific data are lacking. Thiazides are considered mildly diabetogenic since they can induce hyperglycemia (18). Several investigators have noted this effect in pregnant patients treated with thiazides (26–29). Other studies have failed to show maternal hyperglycemia (30, 31). Although apparently at low risk, newborns exposed to thiazide diuretics near term should be observed closely for symptoms of hypoglycemia resulting from maternal hyperglycemia (29).

Neonatal thrombocytopenia has been reported following the use near term of chlorothiazide, hydrochlorothiazide, and methyclothiazide (14, 26, 32–37). Other studies have not found a relationship between thiazide diuretics and platelet counts (38, 39). The positive reports involve only 11 patients, and although the numbers are small, two of the affected infants died (26, 33). The mechanism of the thrombocytopenia is unknown, but the transfer of antiplatelet antibody from the mother to the fetus has been demonstrated (37). Thiazide-induced hemolytic anemia in two newborns was described in 1964 following the use of chlorothiazide and bendroflumethiazide at term (32). Thiazide diuretics may induce severe electrolyte imbalances in the mother's serum and amniotic fluid and in the newborn (40–42). In one case, a stillborn fetus was attributed to electrolyte imbalance and/or maternal hypotension (40). Two hypotonic newborns were discovered to be hyponatremic, a condition believed to have resulted from maternal diuretic therapy (41). Fetal bradycardia, 65–70 beats/min, was shown to be secondary to chlorothiazide-induced maternal hypokalemia (42). In a 1963 study, no relationship was found between neonatal jaundice and chlorothiazide (43). Maternal and fetal death in two cases of acute hemorrhagic pancreatitis were attributed to the use of chlorothiazide in the 2nd and 3rd trimesters (44).

In summary, 1st trimester use of thiazide and related diuretics may cause an increased risk of congenital defects based on the results of one large study. Use in later trimesters does not seem to carry this risk. In addition to malformations, other risk to the fetus or newborn include hypoglycemia, thrombocytopenia, hyponatremia, hypokalemia, and death from maternal complications. Thiazide diuretics may have a direct effect on smooth muscle and inhibit labor. Use of diuretics during pregnancy should be discouraged except for patients with heart disease.

Breast Feeding Summary

Chlorothiazide is excreted into breast milk in low concentrations (45). Following a 500-mg single oral dose, milk levels were less than 1 μg/ml at 1, 2, and 3 hours.

The authors speculated that the risks of pharmacologic effects in nursing infants would be remote. However, it has been stated that thrombocytopenia can occur in the nursing infant if the mother was taking chlorothiazide (46). Documentation of this finding is needed (47). Chlorthalidone has a very low milk:plasma ratio of 0.05 (25).

In one mother taking 50 mg of hydrochlorothiazide daily, peak milk levels of the drug occurred 5–10 hours after a dose and were about 25% of maternal blood concentrations (48). The mean milk concentration of hydrochlorothiazide was about 80 ng/ml. An infant consuming 600 ml of milk per day would thus ingest about 50 µg of the drug, probably an insignificant amount (48). The diuretic could not be detected in the serum of the nursing, 1-month-old infant, and measurements of serum electrolytes, blood glucose, and blood urea nitrogen were all normal.

Thiazide diuretics have been used to suppress lactation (49, 50). Because of this, the American Academy of Pediatrics recommends avoiding thiazide diuretics during the first month of lactation (51).

References

1. Finnerty FA Jr, Buchholz JH, Tuckman J. Evaluation of chlorothiazide (Diuril) in the toxemias of pregnancy. Analysis of 144 patients. JAMA 1958;166:141–4.
2. Zuspan FP, Bell JD, Barnes AC. Balance-ward and double-blind diuretic studies during pregnancy. Obstet Gynecol 1960;16:543–9.
3. Sears RT. Oral diuretics in pregnancy toxaemia. Br Med J 1960;2:148.
4. Assoli NS. Renal effects of hydrochlorothiazide in normal and toxemic pregnancy. Clin Pharmacol Ther 1960;1:48–52.
5. Tatum H, Waterman EA. The prophylactic and therapeutic use of the thiazides in pregnancy. GP 1961;24:101–5.
6. Flowers CE, Grizzle JE, Easterling WE, Bonner OB. Chlorothiazide as a prophylaxis against toxemia of pregnancy. Am J Obstet Gynecol 1962;84:919–29.
7. Weseley AC, Douglas GW. Continuous use of chlorothiazide for prevention of toxemia in pregnancy. Obstet Gynecol 1962;19:355–8.
8. Finnerty FA Jr. How to treat toxemia of pregnancy. GP 1963;27:116–21.
9. Fallis NE, Plauche WC, Mosey LM, Langford HG. Thiazide versus placebo in prophylaxis of toxemia of pregnancy in primagravid patients. Am J Obstet Gynecol 1964;88:502–4.
10. Landesman R, Aguero O, Wilson K, LaRussa R, Campbell W, Penaloza O. The prophylactic use of chlorthalidone, a sulfonamide diuretic, in pregnancy. J Obstet Gynaecol Br Commonw 1965;72:1004–10.
11. Cuadros A, Tatum H. The prophylactic and therapeutic use of bendroflumethiazide in pregnancy. Am J Obstet Gynecol 1964;89:891–7.
12. Finnerty FA Jr, Bepko FJ Jr. Lowering the perinatal mortality and the prematurity rate. The value of prophylactic thiazides in juveniles. JAMA 1966;195:429–32.
13. Kraus GW, Marchese JR, Yen SSC. Prophylactic use of hydrochlorothiazide in pregnancy. JAMA 1966;198:1150–4.
14. Gray MJ. Use and abuse of thiazides in pregnancy. Clin Obstet Gynecol 1968;11:568–78.
15. Heinonen OP, Slone D, Shapiro S. Birth Defects and Drugs in Pregnancy. Littleton:Publishing Sciences Group, 1977:371–3.
16. Ibid, 441.
17. Watt JD, Philipp EE. Oral diuretics in pregnancy toxemia. Br Med J 1960;1:1807.
18. Pitkin RM, Kaminetzky HA, Newton M, Pritchard JA. Maternal nutrition: a selective review of clinical topics. Obstet Gynecol 1972;40:773–85.
19. Lindheimer MD, Katz AI. Sodium and diuretics in pregnancy. N Engl J Med 1973;288:891–4.
20. Christianson R, Page EW. Diuretic drugs and pregnancy. Obstet Gynecol 1976;48:647–52.
21. Lammintausta R, Erkkola R, Eronen M. Effect of chlorothiazide treatment of renin-aldosterone system during pregnancy. Acta Obstet Gynecol Scand 1978;57:389–92.
22. Sibai BM, Grossman RA, Grossman HG. Effects of diuretics on plasma volume in pregnancies with long-term hypertension. Am J Obstet Gynecol 1984;150:831–5.

23. Shoemaker ES, Grant NF, Madden JD, MacDonald PC. The effect of thiazide diuretics on placental function. Tex Med 1973;69:109–15.
24. Garnet J. Placental transfer of chlorothiazide. Obstet Gynecol 1963;21:123–5.
25. Mulley BA, Parr GD, Pau WK, Rye RM, Mould JJ, Siddle NC. Placental transfer of chlorthalidone and its elimination in maternal milk. Eur J Clin Pharmacol 1978;13:129–31.
26. Menzies DN. Controlled trial of chlorothiazide in treatment of early pre-eclampsia. Br Med J 1964;1:739–42.
27. Ladner CN, Pearson JW, Herrick CN, Harrison HE. The effect of chlorothiazide on blood glucose in the third trimester of pregnancy. Obstet Gynecol 1964;23:555–60.
28. Goldman JA, Neri A, Ovadia J, Eckerling B, DeVries A. Effect of chlorothiazide on intravenous glucose tolerance in pregnancy. Am J Obstet Gynecol 1969;105:556–60.
29. Senior B, Slone D, Shapiro S, Mitchell AA, Heinonen OP. Benzothiadiazides and neonatal hypoglycaemia. Lancet 1976;2:377.
30. Lakin N, Zeytinoglu J, Younger M, White P. Effect of chlorothiazide on insulin requirements of pregnant diabetic women. JAMA 1960;173:353–4.
31. Esbenshade JH Jr, Smith RT. Thiazides and pregnancy: a study of carbohydrate tolerance. Am J Obstet Gynecol 1965;92:270–1.
32. Harley JD, Robin H, Robertson SEJ. Thiazide-induced neonatal haemolysis? Br Med J 1964;1:696–7.
33. Rodriguez SU, Leikin SL, Hiller MC. Neonatal thrombocytopenia associated with ante-partum administration of thiazide drugs. N Engl J Med 1964;270:881–4.
34. Leikin SL. Thiazide and neonatal thrombocytopenia. N Engl J Med 1964;271:161.
35. Prescott LF. Neonatal thrombocytopenia and thiazide drugs. Br Med J 1964;1:1438.
36. Jones JE, Reed JF Jr. Renal vein thrombosis and thrombocytopenia in the newborn infant. J Pediatr 1965;67:681–2.
37. Karpatkin S, Strick N, Karpatkin MB, Siskind GW. Cumulative experience in the detection of antiplatelet antibody in 234 patients with idiopathic thrombocytopenic purpura, systemic lupus erythematosus and other clinical disorders. Am J Med 1972;52:776–85.
38. Finnerty FA Jr, Assoli NS. Thiazide and neonatal thrombocytopenia. N Engl J Med 1964;271:160–1.
39. Jerkner K, Kutti J, Victoria L. Platelet counts in mothers and their newborn infants with respect to antepartum administration of oral diuretics. Acta Med Scand 1973;194:473–5.
40. Pritchard JA, Walley PJ. Severe hypokalemia due to prolonged administration of chlorothiazide during pregnancy. Am J Obstet Gynecol 1961;81:1241–4.
41. Alstatt LB. Transplacental hyponatremia in the newborn infant. J Pediatr 1965;66:985–8.
42. Anderson GG, Hanson TM. Chronic fetal bradycardia: possible association with hypokalemia. Obstet Gynecol 1974;44:896–8.
43. Crosland D, Flowers C. Chlorothiazide and its relationship to neonatal jaundice. Obstet Gynecol 1963;22:500–4.
44. Minkowitz S, Soloway HB, Hall JE, Yermakov V. Fatal hemorrhagic pancreatitis following chlorothiazide administration in pregnancy. Obstet Gynecol 1964;24:337–42.
45. Werthmann MW Jr, Krees SV. Excretion of chlorothiazide in human breast milk. J Pediatr 1972;81:781–3.
46. Anonymous. Drugs in breast milk. Med Lett Drugs Ther 1976;16:25–7.
47. Dailey JW. Anticoagulant and cardiovascular drugs. In Wilson JT, ed. Drugs in Breast Milk. Balgowlah, Australia: ADIS Press, 1981:61–4.
48. Miller ME, Cohn RD, Burghart PH. Hydrochlorothiazide disposition in a mother and her breast-fed infant. J Pediatr 1982;101:789–91.
49. Healy M. Suppressing lactation with oral diuretics. Lancet 1961;1:1353–4.
50. Catz CS, Giacoia GP. Drugs and breast milk. Pediatr Clin North Am 1972;19:151–66.
51. Committee on Drugs, American Academy of Pediatrics. The transfer of drugs and other chemicals into human breast milk. Pediatrics 1983;72:375–83.

Name: **CHLOROTRIANISENE**

Class: **Estrogenic Hormone**   Risk Factor: **X$_M$**

Fetal Risk Summary

No data available. Use of estrogenic hormones during pregnancy is contraindicated (see Oral Contraceptives).

Breast Feeding Summary

See Oral Contraceptives.

Name: **CHLORPHENIRAMINE**

Class: **Antihistamine/ Antiemetic**   Risk Factor: **B**

Fetal Risk Summary

The Collaborative Perinatal Project monitored 50,282 mother-child pairs, 1,070 of which had 1st trimester exposure to chlorpheniramine (1). For use anytime during pregnancy, 3,931 exposures were recorded (2). In neither case was evidence found to suggest a relationship to large categories of major or minor malformations. Several possible associations with individual malformations were found but the statistical significance of these is unknown. Independent confirmation is required to determine the actual risk.

Polydactyly in blacks (7 cases in 272 blacks)
Gastrointestinal defects (13 cases)
Eye and ear defects (7 cases)

Hydrocephaly (8 cases)
Congenital dislocation of hip (16 cases)
Malformations of the female genitalia (6 cases)

In a 1971 study, significantly fewer infants with malformations were exposed to antihistamines in the 1st trimester as compared to controls (3). Chlorpheniramine was the sixth most commonly used antihistamine.

A case of infantile malignant osteopetrosis was described in a 4-month-old boy exposed *in utero* on several occasions to Contac (chlorpheniramine, phenylpropranolamine, and belladonna alkaloids), but this is a known genetic defect (4). The boy also had a continual "stuffy" nose.

Breast Feeding Summary

No data available.

References

1. Heinonen OP, Slone D, Shapiro S. *Birth Defects and Drugs in Pregnancy*. Littleton:Publishing Sciences Group, 1977:322–34.
2. *Ibid*, 437, 488.
3. Nelson MM, Forfar JO. Associations between drugs administered during pregnancy and congenital abnormalities of the fetus. Br Med J 1971;1:523–7.
4. Golbus MS, Koerper MA, Hall BD. Failure to diagnose osteopetrosis *in utero*. Lancet 1976;2:1246

Name: **CHLORPROMAZINE**

Class: **Tranquilizer**   Risk Factor: **C**

Fetal Risk Summary

Chlorpromazine is a propylamino phenothiazine. The drug readily crosses the placenta (1–4). In animals, selective accumulation and retention occurs in the fetal pigment epithelium (5). Although delayed ocular damage from high prolonged doses in pregnancy has not been reported in humans, concern has been expressed for this potential toxicity (5, 6).

Chlorpromazine has been used for the treatment of nausea and vomiting of pregnancy during all stages of gestation, including labor, since the mid-1950's (7–9). The drug seems to be safe and effective for this indication. Its use in labor to promote analgesia and amnesia is usually safe, but some patients (up to 18% in one series) have a marked unpredictable fall in blood pressure which could be dangerous to the mother and the fetus (10–14). Use of chlorpromazine during labor should be discouraged because of this adverse effect. One psychiatric patient, who consumed 8,000 mg of chlorpromazine in the last 10 days of pregnancy, delivered a hypotonic, lethargic infant with depressed reflexes and jaundice (4). The adverse effects resolved within 3 weeks.

An extrapyramidal syndrome, which may persist for months, has been observed in some infants whose mothers received chlorpromazine near term (15–19). This reaction is characterized by tremors, increased muscle tone with spasticity, and hyperactive deep tendon reflexes. Hypotenicity has been observed in one newborn and paralytic ileus in two newborns after exposure at term to chlorpromazine (4, 20). However, most reports describing the use chlorpromazine in pregnancy have concluded that it does not adversely affect the fetus or newborn (21–26).

The Collaborative Perinatal Project monitored 50,282 mother-child pairs, 142 of which had 1st trimester exposure to chlorpromazine (27). For use anytime during pregnancy, 284 exposures were recorded. No evidence was found in either group to suggest a relationship to malformations or an effect on perinatal mortality rate, birth weight, or intelligence quotient scores at 4 years of age. Opposite results were found in a prospective French study that compared 304 mothers exposed to phenothiazines during gestation with 10,921 nonexposed controls (28). Malformations were observed in 11 exposed infants (3.5%) and in 178 nonexposed infants (1.6%). Defects observed in four of the exposed infants were:

Syndactyly
Microcephaly, club/foot/hand, muscular
   abdominal aplasia
Endocardial fibroelastosis, brachymesophalangy,
   clinodactyly
Microcephaly

The association was significant ($p < 0.01$) for those phenothiazines with a 3-carbon aliphatic side chain of which chlorpromazine was the principal member. Other phenothiazine groups (2-carbon side chain, piperazine, and piperidine derivatives) were associated with lesser significance ($p < 0.05$). A stillborn fetus delivered at

28 weeks with ectromelia/omphalocele was attributed to the combined use of chloropromazine and meclizine in the 1st trimester (29).

In an *in vitro* study, chlorpromazine was shown to be a potent inhibitor of sperm motility (30). A concentration of 53 μM produced a 50% reduction in motility.

In summary, although one survey found an increased incidence of defects and a report of ectromelia exists, most studies have found chlorpromazine to be safe for both mother and fetus if used occasionally in low doses. Other reviewers have also concluded that the phenothiazines are not teratogenic (24, 31). However, use near term should be avoided due to the danger of maternal hypotension and adverse effects in the newborn.

Breast Feeding Summary

Chlorpromazine is excreted into breast milk in very small concentrations. Following a 1,200-mg oral dose (20 mg/kg), peak milk levels of 0.29 μg/ml were measured at 2 hours (32). This represented a milk:plasma ratio of less than 0.5. The drug could not be detected following a 600-mg oral dose. In a study of four lactating mothers consuming unspecified amounts of the neuroleptic, milk concentrations of chlorpromazine ranged from 7 to 98 ng/ml with maternal serum levels ranging from 16 to 52 ng/ml (33). In two mothers, more drug was found in the milk than in the plasma. Only two of the mothers breast-fed their infants. One infant, consuming milk with a level of 7 ng/ml, showed no ill effects, but the second took milk containing 92 ng/ml and became drowsy and lethargic.

With the one exception described above, there has been a lack of reported adverse effects in breast-fed babies whose mothers were ingesting chlorpromazine (24). Based on this report, however, nursing infants exposed to the agent in milk should be observed for sedation. The American Academy of Pediatrics Committee on Drugs considers the drug compatible with breast-feeding (34).

References

1. Franchi G, Gianni AM. Chlorpromazine distribution in maternal and fetal tissues and biological fluids. Acta Anaesthesiol (Padava) 1957;8:197–207.
2. Moya F, Thorndike V. Passage of drugs across the placenta. Am J Obstet Gynecol 1962;84:1778–98.
3. O'Donoghue SEF. Distribution of pethidine and chlorpromazine in maternal, foetal and neonatal biological fluids. Nature 1971; 229:124–5.
4. Hammond JE, Toseland PA. Placental transfer of chlorpromazine. Arch Dis Child 1970;45:139–40.
5. Ullberg S, Lindquist NG, Sjostrand SE. Accumulation of chorio-retinotoxic drugs in the foetal eye. Nature 1970;227:1257–8.
6. Anonymous. Drugs and the fetal eye. Lancet 1971;1:122.
7. Karp M, Lamb VE, Benaron HBW. The use of chlorpromazine in the obstetric patient: a preliminary report. Am J Obstet Gynecol 1955;69:780–5.
8. Benaron HBW, Dorr EM, Roddick WJ, et al. Use of chlorpromazine in the obstetric patient: a preliminary report. I. In the treatment of nausea and vomiting of pregnancy. Am J Obstet Gynecol 1955; 69:776–9.
9. Sullivan CL. Treatment of nausea and vomiting of pregnancy with chlorpromazine. A report of 100 cases. Postgrad Med 1957;22:429–32.
10. Harer WB. Chlorpromazine in normal labor. Obstet Gynecol 1956;8:1–9.
11. Lindley JE, Rogers SF, Moyer JH. Analgesic-potentiation effect of chlorpromazine during labor; a study of 2093 patients. Obstet Gynecol 1957;10:582–6.
12. Bryans CI Jr, Mulherin CM. The use of chlorpromazine in obstetrical analgesia. Am J Obstet Gynecol 1959;77:406–11.
13. Christhilf SM Jr, Monias MB, Riley RA Jr, Sheehan JC. Chlorpromazine in obstetric analgesia. Obstet Gynecol 1960;15:625–9.

14. Rodgers CD, Wickard CP, McCaskill MR. Labor and delivery without terminal anesthesia. A report of the use of chlorpromazine. Obstet Gynecol 1961;17:92–5.
15. Hill RM, Desmond MM, Kay JL. Extrapyramidal dysfunction in an infant of a schizophrenic mother. J Pediatr 1966;69:589–95.
16. Ayd FJ Jr, ed. Phenothiazine therapy during pregnancy—effects on the newborn infant. Int Drug Ther Newslett 1968;3:39–40.
17. Tamer A, McKay R, Arias D, Worley L, Fogel BJ. Phenothiazine-induced extrapyramidal dysfunction in the neonate. J Pediatr 1969;75:479–80.
18. Levy W, Wisniewski K. Chlorpromazine causing extrapyramidal dysfunction in newborn infant of psychotic mother. NY State J Med 1974;74:684–5.
19 .O'Connor M, Johnson GH, James DI. Intrauterine effect of phenothiazines. Med J Aust 1981;1:416–7.
20. Falterman CG, Richardson J. Small left colon syndrome associated with maternal ingestion of psychotropic drugs. J Pediatr 1980;97:308–10.
21. Kris EB, Carmichael DM. Chlorpromazine maintenance therapy during pregnancy and confinement. Psychiatr Q 1957;31:690–5.
22. Kris EB. Children born to mothers maintained on pharmacotherapy during pregnancy and postpartum. Recent Adv Biol Psychiatr 1962;4:180–7.
23. Sobel DE. Fetal damage due to ECT, insulin coma, chlorpromazine, or reserpine. Arch Gen Psychiatry 1960;2:606–11.
24. Ayd FJ Jr. Children born of mothers treated with chlorpromazine during pregnancy. Clin Med 1964;71:1758–63.
25. Sobel DE. Fetal damage due to ECT, insulin coma, chlorpromazine, or reserpine. Arch Gen Psychiatry 1960;2:606–11.
26. Loke KH, Salleh R. Electroconvulsive therapy for the acutely psychotic pregnant patient: a review of 3 cases. Med J Malaysia 1983;38:131–3.
27. Slone D, Siskind V, Heinonen OP, Monson RR, Kaufman DW, Shapiro S. Antenatal exposure to the phenothiazines in relation to congenital malformations, perinatal mortality rate, birth weight, and intelligence quotient score. Am J Obstet Gynecol 1977;128:486–8.
28. Rumeau-Rouquette C, Goujard J, Huel G. Possible teratogenic effect of phenothiazines in human beings. Teratology 1976;15:57–64.
29. O'Leary JL, O'Leary JA. Nonthalidomide ectromelia; report of a case. Obstet Gynecol 1964;23:17–20.
30. Levin RM, Amsterdam JD, Winokur A, Wein AJ. Effects of psychotropic drugs on human sperm motility. Fertil Steril 1981;36:503–6.
31. Ananth J. Congenital malformations with psychopharmacologic agents. Compr Psychiatry 1975;16:437–45.
32. Blacker KH, Weinstein BJ, Ellman GL. Mother's milk and chlorpromazine. Am J Psychol 1962;114:178–9.
33. Wiles DH, Orr MW, Kolakowska T. Chlorpromazine levels in plasma and milk of nursing mothers. Br J Clin Pharmacol 1978;5:272–3.
34. Committee on Drugs, American Academy of Pediatrics. The transfer of drugs and other chemicals into human breast milk. Pediatrics 1983;72:375–83.

Name: **CHLORPROPAMIDE**

Class: **Oral Hypoglycemic**　　　　　　　　　　Risk Factor: **D***

Fetal Risk Summary

Chlorpropamide is a sulfonylurea used for the treatment of adult-onset diabetes mellitus. It is not indicated for the pregnant diabetic. When administered near term, the drug crosses the placenta and may persist in the neonatal serum for several days (1, 2). One mother, who took 500 mg/day throughout pregnancy, delivered an infant whose serum level was 15.4 mg/100 ml at 77 hours of life (1). Infants of three other mothers, who were consuming 100–250 mg/day at term, had serum levels varying between 1.8 and 2.8 mg/100 ml 8–35 hours after delivery (2). All four infants had prolonged symptomatic hypoglycemia secondary to hyperinsulinism lasting for 4–6 days. In other reports, totaling 69 pregnancies, chlorpropamide in doses of 100–200 mg or more per day either gave no evidence of neonatal hypoglycemia/hyperinsulinism or no constant relationship between daily maternal dosage and neonatal complications (3, 4). However, chlorpropamide should be stopped at least 48 hours before delivery to avoid this potential complication (5).

Although teratogenic in animals, an increased incidence of congenital defects, other than that expected in diabetes mellitus, has not been found with chlorpropamide (6–15). Four malformed infants have been attributed to chlorpropamide but the relationship is unclear (6, 9):

Hand/finger anomalies (6)
Stricture of lower ileum, death (6)
Preauricular sinus (6)
Microcephaly/spastic quadriplegia (9)

Maternal diabetes is known to increase the rate of malformations by 2–4-fold, but the mechanism(s) are not understood (see also Insulin). In spite of the lack of evidence for chlorpropamide teratogenicity, the drug should not be used in pregnancy since it will not provide good control in patients whose disease cannot be controlled by diet alone (5). The manufacturer recommends it not be used in pregnancy (16).

[* Risk Factor C according to manufacturer—Pfizer, 1985.]

Breast Feeding Summary

Chlorpropamide is excreted into breast milk. Following a 500-mg oral dose, the milk concentration in a composite of two samples obtained at 5 hours was 5 μg/ml (17). The effects on a nursing infant from this amount of drug are unknown.

References

1. Zucker P, Simon G. Prolonged symptomatic neonatal hypoglycemia associated with maternal chlorpropamide therapy. Pediatrics 1968;42:824–5.
2. Kemball ML, McIver C, Milnar RDG, Nourse CH, Schiff D, Tiernan JR. Neonatal hypoglycaemia in infants of diabetic mothers given sulphonylurea drugs in pregnancy. Arch Dis Child 1970;45:696–701.
3. Sutherland HW, Stowers JM, Cormack JD, Bewsher PD. Evaluation of chlorpropamide in chemical diabetes diagnosed during pregnancy. Br Med J 1973;3:9–13.
4. Sutherland HW, Bewsher PD, Cormack JD, et al. Effect of moderate dosage of chlorpropamide in pregnancy on fetal outcome. Arch Dis Child 1974;49:283–91.
5. Friend JR. Diabetes. Clin Obstet Gynecol 1981;8:353–82.
6. Soler NG, Walsh CH, Malins JM. Congenital malformations in infants of diabetic mothers. Q J Med 1976;45:303–13.
7. Adam PAJ, Schwartz R. Diagnosis and treatment: should oral hypoglycemic agents be used in pediatric and pregnant patients? Pediatrics 1968;42:819–23.
8. Dignan PSJ. Teratogenic risk and counseling in diabetes. Clin Obstet Gynecol 1981;24:149–59.
9. Campbell GD. Chlorpropamide and foetal damage. Br Med J 1963;1:59–60.
10. Jackson WPU, Campbell GD, Notelovitz M, Blumsohn D. Tolbutamide and chlorpropamide during pregnancy in human diabetes. Diabetes 1962;11(Suppl):98–101.

11. Jackson WPU, Campbell GD. Chlorpropamide and perinatal mortality. Br Med J 1963;2:1652.
12. Macphail I. Chlorpropamide and foetal damage. Br Med J 1963;1:192.
13. Malins JM, Cooke AM, Pyke DA, Fitzgerald MG. Sulphonylurea drugs in pregnancy. Br Med J 1964;2:187.
14. Moss JM, Connor EJ. Pregnancy complicated by diabetes. Report of 102 pregnancies including eleven treated with oral hypoglycemic drugs. Med Ann DC 1965;34;253–60.
15. Douglas CP, Richards R. Use of chlorpropamide in the treatment of diabetes in pregnancy. Diabetes 1967;16:60–1.
16. Product information. Diabinese. Pfizer, 1985.
17. D'Ambrosio GG, Pfizer Laboratories, 1982. Personal communication.

Name: **CHLORPROTHIXENE**

Class: **Tranquilizer**   Risk Factor: **C**

Fetal Risk Summary

Chlorprothixene is structurally and pharmacologically related to chlorpromazine and thiothixene. No specific data on its use in pregnancy have been located (see also Chlorpromazine).

Breast Feeding Summary

No data available.

Name: **CHLORTETRACYCLINE**

Class: **Antibiotic**   Risk Factor: **D**

Fetal Risk Summary

See Tetracycline.

Breast Feeding Summary

Chlortetracycline is excreted into breast milk. Eight patients were given 2–3 g orally per day for 3–4 days (1). Average maternal and milk concentrations were 4.1 and 1.25 μg/ml, respectively, producing a milk:plasma ratio of 0.4. Infant data were not given.

Theoretically, dental staining and inhibition of bone growth could occur in breast-fed infants whose mothers were consuming chlortetracycline. However, this theoretical possibility seems remote since in infants exposed to a closely related antibiotic, tetracycline, serum levels were undetectable (less than 0.05 μg/ml) (2). The American Academy of Pediatrics considers tetracycline compatible with breast-feeding (3). Three potential problems may exist for the nursing infant, even though there are no reports in this regard: modification of bowel flora, direct effects on the infant, and interference with the interpretation of culture results if a fever work-up is required.

References

1. Guilbeau JA, Schoenbach EB, Schuab IG, Latham DV. Aureomycin in obstetrics; therapy and prophylaxis. JAMA 1950;143:520–6.
2. Posner AC, Prigot A, Konicoff NG. Further observations on the use of tetracycline hydrochloride in prophylaxis and treatment of obstetric infections. *Antibiotics Annual 1954–55*, New York:Medical Encyclopedia, 594–8.
3. Committee on Drugs, American Academy of Pediatrics. The transfer of drugs and other chemicals into human breast milk. Pediatrics 1983;72:375–83.

Name: **CHLORTHALIDONE**

Class: **Diuretic**   Risk Factor: **D**

Fetal Risk Summary

Chlorthalidone is structurally related to the thiazide diuretics. See Chlorothiazide.

Breast Feeding Summary

See Chlorothiazide.

Name: **CHLORZOXAZONE**

Class: **Muscle Relaxant**   Risk Factor: **C**

Fetal Risk Summary

No data available.

Breast Feeding Summary

No data available.

Name: **CHOLECALCIFEROL**

Class: **Vitamin**   Risk Factor: **A***

Fetal Risk Summary

Cholecalciferol (vitamin D_3) is converted in the liver to calcifediol which in turn is converted in the kidneys to calcitriol, one of the active forms of vitamin D. See Vitamin D.

[* Risk Factor D if used in doses above the RDA.]

Breast Feeding Summary

See Vitamin D.

Name: **CHOLESTYRAMINE**

Class: **Antilipemic**   Risk Factor: **C**

Fetal Risk Summary

Cholestyramine is a resin used to bind bile acids in a nonabsorbable complex. The resin has been used for the treatment of cholestasis of pregnancy (1–3). No adverse fetal effects were observed. Cholestyramine also binds fat-soluble vitamins and long-term use could result in deficiencies of these agents in either mother or fetus (4). However, in one study, treatment with 9 g daily up to a maximum duration of 12 weeks was not associated with fetal or maternal complications (1).

Breast Feeding Summary

No data available.

References

1. Lutz EE, Margolis AJ. Obstetric hepatosis: treatment with cholestyramine and interim response to steroids. Obstet Gynecol 1969;33:64–71.
2. Heikkinen J, Maentausta O, Ylostalo P, Janne O. Serum bile acid levels in intrahepatic cholestasis of pregnancy during treatment with phenobarbital or cholestyramine. Eur J Obstet Gynecol Reprod Biol 1982;14:153–62.
3. Shaw D, Frohlich J, Wittmann BAK, Willms M. A prospective study of 18 patients with cholestasis of pregnancy. Am J Obstet Gynecol 1982;142:621–5.
4. American Hospital Formulary Service. *Drug Information 1985*. Bethesda:American Society of Hospital Pharmacists, 1985:633–5.

Name: **CIMETIDINE**

Class: **Histamine (H₂ Receptor Antagonist)**   Risk Factor: **B**

Fetal Risk Summary

No reports linking the use of cimetidine with congenital defects have been located. Transient liver impairment has been described in a newborn exposed to cimetidine at term (1). Other reports have not confirmed this toxicity (2–9). The drug has been used at term with antacids to prevent maternal acid aspiration pneumonitis (Mendelson's syndrome) (4–16). No neonatal adverse effects were noted in these studies. At term, cimetidine crosses the placenta, resulting in a peak mean fetal:maternal ratio of 0.84 at 1.5–2 hours (17).

Breast Feeding Summary

Cimetidine is excreted into breast milk and may accumulate in concentrations greater than that found in maternal plasma (18). Following a single 400-mg oral dose a theoretical milk:plasma ratio of 1.6 has been calculated (18). Multiple oral doses of 200 and 400 mg result in milk:plasma ratios of 4.6 to 7.44, respectively. An estimated 6 mg of cimetidine per liter of milk could be ingested by the nursing infant. The clinical significance of this ingestion is unknown, but the drug is considered contraindicated in the lactating woman due to potenital adverse effects on the infant's gastric acidity, inhibition of drug metabolism, and central nervous system stimulation (19).

References

1. Glade G, Saccar CL, Pereira GR. Cimetidine in pregnancy: apparent transient liver impairment in the newborn. Am J Dis Child 1980;134:87–8.
2. McGowan WAW. Safety of cimetidine treatment during pregnancy. J R Soc Med 1979;72:902–7.
3. Zulli P, DiNisio Q. Cimetidine treatment during pregnancy. Lancet 1978;2:945–6.
4. Husemeyer RP, Davenport HT. Prophylaxis for Mendelson's syndrome before elective caesarean sections. A comparison of cimetidine and magnesium trisilicate mixture regimens. Br J Obstet Gynaecol 1980;87:565–70.
5. Pickering BG,, Palahniuk RJ, Cumming M. Cimetidine premedication in elective caesarean section. Can Anaesth Soc J 1980;27:33–5.
6. Dundee JW, Moore J, Johnston JR, McCaughey W. Cimetidine and obstetric anaesthesia. Lancet 1981;2:252.
7. McCaughey W, Howe JP, Moore J, Dundee JW. Cimetidine in elective caesarean section. Effect on gastric acidity. Anaesthesia 1981;36:167–72.
8. Crawford JS. Cimetidine in elective caesarean section. Anaesthesia 1981;36:641–2.
9. McCaughey W, Howe JP, Moore J, Dundee JW. *Ibid*, 642.
10. Hodgkinson R, Glassenberg R, Joyce TH III, Coombs DW, Ostheimer GW, Gibbs CP. Safety and efficacy of cimetidine and antacid in reducing gastric acidity before elective cesarean section. Anesthesiology 1982;57:A408.
11. Ostheimer GW, Morrison JA, Lavoie C, Sepkoski C, Hoffman J, Datta S. The effect of cimetidine on mother, newborn and neonatal neurobehavior. Anesthesiology 1982;57:A405.
12. Hodgkinson R, Glassenberg R, Joyce TH III, Coombs DW, Ostheimer GW, Gibbs CP. Comparison of cimetidine (Tagamet) with antacid for safety and effectiveness in reducing gastric acidity before elective cesarean section. Anesthesiology 1983;59:86–90.
13. Qvist N, Storm K. Cimethidine pre-anesthetic: a prophylactic method against Mendelson's syndrome in cesarean section. Acta Obstet Gynecol Scand 1983;62:157–9.
14. Okasha AS, Motaweh MM, Bali A. Cimetidine-antacid combination as premedication for elective caesarean section. Can Anaesth Soc J 1983;30:593–7.
15. Frank M, Evans M, Flynn P, Aun C. Comparison of the prophylactic use of magnesium trisilicate mixture B.P.C., sodium citrate mixture or cimetidine in obstetrics. Br J Anaesth 1984;56:355–62.
16. McAuley DM, Halliday HL, Johnston JR, Moore J, Dundee JW. Cimetidine in labour: absence of adverse effect on the high-risk fetus. Br J Obstet Gynaecol 1985;92:350–5.
17. Howe JP, McGowan WAW, Moore J, McCaughey W, Dundee JW. The placental transfer of cimetidine. Anaesthesia 1981;36:371–5.
18. Somogyi A, Gugler R. Cimetidine excretion into breast milk. Br J Clin Pharmacol 1979;7:627–9.
19. Committee on Drugs, American Academy of Pediatrics. The transfer of drugs and other chemicals into human breast milk. Pediatrics 1983;72:375–83.

Name: **CINNARIZINE**

Class: **Antihistamine**   Risk Factor: **C**

Fetal Risk Summary

No data available. See Meclizine for representative agent in this class.

Breast Feeding Summary

No data available.

Name: **CINOXACIN**

Class: **Urinary Germicide**   Risk Factor: **B$_M$**

Fetal Risk Summary

No data available. The manufacturer recommends it not be used in pregnancy (1).

Breast Feeding Summary

No data available. The manufacturer recommends it not be used in the lactating woman (1).

References

1. Product information. Cinobac. Dista Products, 1985.

Name: **CISPLATIN**

Class: **Antineoplastic**   Risk Factor: **D**

Fetal Risk Summary

Only one case of cisplatin usage during pregnancy has been located (1). The mother received a single intravenous dose of 50 mg/kg at approximately 10 weeks gestation for carcinoma of the uterine cervix. Two weeks later, a radical hysterectomy was performed. The male fetus was morphologically normal for its developmental age.

Breast Feeding Summary

No data available.

References

1. Jacobs AJ, Marchevsky A, Gordon RE, Deppe G, Cohen CJ. Oat cell carcinoma of the uterine cervix in a pregnant woman treated with cis-diamminedichloroplatinum. Gynecol Oncol 1980;9:405–10.

Name: **CLEMASTINE**

Class: **Antihistamine**   Risk Factor: **C**

Fetal Risk Summary

No data available. See Diphenhydramine for representative agent in this class.

Breast Feeding Summary

Clemastine is excreted into breast milk (1). A 10-week-old girl developed drowsiness, irritability, refusal to feed, neck stiffness, and a high pitched cry 12 hours after the mother began taking the antihistamine, 1 mg twice daily. The mother was also taking phenytoin and carbamazepine. Twenty hours after the last dose, clemastine levels in maternal plasma and milk were 20 and 5–10 ng/ml, respectively, a milk:plasma ratio of 0.25–0.5. The drug could not be detected in the infant's plasma. Symptoms in the baby resolved within 24 hours after the drug was stopped, although breast-feeding was continued. Results of examination 3 weeks later were also normal. Due to the above case report, the American Academy of Pediatrics considers the drug contraindicated during breast-feeding (2).

References

1. Kok THHG, Taitz LS, Bennett MJ, Holt DW. Drowsiness due to clemastine transmitted in breast milk. Lancet 1982;1:914–5.
2. Committee on Drugs, American Academy of Pediatrics. The transfer of drugs and other chemicals into human breast milk. Pediatrics 1983;72:375–83.

Name: **CLIDINIUM**

Class: **Parasympatholytic**   Risk Factor: **C**

Fetal Risk Summary

Clidinium is an anticholinergic quaternary ammonium bromide. In a large prospective study, 2,323 patients were exposed to this class of drugs during the 1st trimester, 4 of whom took clidinium (1). A possible association was found between the total group and minor malformations.

Breast Feeding Summary

No data available (see also Atropine).

References

1. Heinonen OP, Slone D, Shapiro S. *Birth Defects and Drugs in Pregnancy*. Littleton:Publishing Sciences Group, 1977:346–53.

Name: **CLINDAMYCIN**

Class: **Antibiotic**   Risk Factor: **B**

Fetal Risk Summary

No reports linking the use of clindamycin with congenital defects have been located. The drug crosses the placenta, achieving maximum cord serum levels of approximately 50% of the maternal serum (1, 2). Levels in the fetus were considered therapeutic for susceptible pathogens. Fetal tissue levels increase following multiple dosing with the drug concentrating in the fetal liver (1). Maternal serum levels after dosing at various stages of pregnancy were similar to those of nonpregnant patients (2, 3). Clindamycin has been used for prophylactic therapy prior to cesarean section (4).

Breast Feeding Summary

Clindamycin is excreted into breast milk. In two patients receiving 600 mg intravenously every 6 hours, milk levels varied from 2.1 to 3.8 μg/ml (0.2–3.5 hours after drug) (5). When the patients' doses were changed to 300 mg orally every 6 hours, levels varied from 0.7 to 1.8 μg/ml (2–7 hours after drug). Maternal serum levels were not given. Two grossly bloody stools were observed in a nursing infant whose mother was receiving clindamycin and gentamicin (6). No relationship to either drug could be established. However, the condition cleared rapidly when breast-feeding was stopped. Except for this one case, no other adverse effects in nursing infants have been reported. Three potential problems exist for the nursing infant: modification of bowel flora, direct effects on the infant, and interference with the interpretation of culture results if a fever work-up is required. The American Academy of Pediatrics considers clindamycin compatible with breast-feeding (7).

References

1. Philipson A, Sabath LD, Charles D. Transplacental passage of erythromycin and clindamycin. N Engl J Med 1973;288:1219–21.
2. Weinstein AJ, Gibbs RS, Gallagher M. Placental transfer of clindamycin and gentamicin in term pregnancy. Am J Obstet Gynecol 1976;124:688–91.
3. Philipson A, Sabath LD, Charles D. Erythromycin and clindamycin absorption and elimination in pregnant women. Clin Pharmacol Ther 1976;19:68–77.
4. Rehu M, Jahkola M. Prophylactic antibiotics in caesarean section: effect of a short preoperative course of benzyl penicillin or clindamycin plus gentamicin on postoperative infectious morbidity. Ann Clin Res 1980;12:45–8.
5. Smith JA, Morgan JR, Rachlis AR, Papsin FR. Clindamycin in human breast milk. Can Med Assoc J 1975;112:806.
6. Mann CF. Clindamycin and breast-feeding. Pediatrics 1980;66:1030–1.
7. Committee on Drugs, American Academy of Pediatrics. The transfer of drugs and other chemicals into human breast milk. Pediatrics 1983;72:375–83.

Name: **CLOFIBRATE**

Class: **Antilipemic Agent**   Risk Factor: **C**

Fetal Risk Summary

No reports linking the use of clofibrate with congenital defects have been located. There is pharmacologic evidence that clofibrate crosses the rat placenta and reaches measurable levels, but data in humans are lacking (1). The drug is metabolized by glucuronide conjugation and since this system is immature in the newborn, accumulation may occur. Consequently, the use of clofibrate near term is not recommended.

Breast Feeding Summary

No data available. Animal studies suggest that the drug is excreted into milk (1).

References

1. Chhabra S, Kurup CKR. Maternal transport of chlorophenoxyisobutyrate at the foetal and neonatal stages of development. Biochem Pharmacol 1978;27:2063–5.

Name: **CLOMIPHENE**

Class: **Fertility Agent (Nonhormonal)**   Risk Factor: **X_M**

Fetal Risk Summary

Clomiphene is used to induce ovulation and is contraindicated after conception has occurred. Several case reports of neural tube defects have been reported after ovulation stimulation with clomiphene (1–5). However, an association between the drug and these defects has not been established (6–10). In a review by Asch and Greenblatt (6), the percentage of congenital anomalies after clomiphene use was no greater than that in the normal population. Similarly, the study by Kurachi and co-workers (11) of 1,034 pregnancies after clomiphene-induced ovulation found no association with the incidence or type of malformation. Congenital malformations reported in patients who received clomiphene prior to conception include (5, 6, 12–25):

Hydatidiform mole	Retinal aplasia
Syndactyly	Clubfoot
Pigmentation defects	Microcephaly
Congenital heart defects	Cleft lip/palate
Down's syndrome	Ovarian dysplasia
Hypospadias	Polydactyly
Hemangioma	Anencephaly

A single case of hepatoblastoma in a 15-month-old female was thought to be due to the use of clomiphene and follicle-stimulating/luteinizing hormone prior to conception (26).

Inadvertent use of clomiphene early in the 1st trimester has been reported in two patients (18, 24). A ruptured lumbosacral meningomyelocele was observed in one infant exposed during the 4th week of gestation (18). There was no evidence of neurologic defect in the lower limbs or of hydrocephalus. The second infant showed esophageal atresia with fistula, congenital heart defects, hypospadius, and absent left kidney (24). The mother also took methyldopa throughout pregnancy for mild hypertension.

Patients requiring the use of clomiphene should be cautioned that each new course of the drug should be started only after pregnancy has been excluded.

Breast Feeding Summary

No data available.

References

1. Barrett C, Hakim C. Anencephaly, ovulation stimulation, subfertility, and illegitimacy. Lancet 1973;2:916–7.
2. Dyson JL, Kohler HG, Anencephaly and ovulation stimulation. Lancet 1973;1:1256–7.
3. Field B, Kerr C. Ovulation stimulation and defects of neural tube closure. Lancet 1974;2:1511.
4. Sandler B. Anencephaly and ovulation stimulation. Lancet 1973;2:379.
5. Biale Y, Leventhal H, Altaras M, Ben-Aderet N. Anencephaly and clomiphene-induced pregnancy. Acta Obstet Gynecol Scand 1978;57:483–4.
6. Asch RH, Greenblatt RB. Update on the safety and efficacy of clomiphene citrate as a therapeutic agent. J Reprod Med 1976;17:175–180.
7. Harlap S. Ovulation induction and congenital malformations. Lancet 1976;2:961.

8. James WH, Clomiphene, anencephaly, and spina bifida. Lancet 1977;1:603.
9. Ahlgren M, Kallen B, Rannevik G. Outcome of pregnancy after clomiphene therapy. Acta Obstet Gynecol Scand 1976;55:371–5.
10. Elwood JM. Clomiphene and anencephalic births. Lancet 1974;1:31.
11. Kurachi K, Aono T, Minagawa J, Miyake A. Congenital malformations of newborn infants after clomiphene-induced ovulation. Fertil Steril 1983;40:187–9.
12. Miles PA, Taylor HB, Hill WC. Hydatidiform mole in a clomiphene related pregnancy: a case report. Obstet Gynecol 1971;37:358–9.
13. Schneiderman CI, Waxman B. Clomid therapy and subsequent hydatidiform mole formation: a case report. Obstet Gynecol 1972;39:787–8.
14. Wajntraub G, Kamar R, Pardo Y. Hydatidiform mole after treatment with clomiphene. Fertil Steril 1974;25:904.–5.
15. Berman P. Congenital abnormalities associated with maternal clomiphene ingestion. Lancet 1975;2:878.
16. Drew AL. Letter to the editor. Dev Med Child Neurol 1974;16:276.
17. Hack M, Brish M, Serr DM, Insler V, Salomy M, Lunenfeld B. Outcome of pregnancy after induced ovulation. Follow-up of pregnancies and children born after clomiphene therapy. JAMA 1972;220:1329–33.
18. Ylikorkala O. Congenital anomalies and clomiphene. Lancet 1975;2:1262–3.
19. Laing IA, Steer CR, Dudgeon J, Brown JK. Clomiphene and congenital retinopathy. Lancet 1981;2:1107–8.
20. Ford WDA, Little KET. Fetal ovarian dysplasia possibly associated with clomiphene. Lancet 1981;2:1107.
21. Kistner RW. Induction of ovulation with clomiphene citrate. Obstet Gynecol Surv 1965;20:873–99.
22. Goldfarb AF, Morales A, Rakoff AE, Protos P. Critical review of 160 clomiphene-related pregnancies. Obstet Gynecol 1968;31:342–5.
23. Oakely GP, Flynt IW. Increased prevalence of Down's syndrome (mongolism) among the offspring of women treated with ovulation-inducing agents. Teratology 1972;5:264.
24. Singhi M, Singhi S. Possible relationship between clomiphene and neural tube defects. J Pediatr 1978;93:152.
25. Mor-Joseph S, Anteby SO, Granat M, Brzezinsky A, Evron S. Recurrent molar pregnancies associated with clomiphene citrate and human gonadotropins. Am J Obstet Gynecol 1985;151:1085–6.
26. Melamed I, Bujanover Y, Hammer J, Spirer Z. Hepatoblastoma in an infant born to a mother after hormonal treatment for sterility. N Engl J Med 1982;307:820.

Name: **CLOMIPRAMINE**

Class: **Antidepressant**   Risk Factor: **D**

Fetal Risk Summary

The use of clomipramine throughout pregnancy to treat maternal depression has been described in three women (1, 2). All three newborns developed toxic morbidity shortly after birth. Clinical symptoms included lethargy, hypotonia, cyanosis, jitteriness, irregular respirations with respiratory acidosis, and hypothermia. The toxicity was probably due to the anticholinergic properties of the drug (1). The infants were successfully treated with phenobarbital and subsequently developed normally.

Breast Feeding Summary

No data available (see Imipramine).

References

1. Ben Muza A, Smith CS. Neonatal effects of maternal clomipramine therapy. Arch Dis Child 1979;54:405.
2. Ostergaard GZ, Pedersen SE. Neonatal effects of maternal clomipramine treatment. Pediatrics 1982;69:233–4.

Name: **CLOMOCYCLINE**

Class: **Antibiotic**   Risk Factor: **D**

Fetal Risk Summary

See Tetracycline.

Breast Feeding Summary

See Tetracycline.

Name: **CLONAZEPAM** CLONIPEN

Class: **Anticonvulsant**   Risk Factor: **C**

Fetal Risk Summary

Clonazepam is a benzodiazepine anticonvulsant that is chemically and structurally similar to diazepam (1). A 36 weeks gestational age infant, exposed throughout pregnancy to an unspecified amount of clonazepam, developed apnea, cyanosis, lethargy, and hypotonia at 6 hours of age (2). There was no evidence of congenital defects in the 2,750-g newborn. Cord and maternal serum levels of clonazepam were 19 and 32 ng/ml, respectively, a ratio of 0.59. Both levels were within the therapeutic range (5–70 ng/ml) (2). At 18 hours of age, clonazepam level in the infant's serum measured 4.4 ng/ml. Five episodes of prolonged apnea (16–43 seconds per occurrence) were measured by pneumogram over the next 12 hours. Hypotonia and lethargy resolved within 5 days, but overt clinical apnea persisted for 10 days. Follow-up pneumograms demonstrated apnea spells until 10 weeks of age, but the presence of the drug in breast milk may have contributed to the condition (see Breast Feeding Summary). The authors concluded that apnea due to prematurity was not a significant factor. Neurologic development was normal at 5 months.

Breast Feeding Summary

Clonazepam is excreted into breast milk. In a woman treated with an unspecified amount of the anticonvulsant, milk concentrations remained constant between 11 and 13 ng/ml (2). The milk:maternal serum ratio was approximately 0.33. After 7 days of nursing, the infant, described above, had a serum concentration of 2.9 ng/ml. A major portion of this probably resulted from *in utero* exposure, since the elimination half-life of clonazepam in neonates is thought to be prolonged (2). No evidence of drug accumulation after breast-feeding was found. Persistent apnea spells, lasting until 10 weeks of age, were observed, but it was not known if breast-feeding contributed to the condition. Based on this case, the authors recommended that infants exposed *in utero* or during breast-feeding to clonazepam should have serum levels of the drug determined and be closely monitored for central nervous system depression or apnea (2).

References

1. Reith H, Schafer H. Antiepileptic drugs during pregnancy and the lactation period. Pharmacokinetic data. Dtsch Med Wochenschr 1979;104:818–23.
2. Fisher JB, Edgren BE, Mammel MC, Coleman JM. Neonatal apnea associated with maternal clonazepam therapy: a case report. Obstet Gynecol 1985;66(Suppl):34S–5S.

Name: **CLONIDINE**

Class: **Antihypertensive** Risk Factor: **C**

Fetal Risk Summary

No reports linking the use of clonidine with congenital defects have been located. The drug has been used in the 2nd and 3rd trimesters without adverse fetal effects being observed (1–3). Limited use of clonidine during 1st trimester makes assessment of its safety difficult (1).

Breast Feeding Summary

Animal data indicate that clonidine enters breast milk in concentrations exceeding those of maternal blood (1). Following a 150-μg oral dose, human milk concentrations of 1.5 ng/ml may be achieved (milk:plasma ratio 1.5) (1). The significance of this amount is not known.

References

1. Bowers PA, Boehringer Ingelheim Ltd. 1981. Personal communication.
2. Turnbull AC, Ahmed S. Catapres in the treatment of hypertension in pregnancy, a preliminary study. In *Catapres in Hypertension*. Symposium of the Royal College of Surgeons. London, 1970:237–45.
3. Johnston CI, Aickin DR. The control of high blood pressure during labour with clonidine. Med J Aust 1971;2:132.

Name: **CLOTRIMAZOLE**

Class: **Antifungal Antibiotic** Risk Factor: **B**

Fetal Risk Summary

No reports linking the use of clotrimazole with congenital defects have been located. The topical use of the drug in pregnancy has been studied (1–4). No adverse effects attributable to clotrimazole were observed.

Breast Feeding Summary

No data available.

References

1. Tan CG, Good CS, Milne LJR, Loudon JDO. A comparative trial of six day therapy with clotrimazole and nystatin in pregnant patients with vaginal candidiasis. Postgrad Med 1974;50(Suppl 1):102–5.
2. Frerich W, Gad A. The frequency of Candida infections in pregnancy and their treatment with clotrimazole. Curr Med Res Opin 1977;4:640–4.
3. Haram K, Digranes A. Vulvovaginal candidiasis in pregnancy treated with clotrimazole. Acta Obstet Gynecol Scand 1978;57:453–5.
4. Svendsen E, Lie S, Gunderson TH, Lyngstad-Vik I, Skuland J. Comparative evaluation of miconazole, clotrimazole and nystatin in the treatment of candidal vulvo-vaginitis. Curr Ther Res 1978;23:666–72.

Name: **CLOXACILLIN**

Class: **Antibiotic**   Risk Factor: **B$_M$**

Fetal Risk Summary

Cloxacillin is a penicillin antibiotic (see also Penicillin G). No reports linking its use with congenital defects have been located. The Collaborative Perinatal Project monitored 50,282 mother-child pairs, 3,546 of which had 1st trimester exposure to penicillin derivatives (1). For use anytime during pregnancy, 7,171 exposures were recorded (2). In neither case was evidence found to suggest a relationship to large categories of major or minor malformations or to individual defects.

Breast Feeding Summary

No data available (see Penicillin G).

References

1. Heinonen OP, Slone D, Shapiro S. *Birth Defects and Drugs in Pregnancy*. Littleton:Publishing Sciences Group, 1977;297–313.
2. *Ibid*, 435.

Name: **COCAINE**

Class: **Sympathomimetic**   Risk Factor: **C**

Fetal Risk Summary

Cocaine is often used as a topical anesthetic, but reports of this use in pregnancy have not been located. The illicit use of cocaine is also common, and four reports, totaling 27 live-born infants, that provide details of this use during gestation have been located (1–4). In single patient case reports, two mothers who used cocaine during the 1st trimester produced infants with unusual abnormalities (1, 2). Both mothers used other abuse drugs: heroin in one case and marijuana and methaqualone in the other. The anomalies observed were:

Chromosome aneuploidy 45,X; bilaterally absent fifth
toes; features consistent with Turner's syndrome
Multiple defects including hypothalamic hamartoblastoma

In neither of these cases was cocaine established as the causative agent.

A 1985 report described the use of cocaine throughout gestation in 23 pregnancies ending in the birth of live infants (3). The women were divided into two groups and compared to two control groups:

Group I   Cocaine use/no heroin use (12 women)
Group II   Cocaine use/heroin use (15 women)
Group III   No cocaine use/heroin use (15 women)
Group IV   No cocaine use/no heroin use (15 women)

The use of alcohol, marijuana, and cigarettes was similar in the four groups. All patients were enrolled in the study by the 2nd trimester. Those using heroin were converted to methadone and maintained on this drug through delivery.

Only one congenital malformation was observed from the combined total of 53 women (3). A mother in Group I gave birth to an infant with prune-belly syndrome, major anomalies of the genitourinary tract, bilateral hydronephrosis, and bilateral cryptorchidism. The mother had used 4–5 g of cocaine on a single day at 5 weeks gestation.

No statistical differences were discovered among the four groups in birth weights, lengths, or head circumferences (3). Infants exposed *in utero* to cocaine had a greater degree of tremulousness and startle responses. Infants of cocaine-addicted mothers also had depressed interactive abilities and significant impairment of organizational abilities (3). Two neonatal deaths occurred during the 1st month after birth, both from mothers in Group I. One infant died at 2 weeks from sudden infant death syndrome and one from meningitis.

Women in Groups I and II had histories of cocaine use in previous pregnancies, and both groups had significantly increased rates of spontaneous abortions in comparison to the control groups. The study could not determine if a causal relationship existed between cocaine use and abortion. However, during the 3rd trimester, several women reported uterine contractions and increased fetal activity within minutes of using cocaine (3). In addition, onset of labor with abruptio placentae occurred in four women immediately after the use of intravenous cocaine. In an earlier study, abruptio placentae was reported in two women using intravenous and intranasal cocaine (4). The mechanism of this effect may be related to the transient hypertension induced by cocaine (3, 4). The use of intravenous cocaine in sheep produced a mean maximum decrease of 40% in uterine blood flow lasting less than 10 minutes (5). Human studies on the effect of cocaine on uterine perfusion have not been conducted.

Breast Feeding Summary

No data available.

References

1. Kushnick T, Robinson M, Tsao C. 45, X chromosome abnormality in the offspring of a narcotic addict. Am J Dis Child 1972;124:772–3.

2. Huff DS, Fernandes M. Two cases of congenital hypothalamic hamartoblastoma, polydactyly, and other congenital anomalies (Pallister-Hall syndrome). N Engl J Med 1982;306:430–1.
3. Chasnoff IJ, Burns WJ, Schnoll SH, Burns KA. Cocaine use in pregnancy. N Engl J Med 1985;313:666–9.
4. Acker D, Sachs BP, Tracey KJ, Wise WE. Abruptio placentae associated with cocaine use. Am J Obstet Gynecol 1983;146:220–1.
5. Foutz SE, Kotelko DM, Shnider SM, Thigpen JW, Rosen MA, Brookshire GL, Koike M, Levinson G, Elias-Baker B. Placental transfer and effects of cocaine on uterine blood flow and the fetus. Anesthesiology 1983;59:A422 (Abstr).

Name: **CODEINE**

Class: **Narcotic Analgesic/Antitussive**   Risk Factor: **C***

Fetal Risk Summary

The Collaborative Perinatal Project monitored 50,282 mother-child pairs, 563 of which had 1st trimester exposure to codeine (1). No evidence was found to suggest a relationship to large categories of major or minor malformations. Associations were found with six individual defects (1, 2). Only the association with respiratory malformation is statistically significant. The significance of the other associations is unknown and independent confirmation is required.

Respiratory malformations (8 cases)
Genitourinary malformations (other than hypospadias)
    (7 cases)
Down's syndrome (1 case)
Tumors (4 cases)
Umbilical hernia (3 cases)
Inguinal hernia (12 cases)

For use anytime during pregnancy, 2,522 exposures were recorded (3). With the same qualifications, possible associations with four individual defects were found (4):

Hydrocephaly (7 cases)
Pyloric stenosis (8 cases)
Umbilical hernia (7 cases)
Inguinal hernia (51 cases)

In an investigation of 1,427 malformed newborns compared to 3,001 controls, 1st trimester use of narcotic analgesics (codeine most common) was associated with inguinal hernias, cardiac and circulatory system defects, cleft lip and palate, dislocated hip, and other musculoskeletal defects (5). Second trimester use was associated with alimentary tract defects. In a large retrospective Finnish study, the use of opiates (mainly codeine) during the 1st trimester was associated with an increased risk of cleft lip and palate (6, 7). Finally, a survey of 390 infants with congenital heart disease matched with 1,254 normal infants found a higher rate of exposure to several drugs, including codeine, in the offspring with defects (8). Although all four of these studies contain several possible biases that could have affected the results, the data serve a clear warning that indiscriminate use of codeine is not without risk to the fetus.

Use of codeine during labor produces neonatal respiratory depression to the same degree as other narcotic analgesics (9). The first known case of neonatal codeine addiction was described in 1965 (10). The mother had taken analgesic tablets containing 360–480 mg of codeine per day for 8 weeks prior to delivery.

A second report described neonatal codeine withdrawal in two infants of non-addicted mothers (11). The mother of one infant began consuming a codeine cough medication 3 weeks prior to delivery. Approximately 2 weeks before delivery, analgesic tablets with codeine were taken at a frequency of up to 6 tablets/day (48 mg of codeine per day). The second mother was treated with a codeine cough medication and consumed 90–120 mg of codeine per day for the last 10 days of pregnancy. Apgar scores of both infants were 8–10 at 1 and 5 minutes. Typical symptoms of narcotic withdrawal were noted in the infants shortly after birth but not in the mothers.

[* Risk Factor D if used for prolonged periods or in high doses at term.]

Breast Feeding Summary

Codeine passes into breast milk in very small amounts, which are probably insignificant (12–14). The American Academy of Pediatrics considers codeine compatible with breast-feeding (15).

References

1. Heinonen OP, Slone D, Shapiro S. *Birth Defects and Drugs in Pregnancy*. Littleton:Publishing Sciences Group, 1977:287–95.
2. *Ibid*, 471.
3. *Ibid*, 434.
4. *Ibid*, 484.
5. Bracken MB, Holford TR. Exposure to prescribed drugs in pregnancy and association with congenital malformations. Obstet Gynecol 1981;58:336–44.
6. Saxen I. Associations between oral clefts and drugs taken during pregnancy. Int J Epidemiol 1975;4;37–44.
7. Saxen I. Epidemiology of cleft lip and palate: an attempt to rule out chance correlations. Br J Prev Soc Med 1975;29:103–10.
8. Rothman KJ, Fyler DC, Goldblatt A, Kreidberg MB. Exogenous hormones and other drug exposures of children with congenital heart disease. Am J Epidemiol 1979;109:433–9.
9. Bonica JJ. *Principles and Practice of Obstetric Analgesia and Anesthesia*. Philadelphia:FA Davis Co, 1967:245.
10. Van Leeuwen G, Guthrie R, Stange F. Narcotic withdrawal reaction in a newborn infant due to codeine. Pediatrics 1965;36;635–6.
11. Mangurten HH, Benawra R. Neonatal codeine withdrawal in infants of nonaddicted mothers. Pediatrics 1980;65:159–60.
12. Kwit NT, Hatcher RA. Excretion of drugs in milk. Am J Dis Child 1935;49:900–4.
13. Horning MG, Stillwell WG, Nowlin J, Lertratanangkoon K, Stillwell RN, Hill RM. Identification and quantification of drugs and drug metabolites in human breast milk using GC-MS-COM methods. Mod Probl Paediatr 1975;15:73–9.
14. Anonymous. Drugs in breast milk. Med Lett Drugs Ther 1974;16:25–7.
15. Committee on Drugs, American Academy of Pediatrics. The transfer of drugs and other chemicals into human breast milk. Pediatrics 1983;72:375–83.

Name: **COLCHICINE**

Class: **Metaphase Inhibitor**   Risk Factor: **C$_M$**

Fetal Risk Summary

The original reports of colchicine cytogenetic effects have not been confirmed with recent studies (1, 2). Human lymphocytic cultures of cells have shown chromosomal damage when exposed to colchicine. No relationship between teratogenic effects and this damage has been established. Use of colchicine by the father prior to conception has been associated with teratogenicity (atypical Down's syndrome) (1). Other investigators were unable to find teratogenic or cytogenetic effects in 19 male and 19 female subjects (3). Colchicine may or may not cause azoospermia (4, 5). Until colchicine safety is established, the drug should be avoided during the reproductive years.

Breast Feeding Summary

No data available.

References

1. Cestari AN, Vieira Filho JP, Yonenaga Y. A case of human reproductive abnormalities possibly induced by colchicine treatment. Rev Bras Biol 1965;25:253–6.
2. Serreira NR, Buoniconti A. Trisomy after colchicine therapy. Lancet 1968;2:1304.
3. Cohen MM, Levy M, Eliakim M. A cytogenetic evaluation of long-term colchicine therapy in the treatment of familial Mediterranean fever (FMF). Am J Med Sci 1977;274:147–52.
4. Merlin HE. Azoospermia caused by colchicine—a case report. Fertil Steril 1972;23:180–1.
5. Bremer WJ, Paulsen CA. Colchicine and testicular function in man. N Engl J Med 1976;294:1384–5.

Name: **COLISTIMETHATE**

Class: **Antibiotic**   Risk Factor: **B**

Fetal Risk Summary

No reports linking the use of colistimethate with congenital defects have been located. The drug crosses the placenta at term (1).

Breast Feeding Summary

Colistimethate is excreted into breast milk. The milk:plasma ratio is 0.17 to 0.18 (2). While this level is low, three potential problems exist for the nursing infant: modification of bowel flora, direct effects on the infant, and interference with the interpretation of culture results if a fever work-up is required.

References

1. MacAulay MA, Charles D. Placental transmission of colistimethate. Clin Pharmacol Ther 1967;8:578–86.
2. Wilson JT. Milk/plasma ratios and contraindicated drugs. In Wilson JT, ed. *Drugs in Breast Milk*. Balgowlah, Australia: ADIS Press, 1981:78–9.

Name: **CORTICOTROPIN/COSYNTROPIN**

Class: **Corticosteroid-Stimulating Hormone**   Risk Factor: **C**

Fetal Risk Summary

Studies reporting the use of corticotropin in pregnancy have not demonstrated adverse fetal effects (1–4). However, corticosteroids have been suspected of causing malformations (see Cortisone). Since corticotropin stimulates the release of endogenous corticosteroids, this relationship should be considered when prescribing the drug to women in their reproductive years.

Breast Feeding Summary

No data available.

References

1. Johnstone FD, Campbell S. Adrenal response in pregnancy to long-acting tetracosactrin. J Obstet Gynaecol Br Commonw 1974;81:363–7.
2. Simmer HH, Tulchinsky D, Gold EM, et al. On the regulation of estrogen production by cortisol and ACTH in human pregnancy at term. Am J Obstet Gynecol 1974;119:283–96.
3. Aral K, Kuwabara Y, Okinaga S. The effect of adrenocorticotropic hormone and dexamethasone, administered to the fetus in utero, upon maternal and fetal estrogens. Am J Obstet Gynecol 1972;113:316–22.
4. Potert AJ. Pregnancy and adrenalcortical hormones. Br Med J 1962;2:967–72.

Name: **CORTISONE**

Class: **Corticosteroid**   Risk Factor: **D**

Fetal Risk Summary

Since cortisone is often used during pregnancy, reports of congenital defects reflect a much greater utilization of cortisone and not necessarily the fact that cortisone is a more potent teratogen than other glucocorticoids (see Prednisolone, Betamethasone, Dexamethasone, Corticotropin). The Collaborative Perinatal Project monitored 50,282 mother-child pairs, 34 of which had 1st trimester exposure to cortisone (1). No evidence of a relationship to congenital malformations was found. In 35 other reported cases of 1st trimester exposure, congenital defects, including cataracts, cyclopia, intraventricular septal defect, gastroschisis, hydrocephalus, cleft lip, coarctation of the aorta, clubfoot, and undescended testicles, were observed in nine infants (2–7). Concern has been expressed that neonatal adrenal hyperplasia or insufficiency may result from maternal corticosteroid administration (8, 9).

Breast Feeding Summary

No data available.

References

1. Heinonen OP, Slone D, Shapiro S. *Birth Defects and Drugs in Pregnancy*. Littleton:Publishing Sciences Group, 1977:389, 391.

2. Kraus AM. Congenital cataract and maternal steroid ingestion. J Pediatr Ophthalmol 1975;12:107.
3. Khudr G, Olding L. Cyclopia. Am J Dis Child 1973;125:102.
4. deVilliers DM. Kortisoon swangerskap en die ongebore kind. S Afr Med J 1967;41:781–2.
5. Malaps P. Foetal malformation and cortisone therapy. Br Med J 1965;1:795.
6. Harris JWS, Poss IP. Cortisone therapy in early pregnancy. Relation to cleft palate. Lancet 1956;1:1045–7.
7. Wells CN. Treatment of hyperemesis gravidarium with cortisone. I. Fetal results. Am J Obstet Gynecol 1953;66:598–601.
8. Freeman RK, Women's Hospital, Memorial Medical Center, Long Beach, CA, 1982. Unpublished data.
9. Sidhu RK, Hawkins DF. Corticosteroids. Clin Obstet Gynecol 1981;8:383–404.

Name: **COUMARIN DERIVATIVES**

Class: **Anticoagulant**   Risk Factor: **D**

Fetal Risk Summary

The use of coumarin derivatives during pregnancy may result in significant problems for the fetus and newborn. Hall and co-workers (1) have reviewed this subject (167 references). Since this review, several other reports have appeared (2–11). The principal problems confronting the fetus and newborn are:

Embryopathy (fetal warfarin syndrome)
Central nervous system defects
Spontaneous abortion
Stillbirth
Prematurity
Hemorrhage

First trimester use of coumarin derivatives has resulted in 19 known cases of the fetal warfarin syndrome (FWS) (1–3). The common characteristics of the FWS are nasal hypoplasia due to failure of development of the nasal septum and stippled epiphyses. The bridge of the nose is depressed resulting in a flattened, upturned appearance. Other features which may be present are:

Birth weight less than 10th percentile for gestational age
Eye defects (blindness, optic atrophy, microphthalmia)
    when drug used in 2nd and/or 3rd trimesters as well
Development retardation
Laryngeal calcification
Scoliosis
Deafness/hearing loss
Congenital heart disease
Death

The critical period of exposure, based on the review of Hall et al. (1), appears to be the 6th through the 9th weeks of gestation. For all of the known cases of FWS, exposure occurred during at least a portion of these weeks. Exposure outside of the 1st trimester carries the risk of central nervous system defects. No constant grouping of abnormalities was observed nor was there an apparent correlation between time of exposure and the defects, except that all fetuses were exposed in the 2nd and/or 3rd trimesters. Some of the malformations could be related to hemorrhage, but two non-bleeding-related patterns have been identified (1):

Dorsal midline dysplasia characterized by agenesis of corpus callosum, Dandy-Walker malformations, and midline cerebellar atrophy; encephaloceles may be present

Ventral midline dysplasia characterized by optic atrophy (eye anomalies)

Other features of exposure outside the 1st trimester are:

Mental retardation
Hydrocephalus
Spasticity
Seizures
Deafness
Scoliosis
Growth failure
Death

Long-term effects in the child with central nervous system defects are more significant and debilitating than those from the fetal warfarin syndrome (1).

Fetal outcomes for the 463 reported cases of *in utero* exposure to coumarin derivatives are summarized below (1–11):

1ST TRIMESTER EXPOSURE (255):
    Normal infants—167 (65%)
    Spontaneous abortions—41 (16%)
    Stillborn/Neonatal death—17 (7%)
    FWS—19 (8%)
    CNS/Other defects—11 (4%)
2ND/3RD TRIMESTER EXPOSURE (208):
    Normal infants—175 (84%)
    Spontaneous abortions—4 (2%)
    Stillborn/Neonatal death—19 (9%)
    CNS/Other defects—10 (5%)
TOTAL INFANTS EXPOSED (463):
    Normal infants—342 (74%)
    Spontaneous abortions—45 (10%)
    Stillborn/Neonatal death—36 (8%)
    FWS/CNS/Other defects—40 (9%)

Hemorrhage was observed in 11 (3%) of the normal newborns (premature and term). Two of the patients in the 2nd/3rd trimester group were treated with the coumarin derivatives phenprocoumon and nicoumalone. Both infants were normal.

Congenital abnormalities that do not fit the pattern of the FWS or central nervous system defects have been observed in 10 infants (2%) (1, 8). These are thought to be incidental malformations that are probably not related to the use of coumarin derivatives:

Asplenia, two-chambered heart, agenesis of pulmonary artery
Anencephaly, spina bifida, congenital absence of clavicles
Congenital heart disease, death
Fetal distress, focal motor seizures
Bilateral polydactyly
Congenital corneal leukoma
Nonspecified multiple defects
Asplenia, congenital heart disease, incomplete rotation
   of gut, short broad phalanges, hypoplastic nails
Single kidney, toe defects, other anomalies, death
Cleft palate

A 1984 study examined 22 children, with a mean age of 4.0 years, who were exposed *in utero* to warfarin (12). Physical and mental development of the children were comparable to matched controls.

In summary, the use of oral anticoagulants during pregnancy carries with it a significant risk to the fetus. For all cases, only about 70% of pregnancies are expected to result in a normal infant. If the mother's condition requires the use of these agents, she must be informed of the risk and a decision made whether or not to continue the pregnancy.

Breast Feeding Summary

Excretion of coumarin derivatives into breast milk is dependent on the agent used. Three reports on warfarin have been located, totaling 28 lactating women (13–15). Doses ranged between 2 and 12 mg/day in 13 patients with serum levels varying from 1.6 to 8.5 μmol/L (13). Warfarin was not detected in the milk of these patients. Maternal dosages or levels were not provided in the other reports (14, 15). No warfarin was detected in the serum of any of the 28 breast-fed infants. Also, no effects on the bleeding time were found in the 18 infants in whom the test was performed (13–15).

Exposure to ethyl biscoumacetate in milk resulted in bleeding in 5 of 42 exposed infants in one report (16). The maternal dosage was not given. An unidentified metabolite was found in the milk, which may have led to the high complication rate. A 1959 study measured ethyl biscoumacetate levels in 38 milk specimens obtained from four women taking 600–1200 mg/day (17). The drug was detected in only 13 samples, with levels varying from 0.09 to 1.69 μg/ml. No correlation could be found between the milk concentrations and the dosage or time of administration. A total of 22 infants were breast-fed from these and other mothers receiving ethyl biscoumacetate. No adverse effects were observed in the infants, but coagulation tests were not conducted.

Over 1,600 postpartum women were treated with dicumarol to prevent thromboembolic complications in a 1950 study (18). Doses were titrated to adjust the prothrombin clotting time to 40–50% of normal. No adverse effects were noted in any of the nursing infants nor were there any changes in their prothrombin times.

Phenindione use in a lactating woman resulted in a massive scrotal hematoma and wound oozing in a 1½-month-old breast-fed infant shortly after a herniotomy was performed (19). The mother was taking 50 mg every morning and alternating 50 mg/25 mg every night for a suspected pulmonary embolism that developed postpartum. Milk levels varying from 1 to 5 μg/ml have been reported after 50- or

75-mg single doses of phenindione (20). When the dose was 25 mg, only 18 of 68 samples contained detectable amounts of the anticoagulant.

In summary, maternal warfarin consumption apparently does not pose a significant risk to normal, full-term, breast-fed infants. Other oral anticoagulants should be avoided by the lactating woman. The American Academy of Pediatrics considers phenindione contraindicated during breast-feeding because of the risk of hemorrhage in the infant (21). However, warfarin and dicumarol (bishydroxycoumarin) are listed by the Academy as being compatible with breast-feeding (21).

References

1. Hall JG, Pauli RM, Wilson KM. Maternal and fetal sequelae of anticoagulation during pregnancy. Am J Med 1980;68:122–40.
2. Baillie M, Allen ED, Elkington AR. The congenital warfarin syndrome: a case report. Br J Ophthalmol 1980;64:633–5.
3. Harrod MJE, Sherrod PS. Warfarin embryopathy in siblings. Obstet Gynecol 1981;57:673–6.
4. Russo R, Bortolotti U, Schivazappa L, Girolami A. Warfarin treatment during pregnancy: a clinical note. Haemostasis 1979;8:96–8.
5. Biale Y, Cantor A, Lewenthal H, Gueron M. The course of pregnancy in patients with artificial heart valves treated with dipyridamole. Int J Gynaecol Obstet 1980;18:128–32.
6. Moe N. Anticoagulant therapy in the prevention of placental infarction and perinatal death. Obstet Gynecol 1982;59:481–3.
7. Kaplan LC, Anderson GG, Ring BA. Congenital hydrocephalus and Dandy-Walker malformation associated with warfarin use during pregnancy. Birth Defects 1982;18:79–83.
8. Chen WWC, Chan CS, Lee PK, Wang RYC, Wong VCW. Pregnancy in patients with prosthetic heart valves: an experience with 45 pregnancies. Q J Med 1982;51:358–65.
9. Vellenga E, Van Imhoff GW, Aarnoudse JG. Effective prophylaxis with oral anticoagulants and low-dose heparin during pregnancy in an antithrombin III deficient woman. Lancet 1983;2:224.
10. Michiels JJ, Stibbe J, Vellenga E, Van Vliet HHDM. Prophylaxis of thrombosis in antithrombin III-deficient women during pregnancy and delivery. Eur J Obstet Gynecol Reprod Biol 1984;18:149–53.
11. Oakley C. Pregnancy in patients with prosthetic heart valves. Br Med J 1983;286:1680–3.
12. Chong MKB, Harvey D, De Swiet M. Follow-up study of children whose mothers were treated with warfarin during pregnancy. Br J Obstet Gynaecol 1984;91:1070–3.
13. L'E Orme M, Lewis PJ, De Swiet M, Serlin MJ, Sibeon R, Baty JD, Breckenridge AM. May mothers given warfarin breast-feed their infants? Br Med J 1977;1:1564–5.
14. De Swiet M, Lewis PJ. Excretion of anticoagulants in human milk. N Engl J Med 1977;297:1471.
15. McKenna R, Cole ER, Vasan U. Is warfarin sodium contraindicated in the lactating mother? J Pediatr 1983;103:325–7.
16. Gostof, Momolka, Zilenka. Les substances derivees du tromexane dans le lait maternel et leurs actions paradoxales sur la prothrombine. Schweiz Med Wochenschr 1952;30:764–5. As cited in Daily JW. Anticoagulant and cardiovascular drugs. In Wilson JT, ed. *Drugs in Breast Milk.* Australia:ADIS Press, 1981:63.
17. Illingworth RS, Finch E. Ethyl biscoumacetate (Tromexan) in human milk. J Obstet Gynaecol Br Commonw 1959;66:487–8.
18. Brambel CE, Hunter RE. Effect of dicumarol on the nursing infant. Am J Obstet Gynecol 1950;59:1153–9.
19. Eckstein HB, Jack B. Breast-feeding and anticoagulant therapy. Lancet 1970;1:672–3.
20. Goguel M, Noel G, Gillet JY. Therapeutique anticoagulante et allaitement: etude du passage de la phenyl-2-dioxo,1,3 indane dans le lait maternel. Rev Fr Gynecol Obstet 1970;65:409–12. As cited in Anderson PO. Drugs and breast feeding—a review. Drug Intell Clin Pharm 1977;11:208–23.
21. Committee on Drugs, American Academy of Pediatrics. The transfer of drugs and other chemicals into human breast milk. Pediatrics 1983;72:375–83.

Name: **CYCLACILLIN**

Class: **Antibiotic**   Risk Factor: **B_M**

Fetal Risk Summary

Cyclacillin is a penicillin antibiotic (see also Penicillin G). No reports linking its use with congenital defects have been located. The Collaborative Perinatal Project monitored 50,282 mother-child pairs, 3,546 of which had 1st trimester exposure to penicillin derivatives (1). Use of the drug at any time during pregnancy was recorded for 7,171 pairs (2). In neither case was evidence found to suggest a relationship to large categories of major or minor malformations or to individual defects.

Breast Feeding Summary

No data available (see Penicillin G).

References

1. Heinonen OP, Slone D, Shapiro S. *Birth Defects and Drugs in Pregnancy*. Littleton:Publishing Sciences Group, 1977:297–313.
2. *Ibid*, 435.

Name: **CYCLAMATE**

Class: **Sweetener**   Risk Factor: **C**

Fetal Risk Summary

Controlled studies on the effects of cyclamate on the fetus have not been found. The drug crosses the placenta to produce fetal blood levels of about 25% of those in maternal serum (1). Cyclamate has been suspected of causing cytogenetic effects in human lymphocytes (2). One group of investigators attempted to associate these effects with an increased incidence of malformations and behavioral problems, but a causal relationship could not be established (3).

Breast Feeding Summary

No data available.

References

1. Pitkin RM, Reynolds WA, Filer LJ. Placental transmission and fetal distribution of cyclamate in early human pregnancy. Am J Obstet Gynecol 1970;108:1043–50.
2. Bauchinger M. Cytogenetic effect of cyclamate on human peripheral lymphocytes in vivo. Dtsch Med Wochenschr 1970;95:2220–3.
3. Stone D, Matalka E, Pulaski B. Do artificial sweeteners ingested in pregnancy affect the offspring? Nature 1971;231:53.

Name: **CYCLANDELATE**

Class: **Vasodilator**   Risk Factor: **C**

Fetal Risk Summary

No data available.

Breast Feeding Summary

No data available.

Name: **CYCLAZOCINE**

Class: **Narcotic Antagonist**   Risk Factor: **D**

Fetal Risk Summary

Cyclazocine is not available in the United States. In addition to its ability to reverse narcotic overdose, it has been used in the treatment of narcotic dependence (1). Its actions are similar to those of nalorphine (see also Nalorphine).

Breast Feeding Summary

No data available.

References

1. Wade A, ed. *Martindale. The Extra Pharmacopoeia*, ed 27. London:Pharmaceutical Press, 1977:985.

Name: **CYCLIZINE**

Class: **Antihistamine/Antiemetic**   Risk Factor: **B**

Fetal Risk Summary

Cyclizine is a piperazine antihistamine which is used as an antiemetic (see also Buclizine and Meclizine for closely related drugs). The drug is teratogenic in animals but apparently not in humans. In 111 patients given cyclizine during the 1st trimester, no increased malformation rate was observed (1). Similarly, the Collaborative Perinatal Project found no association between 1st trimester cyclizine use and congenital defects, although the number of exposed patients (15) was small compared to the total sample (2). The FDA's OTC Laxative Panel, acting on these data, concluded that cyclizine is not teratogenic (3). In 1974, investigators searching for an association between antihistamines and oral clefts found no relationship between this defect and the cyclizine group (4). Finally, a retrospective study in 1971 found that significantly fewer infants with malformations were exposed to antihistamines/antiemetics in the 1st trimester as compared to controls (5). Cyclizine was the fifth most commonly used antiemetic.

Breast Feeding Summary

No data available.

References

1. Milkovich L, Van den Berg BJ. An evaluation of the teratogenicity of certain antinauseant drugs. Am J Obstet Gynecol 1976;125:244–8.
2. Heinonen OP, Slone D, Shapiro S. *Birth Defects and Drugs in Pregnancy*. Littleton:Publishing Sciences Group, 1977:323.
3. Anonymous. Meclizine; cyclizine not teratogenic. Pink Sheets. F.D.C. Reports 1974:T&G-2.
4. Saxen I. Cleft palate and maternal diphenhydramine intake. Lancet 1974;1:407–8.
5. Nelson MM, Forfar JO. Associations between drugs administered during pregnancy and congenital abnormalities of the fetus. Br Med J 1971;1:523–7.

Name: CYCLOPENTHIAZIDE

Class: **Diuretic**   Risk Factor: **D**

Fetal Risk Summary

See Chlorothiazide.

Breast Feeding Summary

See Chlorothiazide.

Name: CYCLOPHOSPHAMIDE

Class: **Antineoplastic**   Risk Factor: **D**

Fetal Risk Summary

Cyclophosphamide is an alkylating antineoplastic agent. Both normal and malformed newborns have been reported following the use in pregnancy of cyclophosphamide (1–15). Seven malformed infants have resulted from 1st trimester exposure (1–5). Radiation therapy was given to most of the mothers, and at least one patient was treated with other antineoplastics (1, 2, 4). Data on four of these infants are shown below:

Flattened nasal bridge, palate defect, skin tag,
   4 toes each foot, hypoplastic middle phalanx
   5th finger, bilateral inguinal hernia sacs (1)
Toes missing, single coronary artery (2)
Hemangioma, umbilical hernia (3)
Imperforate anus, rectovaginal fistula, growth
   retarded (4)

Pancytopenia occurred in a 1,000-g male infant exposed to cyclophosphamide and five other antineoplastic agents in the 3rd trimester (11). Data from one review indicated that 40% of the patients exposed to anticancer drugs during pregnancy delivered low-birth-weight infants (16). This finding was not related to the timing of exposure. Use of cyclophosphamide in the 2nd and 3rd trimesters does not seem to place the fetus at risk for congenital defects. However, long-term studies of growth and mental development in offspring exposed to cyclophosphamide during the 2nd trimester, the period of neuroblast multiplication, have not been conducted (17).

The long-term effects of cyclophosphamide on male and female germinal epithelium function are unknown (18, 19). Successful pregnancies have been reported following high-dose therapy with this agent (20–25). Of interest, however, is a report associating paternal use of cyclophosphamide and three other antineoplastics prior to conception with congenital anomalies in an infant (26). Defects in the infant included syndactyly of the 1st and 2nd digits of the right foot and Fallot's tetralogy. In a group of men treated over a minimum of 3.5 years with multiple chemotherapy for acute lymphocytic leukemia, one man fathered a normal child while a second fathered two children, one with multiple anomalies (27).

Cyclophosphamide is one of the most common causes of chemotherapy-induced irregular menses, amenorrhea, and azoospermia (18, 21, 22, 28–31). Azoospermia appears to be reversible when the drug is stopped (28–32). Chromosome abnormalities have been demonstrated in patients treated with cyclophosphamide for rheumatoid arthritis and scleroderma (33). Changes in chromosomal structure may lead to an increased incidence of malformations in future offspring. However, the results of chromosome studies were normal in a mother treated during the 2nd and 3rd trimesters and her infant (13).

Breast Feeding Summary

Cyclophosphamide is excreted into breast milk (34). Although the concentrations were not specified, the drug was found in milk up to 6 hours after a single 500-mg intravenous dose. The mother was not nursing. The American Academy of Pediatrics considers cyclophosphamide contraindicated during breast-feeding because of potential adverse effects relating to immune suppression, growth, and carcinogenesis (35).

References

1. Greenberg LH, Tanaka KR. Congenital anomalies probably induced by cyclophosphamide. JAMA 1964;188:423–6.
2. Toledo TM, Harper RC, Moser RH. Fetal effects during cyclophosphamide and irradiation therapy. Ann Intern Med 1971;74:87–91.
3. Coates A. Cyclophosphamide in pregnancy. Aust NZ J Obstet Gynaecol 1970;10:33–4.
4. Murray CL, Reichert JA, Anderson J, Twiggs LB. Multimodal cancer therapy for breast cancer in the first trimester of pregnancy. JAMA 1984;252:2607–8.
5. Sweet DL, Kinzie J. Consequences of radiotherapy and antineoplastic therapy for the fetus. J Reprod Med 1976;17:241–6.
6. Lasher MJ, Geller W. Cyclophosphamide and vinblastine sulfate in Hodgkin's disease during pregnancy. JAMA 1966;195:486–8.
7. Lergier JE, Jimenez E, Maldonado N, Veray F. Normal pregnancy in multiple myeloma treated with cyclophosphamide. Cancer 1974;34:1018–22.
8. Garcia V, San Miguel J, Borrasca AL. Doxorubicin in the first trimester of pregnancy. Ann Intern Med 1981;94:547.
9. Lowenthal RM, Funnell CF, Hope DM, Stewart IG, Humphrey DC. Normal infant after combination chemotherapy including teniposide for Burkitt's lymphoma in pregnancy. Med Pediatr Oncol 1982;10:165–9.

10. Daly H, McCann SR, Hanratty TD, Temperley IJ. Successful pregnancy during combination chemotherapy for Hodgkin's disease. Acta Haematol (Basel) 1980;64:154–6.

11. Pizzuto J, Aviles A, Noriega L, Niz J, Morales M, Romero F. Treatment of acute leukemia during pregnancy: presentation of nine cases. Cancer Treat Rep 1980;64:679–83.

12. Sears HF, Reid J. Granulocytic sarcoma: local presentation of a systemic disease. Cancer 1976;37:1808–13.

13. Falkson HC, Simson IW, Falkson G. Non-Hodgkin's lymphoma in pregnancy. Cancer 1980;45:1679–82.

14. Webb GA. The use of hyperalimentation and chemotherapy in pregnancy: a case report. Am J Obstet Gynecol 1980;137:263–6.

15. Gililland J, Weinstein L. The effects of cancer chemotherapeutic agents on the developing fetus. Obstet Gynecol Surv 1983;38:6–13.

16. Nicholson HO. Cytotoxic drugs in pregnancy: review of reported cases. J Obstet Gynaecol Br Commonw 1968;75:307–12.

17. Dobbing J. Pregnancy and leukaemia. Lancet 1977;1:1155.

18. Schilsky RL, Lewis BJ, Sherins RJ, Young RC. Gonadal dysfunction in patients receiving chemotherapy for cancer. Ann Intern Med 1980;93:109–14.

19. Stewart BH. Drugs that cause and cure male infertility. Drug Ther 1975;5(No. 12):42–8.

20. Card RT, Holmes IH, Sugarman RG, Storb R, Thomas D. Successful pregnancy after high dose chemotherapy and marrow transplantation for treatment of aplastic anemia. Exp Hematol 1980;8:57–60.

21. Schwartz PE, Vidone RA. Pregnancy following combination chemotherapy for a mixed germ cell tumor of the ovary. Gynecol Oncol 1981;12:373–8.

22. Bacon C, Kernahan J. Successful pregnancy in acute leukaemia. Lancet 1975;2:515.

23. Deeg HJ, Kennedy MS, Sanders JE, Thomas ED, Storb R. Successful pregnancy after marrow transplantation for severe aplastic anemia and immunosuppression with cyclosporine. JAMA 1983;250:647.

24. Javaheri G, Lifchez A, Valle J. Pregnancy following removal of and long-term chemotherapy for ovarian malignant teratoma. Obstet Gynecol 1983;61:8S–9S.

25. Rustin GJS, Booth M, Dent J, Salt S, Rustin F, Bagshawe KD. Pregnancy after cytotoxic chemotherapy for gestational trophoblastic tumours. Br Med J 1984;288:103–6.

26. Russell JA, Powles RL, Oliver RTD. Conception and congenital abnormalities after chemotherapy of acute myelogenous leukaemia in two men. Br Med J 1976;1:1508.

27. Evenson DP, Arlin Z, Welt S, Claps ML, Melamed MR. Male reproductive capacity may recover following drug treatment with the L-10 protocol for acute lymphocytic leukemia. Cancer 1984;53:30–6.

28. Qureshji MA, Pennington JH, Goldsmith HJ, Cox PE. Cyclophosphamide therapy and sterility. Lancet 1972;2:1290–1.

29. George CRP, Evans RA. Cyclophosphamide and infertility. Lancet 1972;1:840–1.

30. Sherins RJ, DeVita VT Jr. Effect of drug treatment for lymphoma on male reproductive capacity. Ann Intern Med 1973;79:216–20.

31. Lendon M, Palmer MK, Hann IM, Shalet SM, Jones PHM. Testicular histology after combination chemotherapy in childhood for acute lymphoblastic leukaemia. Lancet 1978;2:439–41.

32. Hinkes E, Plotkin D. Reversible drug-induced sterility in a patient with acute leukemia. JAMA 1973;223:1490–1.

33. Tolchin SF, Winkelstein A, Rodnan GP, Pan SF, Nankin HR. Chromosome abnormalities from cyclophosphamide therapy in rheumatoid arthritis and progressive systemic sclerosis (scleroderma). Arthritis Rheum 1974;17:375–82.

34. Wiernik PH, Duncan JH. Cyclophosphamide in human milk. Lancet 1971;1:912.

35. Committee on Drugs, American Academy of Pediatrics. The transfer of drugs and other chemicals into human breast milk. Pediatrics 1983;72:375–83.

Name: **CYCLOTHIAZIDE**

Class: **Diuretic**   Risk Factor: **D**

Fetal Risk Summary

See Chlorothiazide.

Breast Feeding Summary

See Chlorothiazide.

Name: **CYCRIMINE**

Class: **Parasympatholytic**   Risk Factor: **C**

Fetal Risk Summary

Cycrimine is an anticholinergic agent used in the treatment of parkinsonism. No reports of its use in pregnancy have been located (see also Atropine).

Breast Feeding Summary

No data available (see also Atropine).

Name: **CYPROHEPTADINE**

Class: **Antihistamine/Antiserotonin**   Risk Factor: **B**

Fetal Risk Summary

Cyproheptadine has been used as a serotonin antagonist to prevent habitual abortion in patients with increased serotonin production (1, 2). No congenital defects were observed when the drug was used for this purpose. Two patients, under treatment with cyproheptadine for Cushing's syndrome, conceived while taking the drug (3, 4). Therapy was stopped at 3 months in one patient but continued throughout gestation in the second. Apparently healthy infants were delivered prematurely (33–34 and 36 weeks) from both mothers. The 33–34-week gestational infant, exposed throughout pregnancy to the drug, developed fatal gastroenteritis at 4 months of age (3). In a separate case, a woman with Cushing's syndrome was successfully treated with cyproheptadine and 2 years after stopping the drug, conceived and eventually delivered a healthy male infant (5).

Breast Feeding Summary

No data available. The manufacturer considers cyproheptadine contraindicated in nursing mothers (6).

References

1. Sadovsky E, Pfeifer Y, Polishuk WZ, Sulman FG. A trial of cyproheptadine in habitual abortion. Isr J Med Sci 1972;8:623–5.

2. Sadovsky E. Prevention of hypothalamic habitual abortion by Periactin. Harefuah 1970;78:332–3. As reported in JAMA 1970;212:1253.
3. Kasperlik-Zaluska A, Migdalska B, Hartwig W, Wilczynska J, Marianowski L, Stopinska-Gluszak U, Lozinska D. Two pregnancies in a woman with Cushing's syndrome treated with cyproheptadine. Br J Obstet Gynaecol 1980;87:1171–3.
4. Khir ASM, How J, Bewsher PD. Successful pregnancy after cyproheptadine treatment for Cushing's disease. Eur J Obstet Gynecol Reprod Biol 1982;13:343–7.
5. Griffith DN, Ross EJ. Pregnancy after cyproheptadine treatment for Cushing's disease. N Engl J Med 1981;305:893–4.
6. Product information. Periactin. Merck Sharp and Dohme, 1985.

Name: **CYTARABINE**

Class: **Antineoplastic**   Risk Factor: **D***

Fetal Risk Summary

Normal infants have resulted following *in utero* exposure to cytarabine during all stages of gestation (1–17). However, use during the 1st and 2nd trimesters has been associated with congenital and chromosomal abnormalities (18–20). One leukemic patient treated during the 2nd trimester elected to have an abortion at 24 weeks gestation (18). The fetus had trisomy for group C autosomes without mosaicism. A second pregnancy in the same patient with identical therapy ended normally. Two women, one treated during the 1st trimester and the other treated throughout pregnancy, delivered infants with multiple anomalies:

Bilateral microtia and atresia of external auditory canals,
    right-hand lobster claw with three digits, bilateral lower
    limb defects (19)
Two medial digits of both feet missing, distal phalanges
    of both thumbs missing with hypoplastic remnant of
    of right thumb (20)

Congenital anomalies have also been associated with paternal use of cytarabine plus other antineoplastics prior to conception; the sperm were allegedly damaged, but infertility was not produced in two fathers (21). The results of these pregnancies were:

Fallot's tetralogy, syndactyly of 1st and 2nd digits of
    right foot
Stillborn anencephalic

Cytarabine may produce reversible azoospermia (22, 23). However, male fertility has been demonstrated during maintenance therapy with cytarabine (24). Pancytopenia was observed in a 1,000-g male infant exposed to cytarabine and five other antineoplastic agents during the 3rd trimester (11). Data from one review indicated that 40% of the mothers exposed to antineoplastic drugs during pregnancy delivered low-birth- weight infants (25). This finding was not related to the timing of exposure. Long-term studies of growth and mental development in offspring exposed to cytarabine during the 2nd trimester, the period of neuroblast multiplication, have not been conducted (26).

[* Risk Factor C according to the manufacturer—The Upjohn Co, 1985.]

Breast Feeding Summary

No data available.

References

1. Pawliger DF, McLean FW, Noyes WD. Normal fetus after cytosine arabinoside therapy. Ann Intern Med 1971;74:1012.
2. Au-Yong R, Collins P, Young JA. Acute myeloblastic leukemia during pregnancy. Br Med J 1972;4:493–4.
3. Raich PC, Curet LB. Treatment of acute leukemia during pregnancy. Cancer 1975;36:861–2.
4. Gokal R, Durrant J, Baum JD, Bennett MJ. Successful pregnancy in acute monocytic leukaemia. Br J Cancer 1976;34:299–302.
5. Sears HF, Reid J. Granulocytic sarcoma: local presentation of a systemic disease. Cancer 1976;37:1808–13.
6. Durie BGM, Giles HR. Successful treatment of acute leukemia during pregnancy. Arch Intern Med 1977;137:90–1.
7. Lilleyman JS, Hill AS, Anderton KJ. Consequences of acute myelogenous leukemia in early pregnancy. Cancer 1977;40:1300–3.
8. Moreno H, Castleberry RP, McCann WP. Cytosine arabinoside and 6-thioguanine in the treatment of childhood acute myeloblastic leukemia. Cancer 1977;40:998–1004.
9. Newcomb M, Balducci L, Thigpen JT, Morrison FS. Acute leukemia in pregnancy: successful delivery after cytarabine and doxorubicin. JAMA 1978;239:2691–2.
10. Manoharan A, Leyden MJ. Acute non-lymphocytic leukaemia in the third trimester of pregnancy. Aust NZ J Med 1979;9:71–4.
11. Pizzuto J, Aviles A, Noriega L, Niz J, Morales M, Romero F. Treatment of acute leukemia during pregnancy: presentation of nine cases. Cancer Treat Rep 1980;64:679–83.
12. Colbert N, Najman A, Gorin NC, Blum F, Treisser A, Lasfargues G, Cloup M, Barrat H, Duhamel G. Acute leukaemia during pregnancy: favourable course of pregnancy in two patients treated with cytosine arabinoside and anthracyclines. Nouv Presse Med 1980;9:175–8.
13. Tobias JS, Bloom HJG. Doxorubicin in pregnancy. Lancet 1980;1:776.
14. Taylor G, Blom J. Acute leukemia during pregnancy. South Med J 1980;73:1314–5.
15. Dara P, Slater LM, Armentrout SA. Successful pregnancy during chemotherapy for acute leukemia. Cancer 1981;47:845–6.
16. Plows CW. Acute myelomonocytic leukemia in pregnancy: report of a case. Am J Obstet Gynecol 1982;143:41–3.
17. De Souza JJL, Bezwoda WR, Jetham D, Sonnendecker EWW. Acute leukaemia in pregnancy: a case report and discussion on modern management. S Afr Med J 1982;62:295–6.
18. Maurer LH, Forcier RJ, McIntyre OR, Benirschke K. Fetal group C trisomy after cytosine arabinoside and thioguanine. Ann Intern Med 1971;75:809–10.
19. Wagner VM, Hill JS, Weaver D, Baehner RL. Congenital abnormalities in baby born to cytarabine treated mother. Lancet 1980;2:98–9.
20. Schafer AI. Teratogenic effects of antileukemic chemotherapy. Arch Intern Med 1981;141:514–5.
21. Russell JA, Powles RL, Oliver RTD. Conception and congenital abnormalities after chemotherapy of acute myelogenous leukaemia in two men. Br Med J 1976;1:1508.
22. Lendon M, Palmer MK, Hann IM, Shalet SM, Jones PHM. Testicular histology after combination chemotherapy in childhood for acute lymphoblastic leukaemia. Lancet 1978;2:439–41.
23. Lilleyman JS. Male fertility after successful chemotherapy for lymphoblastic leukaemia. Lancet 1979;2:1125.
24. Matthews JH, Wood JK. Male fertility during chemotherapy for acute leukemia. N Engl J Med 1980;303:1235.
25. Nicholson HO. Cytotoxic drugs in pregnancy: review of reported cases. J Obstet Gynaecol Br Commonw 1968;75:307–12.
26. Dobbing J. Pregnancy and leukaemia. Lancet 1977;1:1155.

Name: **DACARBAZINE**

Class: **Antineoplastic**   Risk Factor: **C_M**

Fetal Risk Summary

No data available (1).

Breast Feeding Summary

No data available.

References

1. Lonergan RC, Miles Pharmaceuticals, 1981. Personal communication.

Name: **DACTINOMYCIN**

Class: **Antineoplastic**   Risk Factor: **C_M**

Fetal Risk Summary

Dactinomycin is an antimitotic antineoplastic agent. Normal pregnancies have followed the use of this drug prior to conception (1–6). Women, however, were less likely to have a live birth following treatment with this drug than with other antineoplastics (5). Three reports of the use of dactinomycin during pregnancy have been located (7, 8). In these cases, dactinomycin was administered during the 2nd and 3rd trimesters and apparently normal infants were delivered.

Data from one review indicated that 40% of the infants exposed to anticancer drugs were of low birth weight (7). This finding was not related to the timing of exposure. Long term studies of growth and mental development in offspring exposed to dactinomycin and other antineoplastic drugs during the 2nd trimester, the period of neuroblast multiplication, have not been conducted (9).

Breast Feeding Summary

No data available.

References

1. Ross GT. Congenital anomalies among children born of mothers receiving chemotherapy for gestational trophoblastic neoplasms. Cancer 1976;37:1043–7.
2. Walden PAM, Bagshawe KD. Pregnancies after chemotherapy for gestational trophoblastic tumours. Lancet 1979;2:1241.
3. Schwartz PE, Vidone RA. Pregnancy following combination chemotherapy for a mixed germ cell tumor of the ovary. Gynecol Oncol 1981;12:373–8.

4. Pastorfide GB, Goldstein DP. Pregnancy after hydatidiform mole. Obstet Gynecol 1973;42:67–70.
5. Rustin GJS, Booth M, Dent J, Salt S, Rustin F, Bagshawe KD. Pregnancy after cytotoxic chemotherapy for gestational trophoblastic tumours. Br Med J 1984;288:103–6.
6. Evenson DP, Arlin Z, Welt S, Claps ML, Melamed MR. Male reproductive capacity may recover following drug treatment with the L-10 protocol for acute lymphocytic leukemia. Cancer 1984;53:30–6.
7. Nicholson HO. Cytotoxic drugs in pregnancy: review of reported cases. J Obstet Gynaecol Br Commonw 1968;75:307–12.
8. Gililland J, Weinstein L. The effects of cancer chemotherapeutic agents on the developing fetus. Obstet Gynecol Survey 1983;38:6–13.
9. Dobbing J. Pregnancy and leukaemia. Lancet 1977;1:1155.

Name: **DANTHRON**
Class: **Purgative**   Risk Factor: **C**

Fetal Risk Summary

Danthron is an anthraquinone purgative. See Cascara Sagrada.

Breast Feeding Summary

No data available. See Cascara Sagrada.

Name: **DAUNORUBICIN**
Class: **Antineoplastic**   Risk Factor: **D$_M$**

Fetal Risk Summary

The use of daunorubicin during pregnancy has been reported in 10 patients, three during the 1st trimester (1–7). No congenital defects were observed in the six live-born infants, but one of these infants was anemic and hypoglycemic and had multiple serum electrolyte abnormalities (7). Results of the remaining pregnancies were two therapeutic abortions (one fetus with enlarged spleen), one intrauterine death, and one stillborn infant with diffuse myocardial necrosis (7).

Data from one review indicated that 40% of the infants exposed to anticancer drugs were of low birth weight (8). This finding was not related to timing of the exposure. Long-term studies of growth and mental development in offspring exposed to anticancer drugs during the 2nd trimester, the period of neuroblast multiplication, have not been conducted (9).

Use of daunorubicin and other antineoplastic drugs in two men was associated with congenital defects in their offspring (10):

Fallot's tetralogy, syndactyly of first and
    second digits, right foot
Stillborn anencephalic

The authors speculated that the drugs damaged the germ cells without producing infertility. In a third man, fertilization occurred during treatment with daunorubicin and resulted in the birth of a healthy infant (11). Successful pregnancies have also been reported in two women after treatment with daunorubicin (12).

Breast Feeding Summary

No data available.

References

1. Sears HF, Reid J. Granulocytic sarcoma: local presentation of a systemic disease. Cancer 1976;37:1808–13.
2. Lilleyman JS, Hill AS, Anderton KJ. Consequences of acute myelogenous leukemia in early pregnancy. Cancer 1977;40:1300–3.
3. Colbert N, Najman A, Gorin NC, et al. Acute leukaemia during pregnancy: favourable course of pregnancy in two patients treated with cytosine arabinoside and anthracyclines. Nouv Presse Med 1980;9:175–8.
4. Tobias JS, Bloom HJG. Doxorubicin in pregnancy. Lancet 1980;1:776.
5. Sanz MA, Rafecas FJ. Successful pregnancy during chemotherapy for acute promyelocytic leukemia. N Engl J Med 1982;306:939.
6. Alegre A, Chunchurreta R, Rodriguez-Alarcon J, Cruz E, Prada M. Successful pregnancy in acute promyelocytic leukemia. Cancer 1982;49:152–3.
7. Gililland J, Weinstein L. The effects of cancer chemotherapeutic agents on the developing fetus. Obstet Gynecol Surv 1983;38:6–13.
8. Nicholson HO. Cytotoxic drugs in pregnancy: review of reported cases. J Obstet Gynaecol Br Commonw 1968;75:307–12.
9. Dobbing J. Pregnancy and leukaemia. Lancet 1977;1:1155.
10. Russell JA, Powles RL, Oliver RTD. Conception and congenital abnormalities after chemotherapy of acute myelogenous leukaemia in two men. Br Med J 1976;1:1508.
11. Matthews JH, Wood JK. Male fertility during chemotherapy for acute leukemia. N Engl J Med 1980;303:1235.
12. Estiu M. Successful pregnancy in leukaemia. Lancet 1977;1:433.

Name: **DECAMETHONIUM**

Class: **Muscle Relaxant**   Risk Factor: **C**

Fetal Risk Summary

Decamethonium is no longer manufactured in the United States. No reports linking the use of decamethonium with congenital defects have been located. The drug has been used at term for maternal analgesia (1).

Breast Feeding Summary

No data available.

References

1. Moya F, Thorndyke V. Passage of drugs across the placenta. Am J Obstet Gynecol 1962;84:1778–98.

Name: **DEFEROXAMINE**

Class: **Heavy Metal Antagonist**   Risk Factor: **C**

Fetal Risk Summary

Deforoxamine is used for the treatment of acute iron intoxication and chronic iron overload. Some animal studies have shown skeletal anomalies at doses close to those used in humans (1). The detailed use of this drug in pregnancy has been described in three pregnant women, two with acute iron overdose and one with transfusion-dependent thalassemia (2–4). Brief mention of three other pregnant patients treated with deferoxamine for acute overdose appeared in an earlier report, but no details were given except that all of the infants were normal (5). The authors have knowledge of a seventh patient treated in the 3rd trimester for overdose with normal outcome (6).

In the thalassemia patient, deferoxamine was given by continuous subcutaneous infusion pump, 2 g every 12 hours, for the first 16 weeks of pregnancy (2). A cesarean section was performed at 33 weeks gestation for vaginal bleeding and premature rupture of the membranes, with delivery of a normal preterm male infant. The neonatal period was complicated by hypoglycemia and prolonged jaundice lasting 6 weeks, but neither problem was thought to be related to deferoxamine.

The iron overdose cases occurred at 15 and 34 weeks, respectively (3, 4). Both women were treated with intramuscular deferoxamine, and one also received the drug nasogastrically. Spontaneous labor with rupture of the membranes occurred 8 hours after iron ingestion in the 34 weeks gestation patient, resulting in the vaginal delivery 6 hours later of a normal male infant (3). The cord blood iron level was 121 μg/100 ml (normal 106–227 μg/100 ml) but fell to 21 μg/100 ml at 12 hours. The infant's clinical course was normal except for low iron levels that required iron supplementation. The authors suggested that the low neonatal iron levels were due to chelation of iron by transplacentally transferred deferoxamine. In the other case, a normal term male infant was delivered without evidence of injury from deferoxamine (4).

Breast Feeding Summary

No data available.

References

1. Product information. Desferal. CIBA Pharmaceutical Co., 1985.
2. Thomas RM, Skalicka AE. Successful pregnancy in transfusion-dependent thalassaemia. Arch Dis Child 1980;55:572–4.
3. Rayburn WF, Donn SM, Wulf ME. Iron overdose during pregnancy: successful therapy with deferoxamine. Am J Obstet Gynecol 1983;147:717–8.
4. Blanc P, Hryhorczuk D, Danel I. Deferoxamine treatment of acute iron intoxication in pregnancy. Obstet Gynecol 1984;64:12S–4S.
5. Strom RL, Schiller P, Seeds AE, Ten Bensel R. Fatal iron poisoning in a pregnant female: case report. Minn Med 1976;59:483–9.
6. Lovett SM. Unpublished data. 1985.

Name: **DEMECARIUM**

Class: **Parasympathomimetic (Cholinergic)**   Risk Factor: **C**

Fetal Risk Summary

Demecarium is used in the eye. No reports of its use in pregnancy have been located. As a quaternary ammonium compound, it is ionized at physiologic pH and transplacental passage in significant amounts would not be expected (see also Neostigmine).

Breast Feeding Summary

No data available.

Name: **DEMECLOCYCLINE**

Class: **Antibiotic**   Risk Factor: **D**

Fetal Risk Summary

See Tetracycline.

Breast Feeding Summary

See Tetracycline.

Name: **DESIPRAMINE**

Class: **Antidepressant**   Risk Factor: **C**

Fetal Risk Summary

Desipramine is an active metabolite of imipramine (see also Imipramine). No reports linking the use of desipramine with congenital defects have been located. Neonatal withdrawal symptoms, including cyanosis, tachycardia, diaphoresis, and weight loss, were observed after desipramine was taken throughout the pregnancy (1).

In an *in vitro* study, desipramine was shown to be a potent inhibitor of sperm motility (2). A concentration of 27 μM produced a 50% reduction in motility.

Breast Feeding Summary

Desipramine enters breast milk in low concentrations (3, 4). In one patient, milk:plasma ratios of 0.4–0.9 were measured with milk levels ranging between 17 and 35 μg/ml (3). No reports of adverse effects have been located. The American Academy of Pediatrics considers desipramine compatible with breast-feeding (5).

References

1. Webster PA. Withdrawal symptoms in neonates associated with maternal antidepressant therapy. Lancet 1973;2:318–9.

2. Levin RM, Amsterdam JD, Winokur A, Wein AJ. Effects of psychotropic drugs on human sperm motility. Fertil Steril 1981;36:503–6.
3. Sovner R, Orsulak PJ. Excretion of imipramine and desipramine in human breast milk. Am J Psychiatry 1979;136:451–2.
4. Erickson SH, Smith GH, Heidrich F. Tricyclics and breast feeding. Am J Psychiatry 1979;136:1483.
5. Committee on Drugs, American Academy of Pediatrics. The transfer of drugs and other chemicals into human breast milk. Pediatrics 1983;72:375–83.

Name: **DESLANOSIDE**

Class: **Cardiac Glycoside**   Risk Factor: **C**

Fetal Risk Summary

See Digitalis.

Breast Feeding Summary

See Digitalis.

Name: **DESMOPRESSIN**

Class: **Pituitary Hormone, Synthetic**   Risk Factor: **B$_M$**

Fetal Risk Summary

Desmopressin is a synthetic polypeptide structurally related to vasopressin. See Vasopressin.

Breast Feeding Summary

See Vasopressin.

Name: **DEXAMETHASONE**

Class: **Corticosteroid**   Risk Factor: **C**

Fetal Risk Summary

No reports linking the use of dexamethasone with congenital defects have been located. Other corticosteroids have been suspected of causing malformations (see Cortisone). Maternal free estriol and cortisol levels are significantly depressed after dexamethasone therapy, but the effects of these changes on the fetus have not been studied (1–3).

Dexamethasone has been used in patients with premature labor at about 26–34 weeks gestation to stimulate fetal lung maturation (4–14). Although this therapy is supported by many clinicians, its use is still controversial since the beneficial effects of steroids are greatest in singleton pregnancies with female fetuses (15–18). These benefits are:

Reduction in incidence of respiratory
     distress syndrome (RDS)
Decreased severity of RDS if it occurs
Decreased incidence of and mortality from
     intracranial hemorrhage
Increased survival of premature infants

Toxicity in the fetus and newborn following the use of dexamethasone is rare.

In studies of women with premature rupture of the membranes, administration of corticosteroids does not always reduce the frequency of RDS or perinatal mortality (19–21). In addition, an increased risk of maternal infection has been observed in patients with premature rupture of the membranes treated with corticosteroids (20, 21). A recent report, however, found no difference in the incidence of maternal complications between treated and nontreated patients (22).

Dexamethasone crosses the placenta to the fetus (23, 24). The drug is partially metabolized (54%) by the perfused placenta to its inactive 11-ketosteroid derivative, more so than betamethasone, but the difference is not statistically significant (24).

Leukocytosis has been observed in infants exposed antenatally to dexamthasone (25, 26). The WBC counts returned to normal in about 1 week.

The use of corticosteroids, including dexamethasone, for the treatment of asthma during pregnancy has not been related to a significantly increased risk of maternal or fetal complications (27). A slight increase in the number of premature births was found, but it could not be determined if this was an effect of the corticosteroids. An earlier study also recorded a shortening of gestation with chronic corticosteroid use (28).

In Rh-sensitized women, the use of dexamethasone may have prevented intra-uterine fetal deterioration and the need for fetal transfusion (29). Five women, in the 2nd and 3rd trimesters, were treated with 24 mg of the steroid weekly for 2–7 weeks resulting, in each case, in a live newborn.

Dexamethasone, 4 mg/day for 15 days, was administered to a woman late in the 3rd trimester for the treatment of autoimmune thrombocytopenic purpura (30). Therapy was given in an unsuccessful attempt to prevent fetal/neonatal thrombocytopenia due to the placental transfer of antiplatelet antibody. Platelet counts in the newborn were 38,000–49,000 /mm^3, but the infant made an uneventual recovery.

The use of dexamethasone for the pharmacologic suppression of the fetal adrenal gland has been described in two women with 21-hydroxylase deficiency (31, 32). This deficiency results in the overproduction of adrenal androgens and the virilization of female fetuses. Dexamethasone, in divided doses of 1 mg/day, was administered from early in the 1st trimester (5th week and 10th week) to term. Normal female infants resulted from both pregnancies.

Although human studies have usually shown a benefit, the use of corticosteroids in animals has been associated with several toxic effects (33, 34):

Reduced fetal head circumference
Reduced fetal adrenal gland weight

Increased fetal liver weight
Reduced fetal thymus weight
Reduced placental weight

Fortunately, none of these effects has been observed in human investigations. Long-term follow-up evaluations of children exposed *in utero* to dexamethasone have shown no adverse effects from this exposure (35, 36).

Breast Feeding Summary

No data available.

References

1. Reck G, Nowostawski, Bredwoldt M. Plasma levels of free estriol and cortisol under ACTH and dexamethasone during late pregnancy. Acta Endocrinol (Copenh) 1977;84:86–7.
2. Kauppilla A. ACTH levels in maternal, fetal and neonatal plasma after short term prenatal dexamethasone therapy. Br J Obstet Gynaecol 1977;84:128–34.
3. Warren JC, Cheatum SG. Maternal urinary estrogen excretion: effect of adrenal suppression. J Clin Endocrinol 1967;27:436–8.
4. Caspi I, Schreyer P, Weinraub Z, Reif R, Levi I, Mundel G. Changes in amniotic fluid lecithin-sphingomyelin ratio following maternal dexamethasone administration. Am J Obstet Gynecol 1975;122:327–31.
5. Spellacy WN, Buhi WC, Riggall FC, Holsinger KL. Human amniotic fluid lecithin/sphingomyelin ratio changes with estrogen or glucocorticoid treatment. Am J Obstet Gynecol 1973;115:216–8.
6. Caspi E, Schreyer P, Weinraub Z, Reif R, Levi I, Mundel G. Prevention of the respiratory distress syndrome in premature infants by antepartum glucocorticoid therapy. Br J Obstet Gynaecol 1976;83:187–93.
7. Ballard RA, Ballard PL. Use of prenatal glucocorticoid therapy to prevent respiratory distress syndrome. Am J Dis Child 1976;130:982–7.
8. Thornfeldt RE, Franklin RW, Pickering NA, Thornfeldt CR, Amell G. The effect of glucocorticoids on the maturation of premature lung membranes: preventing the respiratory distress syndrome by glucocorticoids. Am J Obstet Gynecol 1978;131:143–8.
9. Ballard PL, Ballard RA. Corticosteroids and respiratory distress syndrome: status 1979. Pediatrics 1979;63:163–5.
10. Taeusch HW Jr, Frigoletto F, Kitzmiller J, et al. Risk of respiratory distress syndrome after prenatal dexamethasone treatment. Pediatrics 1979;63:64–72.
11. Caspi E, Schreyer P, Weinraub Z, Lifshitz Y, Goldberg M. Dexamethasone for prevention of respiratory distress syndrome: multiple perinatal factors. Obstet Gynecol 1981;57:41–7.
12. Bishop EH. Acceleration of fetal pulmonary maturity. Obstet Gynecol 1981;58(Suppl):48S–51S.
13. Farrell PM, Engle MJ, Zachman RD, Curet LB, Morrison JC, Rao AV, Poole WK. Amniotic fluid phospholipids after maternal administration of dexamethasone. Am J Obstet Gynecol 1983;145:484–90.
14. Ruvinsky ED, Douvas SG, Roberts WE, Martin JN Jr, Palmer SM, Rhodes PG, Morrison JC. Maternal administration of dexamethasone in severe pregnancy-induced hypertension. Am J Obstet Gynecol 1984;149:722–6.
15. Avery ME. The argument for prenatal administration of dexamethasone to prevent respiratory distress syndrome. J Pediatr 1984;104:240.
16. Sepkowitz S. Prenatal corticosteroid therapy to prevent respiratory distress syndrome. J Pediatr 1984;105:338–9.
17. Avery ME. Reply. J Pediatr 1984;105:339.
18. Levy DL. Maternal administration of dexamethasone to prevent RDS. J Pediatr 1984;105:339.
19. Eggers TR, Doyle LW, Pepperell RJ. Premature rupture of the membranes. Med J Aust 1979;1:209–13.
20. Garite TJ, Freeman RK, Linzey EM, Braly PS, Dorchester WL. Prospective randomized study of corticosteroids in the management of premature rupture of the membranes and the premature gestation. Am J Obstet Gynecol 1981;141:508–15.

21. Garite TJ. Premature rupture of the membranes: the enigma of the obstetrician. Am J Obstet Gynecol 1985;151:1001–5.
22. Curet LB, Morrison JC, Rao AV. Antenatal therapy with corticosteroids and postpartum complications. Am J Obstet Gynecol 1985;152:83–4.
23. Osathanondh R, Tulchinsky D, Kamali H, Fencl MdeM, Taeusch HW Jr. Dexamethasone levels in treated pregnant women and newborn infants. J Pediatr 1977;90:617–20.
24. Levitz M, Jansen V, Dancis J. The transfer and metabolism of corticosteroids in the perfused human placenta. Am J Obstet Gynecol 1978;132:363–6.
25. Otero L, Conlon C, Reynolds P, Duval-Arnould B, Golden SM. Neonatal leukocytosis associated with prenatal administration of dexamethasone. Pediatrics 1981;68:778–80.
26. Anday EK, Harris MC. Leukemoid reaction associated with antenatal dexamethasone administration. J Pediatr 1982;101:614–6.
27. Schatz M, Patterson R, Zeitz S, O'Rourke J, Melam H. Corticosteroid therapy for the pregnant asthmatic patient. JAMA 1975;233:804–7.
28. Jenssen H, Wright PB. The effect of dexamethasone therapy in prolonged pregnancy. Acta Obstet Gynecol Scand 1977;56:467–73.
29. Navot D, Rozen E, Sadovsky E. Effect of dexamethasone on amniotic fluid absorbance in Rh-sensitized pregnancy. Br J Obstet Gynaecol 1982;89:456–8.
30. Yin CS, Scott JR. Unsuccessful treatment of fetal immunologic thrombocytopenia with dexamethasone. Am J Obstet Gynecol 1985;152:316–7.
31. David M, Forest MG. Prenatal treatment of congenital adrenal hyperplasia resulting from 21-hydroxylase deficiency. J Pediatr 1984;105:799–803.
32. Evans MI, Chrousos GP, Mann DW, Larsen JW Jr, Green I, McCluskey J, Loriaux L, Fletcher JC, Koons G, Overpeck J, Schulman JD. Pharmacologic suppression of the fetal adrenal gland in utero. JAMA 1985;253:1015–20.
33. Taeusch HW Jr. Glucocorticoid prophylaxis for respiratory distress syndrome: a review of potential toxicity. J Pediatr 1975;87:617–23.
34. Johnson JWC, Mitzner W, London WT, Palmer AE, Scott R. Betamethasone and the rhesus fetus: multisystemic effects. Am J Obstet Gynecol 1979;133:677–84.
35. Wong YC, Beardsmore CS, Silverman M. Antenatal dexamethasone and subsequent lung growth. Arch Dis Child 1982;57:536–8.
36. Collaborative Group on Antenatal Steroid Therapy. Effects of antenatal dexamethasone administration in the infant: long-term follow-up. J Pediatr 1984;104:259–67.

Name: **DEXBROMPHENIRAMINE**

Class: **Antihistamine**   Risk Factor: **C**

Fetal Risk Summary

Dexbrompheniramine is the *dextro*-isomer of brompheniramine (see Brompheniramine). No reports linking its use with congenital defects have been located.

Breast Feeding Summary

See Brompheniramine.

Name: **DEXCHLORPHENIRAMINE**

Class: **Antihistamine**   Risk Factor: **B$_M$**

Fetal Risk Summary

Dexchlorpheniramine is the *dextro*-isomer of chlorpheniramine (see also Chlorpheniramine). No reports linking its use with congenital defects have been located. One study recorded 14 exposures in the 1st trimester without evidence for an association with malformations (1). Animal studies for chlorpheniramine have not shown a teratogenic effect (2).

Breast Feeding Summary

No data available.

References

1. Heinonen OP, Slone D, Shapiro S. *Birth Defects and Drugs in Pregnancy*. Littleton:Publishing Sciences Group, 1977:323.
2. Product information. Polaramine. Schering Corporation, 1985.

Name: **DEXTROAMPHETAMINE**

Class: **Central Stimulant**   Risk Factor: **D***

Fetal Risk Summary

Contrasting reports on the safety of dextroamphetamine in pregnancy have appeared (1–10). Congenital defects that have been reported with the use of dextroamphetamine include:

Cardiac abnormalities (1, 2)
Bifid exencephaly (3)
Biliary atresia (4)
Multiple eye and central nervous system
    defects (5) (multiple drug use throughout
    pregnancy including LSD)

Amphetamine withdrawal syndrome has been described in a neonate whose mother was self-administering intravenously excessive doses of amphetamine (8). In contrast, two other case reports failed to demonstrate any neonatal effects from the treatment of narcolepsy with large doses of amphetamine (9, 10). Except for the possible indication of narcolepsy, the use of the drug during pregnancy is not recommended.

[* Risk Factor C according to manufacturer—Smith Kline & French, 1985.]

Breast Feeding Summary

Amphetamine, the racemic mixture of *levo*- and *dextro*-amphetamine, is excreted into breast milk (10). After continuous daily dosing of 20 mg, milk concentrations ranged from 55 to 138 ng/ml with milk:plasma ratios varying between 2.8 and 7.5. Amphetamine was found in the urine of the nursing infant. No adverse effects of this exposure were discovered over a 24-month observation period. In a second study, no neonatal insomnia or stimulation was observed in 103 nursing infants whose mothers were taking various amounts of amphetamine (11). A 1983 review article noted irritability and poor sleeping patterns as observed adverse effects from amphetamine exposure in milk, but the number of infants affected and other details were not given (12).

References

1. Nora JJ, Vargo T, Nora A. Dextroamphetamine: a possible environmental trigger of cardiovascular malformations. Lancet 1970;1:1290–1.
2. Gilbert E, Khoury G. Dextroamphetamine and congenital cardiac malformations. J Pediatr 1970;76:638.
3. Matera R, Zabala H, Jimenez A. Bifid exencephalia: teratogen action of amphetamine. Int Surg 1968;50:79–85.
4. Levin J. Amphetamine ingestion with biliary atresia. J Pediatr 1971;79:130–1.
5. Bogdanoff B, Rorke LB, Yanoff M, Warren WS. Brain and eye abnormalities: possible sequelae to prenatal use of multiple drugs including LSD. Am J Dis Child 1972;123:145–8.
6. Nora JJ, McNamara DG, Frazer FC. Dextroamphetamine sulphate and human malformations. Lancet 1967;1:570–1.
7. Milkovich L, van den Berg BJ. Effects of antenatal exposure to anorectic drugs. Am J Obstet Gynecol 1977;129:637–42.
8. Ramer CM. The case of an infant born to an amphetamine addicted mother. Clin Pediatr (Phila) 1974;13:596–7.
9. Briggs GG, Samson JH, Crawford DJ. Lack of abnormalities in a newborn exposed to amphetamine during gestation. Am J Dis Child 1975;129:249–50.
10. Steiner E, Villen T, Hallberg M, Rane A. Amphetamine secretion in breast milk. Eur J Clin Pharmacol 1984;27:123–4.
11. Ayd FJ. Excretion of psychotropic drugs in human milk. Int Drug Ther News Bull 1973;8:33–40.
12. Committee on Drugs, American Academy of Pediatrics. The transfer of drugs and other chemicals into human breast milk. Pediatrics 1983;72:375–83.

Name: **DIATRIZOATE**

Class: **Diagnostic**   Risk Factor: **D**

Fetal Risk Summary

The use of diatrizoate for amniography has been described in several studies (1–10). Except for inadvertent injection of the contrast media into the fetus during amniocentesis, the use of diatrizoate was not thought to result in fetal harm. More recent studies have examined the effect of the drug on fetal thyroid function.

All of the various preparations of diatrizoate contain a high concentration of organically bound iodine. Twenty-eight pregnant women received intra-amniotic injections (50 ml) of diatrizoate for diagnostic indications (11). When compared to nontreated controls, no effect was observed on cord blood levothyroxine (T_4) and liothyronine-resin uptake values regardless of the time interval between injection and delivery. The authors concluded that the iodine remained organically bound until it was eliminated in 2–4 days from the amniotic fluid.

In another report, seven patients within 13 days or less of term were injected intra-amniotically with a mixture of ethiodized oil (12 ml) and diatrizoate (30 ml)(12). Thyrotropin (TSH) levels were determined in the cord blood of five newborns and in the serum of all seven infants on the 5th day of life. TSH was markedly elevated in three of five cord samples and six of seven neonatal samples. Three of the infants had signs and symptoms of hypothyroidism:

Elevated TSH/normal T_4; apathy and jaundice
   clearing immediately with thyroid therapy (1 infant)
Elevated TSH/decreased T_4 (1 infant)
Elevated TSH/decreased T_4 with goiter (1 infant)

In contrast to the initial report, the severity of thyroid suppression seemed greater the longer the time interval between injection and delivery. The explanation offered for these different results was the utilization of the more sensitive TSH serum test and the use of only water-soluble contrast media in the first study.

In summary, diatrizoate may suppress the fetal thyroid gland when administered by intra-amniotic injection. Appropriate measures should be taken to diagnose and treat neonatal hypothyroidism if amniography with diatrizoate is performed.

Breast Feeding Summary

No data available. See also Potassium Iodide.

References

1. McLain CR Jr. Amniography studies of the gastrointestinal motility of the human fetus. Am J Obstet Gynecol 1963;86:1079–87.
2. McLain CR Jr. Amniography, a versatile diagnostic procedure in obstetrics. Obstet Gynecol 1964;23:45–50.
3. McLain CR Jr. Amniography for diagnosis and management of fetal death in utero. Obstet Gynecol 1965;26:233–6.
4. Ferris EJ, Shapiro JH, Spira J. Roentgenologic aspects of intrauterine transfusion. JAMA 1966;196:127–8.
5. Wiltchik SG, Schwarz RH, Emich JP Jr. Amniography for placental localization. Obstet Gynecol 1966;28:641–5.
6. Misenhimer HR. Fetal hemorrhage associated with amniocentesis. Am J Obstet Gynecol 1966;94:1133–5.
7. Blumberg ML, Wohl GT, Wiltchik S, Schwarz R, Emich JP. Placental localization by amniography. AJR 1967;100:688–97.
8. Berner HW Jr. Amniography, an accurate way to localize the placenta. Obstet Gynecol 1967;29:200–6.
9. Creasman WT, Lawrence RA, Thiede HA. Fetal complications of amniocentesis. JAMA 1968;204:949–52.
10. Bottorff MK, Fish SA. Amniography. South Med J 1971;64:1203–6.
11. Morrison JC, Boyd M, Friedman BI, et al. The effects of Renografin-60 on the fetal thyroid. Obstet Gynecol 1973;42:99–103.
12. Rodesch F, Camus M, Ermans AM, Dodion J, Delange F. Adverse effect of amniofetography on fetal thyroid function. Am J Obstet Gynecol 1976;126:723–6.

Name: **DIAZEPAM**

Class: **Sedative**   Risk Factor: **D**

Fetal Risk Summary

Diazepam and its metabolite, n-demethyldiazepam, freely cross the placenta and accumulate in the fetal circulation with newborn levels about 1–3 times greater than maternal serum (1–10). Equilibrium between mother and fetus occurs in 5–10 minutes after intravenous administrations (10). The maternal and fetal serum binding capacity for diazepam is reduced in pregnancy and is not correlated with albumin (11, 12). The plasma half-life in newborns is significantly increased due to a decreased clearance of the drug. Because the transplacental passage is rapid, timing of the intravenous administration with uterine contractions will greatly reduce the amount of drug transferred to the fetus (6).

An association between diazepam and an increased risk of cleft lip and/or palate has been suggested by three studies (13–15). The findings indicated 1st or 2nd trimester use of diazepam, and selected other drugs, is significantly greater among mothers of children born with oral clefts. A mother who took 580 mg of diazepam as a single dose on about the 43rd day of gestation delivered an infant with cleft lip/palate, craniofacial asymmetry, ocular hypertelorism, and bilateral periauricular tags (16). The authors concluded that the drug ingestion was responsible for the defects. Large retrospective studies showing no association between diazepam and cleft lip/palate have also been published (17–19). The results of one of these studies has been criticized and defended (20, 21). Although no association was found with cleft lip/palate, Rosenberg (21) did find a statistically significant association between diazepam and inguinal hernia. This same association, along with others, was found in another investigation. In 1,427 malformed newborns compared to 3,001 controls, 1st trimester use of tranquilizers (diazepam most common) was associated with inguinal hernia, cardiac defects, and pyloric stenosis (22). Second trimester exposure was associated with hemangiomas and cardiac and circulatory defects. The combination of cigarette smoking and tranquilizer use increased the risk of delivering a malformed infant by 3.7-fold as compared to those who smoked but did not use tranquilizers (22). A survey of 390 infants with congenital heart disease matched with 1,254 normal infants found a higher rate of exposure to several drugs, including diazepam, in the offspring with defects (23). Although these studies contained several possible biases that could have affected the results, the data serve as a clear warning against indiscriminate use of diazepam during gestation. Other congenital anomalies reported in infants exposed to diazepam include (24–26):

Absence of both thumbs (2 cases)
Spina bifida (1 case)
Absence of left forearm, syndactyly (1 case)

Many investigators have observed that the use of diazepam during labor is not harmful to the mother or her infant (27–34). A dose response is likely as the frequency of newborn complications rises when doses exceed 30–40 mg or when diazepam is taken for extended periods, allowing accumulation to occur (35–41).

Two major syndromes of neonatal complications have been observed:

Floppy infant syndrome:
   hypotonia
   lethargy
   sucking difficulties
Withdrawal syndrome:
   intrauterine growth retardation
   tremors
   irritability
   hypertonicity
   diarrhea/vomiting
   vigorous sucking

Under miscellaneous effects, diazepam may alter thermogenesis, cause loss of beat-to-beat variability in the fetal heart rate, and decrease fetal movements (42–47).

Breast Feeding Summary

Diazepam and its metabolite, n-demethyldiazepam, enter breast milk (48–52). Lethargy and loss of weight have been reported (51). Milk:plasma ratios varied between 0.2 and 2.7 (50). Diazepam may accumulate in breast-fed infants, and its use in lactating women is not recommended.

References

1. Erkkola R, Kanto J, Sellman R. Diazepam in early human pregnancy. Acta Obstet Gynecol Scand 1974;53:135–8.
2. Kanto J, Erkkola R, Sellman R. Accumulation of diazepam and n-demethyldiazepam in the fetal blood during labor. Ann Clin Res 1973;5:375–9.
3. Idanpaan-Heikkila JE, Jouppila PI, Puolakka JO, Vorne MS. Placental transfer and fetal metabolism of diazepam in early human pregnancy. Am J Obstet Gynecol 1971;109:1011–6.
4. Mandelli M, Morselli PL, Nordio S, Pardi G, Principi N. Sereni F, Tognoni G. Placental transfer of diazepam and its disposition in the newborn. Clin Pharmacol Ther 1975;17:564–72.
5. Gamble JAS, Moore J, Lamke H, Howard PJ. A study of plasma diazepam levels in mother and infant. Br J Obstet Gynaecol 1977;84:588–91.
6. Haram K, Bakke DM, Johannessen KH, Lund T. Transplacental passage of diazepam during labor: influence of uterine contractions. Clin Pharmacol Ther 1978;24:590–9.
7. Bakke OM, Haram K, Lygre T, Wallem G. Comparison of the placental transfer of thiopental and diazepam in caesarean section. Eur J Clin Pharmacol 1981;21:221–7.
8. Haram K, Bakke OM. Diazepam as an induction agent for caesarean section: a clinical and pharmacokinetic study of fetal drug exposure. Br J Obstet Gynaecol 1980;87:506–12.
9. Kanto JH. Use of benzodiazepines during pregnancy, labour and lactation, with particular reference to pharmacokinetic considerations. Drugs 1982;23:354–80.
10. Bakke OM, Haram K. Time-course of transplacental passage of diazepam: influence of injection-delivery interval on neonatal drug concentrations. Clin Pharmacol 1982;7:353–62.
11. Lee JN, Chen SS, Richens A, Menabawey M, Chard T. Serum protein binding of diazepam in maternal and foetal serum during pregnancy. Br J Clin Pharmacol 1982;14:551–4.
12. Ridd MJ, Brown KF, Nation RL, Collier CB. Differential transplacental binding of diazepam: causes and implications. Eur J Clin Pharmacol 1983;24:595–601.
13. Safra JM, Oakley GP. Association between cleft lip with or without cleft palate and neonatal exposure to diazepam. Lancet 1975;2:478–80.
14. Saxen I. Epidemiology of cleft lip and palate. Br J Prev Soc Med 1975;29:103–10.
15. Saxen I. Associations between oral clefts and drugs taken during pregnancy. Int J Epidemiol 1975;4:37–44.

16. Rivas F, Hernandez A, Cantu JM. Acentric craniofacial cleft in a newborn female prenatally exposed to a high dose of diazepam. Teratology 1984;30:179–80.

17. Czeizel A. Diazepam, phenytoin, and etiology of cleft lip and/or cleft palate. Lancet 1976;1:810.

18. Rosenberg L, Mitchell AA, Parsells JL, Pashayan H, Louik C, Shapiro S. Lack of relation of oral clefts to diazepam use during pregnancy. N Engl J Med 1983;309:1282–5.

19. Shiono PH, Mills JL. Oral clefts and diazepam use during pregnancy. N Engl J Med 1984;311:919–20.

20. Entman SS, Vaughn WK. Lack of relation of oral clefts to diazepam use in pregnancy. N Engl J Med 1984;310:1121–2.

21. Rosenberg L et al. Op cit, 1122.

22. Bracken MB, Holford TR. Exposure to prescribed drugs in pregnancy and association with congenital malformations. Obstet Gynecol 1981;58:336–44.

23. Rothman KJ, Fyler DC, Goldblatt A, Kreidberg MB. Exogenous hormones and other drug exposures of children with congenital heart disease. Am J Epidemiol 1979;109:433–9.

24. Istvan EJ. Drug-associated congenital abnormalities. Can Med Assoc J 1970;103:1394.

25. Ringrose CAD. The hazard of neurotrophic drugs in the fertile years. Can Med Assoc J 1972;106:1058.

26. Fourth Annual Report of the New Zealand Committee on Adverse Drug Reactions. NZ Med J 1969;70:118–22.

27. Greenblatt DJ, Shader RI. Effect of benzodiazepines in neonates. N Engl J Med 1975;292:649.

28. Modif M, Brinkman CR, Assali NS. Effects of diazepam on uteroplacental and fetal hemodynamics and metabolism. Obstet Gynecol 1973;41:364–8.

29. Toaff ME, Hezroni J, Toaff R. Effect of diazepam on uterine activity during labor. Isr J Med Sci 1977;13:1007–9.

30. Shannon RW, Fraser GP, Aitken RG, Harper JR. Diazepam in preeclamptic toxaemia with special reference to its effect on the newborn infant. Br J Clin Pract 1972;26:271–5.

31. Yeh SY, Paul RIT, Cordero L, Hon EH. A study of diazepam during labor. Obstet Gynecol 1974;43:363–73.

32. Kasturilal, Shetti RN. Role of diazepam in the management of eclampsia. Curr Ther Res 1975;18:627–30.

33. Eliot BW, Hill JG, Cole AP, Hailey DM. Continuous pethidine/diazepam infusion during labor and its effects on the newborn. Br J Obstet Gynaecol 1975;82:126–31.

34. Lean TH, Retnam SS, Sivasamboo R. Use of benzodiazepines in the management of eclampsia. J Obstet Gynaecol Br Commonw 1968;75:856–62.

35. Scanlon JW. Effect of benzodiazepines in neonates. N Engl J Med 1975;292:649.

36. Gillberg C. "Floppy infant syndrome" and maternal diazepam. Lancet 1977;2:244.

37. Haram K. "Floppy infant syndrome" and maternal diazepam. Lancet 1977;2:612–3.

38. Speight AN. Floppy-infant syndrome and maternal diazepam and/or nitrazepam. Lancet 1977;1:878.

39. Rementeria JL, Bhatt K. Withdrawal symptoms in neonates from intrauterine exposure to diazepam. J Pediatr 1977;90:123–6.

40. Thearle MJ, Dunn PM. Exchange transfusions for diazepam intoxication at birth followed by jejunal stenosis. Proc R Soc Med 1973;66:13–4.

41. Backes CR, Cordero L. Withdrawal symptoms in the neonate from presumptive intrauterine exposure to diazepam: report of case. J Am Osteopath Assoc 1980;79:584–5.

42. Cree JE, Meyer J, Hailey DM. Diazepam in labour: its metabolism and effect on the clinical condition and thermogenesis of the newborn. Br Med J 1973;4:251–5.

43. McAllister CB. Placental transfer and neonatal effects of diazepam when administered to women just before delivery. Br J Anaesth 1980;52:423–7.

44. Owen JR, Irani SF, Blair AW. Effect of diazepam administered to mothers during labour on temperature regulation of neonate. Arch Dis Child 1972;47:107–10.

45. Scher J, Hailey DM, Beard RW. The effects of diazepam on the fetus. J Obstet Gynaecol Br Commonw 1972;79:635–8.

46. van Geijn HP, Jongsma HW, Doesburg WH, Lemmens WA, deHaan J, Eskes TK. The effect of diazepam administration during pregnancy or labor on the heart rate variability of the newborn infant. Eur J Obstet Gynaecol Reprod Biol 1980;10:187–201.

47. Birger M, Homberg R, Insler V. Clinical evaluation of fetal movements. Int J Gynaecol Obstet 1980;18:377–82.

48. van Geijn HP, Kenemans P, Vise T, Vanderkleijn E, Eskes TK. Pharmacokinetics of diazepam and

occurrence in breast milk. In *Proceedings of the Sixth International Congress of Pharmacology,* Helsinki, 1975:514.

49. Hill RM, Nowlin J, Lertratanangkoon K, Stillwell WG, Stillwell RN, Horning MG. The identification and quantification of drugs in human breast milk. Clin Res 1974;22:77A.
50. Cole AP, Hailey DM. Diazepam and active metabolite in breast milk and their transfer to the neonate. Arch Dis Child 1975;50:741–2.
51. Patrick MJ, Tilstone WJ, Reavey P. Diazepam and breast-feeding. Lancet 1972;1:542–3.
52. Catz CS. Diazepam in breast milk. Drug Ther 1973;3:72–3.

Name: **DIAZOXIDE**

Class: **Antihypertensive**   Risk Factor: **C$_M$**

Fetal Risk Summary

Diazoxide readily crosses the placenta and reaches fetal plasma concentrations similar to maternal levels (1). The drug has been used for the treatment of severe hypertension associated with pregnancy (1–12). Some investigators have cautioned against the use of diazoxide in pregnancy (13, 14). In one study, the decrease in maternal blood pressure was sufficient to produce a state of clinical shock and endanger placental perfusion (13). Transient fetal bradycardia has been reported in other studies following a rapid, marked decrease in maternal blood pressure (7, 15). Fatal maternal hypotension have been reported in one patient after diazoxide therapy (16). Thien and co-workers (17) have recommended the infusion technique for administering diazoxide rather than rapid boluses to prevent maternal and fetal complications. However, the use of small bolus doses at frequent intervals (30 mg every 1–2 minutes) has been used to successfully treat maternal hypertension without producing fetal toxicity (18).

Diazoxide is a potent relaxant of uterine smooth muscle and may inhibit uterine contractions if given during labor (2, 3, 5–7, 19–21). The degree and duration of uterine inhibition are dose-dependent (20). Augmentation of labor with oxytocin may be required in patients receiving diazoxide.

Hyperglycemia in the newborn (glucose 500–700 mg/dl) secondary to intravenous diazoxide therapy in a mother just prior to delivery has been observed to persist up to 3 days (22). Neuman and co-workers (13) found hyperglycemia, without ketoacidosis, in all of the mothers and newborns in their series. The glucose levels returned to near normal within 24 hours. The use of oral diazoxide for the last 19–69 days of pregnancy has been associated with alopecia, hypertrichosis lanuginosa, and decreased ossification of the wrist (1). However, long-term oral therapy has not caused similar problems in other newborns exposed *in utero* (4).

Since other antihypertensive drugs are available for severe maternal hypertension and the long-term effects on the infant have not been evaluated, diazoxide should be used with caution, if at all, during pregnancy. If diazoxide is needed after other therapies have failed, small doses are recommended.

Breast Feeding Summary

No data available.

References

1. Milner RDG, Chouksey SK. Effects of fetal exposure to diazoxide in man. Arch Dis Child 1972;47:537–43.
2. Finnerty FA JR, Kakaviatos N, Tuckman J, Magill J. Clinical evaluation of diazoxide: a new treatment for acute hypertension. Circulation 1963;28:203–8.
3. Finnerty FA Jr. Advantages and disadvantages of furosemide in the edematous states of pregnancy. Am J Obstet Gynecol 1969;105:1022–7.
4. Pohl JEF, Thurston H, Davis D, Morgan MY. Successful use of oral diazoxide in the treatment of severe toxaemia of pregnancy. Br Med J 1972;2:568–70.
5. Pennington JC, Picker RH. Diazoxide and the treatment of the acute hypertensive emergency in obstetrics. Med J Aust 1972;2:1051–4.
6. Koch-Weser J. Diazoxide. N Engl J Med 1976;294:1271–4.
7. Morris JA, Arce JJ, Hamilton CJ, et al. The management of severe preeclampsia and eclampsia with intravenous diazoxide. Obstet Gynecol 1977;49:675–80.
8. Keith TA III. Hypertension crisis: recognition and management. JAMA 1977;237:1570–7.
9. MacLean AB, Doig JR, Aickin DR. Hypovolaemia, pre-eclampsia and diuretics. Br J Obstet Gynaecol 1978;85:597–601.
10. Barr PA, Gallery ED. Effect of diazoxide on the antepartum cardiotocograph in severe pregnancy-associated hypertension. Aust NZ J Obstet Gynaecol 1981;21:11–5.
11. MacLean AB, Doig JR, Chatfield WR, Aickin DR. Small-dose diazoxide administration in pregnancy. Aust NZ J Obstet Gynaecol 1981;21:7–10.
12. During VR. Clinical experience obtained from use of diazoxide (Hypertonalum) for treatment of acute intrapartum hypertensive crisis. Zentralbl Gynaekol 1982;104:89–93.
13. Neuman J, Weiss B, Rabello Y, Cabal L, Freeman RK. Diazoxide for the acute control of severe hypertension complicating pregnancy: a pilot study. Obstet Gynecol 1979;53(Suppl):50S–5S.
14. Perkins RP. Treatment of toxemia of pregnancy. JAMA 1977;238:2143–4.
15. Michael CA. Intravenous diazoxide in the treatment of severe preeclamptic toxaemia and eclampsia. Aust NZ J Obstet Gynaecol 1973;13:143–6.
16. Henrich WL, Cronin R, Miller PD, Anderson RJ. Hypotensive sequelae of diazoxide and hydralazine therapy. JAMA 1977;237:264–5.
17. Thien T, Koene RAP, Schijf C, Pieters GFFM, Eskes TKAB, Wijdeveld PGAB. Infusion of diazoxide in severe hypertension during pregnancy. Eur J Obstet Gynaecol Reprod Biol 1980;10:367–74.
18. Dudley DKL. Minibolus diazoxide in the management of severe hypertension in pregnancy. Am J Obstet Gynecol 1985;151:196–200.
19. Barden TP, Keenan WJ. Effects of diazoxide in human labor and the fetus-neonate. Obstet Gynecol 1971;37:631–2 (Abstr).
20. Landesman R, Adeodato de Souza FJ, Countinho EM, Wilson KH, Bomfim de Sousa FM. The inhibitory effect of diazoxide in normal term labor. Am J Obstet Gynecol 1969;103:430–3.
21. Paulissian R. Diazoxide. Int Anesthesiol Clin 1978;16:201–36.
22. Milsap RL, Auld PAM. Neonatal hyperglycemia following maternal diazoxide administration. JAMA 1980;243:144–5.

Name: **DIBENZEPIN**

Class: **Antidepressant**   Risk Factor: **D**

Fetal Risk Summary

No data available. See Imipramine.

Breast Feeding Summary

No data available. See Imipramine.

Name: **DICLOXACILLIN**

Class: **Antibiotic**   Risk Factor: **B$_M$**

Fetal Risk Summary

Dicloxacillin is a penicillin antibiotic (see also Penicillin G). The drug crosses the placenta into the fetal circulation and amniotic fluid. Levels are low compared to other penicillins due to the high degree of maternal protein binding (1, 2). Following a 500-mg intravenous dose, the fetal peak serum level of 3.4 μg/ml occurred at 2 hours (8% of maternal peak) (2). A peak of 1.8 μg/ml was obtained at 6 hours in the amniotic fluid.

No reports linking the use of dicloxacillin with congenital defects have been located. The Collaborative Perinatal Project monitored 50,282 mother-child pairs, 3,546 of which had 1st trimester exposure to penicillin derivatives (3). For use anytime in pregnancy, 7,171 exposures were recorded (4). In neither case was evidence found to suggest a relationship to large categories of major or minor malformations or to individual defects.

Breast Feeding Summary

No data available (see Penicillin G).

References

1. MacAulay M, Berg S, Charles D. Placental transfer of dicloxacillin at term. Am J Obstet Gynecol 1968;102:1162–8.
2. Depp R, Kind A, Kirby W, Johnson W. Transplacental passage of methicillin and dicloxacillin into the fetus and amniotic fluid. Am J Obstet Gynecol 1970;107:1054–7.
3. Heinonen OP, Slone D, Shapiro S. *Birth Defects and Drugs in Pregnancy*. Littleton:Publishing Sciences Group, 1977;297–313.
4. *Ibid*, 435.

Name: **DICUMAROL**

Class: **Anticoagulant**   Risk Factor: **D**

Fetal Risk Summary

See Coumarin Derivatives.

Breast Feeding Summary

See Coumarin Derivatives.

Name: **DICYCLOMINE**

Class: **Parasympatholytic**   Risk Factor: **B**

Fetal Risk Summary

See Doxylamine.

Breast Feeding Summary

See Doxylamine.

Name: **DIENESTROL**

Class: **Estrogenic Hormone**   Risk Factor: **X**

Fetal Risk Summary

Dienestrol is used topically. Estrogens are readily absorbed and intravaginal use can lead to significant concentrations of estrogen in the blood (1, 2). The Collaborative Perinatal Project monitored 614 mother-child pairs with 1st trimester exposure to estrogenic agents, including 36 with exposure to dienestrol (3). An increase in the expected frequency of cardiovascular defects, eye and ear anomalies, and Down's syndrome was found for estrogens as a group but not for dienestrol (3, 4). Use of estrogenic hormones during pregnancy is contraindicated.

Breast Feeding Summary

No reports of adverse effects of dienestrol on the nursing infant have been located. It is possible that decreased milk volume and decreased nitrogen and protein content could occur (see Mestranol and Ethinylestradiol).

References

1. Gilman AG, Goodman LS, Gilman A, eds. *The Pharmacological Basis of Therapeutics*, ed 6. New York:Macmillan Publishing Co, 1980:1428.
2. Rigg LA, Hermann H, Yen SSC. Absorption of estrogens from vaginal creams. N Engl J Med 1978;298:195–7.
3. Heinonen OP, Slone D, Shapiro S. *Birth Defects and Drugs in Pregnancy*. Littleton:Publishing Sciences Group, 1977:389, 391.
4. *Ibid*, 395.

Name: **DIETHYLPROPION**

Class: **Central Stimulant/Anorectant**   Risk Factor: **B**

Fetal Risk Summary

No reports linking the use of diethylpropion with congenital defects have been located. The drug has been studied as an appetite suppressant in 28 pregnant patients and although adverse effects were common in the women, no problems were observed in their offspring (1). A retrospective survey of 1,232 patients exposed to diethylpropion during pregnancy found no difference in the incidence of defects (0.9%) when compared to a matched control group (1.1%) (2). Animal studies have not revealed a teratogenic potential (3).

Breast Feeding Summary

No data available.

References

1. Silverman M, Okun R. The use of an appetite suppressant (diethylpropion hydrochloride) during pregnancy. Curr Ther Res 1971;13:648–53.
2. Bunde CA, Leyland HM. A controlled retrospective survey in evaluation of teratogenicity. J New Drugs 1965;5:193–8.
3. Schardein JL. *Drugs as Teratogens*. Cleveland:CRC Press, 1976:73–5.

Name: **DIETHYLSTILBESTROL**

Class: **Estrogenic Hormone**   Risk Factor: X_M

Fetal Risk Summary

Between 1940 and 1971, an estimated 6 million mothers and their fetuses were exposed to diethylstilbestrol (DES) to prevent reproductive problems such as miscarriage, premature delivery, intrauterine fetal death and toxemia (1–4). Controlled studies have since proven that DES was not successful in preventing these disorders (5, 6). This use has resulted, however, in significant complications of the reproductive system in both female and male offspring (1–12). Two large groups have been established to monitor these complications: the Registry for Research on Hormonal Transplacental Carcinogenesis and the Diethylstilbestrol Adenosis (DESAD) Project (4). The published findings and recommendations of the DESAD project through 1980 plus a number of other studies including the Registry were reviewed in a 1981 National Institutes of Health booklet available from the National Cancer Institute (4). This information was also reprinted in a 1983 journal article (13). The complications identified in female and male children exposed *in utero* to DES are:

FEMALE
  Lower müllerian tract
    Vaginal adenosis
    Vaginal and cervical clear cell adenocarcinoma
    Cervical/vaginal fornix defects (10)
      Cockscomb (hood, transverse ridge of cervix)
      Collar (rim, hood, transverse ridge of cervix)
      Pseudopolyp
      Hypoplastic cervix (immature cervix)
      Altered fornix of vagina
    Vaginal defects (exclusive of fornix) (10)
      Incomplete transverse septum
      Incomplete longitudinal septum
  Upper müllerian tract
    Uterine structural defects
    Fallopian tube structural defects
MALE
  Reproductive dysfunction
  Altered semen analysis
  Infertility

The Registry was established in 1971 to study the epidemiologic, clinical, and pathologic aspects of clear cell adenocarcinoma of the vagina and cervix in DES-exposed women (2). Over 400 cases of clear cell adenocarcinoma have been reported to the registry. Additional reports continue to appear in the literature (14). The risk of carcinoma is apparently higher when DES treatment was given before the 12th week of gestation and is estimated to be 0.14–1.4/1,000 for women under the age of 25 years (2, 4).

A recent report described the first known case of adenosquamous carcinoma of the cervix in an exposed patient (15). In a second case, a 12-year-old exposed girl developed a fatal malignant teratoma of the ovary (16). The relationship between these tumors and DES is unknown.

The frequency of dysplasia and carcinoma *in situ* (CIS) of the cervix and vagina in 3,980 DESAD project patients was significantly increased over controls with an approximate 2–4-fold increase in risk (11). These results were different from earlier studies of these same women which had indicated no increased risk for dysplasia/CIS (17, 18). Robboy and co-workers (11) speculated that the increased incidence now observed was related to the greater amount of squamous metaplasia found in DES-exposed women. Scanning electron microscopy of the cervicovaginal transformation zone has indicated that maturation of epithelium is slowed or arrested at the stage of immature squamous epithelium in some DES-exposed women (19). This process may produce greater susceptibility to such factors as herpesvirus and papillomavirus obtained through early coitus with multiple partners and result in the observed increased rates of dysplasia/CIS (11). Of interest in this regard, a 1983 article reported detectable papillomavirus antigen in the cervical-vaginal biopsies of 16 (43%) of 37 DES-exposed women (20).

The incidence of cervical or vaginal structural changes has been reported to occur in up to 85% of exposed women, although most studies place the incidence in the 22–58% range (2, 3, 5, 7, 12, 21–24). The structural changes are outlined above. The DESAD project reported an incidence of approximately 25% in 1,655 women (10). Selection bias was eliminated by analyzing only those patients identified by record review. Patients referred by physicians and self-referrals had much higher rates of defects, about 49 and 43%, respectively. Almost all of the defects were confined to the cervical-vaginal fornix area with only 14 patients having vaginal changes exclusive of the fornix and nearly all of these being incomplete transverse septums (10).

Reports linking the use of DES with major congenital anomalies have not been located. The Collaborative Perinatal Project monitored 614 mother-child pairs with 1st trimester exposure to estrogens, including 164 with exposure to DES (25). Evidence for an increase in the expected frequency for cardiovascular defects, eye and ear anomalies, and Down's syndrome was found for estrogens as a group, but not for DES (25, 26). Re-evaluation of these data in terms of timing of exposure, vaginal bleeding in early pregnancy, and previous maternal obstetrical history, however, failed to support an association between estrogens and cardiac malformations (27). An earlier study also failed to find any relationship with nongenital malformations (28).

Alterations in the body of the uterus have led to concern regarding increased pregnancy wastage and premature births (8, 22, 29–32). Increased rates of spontaneous abortions, premature births, and ectopic pregnancies are well established by these latter reports, although the relationship to the abnormal changes of the cervix and/or vagina is still unclear (8). Serial observations of vaginal epithelial changes indicate that the frequency of such changes decreases with age (4, 17, 24).

Spontaneous rupture of a term uterus has been described in a 25-year-old primigravida with DES-type changes in her vagina, cervix, and uterus (33). Other reports of this type have not been located.

In a 1984 study, DES exposure had no effect on the age at menarche, first coitus, pregnancy, or live birth, nor on a woman's ability to conceive (34). Kaufman and associates (35) found that although anomalies in the upper genital tract increased the risk for poor pregnancy outcome, they could not relate specific changes to specific types of outcomes.

Hirsutism and irregular menses were found in 72 and 50%, respectively, of 32 DES-exposed women (36). The degree of hirsutism was age-related with the mean ages of severely and mildly hirsute women, being 28.8 and 24.7 years, respectively. Based on various hormone level measurements, the authors concluded that *in utero* DES exposure may result in hypothalamic-pituitary-ovarian dysfunction (36). However, other studies in much larger exposed populations have not observed disturbances of menstruation or excessive hair growth (37).

Data on DES-exposed women who had undergone major gynecologic surgical procedures, excluding cesarean section, were reported in a 1982 study (38). Of 309 exposed women, 33 (11%) had a total of 43 procedures. The authors suggested that DES exposure resulted in an increased incidence of adnexal disease involving adhesions, benign ovarian cysts, and ectopic pregnancies (38). Surgical manipulation of the cervix (cryocautery or conization) in DES-exposed patients results in a high incidence of cervical stenosis and possible development of endometriosis (39, 40). Both studies concluded, however, that the causes of infertility in these patients were comparable to those in a non-DES-exposed population.

Adverse effects in male offspring attributable to *in utero* DES exposure have been reported (1, 5, 41–47). Abnormalities thought to occur at greater frequencies include:

Epididymal cysts
Hypotrophic testis
Microphallus
Variococele
Capsular induration
Altered semen (decreased count, concentration,
      motility, and morphology)

An increase in problems with passing urine and urogenital tract infections has also been observed (41).

DES exposure has been proposed as a possible cause of infertility in male offspring (1). However, in a controlled *in vitro* study, no association was found between exposure to DES and reduced sperm penetration of zona-free hamster eggs (47). In addition, a study of 828 exposed men found no increase over controls for risk of genitourinary abnormalities, infertility, or testicular cancer (48). Based on their data, the authors proposed that previous studies showing a positive relationship may have had selection biases, differences in DES use, or both.

Testicular tumors have been reported in three DES-exposed patients (6, 49). In one case, a teratoma was discovered in a 23-year-old male (6). Two patients, 27 and 28 years of age, were included in the second report (49). Both had left-sided anaplastic seminomas and one had epididymal cysts. A male sibling of one of the patients, also DES-exposed, had severe aligospermia while two exposed sisters had vaginal adenosis and vaginal adenocarcinoma.

Changes in the psychosexual performance of young boys has been attributed to *in utero* exposure to DES and progesterone (50, 51). The mothers received estrogen/progestogen regimens for diabetes. A trend to less heterosexual experience and fewer masculine interests than controls was shown. A 2-fold increase in psychiatric disease, especially depression and anxiety, has been observed in both male and female exposed offspring (6).

Breast Feeding Summary

No data available. Decreased milk volume and nitrogen-protein content may occur if diethylstilbestrol is used during lactation (see Mestranol and Ethinyl Estradiol).

References

1. Stenchever MA, Williamson RA, Leonard J, Karp LE, Ley B, Shy K, Smith D. Possible relationship between in utero diethylstilbestrol exposure and male fertility. Am J Obstet Gynecol 1981;140:186–93.
2. Herbst AL. Diethylstilbestrol and other sex hormones during pregnancy. Obstet Gynecol 1981;58(Suppl):35s–40s.
3. Nordquist SAB, Medhat IA, Ng AB. Teratogenic effects of intrauterine exposure to DES in female offspring. Compr Ther 1979;5:69–74.
4. Robboy SJ, Noller KL, Kaufman RH, Barnes AB, Townsend D, Gundersen JH, Nash S. Information for Physicians. Prenatal diethylstilbestrol (DES) exposure: recommendations of the diethylstilbestrol-adenosis (DESAD) project for the identification and management of exposed individuals. NIH Publication No. 81-2049, 1981.
5. Stillman RJ. In utero exposure to diethylstilbestrol: adverse effects on the reproductive tract and reproductive performance in male and female offspring. Am J Obstet Gynecol 1982;142:905–21
6. Vessey MP, Fairweather DVI, Norman-Smith B, Buckley J. A randomized double-blind controlled trial of the value of stilboestrol therapy in pregnancy: long-term follow-up of mothers and their offspring. Br J Obstet Gynaecol 1983;90:1007–17.
7. Prins RP, Morrow P, Townsend DE, Disaia PJ. Vaginal embryogenesis, estrogens, and adenosis. Obstet Gynecol 1976;48:246–50.
8. Sandberg EC, Riffle NL, Higdon JV, Getman CE. Pregnancy outcome in women exposed to diethylstilbestrol in utero. Am J Obstet Gynecol 1981;140:194–205.
9. Noller KL, Townsend DE, Kaufman RH, Barnes AB, Robboy SJ, Fish CR, Jefferies JA, Bergstralh EJ, O'Brien PC, McGorray SP, Scully R. Maturation of vaginal and cervical epithelium in women exposed in utero to diethylstilbestrol (DESAD Project). Am J Obstet Gynecol 1983;146:279–85.
10. Jefferies JA, Robboy SJ, O'Brien PC, Bergstralh EJ, Labarthe DR, Barnes AB, Noller KL, Hatab PA, Kaufman RH, Townsend DE. Structural anomalies of the cervix and vagina in women enrolled in the diethylstilbestrol adenosis (DESAD) project. Am J Obstet Gynecol 1984;148:59–66.
11. Robboy SJ, Noller KL, O'Brien P, Kaufman RH, Townsend D, Barnes AB, Gundersen J, Lawrence WD, Bergstrahl E, McGorray S, Tilley BC, Anton J, Chazen G. Increased incidence of cervical and vaginal dysplasia in 3,980 diethylstilbestrol-exposed young women. Experience of the National Collaborative Diethylstilbestrol Adenosis Project. JAMA 1984;252:2979–83.
12. Chanen W, Pagano R. Diethylstilboestrol (DES) exposure in utero. Med J Aust 1984;141:491–3.
13. NCI DES Summary. Prenatal diethylstilbestrol (DES) exposure. Clin Pediatr 1983;22:139–43.
14. Kaufman RH, Korhonen MO, Strama T, Adam E, Kaplan A. Development of clear cell adenocarcinoma in DES-exposed offspring under observation. Obstet Gynecol 1982;59(Suppl):68S–72S.
15. Vandrie DM, Puri S, Upton RT, Demeester LJ. Adenosquamous carcinoma of the cervix in a woman exposed to diethylstilbestrol in utero. Obstet Gynecol 1983;61(Suppl):84S–7S.
16. Lazarus KH. Maternal diethylstilboestrol and ovarian malignancy in offspring. Lancet 1984;1:53.

17. O'Brien PC, Noller KL, Robboy SJ, Barnes AB, Kaufman RH, Tilley BC, Townsend DE. Vaginal epithelial changes in young women enrolled in the National Cooperative Diethylstilbestrol Adenosis (DESAD) Project. Obstet Gynecol 1979;53:300–8.

18. Robboy SJ, Kaufman RH, Prat J, Welch WR, Gaffey T, Scully RE, Richart R, Fenoglio CM, Virata R, Tilley BC. Pathologic findings in young women enrolled in the National Cooperative Diethylstilbestrol Adenosis (DESAD) Project. Obstet Gynecol 1979;53:309–17.

19. McDonnell JM, Emens JM, Jordan JA. The congenital cervicovaginal transformation zone in young women exposed to diethylstilboestrol in utero. Br J Obstet Gynaecol 1984;91:574–9.

20. Fu YS, Lancaster WD, Richart RM, Reagan JW, Crum CP, Levine RU. Cervical papillomavirus infection in diethylstilbestrol-exposed progeny. Obstet Gynecol 1983;61:59–62.

21. Ben-Baruch G, Menczer J, Mashiach S, Serr DM. Uterine anomalies in diethylstilbestrol-exposed women with fertility disorders. Acta Obstet Gynecol Scand 1981;60:395–7.

22. Pillsbury SG. Jr. Reproductive significance of changes in the endometrial cavity associated with exposure in utero to diethylstilbestrol. Am J Obstet Gynecol 1980;137:178–82.

23. Professional and Public Relations Committee of the Diethylstilbestrol and Adenosis Pproject of the Division of Cancer Control and Rehabilitation. Exposure in utero to diethylstilbestrol and related synthetic hormones. Association with vaginal and cervical cancers and other abnormalities. JAMA 1976;236:1107–9.

24. Burke L, Antonioli D, Friedman EA. Evolution of diethylstilbestrol-associated genital tract lesions. Obstet Gynecol 1981;57:79–84.

25. Heinonen OP, Slone D, Shapiro S. Birth Defects and Drugs in Pregnancy. Littleton:Publishing Sciences Group, 1977:389,91.

26. Ibid, 395.

27. Wiseman RA, Dodds-Smith IC. Cardiovascular birth defects and antenatal exposure to female sex hormones: a reevaluation of some base data. Teratology 1984;30:359–70.

28. Wilson JG, Brent RL. Are female sex hormones teratogenic? Am J Obstet Gynecol 1981;141:567–80.

29. Herbst AL, Hubby MM, Blough RR, Azizi F. A comparison of pregnancy experience in DES-exposed daughters. J Reprod Med 1980;24:62–9.

30. Barnes AB, Colton T, Gundersen J, Noller KL, Tilley BC, Strama T, Townsend DE, Hatab P, O'Brien PC. Fertility and outcome of pregnancy in women exposed in utero to diethylstilbestrol. N Engl J Med 1980;302:609–13.

31. Veridiano NP, Dilke I, Rogers J, Tancer ML. Reproductive performance of DES-exposed female progeny. Obstet Gynecol 1981;58:58–61.

32. Mangan CE, Borow L, Burnett-Rubin MM, Egan V, Giuntoli RL, Mikuta JJ. Pregnancy outcome in 98 women exposed to diethylstilbestrol in utero, their mothers, and unexposed siblings. Obstet Gynecol 1982; 59:315–9.

33. Williamson HO, Sowell GA, Smith HE. Spontaneous rupture of gravid uterus in a patient with diethylstilbestrol-type changes. Am J Obstet Gynecol 1984;150:158–60.

34. Barnes AB. Menstrual history and fecundity of women exposed and unexposed in utero to diethylstilbestrol. J Reprod Med 1984;29:651–5.

35. Kaufman RH, Noller K, Adam E, Irwin J, Gray M, Jefferies JA, Hilton J. Upper genital tract abnormalities and pregnancy outcome in diethylstilbestrol-exposed progeny. Am J Obstet Gynecol 1984;148:973–84.

36. Peress MR, Tsai CC, Mathur RS, Williamson HO. Hirsutism and menstrual patterns in women exposed to diethylstilbestrol in utero. Am J Obstet Gynecol 1982;144:135–40.

37. Verkauf BS. Discussion. Op cit, 139–40.

38. Schmidt G, Fowler WC Jr. Gynecologic operative experience in women exposed to DES in utero. South Med J 1982;75:260–3.

39. Haney AF, Hammond MG. Infertility in women exposed to diethylstilbestrol in utero. J Reprod Med 1983;28:851–6.

40. Stillman RJ, Miller LC. Diethylstilbestrol exposure in utero and endometriosis in infertile females. Fertil Steril 1984;41:369–72.

41. Henderson BE, Benton B, Cosgrove M, Baptista J, Aldrich J, Townsend D, Hart W, Mack TM. Urogenital tract abnormalities in sons of women treated with diethylstilbestrol. Pediatrics 1976;58:505–7.

42. Gill WB, Schumacher GFB, Bibbo M. Pathological semen and anatomical abnormalities of the genital tract in human male subjects exposed to diethylstilbestrol in utero. J Urol 1977;117:477–80.

43. Gill WB, Schumacher GFB, Bibbo M, Strous FH, Schoenberh HW. Association of diethylstilbestrol exposure in utero with cryptorchidism, testicular hypoplasia and semen abnormalities. J Urol 1979;122:36–9.
44. Gill WB, Schumacher GFB, Bibbo M. Structural and functional abnormalities in the sex organs of male offspring of mothers treated with diethylstilbestrol (DES). J Reprod Med 1976;16:147–53.
45. Driscoll SG, Taylor SM. Effects of prenatal maternal estrogen on the male urogenital system. Obstet Gynecol 1980;56:537–42.
46. Bibbo M, Gill WB, Azizi F, Blough R, Fang VS, Rosenfield RL, Schaumacher GFB, Sleeper K, Sonek MG, Wied GL. Follow-up study of male and female offspring of DES-exposed mothers. Obstet Gynecol 1977;49:1–8.
47. Shy KK, Stenchever MA, Karp LE, Berger RE, Williamson RA, Leonard J. Genital tract examinations and zona-free hamster egg penetration tests from men exposed in utero to diethylstilbestrol. Fertil Steril 1984;42:772–8.
48. Leary FJ, Resseguie LJ, Kurland LT, O'Brien PC, Emslander RF, Noller KL. Males exposed in utero to diethylstilbestrol. JAMA 1984;252:2984–9.
49. Conley GR, Sant GR, Ucci AA, Mitcheson HD. Seminoma and epididymal cysts in a young man with known diethylstilbestrol exposure in utero. JAMA 1983;249:1325–6.
50. Yalom ID, Green R, Fisk N. Prenatal exposure to female hormones. Effect on psychosexual development in boys. Arch Gen Psychiatry 1973;28:554–61.
51. Burke L, Apfel RJ, Fischer S, Shaw J. Observations on the psychological impact of diethylstilbestrol exposure and suggestions on management. J Reprod Med 1980;24:99–102.

Name: **DIGITALIS**

Class: **Cardiac Glycoside**   Risk Factor: **C**

Fetal Risk Summary

No reports linking digitalis or the various digitalis glycosides with congenital defects have been located. Animal studies have failed to show a teratogenic effect (1). Rapid passage to the fetus has been observed after digoxin and digitoxin (2–9). Okita and co-workers (2) found the amount of digitoxin recovered from the fetus was dependent on the length of gestation. In the late 1st trimester, only 0.05–0.10% of the injected dose was recovered from three fetuses. Digitoxin metabolites accounted for 0.18 to 0.33%. At 34 weeks of gestation, digitoxin recovery was 0.85% and metabolites 3.49% from one fetus. Average cord concentrations of digoxin in 3 reports were 50, 81, and 83% of the maternal serum (3, 4, 9). Highest fetal concentrations of digoxin in the 2nd half of pregnancy were found in the heart (5). The fetal heart has only a limited binding capacity for digoxin in the 1st half of pregnancy (5). In animals, amniotic fluid acts as a reservoir for digoxin, but no data are available in humans after prolonged treatment (5). The pharmacokinetics of digoxin in pregnant women have been reported (10, 11). Digoxin has been used for both maternal and fetal indications during all stages of gestation without causing fetal harm (12–23).

Fetal toxicity resulting in neonatal death has been reported after maternal overdose (24). The mother, in her 8th month of pregnancy, took an estimated 8.9 mg of digitoxin as a single dose. Delivery occurred 4 days later. The baby demonstrated digitalis cardiac effects until death at age 3 days from prolonged intrauterine anoxia.

In a series of 22 multiparous patients maintained on digitalis, spontaneous labor occurred more than 1 week earlier than in 64 matched controls (25). The first stage of labor in the treated patients averaged 4.3 hours vs 8 hours in the control group.

In contrast, Ho and co-workers (26) found no effect on duration of pregnancy or labor in 122 patients with heart disease.

Breast Feeding Summary

Digoxin is excreted into breast milk. Data for other cardiac glycosides have not been located. Digoxin milk:plasma ratios have varied from 0.6 to 0.9 (4, 7, 27, 28). Although these amounts seem high, they represent very small amounts of digoxin due to significant maternal protein binding. No adverse effects in the nursing infant have been reported. The American Academy of Pediatrics considers digoxin compatible with breast-feeding (29).

References

1. Shepard TH. *Catalog of Teratogenic Agents*, ed. 3. Baltimore:The Johns Hopkins University Press, 1980:116–7.
2. Okita GT, Plotz EF, Davis ME. Placental transfer of radioactive digitoxin in pregnant women and its fetal distribution. Circ Res 1956;4:376–80.
3. Rogers MC, Willserson JT, Goldblatt A, Smith TW. Serum digoxin concentrations in the human fetus, neonate and infant. N Engl J Med 1972;287:1010–3.
4. Chan V, Tse TF, Wong V. Transfer of digoxin across the placenta and into breast milk. Br J Obstet Gynaecol 1978;85:605–9.
5. Saarikoski S. Placental transfer and fetal uptake of ^{3}H-digoxin in humans. Br J Obstet Gynaecol 1976;83:879–84.
6. Allonen H, Kanto J, Lisalo E. The foeto-maternal distribution of digoxin in early human pregnancy. Acta Pharmacol Toxicol 1976;39:477–80.
7. Finley JP, Waxman MB, Wong PY, Lickrish GM. Digoxin excretion in human milk. J Pediatr 1979;94:339–40.
8. Soyka LF. Digoxin: placental transfer, effects on the fetus, and therapeutic use in the newborn. Clin Perinatol 1975;2:23–35.
9. Padeletti L, Porciani MC, Scimone G. Placental transfer of digoxin (beta-methyl-digoxin) in man. Int J Clin Pharmacol Biopharm 1979;17:82–3.
10. Marzo A, Lo Cicero G, Brina A, Zuliani G, Ghirardi P, Pardi G. Preliminary data on the pharmaco-kinetics of digoxin in pregnancy. Boll Soc Ital Biol Sper 1980;56:219–23.
11. Luxford AME, Kellaway GSM. Pharmacokinetics of digoxin in pregnancy. Eur J Clin Pharmacol 1983;25:117–21.
12. Lingman G, Ohrlander S, Ohlin P. Intrauterine digoxin treatment of fetal paroxysmal tachycardia: case report. Br J Obstet Gynaecol 1980;87:340–2.
13. Kerenyi TD, Gleicher N, Meller J, Brown E, Steinfeld L, Chitkara U, Raucher H. Transplacental cardioversion of intrauterine supraventricular tachycardia with digitalis. Lancet 1980;2:393–4.
14. Harrigan JT, Kangos JJ, Sikka A, Spisso KR, Natarajan N, Rosenfeld D, Leiman S, Korn D. Successful treatment of fetal congestive heart failure secondary to tachycardia. N Engl J Med 1981;304:1527–9.
15. Diro M, Beydoun SN, Jaramillo B, O'Sullivan MJ, Kieval J. Successful pregnancy in a woman with a left ventricular cardiac aneurysm: a case report. J Reprod Med 1983;28:559–63.
16. Heaton FC, Vaughan R. Intrauterine supraventricular tachycardia: cardioversion with maternal digoxin. Obstet Gynecol 1982;60:749–52.
17. Simpson PC, Trudinger BJ, Walker A, Baird PJ. The intrauterine treatment of fetal cardiac failure in a twin pregnancy with an acardiac, acephalic monster. Am J Obstet Gynecol 1983;147:842–4.
18. Spinnato JA, Shaver DC, Flinn GS, Sibai BM, Watson DL, Marin-Garcia J. Fetal supraventricular tachycardia: in utero therapy with digoxin and quinidine. Obstet Gynecol 1984;64:730–5.
19. Bortolotti U, Milano A, Mazzucco A, Valfre C, Russo R, Valente M, Schivazappa L, Thiene G, Gallucci V. Pregnancy in patients with a porcine valve bioprosthesis. Am J Cardiol 1982;50:1051–4.
20. Rotmensch HH, Elkayam E, Frishman W. Antiarrhythmic drug therapy during pregnancy. Ann Intern Med 1983;98:487–97.
21. Gleicher N, Elkayam U. Cardiac problems in pregnancy. II. Fetal aspects: advances in intrauterine diagnosis and therapy. JAMA 1984;252:78–80.

22. Golichowski AM, Caldwell R, Hartsough A, Peleg D. Pharmacologic cardioversion of intrauterine supraventricular tachycardia. A case report. J Reprod Med 1985;30:139–44.
23. Reece EA, Romero R, Santulli T, Kleinman CS, Hobbins JC. In utero diagnosis and management of fetal tachypnea. A case report. J Reprod Med 1985;30:221–4.
24. Sherman JL Jr, Locke RV. Transplacental neonatal digitalis intoxication. Am J Cardiol 1960;6:834–7.
25. Weaver JB, Pearson JF. Influence of digitalis on time of onset and duration of labour in women with cardiac disease. Br Med J 1973;3:519–20.
26. Ho PC, Chen TY, Wong V. The effect of maternal cardiac disease and digoxin administration on labour, fetal weight and maturity at birth. Aust NZ J Obstet Gynaecol 1980;20:24–7.
27. Levy M, Granit L, Laufer N. Excretion of drugs in human milk. N Engl J Med 1977;297:789.
28. Loughnan PM. Digoxin excretion in human breast milk. J Pediatr 1978;92:1019–20.
29. Committee on Drugs, American Academy of Pediatrics. The transfer of drugs and other chemicals into human breast milk. Pediatrics 1983;72:375–85.

Name: **DIGITOXIN**

Class: **Cardiac Glycoside**   Risk Factor: **C$_M$**

Fetal Risk Summary

See Digitalis.

Breast Feeding Summary

See Digitalis.

Name: **DIGOXIN**

Class: **Cardiac Glycoside**   Risk Factor: **C$_M$**

Fetal Risk Summary

See Digitalis.

Breast Feeding Summary

See Digitalis.

Name: **DIHYDROCODEINE BITARTRATE**

Class: **Narcotic Analgesic**   Risk Factor: **B***

Fetal Risk Summary

No reports linking the use of dihydrocodeine with congenital defects have been located. Usage in pregnancy is primarily confined to labor. Respiratory depression in the newborn has been reported to be less than with meperidine, but depression is probably similar when equianalgesic doses are compared (1–3).

[* Risk Factor D if used for prolonged periods or in high doses at term.]

Breast Feeding Summary

No data available.

References

1. Ruch WA, Ruch RM. A preliminary report on dihydrocodeine-scopolamine in obstetrics. Am J Obstet Gynecol 1957;74:1125–7.
2. Myers JD. A preliminary clinical evaluation of dihydrocodeine bitartrate in normal parturition. Am J Obstet Gynecol 1958;75:1096–100.
3. Bonica JJ. *Principles and Practice of Obstetric Analgesia and Anesthesia*. Philadelphia:FA Davis Co, 1967:245.

Name: **DIHYDROTACHYSTEROL**

Class: **Vitamin** Risk Factor: **A***

Fetal Risk Summary

Dihydrotachysterol is a synthetic analogue of vitamin D. It is converted in the liver to 25-hydroxydihydrotachysterol, an active metabolite. See Vitamin D.

[* Risk Factor D if used in doses above the RDA.]

Breast Feeding Summary

See Vitamin D.

Name: **DIMENHYDRINATE**

Class: **Antiemetic** Risk Factor: **B$_M$**

Fetal Risk Summary

Dimenhydrinate is the chlorotheophylline salt of the antihistamine diphenhydramine. A prospective study in 1963 compared dimenhydrinate usage in three groups of patients: 266 with malformed infants and two groups of 266 each without malformed infants (1). No difference in usage of the drug was found between the three groups. The Collaborative Perinatal Project monitored 50,282 mother-child pairs, 319 of which had 1st trimester exposure to dimenhydrinate (2). For use anytime in pregnancy, 697 exposures were recorded (3). In neither case was evidence found to suggest a relationship to large categories of major or minor malformations. Two possible associations with individual malformations were found, but the statistical significance of these are unknown. Independent confirmation is required to determine the actual risk.

Cardiovascular defects (5 cases)
Inguinal hernia (8 cases)

Two reports have described the oxytocic effect of intravenous dimenhydrinate on the full-term uterus (4, 5). When used either alone or with oxytocin, the result was a smoother, shorter labor.

Breast Feeding Summary

No data available.

References

1. Mellin GW, Katzenstein M. Meclozine and fetal abnormalities. Lancet 1963;1:222–3.
2. Heinonen OP, Slone D, Shapiro S. *Birth Defects and Drugs in Pregnancy*. Littleton:Publishing Sciences Group, 1977:367–70.
3. *Ibid*, 440.
4. Watt LO. Oxytocic effects of dimenhydrinate in obstetrics. Can Med Assoc J 1961;84:533–4.
5. Rotter CW, Whitaker JL, Yared J. The use of intravenous Dramamine to shorten the time of labor and potentiate analgesia. Am J Obstet Gynecol 1958:75:1101–4.

Name: **DIMETHINDENE**

Class: **Antihistamine**   Risk Factor: **C**

Fetal Risk Summary

No data available. See Chlorpheniramine for representative agent in this class.

Breast Feeding Summary

No data available.

Name: **DIMETHOTHIAZINE**

Class: **Antihistamine**   Risk Factor: **C**

Fetal Risk Summary

No data available. See Promethazine for representative agent in this class.

Breast Feeding Summary

No data available.

Name: **DIOXYLINE**

Class: **Vasodilator**   Risk Factor: **C**

Fetal Risk Summary

No data available.

Breast Feeding Summary

No data available.

Name: **DIPHEMANIL**

Class: **Parasympatholytic**   Risk Factor: **C**

Fetal Risk Summary

Diphemanil is an anticholinergic quarternary ammonium methylsulfate. No reports of its use in pregnancy have been located (see also Atropine).

Breast Feeding Summary

No data available (see also Atropine).

Name: **DIPHENADIONE**

Class: **Anticoagulant**   Risk Factor: **D**

Fetal Risk Summary

See Coumarin Derivatives.

Breast Feeding Summary

See Coumarin Derivatives.

Name: **DIPHENHYDRAMINE**

Class: **Antihistamine**   Risk Factor: **C**

Fetal Risk Summary

The Collaborative Perinatal Project monitored 50,282 mother-child pairs, 595 of which had 1st trimester exposure to diphenhydramine (1). For use anytime during pregnancy, 2,948 exposures were recorded (2). In neither case was evidence found to suggest a relationship to large categories of major or minor malformations. Several possible associations with individual malformations were found, but the statistical significance of these are unknown (1–3). Independent confirmation is required to determine the actual risk.

Genitourinary malformations (other than hypospadias)
    (5 cases)
Hypospadias (3 cases)
Eye and ear defects (3 cases)

Syndromes (other than Down's syndrome) (3 cases)
Inguinal hernia (13 cases)
Clubfoot (5 cases)
Any ventricular septal defect
    (open or closing) (5 cases)
Malformations of diaphragm (3 cases)

Cleft palate and diphenhydramine usage in the 1st trimester were statistically associated in a 1974 study (4). A group of 599 children with oral clefts were compared to 590 controls without clefts. *In utero* exposures to diphenhydramine in the groups were 20 and 6, respectively, a significant difference. However, in a 1971 report significantly fewer infants with malformations were exposed to antihistamines in the 1st trimester as compared to controls (5). Diphenhydramine was the second most commonly used antihistamine.

Diphenhydramine withdrawal was reported in a newborn infant whose mother had taken 150 mg/day during pregnancy (6). Generalized tremulousness and diarrhea began on the 5th day of life. Treatment with phenobarbital resulted in the gradual disappearance of the symptoms.

Breast Feeding Summary

Diphenhydramine is excreted into human breast milk, but levels have not been reported (7). Although the levels are not thought to be high enough after therapeutic doses to affect the infant, the manufacturer considers the drug contraindicated in nursing mothers. The reason given for this is the increased sensitivity of newborn or premature infants to antihistamines. However, the American Academy of Pediatrics considers diphenhydramine compatible with breast-feeding (8).

References

1. Heinonen OP, Sloan D, Shapiro S. *Birth Defects and Drugs in Pregnancy*. Littleton:Publishing Sciences Group, 1977:323–37.
2. *Ibid*, 437.
3. *Ibid*, 475.
4. Saxen I. Cleft palate and maternal diphenhydramine intake. Lancet 1974;1:407–8.
5. Nelson MM, Forfar JO. Associations between drugs administered during pregnancy and congenital abnormalities of the fetus. Br Med J 1971;1:523–7.
6. Parkin DE. Probable Benadryl withdrawal manifestations in a newborn infant. J Pediatr 1974;85:580.
7. O'Brien TE. Excretion of drugs in human milk. Am J Hosp Pharm 1974;31:844–54.
8. Committee on Drugs, American Academy of Pediatrics. The transfer of drugs and other chemicals into human breast milk. Pediatrics 1983;72:375–83.

Name: **DIPHENOXYLATE**

Class: **Antidiarrheal**   Risk Factor: **C$_M$**

Fetal Risk Summary

Diphenoxylate is a narcotic related to meperidine. It is available only in combination with atropine (to discourage overdosage) for the treatment of diarrhea. No reports linking it with congenital defects have been located. In one study, no malformed infants were observed after 1st trimester exposure in seven patients (1).

Breast Feeding Summary

The manufacturer reports that diphenoxylate is excreted into breast milk, and the effects of that drug and atropine may be evident in the nursing infant (2). One source recommends the drug should not be used in lactating mothers (3). However, the American Academy of Pediatrics considers the combination of diphenoxylate and atropine to be compatible with breast-feeding (4).

References

1. Heinonen OP, Slone D, Shapiro S. *Birth Defects and Drugs in Pregnancy.* Littleton:Publishing Sciences Group, 1977:287.
2. Product information. Lomotil. Searle & Co, 1985.
3. Stewart JJ. Gastrointestinal drugs. In Wilson JT, ed. *Drugs in Breast Milk.* Balgowlah, Australia: ADIS Press, 1981:71.
4. Committee on Drugs, American Academy of Pediatrics. The transfer of drugs and other chemicals into human breast milk. Pediatrics 1983;72:375–83.

Name: **DIPYRIDAMOLE**

Class: **Vasodilator**   Risk Factor: **C**

Fetal Risk Summary

No reports linking the use of dipyridamole with congenital defects have been located. The drug has been used in pregnancy as a vasodilator and to prevent thrombus formation in patients with prosthetic heart valves (1–8). A single intravenous 30-mg dose of dipyridamole was shown to increase uterine perfusion in the 3rd trimester in 10 patients (9). In one pregnancy, a malformed infant was delivered, but the mother was also taking Coumadin (1). The multiple defects in the infant were consistent with the fetal warfarin syndrome (see Coumarin Derivatives). In another report, the only complication was a maternal blood loss of 700 ml, about twice normal, after vaginal delivery (6).

In a randomized, nonblind study to prevent pre-eclampsia, 52 high-risk patients treated from the 13th week of gestation through delivery with daily doses of 300 mg of dipyridamole plus 150 mg of aspirin were compared to 50 high-risk controls (10). Four treated patients were excluded from analysis (spontaneous abortions before 16 weeks) vs five controls (two lost to follow-up plus three spontaneous abortions). Hypertension occurred in 41 patients—19 treated and 22 controls. The outcome of pregnancy was significantly better in treated patients in three areas: pre-eclampsia (none vs 6, $p < 0.01$), fetal and neonatal loss (none vs 5, $p < 0.02$), and severe intrauterine growth retardation (none vs 4, $p < 0.05$). No fetal malformations were observed in either group.

Breast Feeding Summary

Dipyridamole is excreted into breast milk but in levels too low to measure with current techniques (7). The manufacturer knows of no problems in breast-fed infants whose mothers were taking this drug (7).

References

1. Tejani N. Anticoagulant therapy with cardiac valve prosthesis during pregnancy. Obstet Gynecol 1973;42:785–93.

2. Del Bosque MR. Dipiridamol and anticoagulants in the management of pregnant women with cardiac valvular prosthesis. Ginecol Obstet Mex 1973;33:191–8.
3. Littler WA, Bonnar J, Redman CWG, Beilin LJ, Lee GD. Reduced pulmonary arterial compliance in hypertensive patients. Lancet 1973;1:1274–8.
4. Biale Y, Lewenthal H, Gueron M, Beu-Aderath N. Caesarean section in patient with mitral-valve prosthesis. Lancet 1977;1:907.
5. Taguchi K. Pregnancy in patients with a prosthetic heart valve. Surg Gynecol Obstet 1977;145:206–8.
6. Ahmad R, Rajah SM, Mearns AJ, Deverall PB. Dipyridamole in successful management of pregnant women with prosthetic heart valve. Lancet 1976;2:1414–5.
7. Bowers PA, Boehringer Engelheim Ltd, 1981. Personal communication.
8. Biale Y, Cantor A, Lewenthal H, Gueron M. The course of pregnancy in patients with artificial heart valves treated with dipyridamole. Int J Gynaecol Obstet 1980;18:128–32.
9. Lauchkner W, Schwarz R, Retzke U. Cardiovascular action of dipyridamole in advanced pregnancy. Zentralbl Gynaekol 1981;103:220–7.
10. Beaufils M, Uzan S, Donsimoni R, Colau JC. Prevention of pre-eclampsia by early antiplatelet therapy. Lancet 1985;1:840–2.

Name: **DISOPYRAMIDE**

Class: **Antiarrhythmic**   Risk Factor: **C**

Fetal Risk Summary

No reports linking the use of disopyramide with congenital defects in humans or animals have been located. At term, a cord blood level of 0.9 μg/ml (39% of maternal serum) was measured 6 hours after a maternal 200-mg dose (1). Disopyramide has been used throughout pregnancy without evidence of congenital abnormality or growth retardation (1–3). Early onset of labor has been reported in one patient (4). The mother, in her 32nd week of gestation, was given 300 mg orally, followed by 100 or 150 mg every 6 hours for posterior mitral leaflet prolapse. Uterine contractions, without vaginal bleeding or cervical changes, and abdominal pain occurred 1–2 hours after each dose. When disopyramide was stopped, symptoms subsided over the next 4 hours. Oxytocin induction 1 week later resulted in the delivery of a healthy infant. In another patient, use of 200 mg twice daily during the 18th and 19th weeks of pregnancy, was not associated with uterine contractions or other observable adverse effects in the mother or fetus (5).

Breast Feeding Summary

Disopyramide is excreted into breast milk (6). In a woman taking 200 mg three times daily, samples obtained on the 5th–8th day of treatment revealed a mean milk:plasma ratio of 0.9 for disopyramide and 5.6 for the active metabolite. Neither drug was detected in the infant's plasma and no adverse effects were noted. The American Academy of Pediatrics considers disopyramide compatible with breast-feeding (7).

References

1. Shaxted EJ, Milton PJ. Disopyramide in pregnancy: a case report. Curr Med Res Opin 1979;6:70–2.
2. Anderson MS, Searle & Co, 1981. Personal communication.
3. Rotmensch HH, Elkayam U, Frishman W. Antiarrhythmic drug therapy during pregnancy. Ann Intern Med 1983;98:487–97.

4. Leonard RF, Braun TE, Levy AM. Initiation of uterine contractions by disopyramide during pregnancy. N Engl J Med 1978;299:84–5.
5. Stokes IM, Evans J, Stone M. Myocardial infarction and cardiac arrest in the second trimester followed by assisted vaginal delivery under epidural analgesia at 38 weeks gestation. Case report. Br J Obstet Gynaecol 1984;91:197–8.
6. Barnett DB, Hudson SA, McBurney A. Disopyramide and its N-monodesalkyl metabolite in breast milk. Br J Clin Pharmacol 1982;14:310–2.
7. Committee on Drugs, American Academy of Pediatrics. The transfer of drugs and other chemicals into human breast milk. Pediatrics 1983;72:375–83.

Name: **DISULFIRAM**

Class: **Unclassified**   Risk Factor: **X**

Fetal Risk Summary

Disulfiram is used to prevent alcohol consumption in patients with a history of alcohol abuse. The use of disulfiram in pregnancy has been described in seven pregnancies (1, 2). Four of the eight fetuses exposed (one set of twins) had congenital defects and a spontaneous abortion occurred in a fifth fetus. Malformations observed were:

Clubfoot (2 cases) (1)
Multiple anomalies with VACTERL syndrome
   (radial aplasia, vertebral fusion, tracheoesophageal fistula) (1 case) (2)
Phocomelia of lower extremities (1 case) (2)

In the two infants described by Nora and co-workers (2), exposure occurred in the 1st trimester, and the use of other teratogens, including alcohol, was excluded (2). Although controversial, heavy alcohol intake prior to conception has been suspected of producing the fetal alcohol syndrome (3–5). However, the anomalies described in the four infants exposed to disulfiram do not fit the pattern seen with the fetal alcohol syndrome. Based on the above data, termination of pregnancy should be considered if disulfiram is used during the 1st trimester.

Breast Feeding Summary

No data available.

References

1. Favre-Tissot M, Delatour P. Psychopharmacologie et teratogenese a propos du sulfirame: essai experimental. Ann Med-psychol 1965;1:735-40. As cited in Shepard TH. Catalog of Teratogenic Agents, ed. 3. Baltimore:Johns Hopkins University Press, 1980:127.
2. Nora AH, Nora JJ, Blu J. Limb-reduction anomalies in infants born to disulfiram-treated alcoholic mothers. Lancet 1977;2:664.
3. Scheiner AP, Donovan CM, Bartoshesky LE. Fetal alcohol syndrome in child whose parents had stopped drinking. Lancet 1979;1:1077–8.
4. Scheiner AP. Fetal alcohol syndrome in a child whose parents had stopped drinking. Lancet 1979;2:858.
5. Smith DW, Graham JM Jr. Fetal alcohol syndrome in child whose parents had stopped drinking. Lancet 1979;2:527.

Name: **DOBUTAMINE**

Class: **Sympathomimetic (Adrenergic)**   Risk Factor: **C**

Fetal Risk Summary

Dobutamine is structurally related to dopamine. It has not been studied in human pregnancy (see also Dopamine). Short-term use in one patient with a myocardial infarction at 18 weeks gestation was not associated with any known adverse effects (1).

Breast Feeding Summary

No data available.

References

1. Stokes IM, Evans J, Stone M. Myocardial infarction and cardiac arrest in the second trimester followed by assisted vaginal delivery under epidural analgesia at 38 weeks gestation. Case report. Br J Obstet Gynaecol 1984;91:197–8.

Name: **DOCUSATE CALCIUM**

Class: **Laxative**   Risk Factor: **C**

Fetal Risk Summary

See Docusate Sodium.

Breast Feeding Summary

No data available.

Name: **DOCUSATE POTASSIUM**

Class: **Laxative**   Risk Factor: **C**

Fetal Risk Summary

See Docusate Sodium.

Breast Feeding Summary

No data available.

Name: **DOCUSATE SODIUM**

Class: **Laxative**   Risk Factor: **C**

Fetal Risk Summary

No reports linking the use of docusate sodium with congenital defects have been located. Docousate sodium is a common ingredient in many laxative preparations available to the public. In a large prospective study, 116 patients were exposed to this drug during pregnancy (1). No evidence for an association with malformations was found.

Chronic use of 150–250 mg or more per day of docusate sodium throughout pregnancy was suspected of causing hypomagnesemia in a mother and her newborn (2). At 12 hours of age, the neonate exhibited jitteriness which resolved spontaneously. Neonatal serum magnesium levels ranged from 0.9 to 1.1 mg/100 ml between 22 and 48 hours of age with a maternal level of 1.2 mg/100 ml on the 3rd postpartum day. All other laboratory parameters were normal.

Breast Feeding Summary

No data available.

References

1. Heinonen OP, Slone D, Shapiro S. *Birth Defects and Drugs in Pregnancy*. Littleton:Publishing Sciences Group, 1977:442.
2. Schindler AM. Isolated neonatal hypomagnesaemia associated with maternal overuse of stool softener. Lancet 1984;2:822.

Name: **DOPAMINE**

Class: **Sympathomimetic (Adrenergic)**   Risk Factor: **C**

Fetal Risk Summary

Experience with dopamine in human pregnancy is limited. Dopamine has been used to prevent renal failure in nine oligoanuric eclamptic patients by re-establishing diuresis (1). The drug has also been used to treat hypotension in 26 patients undergoing cesarean section (2). No newborn adverse effects attributable to dopamine administration were observed in either study. Since dopamine is indicated only for life-threatening situations, chronic use would not be expected. Animal studies have shown both increases and decreases in uterine blood flow (2). Human studies on uterine perfusion have not been conducted.

Breast Feeding Summary

No data available.

References

1. Gerstner G, Grunberger W. Dopamine treatment for prevention of renal failure in patients with severe eclampsia. Clin Exp Obstet Gynecol 1980;7:219–22.
2. Clark RB, Brunner JA III. Dopamine for the treatment of spinal hypotension during cesarean section. Anesthesiology 1980;53:514–7.

Name: **DOTHIEPIN**

Class: **Antidepressant**   Risk Factor: **D**

Fetal Risk Summary

No data available. See Imipramine.

Breast Feeding Summary

No data available. See Imipramine.

Name: **DOXEPIN**

Class: **Antidepressant**   Risk Factor: **C**

Fetal Risk Summary

No reports linking the use of doxepin with congenital defects have been located (see also Imipramine). Paralytic ileus has been observed in an infant exposed to doxepin at term (1). The condition was thought to be primarily due to chlorpromazine, but the authors speculated that the anticholinergic effects of doxepin worked synergistically with the phenothiazine.

Breast Feeding Summary

No data available. See Imipramine.

References

1. Falterman CG, Richardson CJ. Small left colon syndrome associated with maternal ingestion of psychotropic drugs. J Pediatr 1980;97:308–10.

Name: **DOXORUBICIN**

Class: **Antineoplastic**   Risk Factor: **D**

Fetal Risk Summary

Several reports have described the use of doxorubicin in pregnancy, including three during the 1st trimester (1–14). One of the fetuses exposed during the 1st trimester to doxorubicin, cyclophosphamide, and unshielded radiation was born with an imperforate anus and rectovaginal fistula (14). At about 3 months of age, the infant was small with a head circumference of 46 cm (under the fifth percentile) but was doing well after two corrective surgeries (14). The only other complication observed in exposed infants was transient polycythemia and hyperbilirubinemia in one subject.

The drug was not detected in the amniotic fluid at 20 weeks of gestation, which suggested that the drug was not transferred in measurable amounts to the fetus (1). Placental transfer was demonstrated in a 17-week-old aborted fetus, however, using high-performance liquid chromatography (15). High concentrations were found in fetal liver, kidney, and lung. The drug was not detected in amniotic fluid (<1.66 ng/ml), brain, intestine, or gastrocnemius muscle.

Long-term studies of growth and mental development of offspring exposed to doxorubicin and other antineoplastic agents in the 2nd trimester, the period of neuroblast multiplication, have not been conducted (16). Doxorubicin may cause reversible testicular dysfunction (17, 18). Similarly, normal pregnancies have occurred in women treated before conception with doxorubicin (19).

Breast Feeding Summary

No data available.

References

1. Roboz J, Gleicher N, Wu K, Kerenyi T, Holland J. Does doxorubicin cross the placenta? Lancet 1979;2:1382–3.
2. Khursid M, Saleem M. Acute leukaemia in pregnancy. Lancet 1978;2:534–5.
3. Newcomb M, Balducci L, Thigpen JT, Morrison FS. Acute leukemia in pregnancy: successful delivery after cytarabine and doxorubicin. JAMA 1978;239:2691–2.
4. Hassenstein E, Riedel H. Zur teratogenitat von Adriamycin ein fallbericht. Geburtshilfe Frauenheilkd 1978;38:131–3.
5. Cervantes F, Rozman C. Adriamycina y embarazo. Sangre (Barc) 1980;25:627.
6. Pizzuto J, Aviles A, Noriega L, Niz J, Morales M, Romero F. Treatment of acute leukemia during pregnancy: presentation of nine cases. Cancer Treat Rep 1980;64:679–83.
7. Tobias JS, Bloom HJG. Doxorubicin in pregnancy. Lancet 1980;1:776.
8. Garcia V, San Miguel J, Borrasca AL. Doxorubicin in the first trimester of pregnancy. Ann Intern Med 1981;94:547.
9. Garcia V, San Miguel IJ, Borrasca AL. Adriamycin and pregnancy. Sangre (Barc) 1981;26:129.
10. Dara P, Slater LM, Armentrout SA. Successful pregnancy during chemotherapy for acute leukemia. Cancer 1981;47:845–6.
11. Lowenthal RM, Funnell CF, Hope DM, Stewart IG, Humphrey DC. Normal infant after combination chemotherapy including teniposide for Burkitt's lymphoma in pregnancy. Med Pediatr Oncol 1982;10:165–9.
12. Webb GA. The use of hyperalimentation and chemotherapy in pregnancy: a case report. Am J Obstet Gynecol 1980;137:263–6.
13. Gililland J, Weinstein L. The effects of cancer chemotherapeutic agents on the developing fetus. Obstet Gynecol Surv 1983;38:6–13.
14. Murray CL, Reichert JA, Anderson J, Twiggs LB. Multimodal cancer therapy for breast cancer in the first trimester of pregnancy. A case report. JAMA 1984;252:2607–8.
15. D'Incalci M, Broggini M, Buscaglia M, Pardi G. Transplacental passage of doxorubicin. Lancet 1983;1:75.
16. Dobbing J. Pregnancy and leukaemia. Lancet 1977;1:1155.
17. Lendon M, Palmer MK, Hann IM, Shalet SM, Jones PHM. Testicular histology after combination chemotherapy in childhood for acute lymphoblastic leukaemia. Lancet 1978;2:439–41.
18. Schilsky RL, Lewis BJ, Sherins RJ, Young RC. Gonadal dysfunction in patients receiving chemotherapy for cancer. Ann Intern Med 1980;93:109–14.
19. Rustin GJS, Booth M, Dent J, Salt S, Rustin F, Bagshawe KD. Pregnancy after cytotoxic chemotherapy for gestational trophoblastic tumours. Br Med J 1984;288:103–6.

Name: **DOXYCYCLINE**

Class: **Antibiotic**   Risk Factor: **D**

Fetal Risk Summary

See Tetracycline.

Breast Feeding Summary

Doxycycline is excreted into breast milk. Oral doxycycline, 200 mg, followed after 24 hours by 100 mg, was given to 15 nursing mothers (1). Milk:plasma ratios determined at 3 and 24 hours after the second dose were 0.3 and 0.4, respectively. Mean milk concentrations were 0.77 and 0.38 μg/ml.

Theoretically, dental staining and inhibition of bone growth could occur in breast-fed infants whose mothers were consuming doxycycline. However, this theoretical possibility seems remote, since in infants exposed to a closely related antibiotic, tetracycline, serum levels were undetectable (less than 0.05 μg/ml) (2). The American Academy of Pediatrics considers tetracycline compatible with breast-feeding (3). Three potential problems may exist for the nursing infant even though there are no reports in this regard: modification of bowel flora, direct effects on the infant, and interference with the interpretation of culture results if a fever work-up is required.

References

1. Morganti G, Ceccarelli G, Ciaffi EG. Comparative concentrations of a tetracycline antibiotic in serum and maternal milk. Antibiotica 1968;6:216-23.
2. Posner AC, Prigot A, Konicoff NG. Further observations on the use of tetracycline hydrochloride in prophylaxis and treatment of obstetric infections. In *Antibiotics Annual 1954-55*. New York:Medical Encyclopedia, 594–8.
3. Committee on Drugs, American Academy of Pediatrics. The transfer of drugs and other chemicals into human breast milk. Pediatrics 1983;72:375–83.

Name: **DOXYLAMINE**

Class: **Antiemetic**   Risk Factor: **B**

Fetal Risk Summary

The combination of doxylamine, pyridoxine, and dicyclomine (Bendectin, others) was originally marketed in 1956. The drug was reformulated in 1976 (United States and Canada) to eliminate dicyclomine because that component was not found to contribute to its effectiveness as an antiemetic. Over 33 million women have taken this product during pregnancy, making it one of the most heavily prescribed drugs in this condition. The manufacturer ceased producing the drug combination in 1983 because of litigation over its alleged association with congenital limb defects. Although no longer available as a fixed combination, the individual components are still marketed by various manufacturers.

Over 160 cases of congenital defects have been reported in the literature or to the Food and Drug Administration (FDA) as either "Bendectin-induced" or associated with use of the drug in the 1st trimester (1–6). Defects observed included skeletal, limb, and cardiac anomalies as well as cleft lip or palate. A possible association between doxylamine-pyridoxine and diaphragmatic hernia was reported in 1983 and assumed to reflect earlier findings of a large prospective study (6). Authors of the latter study, however, cautioned that their results were uninterpretable, even when apparently strong associations existed, without independent confirmation (7, 8). In a large case-control study, infants exposed *in utero* to the combination had a slightly greater relative risk (1.40) for congenital defects (9). The risk was more than doubled (2.91) if the mother also smoked. An increased risk for heart value anomalies (2.99) was also found. A significant association was discovered in this study between Bendectin and pyloric stenosis (4.33 to 5.24), representing about a 4-fold increase in risk for this anomaly. Similarly, the Boston

Collaborative Drug Surveillance Programs reported preliminary findings to the FDA indicating a 2.7-fold increase in risk (10). A 1983 case-control study, however, found no association between Bendectin use and the anomaly (11). In evaluating these three reports, the FDA considered them the best available information on the topic but concluded that no definite causal relationship had been shown between Bendectin and pyloric stenosis (10). In addition, the FDA commented that even if there was evidence for an association between the drug and the defect, it did not necessarily constitute evidence of a causal relationship since the nausea and vomiting itself, or the underlying disease causing the condition, could be responsible for the increased risk (10). A 1985 study, which appeared after the above FDA evaluation, found a possible association with pyloric stenosis but could not eliminate the possibility that it was due to other factors (12). A minimal relationship was found between congenital heart disease and doxylamine (Bendectin) use in early pregnancy in another 1985 report comparing 298 cases with 738 controls (13). The authors went to great efforts to assure that their drug histories were accurate. Their findings provided evidence that if an association did exist at all, it was very small.

The evidence indicating that doxylamine/pyridoxine is safe in pregnancy is impressive. A number of large studies, many reviewed by Holmes in 1983 (30), have discovered no relationship between the drug and birth weight, length, head circumference, gestational age, congenital malformations, or other adverse fetal outcome (14–30). The 1985 study by Aselton and co-workers (12) also found no association with defects other than pyloric stenosis. One study was unable to observe chromosomal abnormalities associated with the drug combination while a second study found that use of the drugs was not related to the Poland anomaly (unilateral absence of the pectoralis major muscle with or without epsilateral hand defect) (31, 32).

Although the literature supports the relative safety of this product, when compared to the normal background of malformations, it is not possible to state that it was completely without risk to the fetus (34). As Brent (33) and Holmes (30) have indicated, it is not possible to completely prove a negative effect in the field of teratology.

Breast Feeding Summary

No data available (see also Pyridoxine).

References

1. Korcok M. The Bendectin debate. Can Med Assoc J 1980;123:922–8.
2. Soverchia G, Perri PF. Two cases of malformations of a limb in infants of mothers treated with an antiemetic in a very early phase of pregnancy. Pediatr Med Chir 1981;3:97–9.
3. Donaldson GL, Bury RG. Multiple congenital abnormalities in a newborn boy associated with maternal use of fluphenazine enanthate and other drugs during pregnancy. Acta Paediatr Scand 1982;71:335–8.
4. Grodofsky MP, Wilmott RW. Possible association of use of Bendectin during early pregnancy and congenital lung hypoplasia. N Engl J Med 1984;311:732.
5. Fisher JE, Nelson SJ, Allen JE, Holsman RS. Congenital cystic adenomatoid malformation of the lung. A unique variant. Am J Dis Child 1982;136:1071–4.
6. Bracken MB, Berg A. Bendectin (Debendox) and congenital diaphragmatic hernia. Lancet 1983;1:586.
7. Heinonen OP, Slone D, Shapiro S. Birth Defects and Drugs in Pregnancy. Littleton:Publishing Sciences Group, 1977:474–5.

8. Ohga K, Yamanaka R, Kinumaki H, Awa S, Kobayashi N. Bendectin (Debendox) and congenital diaphragmatic hernia. Lancet 1983;1:930.

9. Eskenazi B, Bracken MB. Bendectin (Debendox) as a risk factor for pyloric stenosis. Am J Obstet Gynecol 1982;144:919–24.

10. FDA Drug Bulletin. Bendectin and pyloric stenosis. 1983;13:14–5.

11. Mitchell AA, Schwingl PJ, Rosenberg L, Louik C, Shapiro S. Birth defects in relation to Bendectin use in pregnancy. II. Pyloric stenosis. Am J Obstet Gynecol 1983;147:737–42.

12. Aselton P, Jick H, Milunsky A, Hunter JR, Stergachis A. First-trimester drug use and congenital disorders. Obstet Gynecol 1985;65:451–5.

13. Zierler S, Rothman KJ. Congenital heart disease in relation to maternal use of Bendectin and other drugs in early pregnancy. N Engl J Med 1985;313:347–52.

14. Milkovich L, van den Berg BJ. An evaluation of the teratogenicity of certain antinauseant drugs. Am J Obstet Gynecol 1976;125:244–8.

15. Shapiro S, Heinonen OP, Siskind V, Kaufman DW, Monson RR, Slone D. Antenatal exposure to doxylamine succinate and dicyclomine hydrochloride (Bendectin) in relation to congenital malformations, perinatal mortality rate, birth weight, intelligence quotient score. Am J Obstet Gynecol 1977;128:480–5.

16. Rothman KJ, Flyer DC, Goldblatt A, Kreidberg MB. Exogenous hormones and other drug exposures of children with congenital heart disease. Am J Epidemiol 1979;109:433–9.

17. Bunde CA, Bowles DM. A technique for controlled survey of case records. Curr Ther Res 1963;5:245–8.

18. Gibson GT, Collen DP, McMichael AJ, Hartshorne JM. Congenital anomalies in relation to the use of doxylamine/dicyclomine and other antenatal factors. An ongoing prospective study. Med J Aust 1981;1:410–4.

19. Correy JF, Newman NM. Debendox and limb reduction deformities. Med J Aust 1981;1:417–8.

20. Clarke M, Clayton DG. Safety of debendox. Lancet 1981;2:659–60.

21. Harron DWG, Griffiths K, Shanks RG. Debendox and congenital malformations in Northern Ireland. Br Med J 1980;4:1379–81.

22. Smithells RW, Sheppard S. Teratogenicity testing in humans: a method demonstrating safety of Bendectin. Teratology 1978;17:31–5.

23. Morelock S, Hingson R, Kayne H, et al. Bendectin and fetal development: a study at Boston City Hospital. Am J Obstet Gynecol 1982;142:209–13.

24. Cordero JF, Oakley GP, Greenberg F, James LM. Is Bendectin a teratogen? JAMA 1981;245:2307–10.

25. Mitchell AA, Rosenberg L, Shapiro S, Slone D. Birth defects related to Bendectin use in pregnancy: I. Oral clefts and cardiac defects. JAMA 1981;245:2311–4.

26. Fleming DM, Knox JDE, Crombie DL. Debendox in early pregnancy and fetal malformation. Br Med J 1981;283:99–101.

27. Greenberg G, Inman WHW, Weatherall JAC, Adelstein AM, Haskey JC. Maternal drug histories and congenital abnormalities. Br Med J 1977;2:853–6.

28. Aselton PJ, Jick H. Additional follow-up of congenital limb disorders in relation to Bendectin use. JAMA 1983;250:33–4.

29. McCredie J, Kricker A, Elliott J, Forrest J. The innocent bystander: doxylamine/dicyclomine/pyridoxine and congenital limb defects. Med J Aust 1984;140:525–7.

30. Holmes LB. Teratogen update: Bendectin. Teratology 1983;27:277–81.

31. Hughes DT, Cavanagh N. Chromosomal studies on children with phocomelia, exposed to Debendox during early pregnancy. Lancet 1983;2:399.

32. David TJ. Debendox does not cause the Poland anomaly. Arch Dis Child 1982;57:479–80.

33. Brent RR. Editorial. The Bendectin saga: another American tragedy. Teratology 1983;27:283–6.

Name: **DROPERIDOL**

Class: **Tranquilizer** Risk Factor: **C**

Fetal Risk Summary

Droperidol is a butyrophenone derivative structurally related to haloperidol (see also Haloperidol). The drug has been used to promote analgesia for cesarean section patients without affecting the respiration of the newborn (1, 2). The placental transfer of droperidol is slow (2). The authors have used the drug as a continuous intravenous infusion for hyperemesis gravidarum during the 2nd and 3rd trimesters without apparent fetal harm (3).

Breast Feeding Summary

No data available.

References

1. Smith AM, McNeil WT. Awareness during anesthesia. Br Med J 1969;1:572–3.
2. Zhdanov GG, Ponomarev GM. The concentration of droperidol in the venous blood of the parturients and in the blood of the umbilical cord of neonates. Anesteziol Reanimatol 1980;4:14–6.
3. Briggs GG, Freeman RK. Unpublished data. 1985.

Name: **DYPHYLLINE**

Class: **Spasmolytic/Vasodilator** Risk Factor: **C$_M$**

Fetal Risk Summary

No data available. See also Theophylline.

Breast Feeding Summary

Dyphylline is excreted into breast milk. In 20 normal lactating women a single 5 mg/kg intramuscular dose produced an average milk:plasma ratio of 2.08 (1). The milk and serum elimination rates were equivalent. The American Academy of Pediatrics considers dyphylline compatible with breast-feeding (2).

References

1. Jarboe CH, Cook LN, Malesic I, Fleischaker J. Dyphylline elimination kinetics in lactating women: blood to milk transfer. J Clin Pharmacol 1981;21:405–10.
2. Committee on Drugs, American Academy of Pediatrics. The transfer of drugs and other chemicals into human breast milk. Pediatrics 1983;72:375–83.

Name: **ECHOTHIOPHATE**

Class: **Parasympathomimetic (Cholinergic)**   Risk Factor: **C**

Fetal Risk Summary

Echothiophate is used in the eye. No reports of its use in pregnancy have been located. As a quaternary ammonium compound, it is ionized at physiologic pH and transplacental passage in significant amounts would not be expected (see also Neostigmine).

Breast Feeding Summary

No data available.

Name: **EDROPHONIUM**

Class: **Parasympathomimetic (Cholinergic)**   Risk Factor: **C**

Fetal Risk Summary

Edrophonium is a quaternary ammonium chloride with anticholinesterase activity used in the diagnosis of myasthenia gravis. The drug has been used in pregnancy without producing fetal malformations (1–7). Because it is ionized at physiologic pH, edrophonium would not be expected to cross the placenta in significant amounts. Caution has been advised against the use in pregnancy of intravenous anticholinesterases since they may cause premature labor (1, 3). This effect on the pregnant uterus increases near term. Intramuscular neostigmine should be used in place of intravenous edrophonium if diagnosis of myasthenia gravis is required in a pregnant patient (3). In one report, however, intravenous edrophonium was given to a woman in the 2nd trimester in an unsuccessful attempt to treat tachycardia secondary to Wolff-Parkinson-White syndrome (6). No effect on the uterus was mentioned, and she continued with an uneventful full-term pregnancy.

Transient muscle weakness has been observed in about 20% of newborns of mothers with myasthenia gravis (8). The neonatal myasthenia is due to transplacental passage of anti-acetylcholine receptor immunoglobulin G antibodies (8).

Breast Feeding Summary

Because it is ionized at physiologic pH, edrophonium would not be expected to be excreted into breast milk (9).

References

1. Foldes FF, McNall PG. Myasthenia gravis: a guide for anesthesiologists. Anesthesiology 1962;23:837–72.
2. Plauche WG. Myasthenia gravis in pregnancy. Am J Obstet Gynecol 1964;88:404–9.
3. McNall PG, Jafarnia MR. Management of myasthenia gravis in the obstetrical patient. Am J Obstet Gynecol 1965;92:518–25.
4. Hay DM. Myasthenia gravis in pregnancy. J Obstet Gynaecol Br Commonw 1969;76:323–9.
5. Heinonen OP, Slone D, Shapiro S. *Birth Defects and Drugs in Pregnancy*. Littleton:Publishing Sciences Group, 1977:345–56.
6. Gleicher N, Meller J, Sandler RZ, Sullum S. Wolff-Parkinson-White syndrome in pregnancy. Obstet Gynecol 1981;58:748–52.
7. Blackhall MI, Buckley GA, Roberts DV, Roberts JB, Thomas BH, Wilson A. Drug-induced neonatal myasthenia. J Obstet Gynaecol Br Commonw 1969;76:157–62.
8. Plauche WG. Myasthenia gravis in pregnancy: an update. Am J Obstet Gynecol 1979;135:691–7.
9. Wilson JT. Pharmacokinetics of drug excretion. In Wilson JT, ed. *Drugs in Breast Milk*. Balgowlah, Australia: ADIS Press, 1981:17.

Name: **EPHEDRINE**

Class: **Sympathomimetic (Adrenergic)** Risk Factor: **C**

Fetal Risk Summary

Ephedrine is a sympathomimetic used widely for bronchial asthma, allergic disorders, hypotension, and the alleviation of symptoms caused by upper respiratory infections. It is a common component of proprietary mixtures containing antihistamines, bronchodilators, and other ingredients. Thus, it is difficult to separate the effects of ephedrine on the fetus from other drugs, disease states, and viruses. Ephedrine-like drugs are teratogenic in some animal species, but human teratogenicity has not been suspected (1, 2). Recent data may require a reappraisal of this opinion. The Collaborative Perinatal Project monitored 50,282 mother-child pairs, 373 of which had 1st trimester exposure to ephedrine (3). For use anytime during pregnancy, 873 exposures were recorded (4). No evidence for a relationship to large categories of major or minor malformations or to individual defects was found. However, an association in the 1st trimester was found between the sympathomimetic class of drugs as a whole and minor malformations (not life-threatening or major cosmetic defects), inguinal hernia, and clubfoot (3). These data are presented as a warning that indiscriminate use of ephedrine, especially in the 1st trimester, is not without risk.

Ephedrine is routinely used to treat or prevent maternal hypotension following spinal anesthesia (5–8). Significant increases in fetal heart rate and beat-to-beat variability may occur (5). These effects are not due to decreases in uterine blood flow and subsequent asphyxia.

Breast Feeding Summary

A single case report has been located describing adverse effects in a 3-month-old nursing infant of a mother consuming a long-acting preparation containing 120 mg of *d*-isoephedrine and 6 mg of dexbrompheniramine (9). The mother had begun taking the preparation on a twice daily schedule 1 or 2 days prior to onset of the infant's symptoms. The infant exhibited irritability, excessive crying, and disturbed sleeping patterns which resolved spontaneously within 12 hours when breast-feeding was stopped.

References

1. Nishimura H, Tanimura T. *Clinical Aspects of the Teratogenity of Drugs*. Amsterdam:Excerpta Medica, 1976:231.
2. Shepard TH. *Catalog of Teratogenic Agents*, ed 3. Baltimore:The Johns Hopkins University Press, 1980:134–5.
3. Heinonen OP, Slone D, Shapiro S. *Birth Defects and Drugs in Pregnancy*. Littleton:Publishing Sciences Group, 1977:345–56.
4. *Ibid*, 439.
5. Wright RG, Shnider SM, Levinson G, Rolbin SH, Parer JT. The effect of maternal administration of ephedrine on fetal heart rate and variability. Obstet Gynecol 1981;57:734–8.
6. Antoine C, Young BK. Fetal lactic acidosis with epidural anesthesia. Am J Obstet Gynecol 1982;142:55–9.
7. Datta S, Alper MH, Ostheimer GW, Weiss JB. Method of ephedrine administration and nausea and hypotension during spinal anesthesia for cesarean section. Anesthesiology 1982;56:68–70.
8. Antoine C, Young BK. Fetal lactic acidosis with epidural anesthesia. Am J Obstet Gynecol 1982;142:55–9.
9. Mortimer EA Jr. Drug toxicity from breast milk? Pediatrics 1977;60:780–1.

Name: **EPINEPHRINE**

Class: **Sympathomimetic (Adrenergic)**   Risk Factor: **C**

Fetal Risk Summary

Epinephrine is a sympathomimetic that is widely used for conditions such as shock, glaucoma, allergic reactions, bronchial asthma, and nasal congestion. Since it occurs naturally in all humans, it is difficult to separate the effects of its administration from effects on the fetus induced by endogenous epinephrine, other drugs, disease states, and viruses. The drug readily crosses the placenta (1). Epinephrine is teratogenic in some animal species, but human teratogenicity has not been suspected (2, 3). Recent data may require a reappraisal of this opinion. The Collaborative Perinatal Project monitored 50,282 mother-child pairs, 189 of which had 1st trimester exposure to epinephrine (4). For use anytime during pregnancy, 508 exposures were recorded (5). A statistically significant association was found between 1st trimester use of epinephrine and major and minor malformations. An association was also found with inguinal hernia after both 1st trimester and anytime use (6). Although not specified, these data may reflect the potentially severe maternal status for which epinephrine administration is indicated. Caution is advised, however, against the indiscriminate use of epinephrine in pregnancy.

Breast Feeding Summary

No data available.

References

1. Morgan CD, Sandler M, Panigel M. Placental transfer of catecholamines in vitro and in vivo. Am J Obstet Gynecol 1972;112:1068–75.
2. Nishimura H, Tanimura T. *Clinical Aspects of the Teratogenicity of Drugs*. Amsterdam:Excerpta Medica, 1976:231.

3. Shepard TH. *Catalog of Teratogenic Agents*, ed 3. Baltimore:The Johns Hopkins University Press, 1980:134–5.
4. Heinonen OP, Slone D, Shapiro S. *Birth Defects and Drugs in Pregnancy*. Littleton:Publishing Sciences Group, 1977:345–56.
5. *Ibid*, 439.
6. *Ibid*, 477, 492.

Name: **ERGOCALCIFEROL**
Class: **Vitamin**   Risk Factor: **A***

Fetal Risk Summary

Ergocalciferol (vitamin D_2) is converted in the liver to 25-hydroxyergocalciferol which in turn is converted in the kidneys to 1,25-dihydroxyergocalciferol, one of the active forms of vitamin D. See Vitamin D.

[* Risk Factor D if used in doses above the RDA.]

Breast Feeding Summary

See Vitamin D.

Name: **ERYTHRITYL TETRANITRATE**
Class: **Vasodilator**   Risk Factor: **C$_M$**

Fetal Risk Summary

See Nitroglycerin or Amyl Nitrite.

Breast Feeding Summary

No data available.

Name: **ERYTHROMYCIN**
Class: **Antibiotic**   Risk Factor: **B**

Fetal Risk Summary

No reports linking the use of erythromycin with congenital defects have been located. The drug crosses the placenta but in concentrations too low to treat most pathogens (1–3). Fetal tissue levels increase after multiple doses (3). However, a case has been described in which erythromycin was used successfully to treat maternal syphilis but failed to adequately treat the fetus (4). During pregnancy, erythromycin serum concentrations vary greatly as compared to normal men and nonpregnant women, which might account for the low levels observed in the fetus (5).

The estolate salt of erythromycin has been observed to induce hepatotoxicity in pregnant patients (6). Approximately 10% of 161 women treated with the estolate form in the 2nd trimester had abnormally elevated levels of SGOT, which returned to normal after therapy was discontinued.

The use of erythromycin in the 1st trimester was reported in a mother who delivered an infant with left absence-of-tibia syndrome (7). The mother was also exposed to other drugs which makes a relationship to the antibiotic unlikely.

The Collaborative Perinatal Project monitored 50,282 mother-child pairs, 79 of which had 1st trimester exposure to erythromycin (8). For use anytime during pregnancy, 230 exposures were recorded (9). No evidence was found to suggest a relationship to large categories of major and minor malformations or to individual defects. Erythromycin, like many other antibiotics, lowers urine estriol concentrations (see also Ampicillin for mechanism and significance) (11). The antibiotic has been used during the 3rd trimester to reduce maternal and infant colonization with group B β-hemolytic streptococcus (12, 13). Erythromycin has also been used during pregnancy for the treatment of genital mycoplasma (14, 15). A reduction in the rates of pregnancy loss and low-birth-weight infants was seen in patients with mycoplasma infection after treatment with erythromycin.

Breast Feeding Summary

Erythromycin is excreted into breast milk (8). Following oral doses of 400 mg every 8 hours, milk levels ranged from 0.4 to 1.6 μg/ml. Oral doses of 2 g/day produced milk concentrations of 1.6–3.2 μg/ml. The milk:plasma ratio in both groups was 0.5. No reports of adverse effects in infants exposed to erythromycin in breast milk have been located. However, three potential problems exist for the nursing infant: modification of bowel flora, direct effects on the infant, and interference with the interpretation of culture results if a fever work-up is required.

References

1. Heilman FR, Herrell WE, Wellman WE, Geraci JE. Some laboratory and clinical observations on a new antibiotic, erythromycin (Ilotycin). Proc Staff Meet Mayo Clin 1952;27:285–304.
2. Kiefer L, Rubin A, McCoy JB, Foltz EL. The placental transfer of erythromycin. Am J Obstet Gynecol 1955;69:174–7.
3. Philipson A, Sabath LD, Charles D. Transplacental passage of erythromycin and clindamycin. N Engl J Med 1973;288:1219–20.
4. Fenton LJ, Light LJ. Congenital syphilis after maternal treatment with erythromycin. Obstet Gynecol 1976;47:492–4.
5. Philipson A, Sabath LD, Charles D. Erythromycin and clindamycin absorption and elimination in pregnant women. Clin Pharmacol Ther 1976;19:68–77.
6. McCormack WM, George H, Donner A, Kodgis LF, Albert S, Lowe EW, Kass EH. Hepatotoxicity of erythromycin estolate during pregnancy. Antimicrob Agents Chemother 1977;12:630–5.
7. Jaffe P, Liberman MM, McFadyen I, Valman HB. Incidence of congenital limb-reduction deformities. Lancet 1975;1:526–7.
8. Heinonen OP, Slone D, Shapiro S. *Birth Defects and Drugs in Pregnancy*. Littleton:Publishing Sciences Group, 1977:297–313.
9. *Ibid*, 435.
10. Knowles JA. Drugs in milk. Ped Currents 1972;21:28–32.
11. Gallagher JC, Ismail MA, Aladjem S. Reduced urinary estriol levels with erythromycin therapy. Obstet Gynecol 1980;56:381–2.

12. Merenstein GB, Todd WA, Brown G, Yost CC, Luzier T. Group B β-hemolytic streptococcus: randomized controlled treatment study at term. Obstet Gynecol 1980;55:315–8.
13. Easmon CSF, Hastings MJG, Deeley J, Bloxham B, Rivers RPA, Marwood R. The effect of intrapartum chemoprophylaxis on the vertical transmission of group B streptococci. Br J Obstet Gynaecol 1983;90:633–5.
14. Quinn PA, Shewchuk AB, Shuber J, Lie KI, Ryan E, Chipman ML, Nocilla DM. Efficacy of antibiotic therapy in preventing spontaneous pregnancy loss among couples colonized with genital myco-plasmas. Am J Obstet Gynecol 1983;145:239–44.
15. Kass EH, McCormack WM. Genital mycoplasma infection and perinatal morbidity. N Engl J Med 1984;311:258.

Name: **ESTRADIOL**

Class: **Estrogenic Hormone** Risk Factor: **X**

Fetal Risk Summary

Estradiol and its salts (cypionate, valerate) are used for treatment of menopausal symptoms, female hypogonadism and primary ovarian failure. The Collaborative Perinatal Project monitored 614 mother-child pairs with 1st trimester exposure to estrogenic agents (including 48 with exposure to estradiol) (1). An increase in the expected frequency of cardiovascular defects, eye and ear anomalies, and Down's syndrome was found for estrogens as a group but not for estradiol (1, 2). Re-evaluation of these data in terms of timing of exposure, vaginal bleeding in early pregnancy, and previous maternal obstetrical history, however, failed to support an association between estrogens and cardiac malformations (3). An earlier study also failed to find any relationship with nongenital malformations (4).

Developmental changes in the psychosexual performance of boys has been attributed to *in utero* exposure to estradiol and progesterone (5). The mothers received an estrogen/progestogen regimen for their diabetes. Hormone-exposed males demonstrated a trend to have less heterosexual experience and fewer masculine interests than controls. Estradiol has been administered to women in labor in an attempt to potentiate the cervical ripening effects of prostaglandins (6). No detectable effect was observed. Use of estrogenic hormones during pregnancy is contraindicated.

Breast Feeding Summary

Estradiol is used to suppress postpartum breast engorgement in patients who do not desire to breast-feed. Following the administration of vaginal suppositories containing 50 or 100 mg of estradiol in six lactating women, less than 10% of the dose appeared in breast milk (7).

References

1. Heinonen OP, Slone D, Shapiro S. *Birth Defects and Drugs in Pregnancy*. Littleton:Publishing Sciences Group, 1977:389,391.
2. *Ibid*, 395.
3. Wiseman RA, Dodds-Smith IC. Cardiovascular birth defects and antenatal exposure to female sex hormones: a reevaluation of some base data. Teratology 1984;30:359–70.
4. Wilson JG, Brent RL. Are female sex hormones teratogenic? Am J Obstet Gynecol 1981;141:567–80.

5. Yalom ID, Green R, Fisk N. Prenatal exposure to female hormones. Effect of psychosexual development in boys. Arch Gen Psychiatry 1973;28:554–61.
6. Luther ER, Roux J, Popat R, Gardner A, Gray J, Soubiran E, Korcaz Y. The effect of estrogen priming on induction of labor with prostaglandins. Am J Obstet Gynecol 1980;137:351–7.
7. Nilsson S, Nygren KG, Johansson EDB. Transfer of estradiol to human milk. Am J Obstet Gynecol 1978;132:653–7.

Name: ESTROGENS, CONJUGATED

Class: **Estrogenic Hormone**   Risk Factor: X_M

Fetal Risk Summary

Conjugated estrogens are a mixture of estrogenic substances (primarily estrone). The Collaborative Perinatal Project monitored 13 mother-child pairs who were exposed to conjugated estrogens during the 1st trimester (1). An increased risk for malformations was found, although identification of the malformations was not provided. Estrogenic agents as a group were monitored in 614 mother-child pairs. An increase in the expected frequency of cardiovascular defects, eye and ear anomalies, and Down's syndrome was reported (2). Re-evaluation of these data in terms of timing of exposure, vaginal bleeding in early pregnancy, and previous maternal obstetrical history, however, failed to support an association between estrogens and cardiac malformations (3). An earlier study also failed to find any relationship with nongenital malformations (4). No adverse effects were observed in one infant exposed during the 1st trimester to conjugated estrogens (5). However, in a second infant exposed during the 4th–7th weeks of gestation, multiple anomalies were found (6):

> Cleft palate, wormian bones, heart defect, dislocated
>   hips, absent tibiae, polydactyly, and abnormal
>   dermal pattern

Conjugated estrogens have been used to induce ovulation in anovulatory women (7). They have also been used as partially successful contraceptives when given within 72 hours of unprotected, midcycle coitus (8). No fetal adverse effects were mentioned in either of these reports.

Breast Feeding Summary

No reports of adverse effects from conjugated estrogens in the nursing infant have been located. It is possible that decreased milk volume and decreased nitrogen and protein content could occur (see Mestranol, Ethinyl Estradiol).

References

1. Heinonen OP, Slone D, Shapiro S. *Birth Defects and Drugs in Pregnancy*. Littleton:Publishing Sciences Group, 1977:389,391.
2. *Ibid*, 395.
3. Wiseman RA, Dodds-Smith IC. Cardiovascular birth defects and antenatal exposure to female sex hormones: a reevaluation of some base data. Teratology 1984;30:359–70.

4. Wilson JG, Brent RL. Are female sex hormones teratogenic? Am J Obstet Gynecol 1981;141:567–80.
5. Hagler S, Schultz A, Hankin H, Kunstadter RH. Fetal effects of steroid therapy during pregnancy. Am J Dis Child 1963;106:586–90.
6. Ho CK, Kaufman RL, McAlister WH. Congenital malformations. Am J Dis Child 1975;129:714–6.
7. Price R. Pregnancies using conjugated oestrogen therapy. Med J Aust 1980;2:341–2.
8. Dixon GW, Schlesselman JJ, Ory HW, Blye RP. Ethinyl estradiol and conjugated estrogens as postcoital contraceptives. JAMA 1980;244:1336–9.

Name: **ESTRONE**

Class: **Estrogenic Hormone**   Risk Factor: **X**

Fetal Risk Summary

See Estrogens, Conjugated.

Breast Feeding Summary

See Estrogens, Conjugated.

Name: **ETHACRYNIC ACID**

Class: **Diuretic**   Risk Factor: **D**

Fetal Risk Summary

Ethacrynic acid is a potent diuretic. It has been used for toxemia, pulmonary edema, and diabetes insipidus during pregnancy (1–10). Although it is not an animal teratogen and limited 1st trimester human experience has not shown an increased incidence of malformations, ethacrynic acid is not recommended for use in pregnant women (11, 12). Diuretics do not prevent or alter the course of toxemia, and they may decrease placental perfusion (see also Chlorothiazide) (13–15). Ototoxicity has been observed in a mother and her newborn following the use of ethacrynic acid and kanamycin during the 3rd trimester (16).

Breast Feeding Summary

No data available (see also Chlorothiazide). The manufacturer considers ethacrynic acid contraindicated in nursing mothers (11).

References

1. Delgado Urdapilleta J, Dominguez Robles H, Villalobos Roman M, Perez Diaz A. Ethacrynic acid in the treatment of toxemia of pregnancy. Ginecol Obstet Mex 1968;23:271–80.
2. Felman D, Theoleyre J, Dupoizat H. Investigation of ethacrynic acid in the treatment of excessive gain in weight and pregnancy arterial hypertension. Lyon Med 1967;217:1421–8.
3. Sands RX, Vita F. Ethacrynic acid (a new diuretic), pregnancy, and excessive fluid retention. Am J Obstet Gynecol 1968;101:603–9.
4. Kittaka S, Aizawa M, Tokue I, Shimizu M. Clinical results in edecril tablet in the treatment of toxemia of late pregnancy. Obstet Gynecol (Jpn) 1968;36:934–7.

5. Mahon R, Dubecq JP, Baudet E, Coqueran J. Use of edecrin in obstetrics. Bull Fed Soc Gynecol Obstet Lang Fr 1968;20:440–2.
6. Imaizumi S, Suzuoki Y, Torri M, et al. Clinical trial of ethacrynic acid (Edecril) for toxemia of pregnancy. Jpn J Med Consult New Remedies 1969;6:2364–8.
7. Young BK, Haft JI. Treatment of pulmonary edema with ethacrynic acid during labor. Am J Obstet Gynecol 1970;107:330–1.
8. Harrison KA, Ajabor LN, Lawson JB. Ethacrynic acid and packed-blood-cell transfusion in treatment of severe anaemia in pregnancy. Lancet 1971;1:11–4.
9. Fort AT, Morrison JC, Fisk SA. Iatrogenic hypokalemia of pregnancy by furosemide and ethacrynic acid: two case reports. J Reprod Med 1971;6:21–2.
10. Pico I, Greenblatt RB. Endocrinopathies and infertility. IV. Diabetes insipidus and pregnancy. Fertil Steril 1969;20:384–92.
11. Product information. Edecrin. Merck Sharp & Dohme, 1985.
12. Wilson AL, Matzke GR. The treatment of hypertension in pregnancy. Drug Intell Clin Pharm 1981;15:21–6.
13. Pitkin RM, Kaminetzky HA, Newton M, Pritchard JA. Maternal nutrition: a selective review of clinical topics. Obstet Gynecol 1972;40:773–85.
14. Lindheimer MD, Katz AI. Sodium and diuretics in pregnancy. N Engl J Med 1973;288:891–4.
15. Christianson R, Page EW. Diuretic drugs and pregnancy. Obstet Gynecol 1976;48:647–52.
16. Jones HC. Intrauterine ototoxicity: a case report and review of literature. J Natl Med Assoc 1973;65:201–3.

Name: **ETHAMBUTOL**

Class: **Antituberculosis Agent**　　　　　　　　Risk Factor: **B**

Fetal Risk Summary

No reports linking the use of ethambutol with congenital defects have been located. The literature supports the safety of ethambutol in combination with isoniazid during pregnancy (1–4). Bobrowitz (1) studied 38 patients (42 pregnancies) receiving antitubercular therapy of two to five drug regimens. The minor abnormalities noted were within the expected frequency of occurrence. Lewit and co-workers (2) observed six aborted fetuses at 5–12 weeks of age. Embryonic optic systems were specifically examined and were found normal. However, long-term follow-up examinations for ocular damage have not been reported, and this has caused concern in some clinicians (5).

Breast Feeding Summary

No reports have been located describing the use of ethambutol in lactating women. The American Academy of Pediatrics considers ethambutol compatible with breast-feeding (6).

References

1. Bobrowitz ID. Ethambutol in pregnancy. Chest 1974;66:20–4.
2. Lewit T, Nebel L, Terracina S, Karman S. Ethambutol in pregnancy: observations on embryogenesis. Chest 1974;66:25–6.
3. Snider DE, Layde PM, Johnson MW, Lyle MA. Treatment of tuberculosis during pregnancy. Am Rev Respir Dis 1980;122:65–79.
4. Brock PG, Roach M. Antituberculous drugs in pregnancy. Lancet 1981;1:43.
5. Wall MA. Treatment of tuberculosis during pregnancy. Am Rev Respir Dis 1980;122:989.

6. Committee on Drugs, American Academy of Pediatrics. The transfer of drugs and other chemicals into human breast milk. Pediatrics 1983;72:375–83.

Name: **ETHANOL**

Class: **Sedative** Risk Factor: **D***

Fetal Risk Summary

The teratogenic effects of ethanol (alcohol) have been recognized since antiquity, but this knowledge gradually fell into disfavor and was actually dismissed as superstition in the 1940's (1). Approximately three decades later, the characteristic pattern of anomalies that came to be known as the fetal alcohol syndrome (FAS) were rediscovered, first in France and then in the United States (2–5). By 1981, over 800 clinical and research papers on the FAS had been published (6).

Mild FAS (low birth weight) has been induced by the daily consumption of as few as two drinks (1 ounce of absolute alcohol) in early pregnancy, but the complete syndrome is usually seen when maternal consumption is four to five drinks (2–2.5 ounces of absolute alcohol) per day or more. The Council on Scientific Affairs of the American Medical Association and the American Council on Science and Health have each published reports on the consequences of maternal alcohol ingestion during pregnancy (7, 8). The incidence of the FAS, depending upon the population studied, is estimated to be between 1/300 and 1/2,000 live births with 30–40% of the offspring of alcoholic mothers expected to show the complete syndrome (7). The true incidence may be even higher since the diagnosis of FAS can be delayed for many years (9).

Heavy alcohol intake by the father prior to conception has been suspected of producing the FAS (10, 11). However, this association has been challenged (12). The report by the AMA Council states that growth retardation and some adverse aspects of fetal development may be due to paternal influence, but conclusive evidence for the full-blown FAS is lacking (7).

The mechanism of the teratogenic effect of ethanol is unknown but may be related to acetaldehyde, a metabolic by-product of ethanol (7). One researcher reported higher blood levels of acetaldehyde in mothers of children with FAS than in alcoholics who delivered normal children (13). However, the analysis techniques used in that study have been questioned and the high concentrations may have been due to artifactual formation of acetaldehyde (14). At the cellular level, alcohol, or one of its metabolites, may disrupt protein synthesis, resulting in cellular growth retardation with serious consequences for fetal brain development (15).

The complete FAS consists of abnormalities in three areas with a fourth area often involved: 1) craniofacial dysmorphology, 2) prenatal and antenatal growth deficiencies, 3) central nervous system dysfunction, and 4) various other abnormalities (7, 8). Problems occurring in the latter area include cardiac and renogenital defects and hemangiomas in about one-half of the cases (3–5, 16). Sandor and co-workers (17) described cardiac malformations in 43 patients (57%) in a series of 76 children with the FAS evaluated for 0–6 years (age: birth to 18 years). Functional murmurs (12 cases, 16%) and ventricular septal defects (20 patients,

26%) accounted for the majority of anomalies. Other cardiac lesions present, in descending order of frequency, were: double outlet right ventricle and pulmonary atresia, dextrocardia (with ventricular septal defect), patent ductus arteriosus with secondary pulmonary hypertension, and cor pulmonale. Liver abnormalities have also been reported (18, 19). Behavioral problems, including minimal brain dysfunction, are long-term effects of the FAS (1).

ANOMALIES ASSOCIATED WITH FETAL ALCOHOL SYNDROME (2–12, 16–28)
Craniofacial
    Eyes: short palpebral fissures, ptosis, strabismus,
        epicanthal folds, myopia, microphthalmia,
        blepharophimosis
    Ears: poorly formed conchae, posterior rotation
    Nose: short, upturned hypoplastic philtrum
    Mouth: prominent lateral palatine ridges, thinned upper
        vermilion, retrognathia in infancy, micrognathia or
        relative prognathia in adolescence, cleft lip or palate,
        small teeth with faulty enamel
    Maxilla: hypoplastic
Central nervous system
    Dysfunction demonstrated by mild to moderate
        retardation, microcephaly, poor coordination,
        hypotonia, irritability in infancy and
        hyperactivity in childhood
Growth
    Prenatal (affecting body length more than weight)
        and postnatal deficiency
Cardiac
    Murmurs, atrial septal defect, ventricular septal
        defect, great vessel anomalies, tetralogy of Fallot
Renogenital
    Labial hypoplasia, hypospadias, renal defects
Cutaneous
    Hemangiomas, hirsutism in infancy
Skeletal
    Abnormal palmar creases, pectus excavatum,
        restriction of joint movement, nail hypoplasia,
        radioulnar synostosis, pectus carinatum,
        bifid xiphoid, Klippel-Feil anomaly,
        scoliosis
Muscular
    Hernias of diaphragm, umbilicus or groin,
        diastasis recti

A strong association between moderate drinking (>1 ounce absolute alcohol twice per week) and 2nd trimester (15–27 weeks) spontaneous abortions has been found (20, 21). Alcohol consumption at this level may increase the risk of miscarriage by 2–4-fold, apparently by acting as an acute fetal toxin.

Two reports have described neural tube defects in six infants exposed to heavy amounts of alcohol during early gestation (29, 30). Lumbosacral meningomyelocele was observed in five of the newborns and anencephaly in one. One of the infants also had a dislocated hip and clubfeet (29).

A possible association between maternal drinking and clubfoot was proposed in a short 1985 report (31). Three of 43 infants, delivered from maternal alcoholics, had fetal talipes equinovarus (clubfoot), an incidence significantly greater than expected ($p < 0.00001$).

Gastroschisis has been observed in dizygotic twins delivered from a mother who consumed 5–6 ounces of absolute ethanol per day during the first 10 weeks of gestation (32). Although an association could not be proven, the authors speculated the defects resulted from the heavy alcohol ingestion.

A 1982 report described four offspring of alcoholic mothers with clinical and laboratory features of combined FAS and DiGeorge syndrome (33). Several characteristics of the two syndromes are similar, including craniofacial, cardiac, central nervous system, renal, and immune defects (33). Features not shared are hypoparathyroidism (part of DiGeorge syndrome) and skeletal anomalies (part of FAS). A possible causative relationship was suggested between maternal alcoholism and the DiGeorge syndrome.

An unusual chromosome anomaly was discovered in a 2-year-old girl whose mother drank heavily during early gestation (34). The infant's karotype revealed an isochromosome for the long arm of number 9: 46,XX,-9,+i(9q). The infant had several characteristics of the FAS, including growth retardation. The relationship between the chromosome defect and alcohol is unknown.

Prospective analysis of 31,604 pregnancies found that the percentage of newborns below the 10th percentile of weight for gestational age increased sharply as maternal alcohol intake increased (35). In comparison to nondrinkers, mean birth weight was reduced 14 g in those drinking less than one drink per day and 165 g in those drinking three to five drinks per day. The risk for growth retardation was markedly increased by the ingestion of one to two drinks each day. Another study discovered that women drinking more than 100 g of absolute alcohol per week at the time of conception had an increased risk of delivering a growth-retarded infant (36). The risk was twice that of women ingesting less than 50 g/week. Of special significance, the risk for growth retardation was not reduced if drinking was reduced later in pregnancy. However, a 1983 report found that if heavy drinkers reduced their consumption in midpregnancy, growth impairment was also reduced, although an increased incidence of congenital defects was still evident (37). Significantly smaller head circumferences have been measured in offspring of mothers who drank more than an average of 20 ml of alcohol per day compared to nondrinkers (38). In this same study, the incidence of major congenital anomalies in drinkers and nondrinkers was 1.2% vs none (38). These authors concluded that there was no safe level of alcohol consumption in pregnancy.

Infant development is impaired by exposure to alcohol during gestation. A significant correlation was found between heavy maternal alcohol intake and effects in the infant, including delayed mental and motor development, congenital anomalies, and growth retardation (39). Adverse effects after even short exposure were shown in an evaluation of 25 children 4–7 years of age whose mothers had been treated with alcohol infusions to prevent preterm labor (40). In comparison with matched controls, seven children born during or within 15 hours of termination of the infusion had significant pathologic conditions in developmental and personality evaluations.

Alcohol ingestion has been shown to abolish fetal breathing (41). Eleven women, at 37–40 weeks gestation, were given 0.25 g/kg of ethanol. Within 30 minutes, fetal breathing movements were almost abolished and remained so for 3 hours. No effect on gross fetal body movements or fetal heart rate was observed.

Neonatal alcohol withdrawal has been demonstrated in offspring of mothers ingesting a mean of 21 ounces of alcohol per week during pregnancy (42). In comparison to infants exposed to an equivalent amount of ethanol only during early gestation or to infants whose mothers never drank, the heavily exposed infants had significantly more withdrawal symptoms. No differences were found between the infants exposed only during early gestation and those never exposed. Electroencephalogram (EEG) testing of infants at 4–6 weeks of age indicated that irritability and tremors may be due to a specific effect of ethanol on the fetal brain and not due to withdrawal or prematurity (43). Persistent EEG hypersynchrony was observed in those infants delivered from mothers who drank more than 2 ounces of alcohol per day during pregnancy. The EEG findings were found in the absence of dysmorphology and as a result, the authors suggested this symptom should be added to the definition of the FAS (43).

Combined fetal alcohol and hydantoin syndromes have been described in several reports (44–47). The infants exhibited numerous similar features from exposure to alcohol and phenytoin. The possibility that the agents are also carcinogenic *in utero* has been suggested by the finding of ganglioneuroblastoma in a 35-month-old boy and Hodgkin's disease in a 45-month-old girl, both with the combined syndromes (see also Phenytoin) (45–47). Adrenal carcinoma in a 13-year-old girl with FAS has also been reported (48). These findings may be fortuitous but long-term follow-up of children with the FAS is needed.

In summary, ethanol is a teratogen and its use during pregnancy is associated with significant risk to the fetus and newborn. Heavy maternal use is related to a spectrum of defects collectively termed the fetal alcohol syndrome. Even moderate use may be related to spontaneous abortions, and developmental and behavioral dysfunction in the infant. A safe level of maternal alcohol consumption has not been established (7, 8, 49). Based on practical considerations, the American Council on Science and Health recommends that pregnant women limit their alcohol consumption to no more than two drinks daily (1 ounce of absolute alcohol) (8). However, the safest course for women who are pregnant, or who are planning to become pregnant, is abstinence (7, 49).

[* Risk Factor X if used in large amounts or for prolonged periods.]

Breast Feeding Summary

Although alcohol passes freely into breast milk, reaching concentrations approximating maternal serum levels, the effect on the infant is probably insignificant except in rare cases or at very high concentrations (50). The toxic metabolite of ethanol, acetaldehyde, apparently does not pass into milk even though considerable levels can be measured in the mother's blood (51). One report calculated the amount of alcohol received in a single feeding from a mother with a blood concentration of 100 mg/dl (equivalent to a heavy, habitual drinker) as 164 mg, an insignificant amount (52). Maternal blood alcohol levels have to reach 300 mg/dl before mild sedation might be seen in the baby.

Potentiation of severe hypoprothrombic bleeding, a pseudo-Cushing syndrome, and an effect on the milk-ejecting reflex have been reported in nursing infants of alcoholic mothers (53–55). The American Academy of Pediatrics considers maternal ethanol use compatible with breast-feeding, although adverse effects may occur (56).

References

1. Shaywitz BA. Fetal alcohol syndrome: an ancient problem rediscovered. Drug Ther 1978;8:95–108.
2. Lemoine P, Harroussean H, Borteyrn JP. Les enfants de parents alcooliques: anomalies observees. A propos de 127 cas. Quest Med 1968;25:477–82.
3. Ulleland CN. The offspring of alcoholic mothers. Ann NY Acad Sci 1972;197:167–9.
4. Jones KL, Smith DW, Ulleland CN, Streissguth AP. Pattern of malformation in offspring of chronic alcoholic mothers. Lancet 1973;1:1267–71.
5. Jones KL, Smith DW. Recognition of the fetal alcohol syndrome in early infancy. Lancet 1973;2:999–1001.
6. Abel EL. *Fetal Alcohol Syndrome, vol 1: An Annotated and Comprehensive Bibliography*. Boca Raton, FL: CRC Press, 1981. As cited in Anonymous. Alcohol and the fetus—is zero the only option? Lancet 1983;1:682–3.
7. Council on Scientific Affairs, American Medical Association. Fetal effects of maternal alcohol use. JAMA 1983;249:2517–21.
8. Alcohol use during pregnancy. A report by the American Council on Science and Health. As reprinted in Nutr Today 1982;17:29–32.
9. Lipson AH, Walsh DA, Webster WS. Fetal alcohol syndrome. A great paediatric imitator. Med J Aust 1983;1:266–9.
10. Scheiner AP, Donovan CM, Burtoshesky LE. Fetal alcohol syndrome in child whose parents had stopped drinking. Lancet 1979;1:1077–8.
11. Scheiner AP. Fetal alcohol syndrome in a child whose parents had stopped drinking. Lancet 1979;2:858.
12. Smith DW, Graham JM Jr. Fetal alcohol syndrome in child whose parents had stopped drinking. Lancet 1979;2:527.
13. Veghelyi PV. Fetal abnormality and maternal ethanol metabolism. Lancet 1983;2:53–4.
14. Ryle PR, Thomson AD. Acetaldehyde and the fetal alcohol syndrome. Lancet 1983;2:219–20.
15. Kennedy LA. The pathogenesis of brain abnormalities in the fetal alcohol syndrome: an integrating hypothesis. Teratology 1984;29:363–8.
16. FDA Drug Bulletin, *Fetal Alcohol Syndrome*, vol. 7. National Institute on Alcohol Abuse and Alcoholism, 1977:4.
17. Sandor GGS, Smith DF, MacLeod PM. Cardiac malformations in the fetal alcohol syndrome. J Pediatr 1981;98:771–3.
18. Habbick BF, Casey R, Zaleski WA, Murphy F. Liver abnormalities in three patients with fetal alcohol syndrome. Lancet 1979;1:580–1.
19. Khan A, Bader JL, Hoy GR, Sinks LF. Hepatoblastoma in child with fetal alcohol syndrome. Lancet 1979;1:1403–4.
20. Harlap S, Shiono PH. Alcohol, smoking and incidence of spontaneous abortions in the first and second trimester. Lancet 1980;2:173–6.
21. Kline J, Shrout P, Stein Z, Susser M, Warburton D. Drinking during pregnancy and spontaneous abortion. Lancet 1980;2:176–80.
22. Hanson JW, Jones KL, Smith DW. Fetal alcohol syndrome experience with 41 patients. JAMA 1976;235:1458–60.
23. Goetzman BW, Kagan J, Blankenship WJ. Expansion of the fetal alcohol syndrome. Clin Res 1975;23:100A.
24. DeBeukelaer MM, Randall CL, Stroud DR. Renal anomalies in the fetal alcohol syndrome. J Pediatr 1977;91:759–60.
25. Qazi Q, Masakawa A, Milman D, McGann B, Chua A, Haller J. Renal anomalies in fetal alcohol syndrome. Pediatrics 1979;63:886–9.

26. Steeg CN, Woolf P. Cardiovascular malformations in the fetal alcohol syndrome. Am Heart J 1979;98:636–7.
27. Halliday HL, Reid MM, McClure G. Results of heavy drinking in pregnancy. Br J Obstet Gynaecol 1982;89:892–5.
28. Beattie JO, Day RE, Cockburn F, Garg RA. Alcohol and the fetus in the west of Scotland. Br Med J 1983;287:17–20.
29. Friedman JM. Can maternal alcohol ingestion cause neural tube defects? J Pediatr 1982;101:232–4.
30. Castro-Gago M, Rodriguez-Cervilla J, Ugarte J, Novo I, Pombo M. Maternal alcohol ingestion and neural tube defects. J Pediatr 1984;104:796–7.
31. Halmesmaki E, Raivio K, Ylikorkala O. A possible association between maternal drinking and fetal clubfoot. N Engl J Med 1985;312:790.
32. Sarda P, Bard H. Gastroschisis in a case of dizygotic twins: the possible role of maternal alcohol consumption. Pediatrics 1984;74:94–6.
33. Ammann AJ, Wara DW, Cowan MJ, Barrett DJ, Stiehm ER. The DiGeorge syndrome and the fetal alcohol syndrome. Am J Dis Child 1982;136:906–8.
34. Gardner LI, Mitter N, Coplan J, Kalinowski DP, Sanders KJ. Isochromosome 9q in an infant exposed to ethanol prenatally. N Engl J Med 1985;312:1521.
35. Mills JL, Graubard BI, Harley EE, Rhoads GG, Berendes HW. Maternal alcohol consumption and birth weigh. How much drinking during pregnancy is safe? JAMA 1984;252:1875–9.
36. Wright JT, Waterson EJ, Barrison IG, Toplis PJ, Lewis IG, Gordon MG, MacRae KD, Morris NF, Murray-Lyon IM. Alcohol consumption, pregnancy, and low birthweight. Lancet 1983;1:663–5.
37. Rosett HL, Weiner L, Lee A, Zuckerman B, Dooling E, Oppenheimer E. Patterns of alcohol consumption and fetal development. Obstet Gynecol 1983;61:539–46.
38. Davis PJM, Partridge JW, Storrs CN. Alcohol consumption in pregnancy. How much is safe? Arch Dis Child 1982;57:940–3.
39. Golden NL, Sokol RJ, Kuhnert BR, Bottoms S. Maternal alcohol use and infant development. Pediatrics 1982;70:931–4.
40. Sisenwin FE, Tejani NA, Boxer HS, DiGiuseppe R. Effects of maternal ethanol infusion during pregnancy on the growth and development of children at four to seven years of age. Am J Obstet Gynecol 1983;147:52–6.
41. McLeod W, Brien J, Loomis C, Carmichael L, Probert C, Patrick J. Effect of maternal ethanol ingestion on fetal breathing movements, gross body movements, and heart rate at 37 to 40 weeks' gestational age. Am J Obstet Gynecol 1983;145:251–7.
42. Coles CD, Smith IE, Fernhoff PM, Falek A. Neonatal ethanol withdrawal: characteristics in clinically normal, nondysmorphic neonates. J Pediatr 1984;105:445–51.
43. Ioffe S, Childiaeva R, Chernick V. Prolonged effects of maternal alcohol ingestion on the neonatal electroencephalogram. Pediatrics 1984;74:330–5.
44. Wilker R, Nathenson G. Combined fetal alcohol and hydantoin syndromes. Clin Pediatr 1982;21:331–4.
45. Seeler RA, Israel JN, Royal JE, Kaye CI, Rao S, Abulaban M. Ganglioneuroblastoma and fetal hydantoin-alcohol syndromes. Pediatrics 1979;63:524–7.
46. Ramilo J, Harris VJ. Neuroblastoma in a child with the hydantoin and fetal alcohol syndrome. The radiographic features. Br J Radiol 1979;52:993–5.
47. Bostrom B, Nesbit ME Jr. Hodgkin disease in a child with fetal alcohol-hydantoin syndrome. J Pediatr 1983;103:760–2.
48. Hornstein L, Crowe C, Gruppo R. Adrenal carcinoma in child with history of fetal alcohol syndrome. Lancet 1977;2:1292–3.
49. Anonymous. Alcohol and the fetus—is zero the only option? Lancet 1983;1:682–3.
50. Anonymous. Update: drugs in breast milk. Med Lett Drugs Ther 1979;21:21.
51. Kesaniemi YA. Ethanol and acetaldehyde in the milk and peripheral blood of lactating women after ethanol administration. J Obstet Gynaecol Br Commonw 1974;81:84–6.
52. Wilson JT, Brown RD, Cherek DR, Dailey JW, Hilman B, Jobe PC, Manno BR, Manno JE, Redetzki HM, Stewart JJ. Drug excretion in human breast milk. Principles, pharmacokinetics and projected consequences. Clin Pharmacol 1980;5:1–66.
53. Hoh TK. Severe hypoprothrombinaemic bleeding in the breast-fed young infant. Singapore Med J 1969;10:43–9.
54. Binkiewicz A, Robinson MJ, Senior B. Pseudo-Cushing syndrome caused by alcohol in breast milk. J Pediatr 1978;93:965.

55. Cobo E. Effect of different doses of ethanol on the milk-ejecting reflex in lactating women. Am J Obstet Gynecol 1973;115:817–21.
56. Committee on Drugs, American Academy of Pediatrics. The transfer of drugs and other chemicals into human breast milk. Pediatrics 1983;72:375–83.

Name: **ETHCHLORVYNOL**

Class: **Hypnotic**   Risk Factor: **C_M**

Fetal Risk Summary

No reports linking the use of ethchlorvynol with congenital defects have been located. The Collaborative Perinatal Project reported 68 patients with 1st trimester exposure to nonbarbiturate sedatives, 12 of which had been exposed to ethchlorvynol (1). For the group as a whole, a slight increase in the expected frequency of malformations was found. Specific data for the ethchlorvynol-exposed infants were not given. Animal data indicate that rapid equilibrium occurs between maternal and fetal blood with maximum fetal blood levels measured within 2 hours of maternal ingestion (2). The authors concluded that following maternal ingestion of a toxic or lethal dose, delivery should be accomplished before equilibrium occurs. Neonatal withdrawal symptoms consisting of mild hypotonia, poor suck, absent rooting, poor grasp, and delayed onset jitteriness have been reported (3). The mother had been taking 500 mg daily during the 3rd trimester.

Breast Feeding Summary

No data available.

References

1. Heinonen OP, Slone D, Shapiro S. *Birth Defects and Drugs in Pregnancy*. Littleton:Publishing Sciences Group, 1977:336–7.
2. Hume AS, Williams JM, Douglas BH. Disposition of ethchlorvynol in maternal blood, fetal blood, amniotic fluid, and chorionic fluid. J Reprod Med 1971;6:54–6.
3. Rumack BH, Walravens PA, Department of Pediatrics, University of Colorado Medical Center, 1981. Personal communication.

Name: **ETHINYL ESTRADIOL**

Class: **Estrogenic Hormone**   Risk Factor: **X**

Fetal Risk Summary

Ethinyl estradiol is used frequently in combination with progestins for oral contraception (see Oral Contraceptives). The Collaborative Perinatal Project monitored 89 mother-child pairs who were exposed to ethinyl estradiol during the 1st trimester (1). An increased risk for malformations was found, although identification of the malformations was not provided. Estrogenic agents as a group were monitored in 614 mother-child pairs. An increase in the expected frequency of cardiovascular defects, eye and ear anomalies, and Down's syndrome was reported (2). Reevaluation of these data in terms of timing of exposure, vaginal bleeding in early pregnancy, and previous maternal obstetrical history, however, failed to support an association between estrogens and cardiac malformations (3). An earlier study also failed to find any relationship with nongenital malformations. In a smaller study, 12 mothers were exposed to ethinyl estradiol during the 1st trimester (5). No fetal abnormalities were observed. Ethinyl estradiol has also been used as a contraceptive when given with 72 hours of unprotected midcycle coitus (6). Use of estrogenic hormones during pregnancy is contraindicated.

Breast Feeding Summary

Estrogens are frequently used for suppression of postpartum lactation (7, 8). Very small amounts are excreted in milk (8). Ethinyl estradiol, when used in oral contraceptives, has been associated with decreased milk production and decreased composition of nitrogen and protein content in human milk (9). Although the magnitude of these changes is low, the differences in milk production and composition may be of nutritional importance to nursing infants of malnourished mothers. If breast feeding is desired, the lowest dose of oral contraceptives should be chosen. Monitoring of infant weight gain and the possible need for nutritional supplementation should be considered (see Oral Contraceptives).

References

1. Heinonen OP, Slone D, Shapiro S. *Birth Defects and Drugs in Pregnancy*. Littleton:Publishing Sciences Group, 1977:389,391.
2. *Ibid*,395.
4. Wiseman RA, Dodds-Smith IC. Cardiovascular birth defects and antenatal exposure to female sex hormones: a reevaluation of some base data. Teratology 1984;30:359–70.
4. Wilson JG, Brent RL. Are female sex hormones teratogenic? Am J Obstet Gynecol 1981;141:567–80.
5. Hagler S, Schultz A, Hankin H, Kunstadler RH. Fetal effects of steroid therapy during pregnancy. Am J Dis Child 1963;106:586–90.
6. Dixon GW, Schlesselman JJ, Ory HW, Blye RP. Ethinyl estradiol and conjugated estrogens as postcoital contraceptives. JAMA 1980;244:1336–9.
7. Gilman AG, Goodman LS, Gilman A, eds. *The Pharmacological Basis of Therapeutics*, ed 6. New York:Macmillan Publishing Co, 1980:1431.
8. Klinger G, Claussen C, Schroder S. Excretion of ethinyloestradiol sulfonate in the human milk. Zentralbl Gynaekol 1981;103:91–5.
9. Lonnerdal B, Forsum E, Hambraeus L. Effect of oral contraceptives on composition and volume of breast milk. Am J Clin Nutr 1980;33:816–24.

Name: **ETHIODIZED OIL**

Class: **Diagnostic**   Risk Factor: **D**

Fetal Risk Summary

Ethiodized oil contains a high concentration of organically bound iodine. Use of this agent close to term has been associated with neonatal hypothyroidism (see Diatrizoate).

Breast Feeding Summary

See Potassium Iodide.

Name: **ETHISTERONE**

Class: **Progestogenic Hormone**   Risk Factor: **D**

Fetal Risk Summary

The Food and Drug Administration mandated deletion of pregnancy-related indications for all progestins because of a possible association with congenital anomalies. No reports linking the use of ethisterone alone with congenital defects have been located. The Collaborative Perinatal Project monitored 866 mother-child pairs with 1st trimester exposure to progestational agents (including two with exposure to ethisterone) (1). An increase in the expected frequency of cardiovascular defects and hypospadias was observed for the progestational agents as a group, but not for ethisterone as a single agent (2). In a subsequent report from the Collaborative Study, a single case of tricuspid atresia and ventricular septal defect was identified with 3rd trimester exposure to ethisterone and ethinyl estradiol (3). Re-evaluation of these data in terms of timing of exposure, vaginal bleeding in early pregnancy, and previous maternal obstetrical history, however, failed to support an association between female sex hormones and cardiac malformations (4). An earlier study also failed to find any relationship with nongenital malformations (5). (See also Hydroxyprogesterone and Medroxyprogesterone.)

Breast Feeding Summary

See Oral Contraceptives.

References

1. Heinonen OP, Slone D, Shapiro S. *Birth Defects and Drugs in Pregnancy*. Littleton:Publishing Sciences Group, 1977:389,91.
2. *Ibid*, 394.
3. Heinonen OP, Slone D, Monson RR, Hook EB, Shapiro S. Cardiovascular birth defects and antenatal exposure to female sex hormones. N Engl J Med 1977;296:67–70.
4. Wiseman RA, Dodds-Smith IC. Cardiovascular birth defects and antenatal exposure to female sex hormones: a reevaluation of some base data. Teratology 1984;30:359–70.
5. Wilson JG, Brent RL. Are female sex hormones teratogenic? Am J Obstet Gynecol 1981;141:567–80.

Name: **ETHOHEPTAZINE**

Class: **Analgesic**   Risk Factor: **C**

Fetal Risk Summary

The Collaborative Perinatal Project monitored 50,282 mother-child pairs, 60 of which had 1st trimester exposure to ethoheptazine (1). For use anytime during pregnancy, 300 exposures were recorded (2). Although the numbers were small, a possible relationship may exist between this drug and major or minor malformations. Further, a possible association with individual defects was observed (3). The statistical significance of these associations is unknown, and independent confirmation is required.

Congenital dislocation of the hip (3 cases)
Umbilical hernia (3 cases)
Inguinal hernia (8 cases)

Breast Feeding Summary

No data available.

References

1. Heinonen OP, Slone D, Shapiro S. *Birth Defects and Drugs in Pregnancy*. Littleton:Publishing Sciences Group, 1977:287–95.
2. *Ibid*, 434.
3. *Ibid*, 485.

Name: **ETHOPROPAZINE**

Class: **Parasympatholytic (Anticholinergic)**   Risk Factor: **C**

Fetal Risk Summary

Ethopropazine is a phenothiazine compound with anticholinergic activity that is used in the treatment of parkinsonism (see also Atropine and Promethazine). No reports of its use in pregnancy have been located.

Breast Feeding Summary

No data available (see also Atropine and Promethazine).

Name: **ETHOSUXIMIDE**

Class: **Anticonvulsant**   Risk Factor: **C**

Fetal Risk Summary

Ethosuximide is a succinimide anticonvulsant used in the treatment of petit mal epilepsy. The use of ethosuximide during pregnancy has been reported in 163 pregnancies (1–11). Due to the lack of specific information on the observed malformations, multiple drug therapies, and differences in study methodology, conclusions linking the use of ethosuximide with congenital defects are difficult. Spontaneous hemorrhage in the neonate following *in utero* exposure to ethosuximide has been reported (see also Phenytoin and Phenobarbital) (6). Abnormalities identified with ethosuximide use in 10 pregnancies include:

Patent ductus arteriosus (8 cases)
Cleft lip and/or palate (7 cases)
Mongoloid facies, short neck, altered palmar
    crease, and an accessory nipple (1 case)
Hydrocephalus (1 case)

Ethosuximide has a much lower teratogenic potential than the oxazolidinedione class of anticonvulsants (see also Trimethadione and Paramethadione) (11, 12). The succinimide anticonvulsants should be considered the anticonvulsants of choice for the treatment of petit mal epilepsy during the 1st trimester.

Breast Feeding Summary

Ethosuximide freely enters the breast milk in concentrations similar to those in the maternal serum (13–15). Two reports measured similar milk:plasma ratios of 1.0 and 0.78 (13, 14). No adverse effects on the nursing infant have been reported. The American Academy of Pediatrics considers ethosuximide compatible with breast-feeding (16).

References

1. Speidel BD, Meadow SR. Maternal epilepsy and abnormalities of the fetus and newborn. Lancet 1972;2:839–43.
2. Fedrick J. Epilepsy and pregnancy: A report from the Oxford Record Linkage Study. Br Med J 1973;2:442–8.
3. Lowe CR. Congenital malformations among infants born to epileptic women. Lancet 1973;1:9–10.
4. Starreveld-Zimmerman AAE, van der Kolk WJ, Meinardi H, Elshve J. Are anticonvulsants teratogenic? Lancet 1973;2:48–9.
5. Kuenssberg EV, Knox JDE. Teratogenic effect of anticonvulsants. Lancet 1973;2:198.
6. Speidel BD, Meadow SR. Epilepsy, anticonvulsants and congenital malformations. Drugs 1974;8:354–65.
7. Janz D. The teratogenic risk of antiepileptic drugs. Epilepsia 1975;16:159–69.
8. Nakane Y, Okuma T, Takahashi R, et al. Multi-institutional study on the teratogenicity and fetal toxicity of antiepileptic drugs: a report of a collaborative study group in Japan. Epilepsia 1980;21:663–80.
9. Heinonen OP, Slone D, Shapiro S. *Birth Defects and Drugs in Pregnancy*. Littleton:Publishing Sciences Group, 1977:358–9.
10. Dansky L, Andermann E, Andermann F. Major congenital malformations on the offspring of epileptic patients: genetic and environment risk factors. In *Epilepsy, Pregnancy and the Child*. Proceedings of a Workshop in Berlin, September 1980. New York:Raven Press, 1981.
11. Fabro S, Brown NA. Teratogenic potential of anticonvulsants. N Engl J Med 1979;300:1280–1.
12. The National Institutes of Health. Anticonvulsants found to have teratogenic potential. JAMA 1981;241:36.
13. Koup JR, Rose JQ, Cohen ME. Ethosuximide pharmacokinetics in pregnant patient and her newborn. Epilepsia 1978;19:535.
14. Kaneko S, Sato T, Suzuki K. The levels of anticonvulsants in breast milk. Br J Clin Pharmacol 1979;7:624–6.
15. Horning MG, Stillwell WG, Nowlin J, Lertratanangkoon K, Stillwill RN, Hill RM. Identification and quantification of drugs and drug metabolites in human breast milk using GC-MS-COM methods. Mod Prob Paediatr 1975;15:73–9.
16. Committee on Drugs, American Academy of Pediatrics. The transfer of drugs and other chemicals into human breast milk. Pediatrics 1983;72:375–83.

Name: ETHOTOIN

Class: **Anticonvulsant**   Risk Factor: **D**

Fetal Risk Summary

Ethotoin is a low-potency hydantoin anticonvulsant (1). The fetal hydantoin syndrome has been associated with the use of the more potent phenytoin (see Phenytoin). Only six reports describing the use of ethotoin during the 1st trimester have been located (2–4). Congenital malformations observed in two of these cases included cleft lip/palate and patent ductus arteriosus (3, 4). No cause and effect relationship was established. Although the toxicity of ethotoin appears to be lower than the more potent phenytoin, the occurrence of congenital defects in two fetuses exposed to ethantoin suggests that a teratogenic potential may exist.

Breast Feeding Summary

No data available.

References

1. Schmidt RP, Wilder BJ. Epilepsy. In *Contemporary Neurology Services*, vol. 2. Philadelphia, FA Davis Co., 1968:154.
2. Heinonen OP, Slone D, Shapiro S. *Birth Defects and Drugs in Pregnancy*. Littleton:Publishing Sciences Group, 1977:358–9.
3. Zablen M, Brand N. Cleft lip and palate with the anticonvulsant ethantoin. N Engl J Med 1978;298:285.
4. Nakane Y, Okuma T, Takahashi R, et al. Multi-institutional study on the teratogenicity and fetal toxicity of antiepileptic drugs: a report of a collaborative study group in Japan. Epilepsia 1980;21:663–80.

Name: **ETHYL BISCOUMACETATE**

Class: **Anticoagulant**   Risk Factor: **D**

Fetal Risk Summary

See Coumarin Derivatives.

Breast Feeding Summary

See Coumarin Derivatives.

Name: **ETHYNODIOL**

Class: **Progestogenic Hormone**   Risk Factor: **D**

Fetal Risk Summary

Ethynodiol is used primarily in oral contraceptive products (see Oral Contraceptives).

Breast Feeding Summary

See Oral Contraceptives.

Name: **EVAN'S BLUE**

Class: **Dye**   Risk Factor: **C**

Fetal Risk Summary

No reports linking the use of Evan's blue with congenital defects have been located. The dye is teratogenic in some animal species (1). Evan's blue has been injected intra-amniotically for diagnosis of ruptured membranes without apparent effect on the fetus except for temporary staining of the skin (2, 3). The use of Evan's blue during pregnancy for plasma volume determinations is routine (4–7). No problems in the fetus or newborn have been attributed to this use.

Breast Feeding Summary

No data available.

References

1. Wilson JG. Teratogenic activity of several azo dyes chemically related to trypan blue. Anat Rec 1955;123:313–34.
2. Atley RD, Sutherst JR. Premature rupture of the fetal membranes confirmed by intraamniotic injection of dye (Evans blue T-1824). Am J Obstet Gynecol 1970;108:993–4.
3. Morrison L, Wiseman HJ. Intra-amniotic injection of Evans blue dye. Am J Obstet Gynecol 1972;113:1147.
4. Quinlivan WLG, Brock JA, Sullivan H. Blood volume changes and blood loss associated with labor. I. Correlation of changes in blood volume measured by I^{131}-albumin and Evans blue dye, with measured blood loss. Am J Obstet Gynecol 1970;106:843–9.
5. Sibai BM, Abdella TN, Anderson GD, Dilts PV Jr. Plasma volume findings in pregnant women with mild hypertension: therapeutic considerations. Am J Obstet Gynecol 1983;145:539–44.
6. Goodlin RC, Anderson JC, Gallagher TF. Relationship between amniotic fluid volume and maternal plasma volume expansion. Am J Obstet Gynecol 1983;146:505–11.
7. Hays PM, Cruikshank DP, Dunn LJ. Plasma volume determination in normal and preeclamptic pregnancies. Am J Obstet Gynecol 1985;151:958–66.

Name: **FENFLURAMINE**

Class: **Central Stimulant/Anorectant**   Risk Factor: **C_M**

Fetal Risk Summary

No data available (see Diethylpropion, Dextroamphetamine).

Breast Feeding Summary

No data available.

Name: **FENOPROFEN**

Class: **Nonsteroidal Anti-inflammatory**   Risk Factor: **B***

Fetal Risk Summary

No reports linking the use of fenoprofen with congenital defects have been located. The drug was used during labor in one study (1). No data were given except that the drug could not be detected in cord blood or amniotic fluid. If the drug did reach the fetus, fenoprofen, a prostaglandin synthetase inhibitor, could theoretically cause constriction of the ductus arteriosus *in utero* (2). Persistent pulmonary hypertension of the newborn should also be considered (2). Drugs in this class have been shown to inhibit labor and prolong pregnancy (3). The manufacturer recommends the drug not be used during pregnancy (4).

[* Risk Factor D if used in the 3rd trimester or near delivery.]

Breast Feeding Summary

Fenoprofen passes into breast milk in very small quantities. The milk:plasma ratio in nursing mothers given 600 mg every 6 hours for 4 days was approximately 0.017 (1). The clinical significance of this amount is unknown.

References

1. Rubin A, Chernish SM, Crabtree R, et al. A profile of the physiological disposition and gastrointestinal effects of fenoprofen in man. Curr Med Res Opin 1974;2:529–44.
2. Levin DL. Effects of inhibition of prostaglandin synthesis on fetal development, oxygenation, and the fetal circulation. Semin Perinatol 1980;4:35–44.
3. Fuchs F. Prevention of prematurity. Am J Obstet Gynecol 1976;126:809–20.
4. Product information. Nalfon. Dista Products Co, 1985.

Name: **FENOTEROL**

Class: **Sympathomimetic (Adrenergic)**   Risk Factor: **B**

Fetal Risk Summary

No reports linking the use of fenoterol with congenital defects have been located. Fenoterol, a β-sympathomimetic, has been used to prevent premature labor (1, 2). The effects in the mother, fetus, and newborn are similar to those of the parent compound (see Metaproterenol). Fenoterol has been shown to inhibit prostaglandin-induced uterine activity at term (3).

Fenoterol was administered to 11 patients 30 minutes prior to cesarean section under general anesthesia at an infusion rate of 3 μg/min (4). No adverse effects were seen in the mother, fetus, or newborn after this short exposure. Infusion in hypertensive pregnant patients caused a greater drop in diastolic blood pressure than the same dose in normotensive pregnant women (5). Other cardiovascular parameters in the mothers and fetuses were comparable between the two groups.

Breast Feeding Summary

No data available.

References

1. Lipshitz J, Baillie P, Davey DA. A comparison of the uterine beta-2-adrenoreceptor selectivity of fenoterol, hexoprenaline, ritodrine and salbutamol. S Afr Med J 1976;50:1969–72.
2. Lipshitz J. The uterine and cardiovascular effects of oral fenoterol hydrochloride. Br J Obstet Gynaecol 1977;84:737–9.
3. Lipshitz J, Lipshitz EM. Uterine and cardiovascular effects of fenoterol and hexoprenaline in prostaglandin F_{2a}-induced labor in humans. Obstet Gynecol 1984;63:396–400.
4. Jouppila R, Kauppila A, Tuimala R, Pakarinen A, Moilunen K. Maternal, fetal and neonatal effects of beta-adrenergic stimulation in connection with cesarean section. Acta Obstet Gynecol Scand 1980;59:489–93.
5. Oddoy UA, Joschko K. Effects of fenoterol on blood pressure, heart rate, and cardiotocogram of hypertensive and normotensive women in advanced pregnancy. Zentralbl Gynaekol 1982;104:415–21.

Name: **FENTANYL**

Class: **Narcotic Analgesic**   Risk Factor: **B***

Fetal Risk Summary

No reports linking the use of fentanyl with congenital defects have been located. Use of the drug during labor should be expected to produce neonatal respiratory depression to the same degree as other narcotic analgesics. Respiratory depression has been observed in one infant whose mother received epidural fentanyl during labor (1). Fentanyl given during general anesthesia may produce loss of fetal heart rate variability without causing fetal hypoxia (2). The narcotic has been combined with bupivacaine for spinal anesthesia during labor (3, 4).

[* Risk Factor D if used for prolonged periods or in high doses at term.]

Breast Feeding Summary

No data available.

References

1. Carrie LES, O'Sullivan GM, Seegobin R. Epidural fentanyl in labour. Anaesthesia 1981;36:965–9.
2. Johnson ES, Colley PS. Effects of nitrous oxide and fentanyl anesthesia on fetal heart-rate variability intra- and postoperatively. Anesthesiology 1980;52:429–30.
3. Justins DM, Francis D, Houlton PG, Reynolds F. A controlled trial of extradural fentanyl in labour. Br J Anaesth 1982;54:409–13.
4. Milon D, Bentue-Ferrer D, Noury D, Reymann JM, Sauvage J, Allain H, Saint-Marc C, van den Driessche J. Peridural anesthesia for cesarean section employing a bupivacaine-fentanyl combination. Ann Fr Anesth Reanim 1983;2:273–9.

Name: **FLUCYTOSINE**

Class: **Antifungal**   Risk Factor: **C**

Fetal Risk Summary

Flucytosine is embryotoxic and teratogenic in some species of animals, but its use in human pregnancy has not been studied. Following oral administration, about 4% of the drug is metabolized to 5-fluorouracil, an antineoplastic agent (1). Fluorouracil is suspected of producing congenital defects in humans (see Fluorouracil). Three case reports of pregnant patients treated in the 2nd and 3rd trimesters with flucytosine have been located (2–4). No defects were observed in the newborns.

Breast Feeding Summary

No data available.

References

1. Diasio RB, Lakings DE, Bennett JE. Evidence for conversion of 5-fluorocytosine to 5-fluorouracil in humans: possible factor in 5-fluorocytosine clinical toxicity. Antimicrob Agents Chemother 1978;14:903–8.
2. Philpot CR, Lo D. Cryptococcal meningitis in pregnancy. Med J Aust 1972;2:1005–7.
3. Schonebeck J, Segerbrand E. Candida albicans septicaemia during first half of pregnancy successfully treated with 5-fluorocytosine. Br Med J 1973;4:337–8.
4. Curole DN. Cryptococcal meningitis in pregnancy. J Reprod Med 1981;26:317–9.

Name: **FLUNITRAZEPAM**

Class: **Hypnotic**   Risk Factor: **C**

Fetal Risk Summary

Flunitrazepam is a benzodiazepine (see also Diazepam). No reports linking the use of flunitrazepam with congenital defects have been located, but other drugs in this group have been suspected of causing fetal malformations (see also Diazepam or

Chlordiazepoxide). In contrast to other benzodiazepines, flunitrazepam crosses the placenta slowly (1, 2). About 12 hours after a 1-mg oral dose, cord:maternal blood ratios in early and late pregnancy were about 0.5 and 0.22, respectively. Amniotic fluid:maternal serum ratios were in the 0.02–0.07 range in both cases. Accumulation in the fetus may occur after repeated doses (1).

Breast Feeding Summary

Flunitrazepam is excreted into breast milk. Following a single 2-mg oral dose in five patients, mean milk:plasma ratios at 11, 15, 27, and 39 hours were 0.61, 0.68, 0.9, and 0.75, respectively (1, 2). The effects of these levels on the nursing infant are unknown, but they are probably insignificant.

References

1. Kanto J, Aaltonen L, Kangas L, Erkkola R, Pitkanen Y. Placental transfer and breast milk levels of flunitrazepam. Curr Ther Res 1979;26:539–46.
2. Kanto JH. Use of benzodiazepines during pregnancy, labour and lactation, with special reference to pharmacokinetic considerations. Drugs 1982;23:354–80.

Name: **FLUOROURACIL**

Class: **Antineoplastic**   Risk Factor: **D**

Fetal Risk Summary

Experience with fluorouracil during pregnancy is limited. Following systemic therapy in the 1st trimester, multiple defects were observed in an aborted fetus (1):

> Radial aplasia, absent thumbs and three fingers, hypoplasia of lungs, aorta, thymus, and bile duct, aplasia of esophagus, duodenum, and ureters, single umbilical artery, absent appendix, imperforate anus, and a cloaca (also exposed to 5 rad of irradiation)

Toxicity consisting of cyanosis and jerking extremities has been reported in a newborn exposed to fluorouracil in the 3rd trimester (2). There are no reports of fetal effects after topical use of the drug.

Data from one review indicated that 40% of the infants exposed to anticancer drugs were of low birth weight (3). Long-term studies of growth and mental development in offspring exposed to fluorouracil and other antineoplastic drugs during the 2nd trimester, the period of neuroblast multiplication, have not been conducted (4).

Amenorrhea has been observed in women treated with fluorouracil for breast cancer, but this was probably due to concurrent administration of melphalan (see also Melphalan) (5, 6).

Breast Feeding Summary

No data available.

References

1. Stephens JD, Golbus MS, Miller TR, Wilber RR, Epstein CJ. Multiple congenital anomalies in a fetus exposed to 5-fluorouracil during the first trimester. Am J Obstet Gynecol 1980;137:747–9.

2. Stadler HE, Knowles J. Fluorouracil in pregnancy: effect on the neonate. JAMA 1971;217:214–5.
3. Nicholson HO. Cytotoxic drugs in pregnancy: review of reported cases. J Obstet Gynaecol Br Commonw 1968;75:307–12.
4. Dobbing J. Pregnancy and leukaemia. Lancet 1977;1:1155.
5. Fisher B, Sherman B, Rockette H, Redmond C, Margolese K, Fisher ER. L-Phenylalanine (L-PAM) in the management of premenopausal patients with primary breast cancer. Cancer 1979;44:847–57.
6. Schilsky RL, Lewis BJ, Sherins RJ, Young RC. Gonadal dysfunction in patients receiving chemotherapy for cancer. Ann Intern Med 1980;93:109–14.

Name: **FLUPENTHIXOL**

Class: **Tranquilizer**   Risk Factor: **C**

Fetal Risk Summary

Flupenthixol crosses the placenta with cord blood levels averaging 24% of maternal serum (1). Amniotic fluid concentrations were similar to those of cord blood. No effects on the infants were observed.

Breast Feeding Summary

Flupenthixol is excreted into breast milk with concentrations about 30% higher than those of maternal serum (1). However, these amounts are still very low and probably are not clinically significant (1).

References

1. Kirk L, Jorgensen A. Concentrations of cis(z)-flupentixol in maternal serum, amniotic fluid, umbilical cord serum, and milk. Psychopharmacology (Berlin) 1980;72:107–8.

Name: **FLUPHENAZINE**

Class: **Tranquilizer**   Risk Factor: **C**

Fetal Risk Summary

Fluphenazine is a piperazine phenothiazine in the same group as prochlorperazine. Phenothiazines readily cross the placenta (1). Extrapyramidal symptoms in the newborn have been attributed to *in utero* exposure to fluphenazine (see also Chlorpromazine) (2). An infant with multiple anomalies was born to a mother treated with fluphenazine enanthate injections throughout pregnancy (3). The mother also took Debendox (see Doxylamine) during the 1st trimester. The anomalies included:

Ocular hypertelorism with telecanthus, cleft lip and palate, imperforate anus, hypospadias of penoscrotal type, jerky, roving eye movements, episodic rapid nystagmoid movements, rectourethral fistula, poor ossification of frontal skull bone

Other reports have indicated that the phenothiazines are relatively safe during pregnancy (see also Prochlorperazine).

Breast Feeding Summary

No data available. See also Prochlorperazine.

References

1. Moya F, Thorndike V. Passage of drugs across the placenta. Am J Obstet Gynecol 1962;84:1778–98.
2. Cleary MF. Fluphenazine decanoate during pregnancy. Am J Psychiatry 1977;134:815–6.
3. Donaldson GL, Bury RG. Multiple congenital abnormalities in a newborn boy associated with maternal use of fluphenazine enanthate and other drugs during pregnancy. Acta Paediatr Scand 1982;71:335–8.

Name: **FOLIC ACID**

Class: **Vitamin** Risk Factor: **A***

Fetal Risk Summary

Folic acid, a water-soluble B complex vitamin, is essential for nucleoprotein synthesis and the maintenance of normal erythropoiesis (1). The American RDA for folic acid in pregnancy is 0.8 mg (2).

Rapid transfer of folic acid to the fetus occurs in pregnancy (3–5). One investigation indicated that the placenta stores folic acid and transfer occurs only after placental tissue vitamin receptors are saturated (6). Results compatible with this hypothesis were found in a 1975 study using radiolabeled folate in women undergoing 2nd trimester abortions (7).

Folic acid deficiency is common during pregnancy (8–10). If not supplemented, maternal serum and RBC folate values decline during pregnancy (8, 11–15). Even with vitamin supplements, however, maternal folate hypovitaminemia may result (8). This depletion is thought to result from preferential uptake of folic acid by the fetal circulation such that at birth, newborn levels are significantly higher than maternal levels (8, 14–17). At term, mean serum folate level in 174 mothers was 5.6 ng/ml (range 1.5–7.6) and in their newborns 18 ng/ml (range 5.5–66.0) (8). In an earlier study, similar serum values were measured, with RBC folate level decreasing from 157 ng/ml at 15 weeks gestation to 118 ng/ml at 38 weeks (11). Folic acid supplementation prevented the decrease in both serum and RBC folate levels.

The most common complication of maternal folic acid deficiency is megaloblastic anemia (9, 18–27). The three main factors involved in the pathogenesis of megaloblastic anemia of pregnancy are depletion of maternal folic acid stores by the fetus, inadequate maternal intake of the vitamin, and faulty absorption (24). Multiple pregnancy, hemorrhage, and hemolytic anemia hasten the decline of maternal levels (12, 24). A 1969 study used 1-mg daily supplements to uniformly produce a satisfactory hematologic response in these conditions (26).

The effects on the mother and fetus resulting from folate deficiency are controversial. These effects can be summarized as:

Fetal anomalies
Placental abruption
Pregnancy-induced hypertension (PIH, toxemia, pre-eclampsia)
Abortions
Placenta previa
Low birth weight
Premature delivery

Folic acid deficiency is a well known experimental animal teratogen (28). In humans, the relationship between fetal defects and folate deficiency is less clear. Several reports have claimed an increase in congenital malformations associated with low levels of this vitamin (9, 21–23, 29–32). Other investigators have stated that maternal deficiency does not result in fetal anomalies (19, 20, 33–39). Scott and co-workers (33) found the folate status of mothers giving birth to severely malformed fetuses to be no different from that of the general obstetric population and much better than that of mothers with overt megaloblastic anemia. Similar results were found in other series (37–39). In one of these, 10 mg/day of folic acid was given to one patient from about the 6th week through term (37). The mother, who had a history of giving birth to children with neural tube defects (NTD), gave birth to a child with spina bifida and craniolacunia. A subsequent pregnancy in this woman, without supplementation, resulted in a healthy infant. The data of Laurence et al (29), however, suggest a relationship between folic acid and NTD (See also Vitamins, Multiple). In their randomized double-blind trial to prevent recurrences of NTD, 44 women took 4 mg of folic acid per day from before conception through early pregnancy. There were no recurrences in this group. A group of 51 women given placebos plus 16 noncompliant patients from the treated group had four and two recurrences, respectively. The difference between the supplemented and nonsupplemented patients was significant ($p = 0.04$). Smithells and co-workers (40) reported significantly lower RBC folate levels in mothers of infants with NTD than in mothers of normal infants, but not all of the affected group had low serum folate levels. In a subsequent report by those investigators, very low vitamin B_{12} concentrations were found, suggesting that the primary deficiency may have been due to this latter vitamin with resulting depletion of RBC and tissue folate (41). A large retrospective study found a protective effect with folate administration during pregnancy, leading to a possible conclusion that deficiency of this vitamin could be teratogenic (32).

The strongest evidence for an association between folic acid and fetal defects comes from examination of patients treated with drugs that are either folic acid antagonists or induce folic acid deficiency, although agreement with the latter is not universal (36, 42, 43). The folic acid antagonists, aminopterin and methotrexate, are known teratogens (see Aminopterin and Methotrexate). A very high incidence of defects resulted when aminopterin was used as an unsuccessful abortifacient in the 1st trimester. These antineoplastic agents may cause fetal injury by blocking the conversion of folic acid to tetrahydrofolic acid in both the fetus and the mother. In contrast, certain anticonvulsants, such as phenytoin and phenobarbital, induce maternal folic acid deficiency possibly by impairing gastrointestinal absorption or increasing hepatic metabolism of the vitamin (36, 42, 43). Whether these agents also induce folic acid deficiency in the fetus is less certain since the fetus seems to be efficient in drawing on available maternal stores of folic acid. Low maternal folate levels, however, have been proposed as a mechanism for the increased incidence of defects observed in infants exposed *in utero* to anticonvulsants. Biale and Lewenthal, in a 1984 article (42), reported research on the relationship between folic acid, anticonvulsants, and fetal defects. In the retrospective part of this study, a group of 24 women treated with phenytoin and other anticonvulsants produced 66 infants, of which 10 (15%) had major anomalies. Two of the mothers with affected infants had markedly low RBC folate concentrations. A second group of 22 epileptic women were then given supplements of daily folic acid, 2.5–5.0 mg, starting before conception in 26 pregnancies and within the first 40 days in six. This group produced 33 newborns (32 pregnancies—1 set of twins) with no defects, a significant difference from the group not receiving supplementation. Negative associations between anticonvulsant-induced folate deficiency and birth defects have also been reported (36, 43). Pritchard and co-workers studied a group of epileptic women taking anticonvulsants and observed only two defects (2.9%) in pregnancies producing a live baby, a rate similar to that expected in a healthy population (36). Although folate levels were not measured in this retrospective survey, maternal folate deficiency was predicted by the authors, based on their current research with folic acid in patients taking anticonvulsants. Hiilesmaa and co-workers (43) observed 20 infants (15%) with defects from 133 women taking anticonvulsants. No neural tube defects were found, but this defect is rare in Finland and an increase in the anomaly could have been missed (43). All of the women were given supplements of 0.1–1.0 mg (average 0.5 mg) of folate/day from the 6th to 16th week of gestation until delivery. Folate levels were usually within the normal range (normal levels considered to be: serum >1.8 ng/ml, RBC >203 ng/ml).

Maternal folic acid status may be associated with placental abruption (22, 23, 25, 31, 44). Hibbard and Jeffcoate (44), in their review and analysis of 506 consecutive cases of abruptio placentae, found defective folate metabolism as a predisposing factor in 97.5% of the cases. They theorized that folic acid deficiency early in pregnancy caused irreversible damage to the fetus, chorion, and decidua, leading to abruption, abortion, premature delivery, low birth weight, and fetal malformations. Stone and co-workers (45) discovered that 60% of their patients with abruption had folate deficiencies, but their numbers were too small for statistical analysis. In other series, no correlation was found between low levels of folic acid and this complication (15, 35, 46).

A relationship between folate deficiency and PIH is doubtful. Gatenby and Lillie (19) found PIH in 14% of their patients with megaloblastic anemia as compared to the predicted incidence of 6% in that group. In another report, although 22 of 36 PIH patients had folate deficiency, the authors were unable to conclude that a positive association existed (31, 45). Neither Pritchard et al (20) nor Giles (24) found any relationship between low levels of the vitamin and PIH. In Giles' study (24), the incidence of PIH in megaloblastic anemia was 12.2% compared to 14.0% in normoblastic anemia. Whalley and co-workers (47) studied folate levels in 101 pre-eclamptic and 17 eclamptic women and compared them to 52 normal controls and 29 women with overt megaloblastic anemia. No correlation was found between levels of folic acid and the complications.

Several papers have associated folic acid deficiency with abortion (22, 23, 31,

44, 48–50). The etiology of some abortions, as proposed by Hibbard and Jeffcoate (44), is faulty folate metabolism in early pregnancy, producing irreversible injury to the fetus and placenta. Others have been unable to detect any significant relationship between serum and RBC folate levels and abortion (11, 34, 51). In the series of 66 patients with early spontaneous abortions studied by Streiff and Little (51), the incidence of folate deficiency was the same as in those with uncomplicated pregnancies. These researchers did find a relationship between low folic acid levels and placenta previa. However, Chanarin and co-workers (11) found no evidence of an association between folate deficiency and either abortion or antepartum hemorrhage.

The relationship between prematurity, low birth weight, and folic acid levels has been investigated. Baker and co-workers (17) measured significantly lower folate levels in the blood of low-birth-weight neonates as compared to normal-weight infants. The incidences of premature delivery and birth weight under 2,500 g were both raised in folate-deficient mothers in a report by Gatenby amd Lillie (19). These patients all had severe megaloblastic anemia and a poor standard of nutrition. In the study by Hibbard and Jeffcoate (44) of 510 infants from folate-deficient mothers, 276 (56%) weighed 2,500 g or less compared to a predicted incidence of 8.6%. Martin and co-workers (50) studied a group of women with uterine bleeding during pregnancy and found a significant association between serum folate level and low birth weight. Similarly, the study by Whiteside and co-workers (52) indicated a significant relationship between folate levels at the end of the 2nd trimester and newborn birth weight. In contrast to the above, others have found no association between folic acid deficiency and prematurity (24, 35, 53, 54), nor an association between serum folate and birth weight (11, 35, 55, 56).

Two reports have alluded to problems with high folic acid levels in the mother during pregnancy (57, 58). An isolated case report has described an anencephalic fetus whose mother was under psychiatric care (57). She had been treated with very high doses of folic acid and vitamins B_1, B_6, and C. The relationship between the vitamins and the defect is unknown. Mukherjee and co-workers (58) examined the effect of folic acid, zinc, and other nutrients on pregnancy outcome. Total complications of pregnancy (infection, bleeding, fetal distress, prematurity or death, PIH, and tissue fragility) were associated with high serum folate and low serum zinc levels. The explanation offered for these surprising findings was that folate inhibits intestinal absorption of zinc, which, they proposed, was responsible for the complications. This study also found an association between low folate level and abortion.

In summary, folic acid deficiency during pregnancy is a common problem in undernourished women and women not receiving supplements. The relationship between folic acid levels and various maternal or fetal complications appears to be complex. Evidence has accumulated that interference with folic acid metabolism by some drugs early in pregnancy will result in congenital anomalies. Whether simple maternal folic acid deficiency can also induce fetal malformations is presently uncertain. The timing of folic acid deficiency (i.e., very early 1st trimester vs later 1st trimester) may be important but further studies are required. A clinical trial is currently being conducted in the United Kingdom to answer this question (see Multiple Vitamins for details). For other complications, it is probable that a number of factors, of which folic acid is only one, contribute to poor pregnancy outcome.

Consequently, to assure good maternal and fetal health, supplementation of the pregnant woman with the folic acid RDA or sufficient amounts to maintain normal maternal folate levels is recommended.

[* Risk Factor C if used in doses above the RDA.]

Breast Feeding Summary

Folic acid is actively excreted in human breast milk (59–68). Accumulation of folate in milk takes precedence over maternal folate needs (59). Levels of folic acid are relatively low in colostrum, but as lactation proceeds, concentrations of the vitamin rise (60–62). Folate levels in newborns and breast-fed infants are consistently higher than those in mothers and normal adults (63, 64). In Japanese mothers, mean breast milk folate concentrations were 141.4 ng/ml, resulting in a total intake by the infant of 14–25 μg/kg/day (64). Much lower mean levels were measured in pooled human milk in an English study examining preterm (26 mothers: 29–34 weeks) and term (35 mothers: 39 weeks or longer) patients (61). Preterm milk levels rose from 10.6 ng/ml (colostrum) to 30.5 ng/ml (16–196 days) while term milk levels increased over the same period from 17.6 to 42.3 ng/ml.

Supplementation with folic acid is apparently not needed in mothers with good nutritional habits (62–66). Folic acid deficiency and megaloblastic anemia did not develop in women not receiving supplements even when lactation exceeded I year (62, 63). In another study, maternal serum and red blood cell folate levels increased significantly after 1 mg of folic acid per day for 4 weeks, but milk folate level remained unchanged (64). Thomas and co-workers (65) gave well-nourished lactating women a multivitamin preparation containing 0.8 mg of folic acid. At 6 months postpartum, milk concentrations of folate did not differ significantly from those of controls not receiving supplements. Smith and co-workers (66) measured more than adequate blood folate levels in American breast-fed infants during the first year of life. The mean milk concentration of folate consumed by these infants was 85 ng/ml.

In patients with poor nutrition, lactation may lead to severe maternal folic acid deficiency and megaloblastic anemia (59). For these patients, there is evidence that low folate levels, as part of the total nutritional status of the mother, are related to the length of the lactation period (62). Lactating mothers with megaloblastic anemia were treated by Cooperman and co-workers (60) with 5 mg of folic acid per day for 3 days. Breast milk folate rose from 7–9 to 15–40 ng/ml 1 day after treatment began. The elevated levels were maintained for 3 weeks without further treatment. Sneed and co-workers (67) compared nine low socioeconomic women treated with multivitamins containing 0.8 mg of folic acid with seven untreated controls. Breast milk folate level was significantly higher in the treated women. In another study of lactating women with low nutritional status, supplementation with folic acid, 0.2–10.0 mg/day, resulted in mean milk concentrations of 2.3–5.6 ng/ml (68). Milk concentrations were directly proportional to dietary intake.

Folic acid concentrations were determined in preterm and term milk in a study to determine the effect of storage time and temperature (69). Storage of milk in a freezer resulted in progressive decreases over 3 months such that the RDA of folate for infants could not be provided from milk stored for this length of time. Storage in a refrigerator for 24 hours did not affect folate levels.

The American RDA for folic acid during lactation is 0.5 mg (2). If the lactating woman's diet adequately supplies this amount, maternal supplementation with folic acid is not needed. Maternal supplementation with the RDA for folic acid is recommended for those patients with inadequate nutritional intake.

References

1. American Hospital Formulary Service. *Drug Information 1985*. Bethesda:American Society of Hospital Pharmacists, 1985:1683–4.
2. *Recommended Dietary Allowances*, 9th ed. Washington, DC:National Academy of Sciences, 1980.
3. Frank O, Walbroehl G, Thomson A, Kaminetzky H, Kubes Z, Baker H. Placental transfer: fetal retention of some vitamins. Am J Clin Nutr 1970;23:662–3.
4. Kaminetzky HA, Baker H, Frank O, Langer A. The effects of intravenously administered water-soluble vitamins during labor in normovitaminemic and hypovitaminemic gravidas on maternal and neonatal blood vitamin levels at delivery. Am J Obstet Gynecol 1974;120:697–703.
5. Hill EP, Longo LD. Dynamics of maternal-fetal nutrient transfer. Fed Proc 1980;39:239–44.
6. Baker H, Frank O, Deangelis B, Feingold S, Kaminetzky HA. Role of placenta in maternal-fetal vitamin transfer in humans. Am J Obstet Gynecol 1981;141:792–6.
7. Landon MJ, Eyre DH, Hytten FE. Transfer of folate to the fetus. Br J Obstet Gynaecol 1975;82:12–9.
8. Baker H, Frank O, Thomason AD, Langer A, Munves ED, De Angelis B, Kaminetzky HA. Vitamin profile of 174 mothers and newborns at parturition. Am J Clin Nutr 1975;28:59–65.
9. Kaminetzky HA, Baker H. Micronutrients in pregnancy. Clin Obstet Gynecol 1977;20:263–80.
10. Dostalova L. Correlation of the vitamin status between mother and newborn during delivery. Dev Pharmacol Ther 1982;4 (Suppl 1):45–57.
11. Chanarin I, Rothman D, Ward A, Perry J. Folate status and requirement in pregnancy. Br Med J 1968;2:390–4.
12. Ball EW, Giles C. Folic acid and vitamin B_{12} levels in pregnancy and their relation to megaloblastic anemia. J Clin Pathol 1964;17:165–74.
13. Ek J, Magnus EM. Plasma and red blood cell folate during normal pregnancies. Acta Obstet Gynecol Scand 1981;60:247–51.
14. Baker H, Ziffer H, Pasher I, Sobotka H. A Comparison of maternal and foetal folic acid and vitamin B_{12} at parturition. Br Med J 1958;1:978–9.
15. Avery B, Ledger WJ. Folic acid metabolism in well-nourished pregnant women. Obstet Gynecol 1970;35:616–24.
16. Ek J. Plasma and red cell folate values in newborn infants and their mothers in relation to gestational age. J Pediatr 1980;97:288–92.
17. Baker H, Thind IS, Frank O, DeAngelis B, Caterini H, Lquria DB. Vitamin levels in low-birth-weight newborn infants and their mothers. Am J Obstet Gynecol 1977;129:521–4.
18. Chanarin I, MacGibbon BM, O'Sullivan WJ, Mollin DL. Folic-acid deficiency in pregnancy: the pathogenesis of megaloblastic anaemia of pregnancy. Lancet 1959;2:634–9.
19. Gatenby PBB, Lillie EW. Clinical analysis of 100 cases of severe megaloblastic anaemia of pregnancy. Br Med J 1960;2:1111–4.
20. Pritchard JA, Mason RA, Wright MR. Megaloblastic anemia during pregnancy and the puerperium. Am J Obstet Gynecol 1962;83:1004–20.
21. Fraser JL, Watt HJ. Megaloblastic anemia in pregnancy and the puerperium. Am J Obstet Gynecol 1964;89:532–4.
22. Hibbard BM. The role of folic acid in pregnancy: with particular reference to anaemia, abruption and abortion. J Obstet Gynaecol Br Commonw 1964;71:529–42.
23. Hibbard BM, Hibbard ED, Jeffcoate TNA. Folic acid and reproduction. Acta Obstet Gynecol Scand 1965;44:375–400.
24. Giles C. An account of 335 cases of megaloblastic anaemia of pregnancy and the puerperium. J Clin Pathol 1966;19:1–11.
25. Streiff RR, Little AB. Folic acid deficiency in pregnancy. N Engl J Med 1967;276:776–9.
26. Pritchard JA, Scott DE, Whalley PJ. Folic acid requirements in pregnancy-induced megaloblastic anemia. JAMA 1969;208:1163–7.
27. Rothman D. Folic acid in pregnancy. Am J Obstet Gynecol 1970;108:149–75.

28. Shepard TH. *Catalog of Teratogenic Agents*, ed 3. Baltimore:The Johns Hopkins University Press, 1980:153–4.
29. Laurence KM, James N, Miller MH, Tennant GB, Campbell H. Double-blind randomised controlled trial of folate treatment before conception to prevent recurrence of neural-tube defects. Br Med J 1981;282:1509–11.
30. Hibbard ED, Smithells RW. Folic acid metabolism and human embryopathy. Lancet 1965;1:1254.
31. Stone ML. Effects on the fetus of folic acid deficiency in pregnancy. Clin Obstet Gynecol 1968;11:1143–53.
32. Nelson MM, Forfar JO. Associations between drugs administered during pregnancy and congenital abnormalities of the fetus. Br Med J 1971;1:523–7.
33. Scott DE, Whalley PJ, Pritchard JA. Maternal folate deficiency and pregnancy wastage. II. Fetal malformation. Obstet Gynecol 1970;36:26–8.
34. Pritchard JA, Scott DE, Whalley PJ, Haling RF Jr. Infants of mothers with megaloblastic anemia due to folate deficiency. JAMA 1970;211:1982–4.
35. Kitay DZ, Hogan WJ, Eberle B, Mynt T. Neutrophil hypersegmentation and folic acid deficiency in pregnancy. Am J Obstet Gynecol 1969;104:1163–73.
36. Pritchard JA, Scott DE, Whalley PJ. Maternal folate deficiency and pregnancy wastage. IV. Effects of folic acid supplements, anticonvulsants, and oral contraceptives. Am J Obstet Gynecol 1971;109:341–6.
37. Emery AEH, Timson J, Watson-Williams, EJ. Pathogenesis of spina bifida. Lancet 1969;2:909–10.
38. Hall MH. Folates and the fetus. Lancet 1977;1:648–9.
39. Emery AEH. Folates and fetal central-nervous-system malformations. Lancet 1977;1:703.
40. Smithells RW, Sheppard S, Schorah CJ. Vitamin deficiencies and neural tube defects. Arch Dis Child 1976;51:944–50.
41. Schorah CJ, Smithells RW, Scott J. Vitamin B_{12} and anencephaly. Lancet 1980;1:880.
42. Biale Y, Lewenthal H. Effect of folic acid supplementation on congenital malformations due to anticonvulsive drugs. Eur J Obstet Gynecol Reprod Biol 1984;18:211–6.
43. Hiilesmaa VK, Teramo K, Granstrom M-L, Bardy AH. Serum folate concentrations during pregnancy in women with epilepsy: relation to antiepileptic drug concentrations, number of seizures, and fetal outcome. Br Med J 1983;287:577–9.
44. Hibbard BM, Jeffcoate TNA. Abruptio placentae. Obstet Gynecol 1966;27:155–67.
45. Stone ML, Luhby AL, Feldman R, Gordon M, Cooperman JM. Folic acid metabolism in pregnancy. Am J Obstet Gynecol 1967;99:638–48.
46. Whalley PJ, Scott DE, Pritchard JA. Maternal folate deficiency and pregnancy wastage. I. Placental abruption. Am J Obstet Gynecol 1969;105:670–8.
47. Whalley PJ, Scott DE, Pritchard JA. Maternal folate deficiency and pregnancy wastage. III. Pregnancy-induced hypertension. Obstet Gynecol 1970;36:29–31.
48. Martin JD, Davis RE. Serum folic acid activity and vaginal bleeding in early pregnancy. J Obstet Gynaecol Br Commonw 1964;71:400–3.
49. Martin RH, Harper TA, Kelso W. Serum-folic-acid in recurrent abortions. Lancet 1965;1:670–2.
50. Martin JD, Davis RE, Stenhouse N. Serum folate and vitamin B12 levels in pregnancy with particular reference to uterine bleeding and bacteriuria. J Obstet Gynaecol Br Commonw 1967;74:697–701.
51. Streiff RR, Little B. Folic acid deficiency as a cause of uterine hemorrhage in pregnancy. J Clin Invest 1965;44:1102.
52. Whiteside MG, Ungar B, Cowling DC. Iron, folic acid and vitamin B_{12} levels in normal pregnancy, and their influence on birth-weight and the duration of pregnancy. Med J Aust 1968;1:338–42.
53. Husain OAN, Rothman D, Ellis L. Folic acid deficiency in pregnancy. J Obstet Gynaecol Br Commonw 1963;70:821–7.
54. Abramowicz M, Kass EH. Pathogenesis and prognosis of prematurity (continued). N Engl J Med 1966;275:938–43.
55. Scott KE, Usher R. Fetal malnutrition: its incidence, causes, and effects. Am J Obstet Gynecol 1966;94:951–63.
56. Varadi S, Abbott D, Elwis A. Correlation of peripheral white cell and bone marrow changes with folate levels in pregnancy and their clinical significance. J Clin Pathol 1966;19:33–6.
57. Averback P. Anencephaly associated with megavitamin therapy. Can Med Assoc J 1976;114:995.
58. Mukherjee MD, Sandstead HH, Ratnaparkhi MV, Johnson LK, Milne DB, Stelling HP. Maternal zinc, iron, folic acid, and protein nutriture and outcome of human pregnancy. Am J Clin Nutr 1984;40:496–507.

59. Metz J. Folate deficiency conditioned by lactation. Am J Clin Nutr 1970;23:843–7.
60. Cooperman JM, Dweck HS, Newman LJ, Garbarino C, Lopez R. The folate in human milk. Am J Clin Nutr 1982;36:576–80.
61. Ford JE, Zechalko A, Murphy J, Brooke OG. Comparison of the B vitamin composition of milk from mothers of preterm and term babies. Arch Dis Child 1983;58:367–72.
62. Ek J. Plasma, red cell, and breast milk folacin concentrations in lactating women. Am J Clin Nutr 1983;38:929–35.
63. Ek J, Magnus EM. Plasma and red blood cell folate in breastfed infants. Acta Paediatr Scand 1979;68:239–43.
64. Tamura T, Yoshimura Y, Arakawa T. Human milk folate and folate status in lactating mothers and their infants. Am J Clin Nutr 1980;33:193–7.
65. Thomas MR, Sneed SM, Wei C, Nail PA, Wilson M, Sprinkle EE III. The effects of vitamin C, vitamin B_6, vitamin B_{12}, folic acid, riboflavin, and thiamine on the breast milk and maternal status of well-nourished women at 6 months postpartum, Am J Clin Nutr 1980;33:2151–6.
66. Smith AM, Picciano MF, Deering RH. Folate intake and blood concentrations of term infants. Am J Clin Nutr 1985;41:590–8.
67. Sneed SM, Zane C, Thomas MR. The effects of ascorbic acid, vitamin B_6, vitamin B_{12}, and folic acid supplementation on the breast milk and maternal nutritional status of low socioeconomic lactating women. Am J Clin Nutr 1981;34:1338–46.
68. Deodhar AD, Rajalakshmi R, Ramakrishnan CV. Studies on human lactation. Part III. Effect of dietary vitamin supplementation on vitamin contents of breast milk. Acta Paediatr (Stockholm) 1964;53:42–8.
69. Bank MR, Kirksey A, West K, Giacoia G. Effect of storage time and temperature on folacin and vitamin C levels in term and preterm human milk. Am J Clin Nutr 1985;41:235–42.

Name: **FURAZOLIDONE**

Class: **Anti-infective**   Risk Factor: **C**

Fetal Risk Summary

No reports linking the use of furazolidone with congenital defects have been located. The Collaborative Perinatal Project monitored 50,282 mother-child pairs, 132 of which had 1st trimester exposure to furazolidone (1). No association with malformations was found. Theoretically, furazolidone could produce hemolytic anemia in a glucose-6-phosphate-dehydrogenase-deficient newborn if given at term. Placental passage of the drug has not been reported.

Breast Feeding Summary

No data available.

References

1. Heinonen OP, Slone D, Shapiro S. *Birth Defects and Drugs in Pregnancy*. Littleton:Publishing Sciences Group, 1977:299–302.

Name: **FUROSEMIDE**

Class: **Diuretic**   Risk Factor: **C$_M$**

Fetal Risk Summary

Furosemide is a potent diuretic. Cardiovascular disorders such as pulmonary edema, severe hypertension, or congestive heart failure are probably the only valid indications for this drug in pregnancy. Furosemide crosses the placenta (1). Following oral doses of 25–40 mg, peak concentrations in cord serum of 330 ng/ml were recorded at 9 hours. Maternal and cord levels were equal at 8 hours. Increased fetal urine production after maternal furosemide therapy has been observed (2, 3). Administration of furosemide to the mother has been used to assess fetal kidney function by provoking urine production, which is then visualized by ultrasonic techniques (4, 5). Diuresis was found more often in newborns exposed to furosemide shortly before birth than in controls (6). Urinary sodium and potassium levels in the treated newborns were significantly greater than those in the nonexposed controls.

Furosemide is rarely given during the 1st trimester. After the 1st trimester, furosemide has been used for edema, hypertension, and toxemia of pregnancy without causing fetal or newborn adverse effects (7–29). Many investigators now consider diuretics contraindicated in pregnancy, except for patients with cardiovascular disorders, since they do not prevent or alter the course of toxemia and they may decrease placental perfusion (30–33). A 1984 study determined that the use of diuretics for hypertension in pregnancy prevented normal plasma volume expansion and did not change perinatal outcome (34).

Administration of the drug during pregnancy does not significantly alter amniotic fluid volume (28). Serum uric acid levels, which are increased in toxemia, are further elevated by furosemide (35). No association was found in a 1973 study between furosemide and low platelet counts in the neonate (36). Unlike the thiazide diuretics, neonatal thrombocytopenia has not been reported for furosemide.

Breast Feeding Summary

Furosemide is excreted into breast milk (37). While no reports of adverse effects in nursing infants have been found, the manufacturer recommends against breast-feeding if furosemide must be given to the mother (37). Thiazide diuretics have been used to suppress lactation (see Chlorothiazide).

References

1. Beermann B, Groschinsky-Grind M, Fahraeus L, Lindstroem B. Placental transfer of furosemide. Clin Pharmacol Ther 1978;24:560–2.
2. Wladimiroff JW. Effect of frusemide on fetal urine production. Br J Obstet Gynaecol 1975;82:221–4.
3. Stein WW, Halberstadt E, Gerner R, Roemer E. Affect of furosemide on fetal kidney function. Arch Gynekol 1977;224:114–5.
4. Barrett RJ, Rayburn WF, Barr M Jr. Furosemide (Lasix) challenge test in assessing bilateral fetal hydronephrosis. Am J Obstet Gynecol 1983;147:846–7.
5. Harman CR. Maternal furosemide may not provoke urine production in the compromised fetus. Am J Obstet Gynecol 1984;150:322–3.
6. Pecorari D, Ragni N, Autera C. Administration of furosemide to women during confinement, and its action on newborn infants. Acta Biomed Ateneo Parmense 1969;40:2–11.

7. Pulle C. Diuretic therapy in monosymptomatic edema of pregnancy. Minerva Med 1965;56:1622–3.

8. DeCecco L. Furosemide in the treatment of edema in pregnancy. Minerva Med 1965;56:1586–91.

9. Bocci A, Pupita F, Revelli E, Bartoli E, Molaschi M, Massobrio A. The water-salt metabolism in obstetrics and gynecology. Minerva Ginecol 1965;17:103–10.

10. Sideri L. Furosemide in the treatment of oedema in gynaecology and obstetrics. Clin Ter 1966;39:339–46.

11. Wu CC, Lee TT, Kao SC. Evaluation of new diuretic (furosemide) on pregnant women. A pilot study. J Obstet Gynecol Republic China 1966;5:318–20.

12. Loch EG. Treatment of gestosis with diuretics. Med Klin 1966;61:1512–5.

13. Buchheit M, Nicolai. Influence of furosemide (Lasix) on gestational edemas. Med Klin 1966;61:1515–8.

14. Tanaka T. Studies on the clinical effect of Lasix in edema of pregnancy and toxemia of pregnancy. Sanka To Fujinka 1966;41:914–20.

15. Merger R, Cohen J, Sadut R. Study of the therapeutic effects of furosemide in obstetrics. Rev Fr Gynecol 1967;62:259–65.

16. Nascimento R, Fernandes R, Cunha A. Furosemide as an accessory in the therapy of the toxemia of pregnancy. Hospital (Portugal) 1967;71:137–40.

17. Finnerty FA Jr. Advantages and disadvantages of furosemide in the edematous states of pregnancy. Am J Obstet Gynecol 1969;105:1022–7.

18. Das Gupta S. Frusemide in blood transfusion for severe anemia in pregnancy. J Obstet Gynaecol India 1970;20:521–5.

19. Kawathekar P, Anusuya SR, Sriniwas P, Lagali S. Diazepam (Calmpose) in eclampsia: a preliminary report of 16 cases. Curr Ther Res 1973;15:845–55.

20. Pianetti F. Our results in the treatment of parturient patients with oedema during the five years 1966–1970. Atti Accad Med Lombarda 1973;27:137–40.

21. Azcarte Sanchez S, Quesada Rocha T, Rosas Arced J. Evaluation of a plan of treatment in eclampsia (first report). Ginecol Obstet Mex 1973;34:171–86.

22. Bravo Sandoval J. Management of pre-eclampsia-eclampsia in the third gyneco-obstetrical hospital. Cir Cirujanos 1973;41:487–94.

23. Franck H, Gruhl M. Therapeutic experience with nortensin in the treament of toxemia of pregnancy. Münch Med Wochenschr 1974;116:521–4.

24. Cornu P, Laffay J, Ertel M, Lemiere J. Resuscitation in eclampsia. Rev Prat 1975;25:809–30.

25. Finnerty FA Jr. Management of hypertension in toxemia of pregnancy. Hosp Med 1975;11:52–65.

26. Saldana-Garcia RH. Eclampsia: maternal and fetal mortality. Comparative study of 80 cases. In *VIII World Congress of Gynecology and Obstetrics*. Int Cong Ser 1976;396:58–9.

27. Palot M, Jakob L, Decaux J, Brundis JP, Quereux C, Wahl P. Arterial hypertensions of labor and the postpartum period. Rev Fr Gynecol Obstet 1979;74:173–6.

28. Votta RA, Parada OH, Windgrad RH, Alvarez OH, Tomassinni TL, Patori AA. Furosemide action on the creatinine concentration of amniotic fluid. Am J Obstet Gynecol 1975;123:621–4.

29. Clark AD, Sevitt LH, Hawkins DF. Use of furosemide in severe toxaemia of pregnancy. Lancet 1972;1:35–6.

30. Pitkin RM, Kaminetzky HA, Newton M, Pritchard JA. Maternal nutrition: a selective review of clinical topics. Obstet Gynecol 1972;40:773–85.

31. Lindheimer MD, Katz AI. Sodium and diuretics in pregnancy. N Engl J Med 1973;288:891–4.

32. Christianson R, Page EW. Diuretic drugs and pregnancy. Obstet Gynecol 1976;48:647–52.

33. Gant NF, Madden JD, Shteri PK, MacDonald PC. The metabolic clearance rate of dehydroisoandrosterone sulfate. IV. Acute effects of induced hypertension, hypotension, and natriuresis in normal and hypertensive pregnancies. Am J Obstet Gynecol 1976;124:143–8.

34. Sibai BM, Grossman RA, Grossman HG. Effects of diuretics on plasma volume in pregnancies with long-term hypertension. Am J Obstet Gynecol 1984;150:831–5.

35. Carswell W, Semple PF. The effect of furosemide on uric acid levels in maternal blood, fetal blood and amniotic fluid. J Obstet Gynaecol Br Commonw 1974;81:472–4.

36. Jerkner K, Kutti J, Victorin L. Platelet counts in mothers and their newborn infants with respect to antepartum administration of oral diuretics. Acta Med Scand 1973;194:473–5.

37. Product information. Lasix. Hoechst-Roussel Pharmaceuticals, 1985.

Name: **GENTAMICIN**

Class: **Antibiotic**   Risk Factor: **C**

Fetal Risk Summary

Gentamicin is an aminoglycoside antibiotic. The drug rapidly crosses the placenta into the fetal circulation and amniotic fluid (1–8). Following 40–80-mg intramuscular doses given to patients in labor, peak cord serum levels averaging 34–44% of maternal levels were obtained at 1–2 hours (1, 4, 8). No toxicity attributable to gentamicin was seen in any of the newborns. Patients undergoing 1st and 2nd trimester abortions were given 1 mg/kg intramuscularly (5). Gentamicin could not be detected in their cord serum before 2 hours. Amniotic fluid levels were undetectable at this dosage up to 9 hours postinjection. Doubling the dose to 2 mg/kg allowed detectable levels in the fluid in one of two samples 5 hours postinjection.

Intra-amniotic instillations of gentamicin were given to 11 patients with premature rupture of the membranes (9). Ten patients received 25 mg every 12 hours and one received 25 mg every 8 hours, for a total of 1–19 doses per patient. Maternal gentamicin serum levels ranged from 0.063 to 6 μg/ml (all but one were less than 0.6 μg/ml and that one was believed to be due to error). Cord serum levels varied from 0.063 to 2 μg/ml (all but two were less than 0.6 μg/ml). No harmful effects were seen in the newborns after prolonged exposure to high local concentrations of gentamicin.

No reports linking the use of gentamicin to congenital defects have been located. Ototoxicity, which is known to occur after gentamicin therapy, has not been reported as an effect of *in utero* exposure. However, eighth cranial nerve toxicity in the fetus is well known following exposure to other aminoglycosides (see Kanamycin and Streptomycin) and may potentially occur with gentamicin. Potentiation of $MgSO_4$-induced neuromuscular weakness has been reported in a neonate exposed during the last 32 hours of pregnancy to 24 g of $MgSO_4$ (10). The depressed infant was treated with gentamicin for sepsis at 12 hours of age. After the second dose, the infant's condition worsened, with rapid onset of respiratory arrest. Emergency treatment was successful, and no lasting effects of the toxic interaction were noted.

Breast Feeding Summary

Data on the excretion of gentamicin into breast milk are lacking. In one case report, a nursing infant developed two grossly bloody stools while his mother was receiving gentamicin and clindamycin (10). The condition cleared rapidly when breast-feeding was discontinued. Clindamycin is known to be excreted into breast milk as are the aminoglycosides (see Amikacin, Kanamycin, Streptomycin, and Tobramycin).

References

1. Percetto G, Baratta A, Menozzi M. Observations on the use of gentamicin in gynecology and obstetrics. Minerva Ginecol 1969;21:1–10.

2. von Kobyletzki D. Experimental studies on the transplacental passage of gentamicin. Paper presented at Fifth International Congress on Chemotherapy, Vienna, 1967.
3. von Koblyetzki D, Wahlig H, Gebhardt F. Pharmacokinetics of gentamicin during delivery. In *Proceedings of the Sixth International Congress on Chemotherapy*, Tokyo. Antimicrob Anticancer Chemother 1969;1:650–2.
4. Yoshioka H, Monma T, Matsuda S. Placental transfer of gentamicin. J Pediatr 1972;80:121–3.
5. Garcia S, Ballard C, Martin C, Ivler D, Mathies A, Bernard B. Perinatal pharmacology of gentamicin. Clin Res 1972;20:252 (Abstr).
6. Daubenfeld O, Modde H, Hirsch H. Transfer of gentamicin to the foetus and the amniotic fluid during a steady state in the mother. Arch Gynecol 1974;217:233–40.
7. Kauffman R, Morris J, Azarnoff D. Placental transfer and fetal urinary excetion of gentamicin during constant rate maternal infusion. Pediatr Res 1975;9:104–7.
8. Weistein A, Gibbs R, Gallagher M. Placental transfer of clindamycin and gentamicin in term pregnancy. Am J Obstet Gynecol 1976;124:688–91.
9. Freeman D, Matsen J, Arnold N. Amniotic fluid and maternal and cord serum levels of gentamicin after intra-amniotic instillation in patients with premature rupture of the membranes. Am J Obstet Gynecol 1972;113:1138–41.
10. L'Hommedieu CS, Nicholas D, Armes DA, Jones P, Nelson T, Pickering LK. Potentiation of magnesium sulfate-induced neuromuscular weakness by gentamicin, tobramycin, and amikacin. J Pediatr 1983;102:629–31.
11. Mann CF. Clindamycin and breast-feeding. Pediatrics 1980;66:1030–1.

Name: **GENTIAN VIOLET**

Class: **Disinfectant/Anthelmintic**   Risk Factor: **C**

Fetal Risk Summary

The Collaborative Perinatal Project monitored 50,282 mother-child pairs, 40 of which had 1st trimester exposure to gentian violet (1). Evidence was found to suggest a relationship to malformations based on defects in four patients. Independent confirmation is required to determine the actual risk.

Breast Feeding Summary

No data available.

References

1. Heinonen OP, Slone D, Shapiro S. *Birth Defects and Drugs in Pregnancy*. Littleton:Publishing Sciences Group, 1977:302.

Name: **GITALIN**

Class: **Cardiac Glycoside**   Risk Factor: **C**

Fetal Risk Summary

See Digitalis.

Breast Feeding Summary

See Digitalis.

Name: **GLYCERIN**

Class: **Diuretic**   Risk Factor: **C**

Fetal Risk Summary

No data available.

Breast Feeding Summary

No data available.

Name: **GLYCOPYRROLATE**

Class: **Parasympatholytic (Anticholinergic)**   Risk Factor: **B$_M$**

Fetal Risk Summary

Glycopyrrolate is an anticholinergic agent. In a large prospective study, 2,323 patients were exposed to this class of drugs during the 1st trimester, only four of whom took glycopyrrolate (1). A possible association was found between the total group and minor malformations. Glycopyrrolate has been used prior to cesarean section to decrease gastric secretions (2–5). Maternal heart rate, but not blood pressure, was increased. Uterine activity increased as expected for normal labor. Fetal heart rate and variability were not changed significantly, confirming the limited placental transfer of this quaternary ammonium compound. No effects in the newborns were observed.

Breast Feeding Summary

No data available (see also Atropine).

References

1. Heinonen OP, Slone D, Shapiro S. *Birth Defects and Drugs in Pregnancy*. Littleton:Publishing Sciences Group, 1977:346–53.
2. Diaz DM, Diaz SF, Marx GF. Cardiovascular effects of glycopyrrolate and belladonna derivatives in obstetric patients. Bull NY Acad Med 1980;56:245–8.
3. Abboud TK, Read J, Miller F, Chen T, Valle R, Henriksen EH. Use of glycopyrrolate in the parturient: effect on the maternal and fetal heart and uterine activity. Obstet Gynecol 1981;57:224–7.
4. Roper RE, Salem MG. Effects of glycopyrrolate and atropine combined with antacid on gastric acidity. Br J Anaesth 1981;53:1277–80.
5. Abboud T, Raya J, Sadri S, Grobler N, Stine L, Miller F. Fetal and maternal cardiovascular effects of atropine and glycopyrrolate. Anesth Analg 1983;62:426–30.

Name: **GOLD SODIUM THIOMALATE**

Class: **Gold Compound**   Risk Factor: **C**

Fetal Risk Summary

Gold compounds have been used for the treatment of maternal rheumatoid arthritis and other conditions in a small number of pregnancies (1–4). Freyberg and co-workers (1) noted that several pregnant patients had been treated with gold salts without harmful effects observed in the newborns. In a Japanese report, 119 patients were treated during the 1st trimester with gold, 26 of whom received the drug throughout pregnancy (2). Two anomalies were observed in the newborns: dislocated hip in one infant and a flattened acetabulum in another.

Gold compounds cross the placenta. A patient who had received a total dose of 570 mg of gold sodium thiomalate from before conception through the 20th week of gestation elected to terminate her pregnancy (3). No obvious fetal abnormalities were observed, but gold deposits were found in the fetal liver and kidneys. A second patient received monthly 100-mg injections of gold throughout pregnancy (4). The last dose, given 3 days prior to delivery, produced a cord serum concentration of 2.25 μg/ml, 57% of the simultaneous maternal serum level. No anomalies were observed in the infant.

Although gold compounds apparently do not pose a major risk to the fetus, the clinical experience is limited and long-term follow-up studies of exposed fetuses have not been reported.

Breast Feeding Summary

Gold is excreted in milk (5, 6). A woman received a total aurothioglucose dose of 135 mg in the postpartum period (5). Gold levels in two milk samples collected a week apart were 8.64 and 9.97 μg/ml. The validity of these figures has been challenged on a mathematical basis, so the exact amount excreted is open to question (6). In addition, the timing of the samples in relation to the dose was not given. Of interest, however, was the demonstration of gold levels in the infant's red blood cells (0.354 μg/ml) and serum (0.712 μg/ml) obtained on the same date as the second milk sample. The author speculated that this unexpected oral absorption may have been the cause of various unexplained adverse reactions noted in nursing infants of mothers receiving gold injections, such as rashes, nephritis, hepatitis, and hematologic abnormalities (5). A separate report described a lactating woman who was treated with 50 mg of gold sodium thiomalate weekly for 7 weeks after an initial 20-mg dose (total dose 370 mg) (7). Milk and infant urine samples collected 66 hours after the last dose yielded gold levels of 0.022 and 0.0004 μg/ml, respectively. Repeat samples collected 7 days after an additional 25-mg dose produced milk and urine levels of 0.04 and <0.0004 μg/ml, respectively. No explanation was found for the higher milk concentration following the lower dose. Three months after cessation of therapy, transient facial edema was observed in the nursing infant, but it was not known if this was related to the maternal gold administration.

In summary, although two studies have found markedly different levels, gold is excreted in milk and small amounts are absorbed by the infant. Adverse effects in the nursing infant have been suggested but not proven. However, due to the prolonged maternal elimination time after gold administration and the potential for severe toxicity in the nursing infant, nursing should be avoided. The American Academy of Pediatrics considers gold salts contraindicated during breast-feeding because of their potential for producing rashes and inflammation of the kidney and liver (8, 9).

References

1. Freyberg RH, Ziff M, Baum J. Gold therapy for rheumatoid arthritis. In Hollander JL, McCarty DJ Jr, eds. *Arthritis and Allied Conditions*, ed 8. Philadelphia:Lea & Febiger, 1972:479.
2. Miyamoto T, Miyaji S, Horiuchi Y, Hara M, Ishihara K. Gold therapy in bronchial asthma—special emphasis upon blood level of gold and its teratogenicity. J Jpn Soc Intern Med 1974;63:1190–7.
3. Rocker I, Henderson WJ. Transfer of gold from mother to fetus. Lancet 1976;2:1246.
4. Cohen DL, Orzel J, Taylor A. Infants of mothers receiving gold therapy. Arthritis Rheum 1981;24:104–5.
5. Blau SP. Metabolism of gold during lactation. Arthritis Rheum 1973;16:777–8.
6. Gottlieb NL. Suggested errata. Arthritis Rheum 1974;17:1057.
7. Bell RAF, Dale IM. Gold secretion in maternal milk. Arthritis Rheum 1976;19:1374.
8. Committee on Drugs, American Academy of Pediatrics. The transfer of drugs and other chemicals into human breast milk. Pediatrics 1983;72:375–83.
9. Hill RM, Tennyson LM. The lactating allergic patient: which drugs cause concern for the infant?. Immunol Allergy Prac 1984;6:221–7.

Name: **GRISEOFULVIN**

Class: **Antifungal**   Risk Factor: **C**

Fetal Risk Summary

Griseofulvin is embryotoxic and teratogenic in some species of animals, but its use in human pregnancy has not been studied. Because of the animal toxicity, at least one publication believes it should not be given during pregnancy (1). Placental transfer of griseofulvin has been demonstrated at term (2).

A possible interaction between oral contraceptives and griseofulvin has been reported in 22 women (3). Transient intermenstrual bleeding in 15, amenorrhea in 5, and unintended pregnancies in 2 were described.

Breast Feeding Summary

No data available.

References

1. Anonymous. Griseofulvin: a new formulation and some old concerns. Med Lett Drugs Ther 1976;18:17.
2. Rubin A, Dvornik D. Placental transfer of griseofulvin. Am J Obstet Gynecol 1965;92:882–3.
3. van Dijke CPH, Weber JCP. Interaction between oral contraceptives and griseofulvin. Br Med J 1984;288:1125–6.

Name: **GUAIFENESIN**

Class: **Expectorant**   Risk Factor: **C**

Fetal Risk Summary

The Collaborative Perinatal Project monitored 197 mother-child pairs with 1st trimester exposure to guaifenesin (1). An increase in the expected frequency of inguinal hernias was found. For use anytime during pregnancy, 1,336 exposures were recorded (2). In this latter case, no evidence for an association with malformations was found. In another large study in which 241 women were exposed to the drug during pregnancy, no strong association was found between guaifenesin and congenital defects (3).

A 1981 report described a woman who consumed, throughout pregnancy, 480–840 ml/day of a cough syrup (4). The potential maximum daily doses based on 840 ml of syrup were: 16.8 g of guaifenesin, 5.0 g of pseudoephedrine, 1.68 g of dextromethorphan, and 79.8 ml of ethanol. The infant had features of the fetal alcohol syndrome (see Ethanol) and displayed irritability, tremors, and hypertonicity. It is not known if guaifenesin or the other drugs, other than ethanol, were associated with the adverse effects observed in the infant.

Breast Feeding Summary

No data available.

References

1. Heinonen OP, Slone D, Shapiro S. *Birth Defects and Drugs in Pregnancy*. Littleton:Publishing Sciences Group, 1977:478.
2. *Ibid*, 442.
3. Aselton P, Jick H, Milunsky A, Hunter JR, Stergachis A. First-trimester drug use and congenital disorders. Obstet Gynecol 1985;65:451–5.
4. Chasnoff IJ, Diggs G, Schnoll SH. Fetal alcohol effects and maternal cough syrup abuse. Am J Dis Child 1981;135:968.

Name: **HALOPERIDOL**

Class: **Tranquilizer**   Risk Factor: **C**

Fetal Risk Summary

Two reports describing limb reduction malformations after 1st trimester use of haloperidol have been located (1, 2). In one of these cases, high doses (15 mg/day) were used (2). Other investigations have not found these defects (3–7). Defects observed in the two infants were:

Ectrophocomelia (1)
Multiple upper and lower limb defects, aortic valve defect, death (2)

In 98 of 100 patients treated with haloperidol for hyperemesis gravidarum in the 1st trimester, no effects were produced on birth weight, duration of pregnancy, sex ratio, fetal or neonatal mortality, and no malformations were found in abortuses, stillborn, or liveborn infants (3). Two of the patients were lost to follow-up. In 31 infants with severe reduction deformities born over a 4-year period, none of the mothers remembered taking haloperidol (4). Haloperidol has been used for the control of chorea gravidarum and manic-depressive illness during the 2nd and 3rd trimesters (8, 9). During labor, the drug has been administered to the mother without causing neonatal depression or other effects in the newborn (5).

Breast Feeding Summary

Haloperidol is excreted into breast milk. In one patient receiving an average of 29.2 mg/day, a milk level of 5 ng/ml was detected (10). When the dose was decreased to 12 mg, a level of 2 ng/ml was measured. In a second patient taking 10 mg daily, milk levels up to 23.5 ng/ml were found (11). A milk:plasma ratio of 0.6–0.7 was calculated. No adverse effects were noted in the nursing infant. The American Academy of Pediatrics considers haloperidol compatible with breast-feeding (12).

References

1. Dieulangard P, Coignet J, Vidal JC. Sur un cas d'ectro-phocomelie peut-etre d'origine medicamenteuse. Bull Fed Gynecol Obstet 1966;18:85–7.
2. Kopelman AE, McCullar FW, Heggeness L. Limb malformations following maternal use of haloperidol. JAMA 1975;231:62–4.
3. Van Waes A, Van de Velde E. Safety evaluation of haloperidol in the treatment of hyperemesis gravidarum. J Clin Pharmacol 1969;9:224–7.
4. Hanson JW, Oakley GP. Haloperidol and limb deformity. JAMA 1975;231:26.
5. Ayd FJ Jr. Haloperidol: fifteen years of clinical experience. Dis Nerv Syst 1972;33:459–69.
6. Magnier P. On hyperemesis gravidarum; a therapeutical study of R 1625. Gynecol Prat 1964;15:17–23.
7. Loke KH, Salleh R. Electroconvulsive therapy for the acutely psychotic pregnant patient: a review of 3 cases. Med J Malaysia 1983;38:131–3.

8. Donaldson JO. Control of chorea gravidarum with haloperidol. Obstet Gynecol 1982;59:381–2.

9. Nurnberg HG. Treatment of mania in the last six months of pregnancy. Hosp Community Psychiatry 1980;31:122–6.

10. Stewart RB, Karas B, Springer PK. Haloperidol excretion in human milk. Am J Psychiatry 1980;137:849–50.

11. Whalley LJ, Blain PG, Prime JK. Haloperidol secreted in breast milk. Br Med J 1981;282:1746–7.

12. Committee on Drugs, American Academy of Pediatrics. The transfer of drugs and other chemicals into human breast milk. Pediatrics 1983;72:375–83.

Name: **HEPARIN**

Class: **Anticoagulant**   Risk Factor: **C**

Fetal Risk Summary

No reports linking the use of heparin during gestation with congenital defects have been located. Other problems, at times lethal to the fetus or neonate, may be related to heparin or to the severe maternal disease necessitating anticoagulant therapy. Hall and co-workers (1) reviewed the use of heparin and other anticoagulants during pregnancy (167 references) (see also Coumarin Derivatives). They concluded from the published cases in which heparin was used without other anticoagulants that significant risks existed for the mother and fetus and that heparin was not a clearly superior form of treatment for anticoagulation during pregnancy. Nageotte and co-workers (2) analyzed the same data to arrive at a different conclusion.

	Hall	Nageotte
Total number of cases	135	120
Term liveborn—no complications	86	86
Premature—survived without complications	19	19
Liveborn—complications (not specified)	1	1
Premature—expired		
Heparin therapy appropriate*	10	5
Heparin therapy not appropriate*	—	4[a]
Severe maternal disease making successful outcome of pregnancy unlikely		1[b]
Spontaneous abortions		
Unknown cause	2	1
Maternal death due to pulmonary embolism	—	1
Stillbirths		
Heparin therapy appropriate*	17	8
Heparin therapy not appropriate*	—	7[c]
Heparin and Coumadin used	—	2

* Appropriateness as determined by current standards
[a] Hypertension of pregnancy (4)
[b] Tricuspid atresia (1)
[c] Hypertension of pregnancy (6); proliferative glomerulonephritis (1)

By eliminating the 15 cases in which maternal disease or other drugs were the most likely cause of the fetal problem, the analysis of Nageotte et al results in a 13% (15 of 120) unfavorable outcome vs the 22% (30 of 135) of Hall et al. This new value appears to be significantly better than the 31% (133 of 426) abnormal outcome reported for coumarin derivatives (see Coumarin Derivatives). Further, in contrast to coumarin derivatives where a definitive drug-induced pattern of malformations has been observed (fetal warfarin syndrome), heparin has not been related to congenital defects nor does it cross the placenta (3–5). Consequently, the mechanism of heparin's adverse effect on the fetus, if it exists, must be indirect. Hall et al (1) theorized that fetal effects may be due to calcium (or other cation) chelation, resulting in the deficiency of that ion(s) in the fetus. A more likely explanation, in light of the report of Nageotte et al, is severe maternal disease that could be relatively independent of heparin use. Thus, heparin appears to have major advantages over oral anticoagulants as the treatment of choice during pregnancy.

Long-term heparin therapy during pregnancy has been associated with maternal osteopenia (14–18). Both low-dose (10,000 units/day) and high-dose heparin have been implicated, but the latter is more often related to this complication. One study found bone demineralization to be dose-related, with more severe changes occurring after long-term therapy (>25 weeks) and in patients who had also received heparin in a previous pregnancy (17). The significant decrease in 1,25-dihydroxy-vitamin D levels measured in heparin-treated pregnant patients may be related to the pathogenesis of this adverse effect (15, 16). Similar problems have not been reported in newborns.

Breast Feeding Summary

Heparin is not excreted into breast milk due to its high molecular weight (15,000) (19).

References

1. Hall JG, Pauli RM, Wilson KM. Maternal and fetal sequelae of anticoagulation during pregnancy. Am J Med 1980;68:122–40.
2. Nageotte MP, Freeman RK, Garite TJ, Block RA. Anticoagulation in pregnancy. Am J Obstet Gynecol 1981;141:472.
3. Flessa HC, Kapstrom AB, Glueck HI, Will JJ, Miller MA, Brinker B. Placental transport of heparin. Am J Obstet Gynecol 1965;93:570–3.
4. Russo R, Bortolotti U, Schivazappa L, Girolami A. Warfarin treatment during pregnancy: a clinical note. Haemostasis 1979;8:96–8.
5. Moe N. Anticoagulant-therapy in the prevention of placental infarction and perinatal death. Obstet Gynecol 1982;59:481–3.
6. Hellgren M, Nygards EB. Long-term therapy with subcutaneous heparin during pregnancy. Gynecol Obstet Invest 1982;13:76. As cited in Obstet Gynecol Surv 1982;37:615–6.
7. Cohen AW, Gabbe SG, Mennuti MT. Adjusted-dose heparin therapy by continuous intravenous infusion for recurrent pulmonary embolism during pregnancy. Am J Obstet Gynecol 1983;146:463–4.
8. Howell R, Fidler J, Letsky E. The risks of antenatal subcutaneous heparin prophylaxis: a controlled trial. Br J Obstet Gynaecol 1983;90:1124–8.
9. Vellenga E, van Imhoff GW, Aarnoudse JG. Effective prophylaxis with oral anticoagulants and low-dose heparin during pregnancy in an antithrombin III deficient woman. Lancet 1983;2:224.
10. Bergqvist A, Bergqvist D, Hallbook T. Deep vein thrombosis during pregnancy. Acta Obstet Gynecol Scand 1983;62:443–8.
11. Michiels JJ, Stibbe J, Vellenga E, van Vliet HHDM. Prophylaxis of thrombosis in antithrombin III-deficient women during pregnancy and delivery. Eur J Obstet Gynecol Reprod Biol 1984;18:149–53.
12. Nelson DM, Stempel LE, Fabri PJ, Talbert M. Hickman catheter use in a pregnant patient requiring therapeutic heparin anticoagulation. Am J Obstet Gynecol 1984;149:461–2.
13. Romero R, Duffy TP, Berkowitz RL, Chang E, Hobbins JC. Prolongation of a preterm pregnancy

complicated by death of a single twin in utero and disseminated intravascular coagulation: effects of treatment with heparin. N Engl J Med 1984;310:772–4.

14. Wise PH, Hall AJ. Heparin-induced osteopenia in pregnancy. Br Med J 1980;281:110–1.
15. Aarskog D, Aksnes L, Lehmann V. Low 1,25-dihydroxyvitamin D in heparin-induced osteopenia. Lancet 1980;2:650–1.
16. Aarskog D, Aksnes L, Markestad T, Ulstein M, Sagen N. Heparin-induced inhibition of 1,25-dihydroxyvitamin D formation. Am J Obstet Gynecol 1984;148:1141–2.
17. De Swiet M, Dorrington Ward P, Fidler J, Horsman A, Katz D, Letsky E, Peacock M, Wise PH. Prolonged heparin therapy in pregnancy causes bone demineralization. Br J Obstet Gynaecol 1983;90:1129–34.
18. Griffiths HT, Liu DTY. Severe heparin osteoporosis in pregnancy. Postgrad Med J 1984;60:424–5.
19. O'Reilly RA. Anticoagulant, antithrombotic, and thrombolytic drugs. In Gilman AG, Goodman LS, Gilman A, eds. *The Pharmacological Basis of Therapeutics*, ed 6. New York: Macmillan Publishing Co, 1980:1350.

Name: **HEROIN**

Class: **Narcotic Analgesic**   Risk Factor: **B***

Fetal Risk Summary

In the United States, heroin exposure during pregnancy is confined to illicit use as opposed to other countries, such as Great Britain, where the drug is commercially available. The documented fetal toxicity of heroin derives from the illicit use and resulting maternal-fetal addiction. In the form available to the addict, heroin is adulterated with various substances such as lactose, glucose, mannitol, starch, quinine, amphetamines, strychnine, procaine, or lidocaine or contaminated with bacteria, viruses or fungi (1, 2). Maternal use of other drugs, both abuse and nonabuse, is likely. It is, therefore, difficult to separate entirely the effects of heroin on the fetus from the possible effects of other chemical agents, multiple diseases with addiction, and life-style.

Heroin rapidly crosses the placenta, entering fetal tissues within 1 hour of administration. Withdrawal of the drug from the mother causes the fetus to undergo simultaneous withdrawal. Intrauterine death may occur from meconium aspiration (3, 4).

Assessment of fetal maturity and status is often difficult due to uncertain dates and an accelerated appearance of mature lecithin/sphingomyelin ratios (5).

Until recently, the incidence of congenital anomalies was not thought to be increased (6–8). Current data, however, suggest that a significant increase in major anomalies can occur (9). In a group of 830 heroin-addicted mothers, the incidence of infants with congenital abnormalities was significantly greater than that in a group of 400 controls (9). Higher rates of jaundice, respiratory distress syndrome, and low Apgar scores were also found. Malformations reported with heroin are multiple and varied with no discernible patterns of defects evident (6–13). In addition, all of the mothers in the studies reporting malformed infants were consuming numerous other drugs, including drugs of abuse.

Characteristics of the infant delivered from a heroin-addicted mother may be (14):

Accelerated liver maturity with a lower incidence of jaundice (8, 15)
Lower incidence of hyaline membrane disease after 32 weeks gestation (5, 16)
Normal Apgar scores (6)

(*Note*: The findings of Ostrea and Chavez (9) are in disagreement with the above statements.)

Low birth weight; up to 50% weigh less than 2,500 g
Small size for gestational age
Narcotic withdrawal in about 85% (58–91%); symptoms apparent usually within
the first 48 hours with some delaying up to 6 days; incidence is directly
related to daily dose and length of maternal addiction; hyperactivity, respiratory distress, fever, diarrhea, mucus secretion, sweating, convulsions, yawn-
ing and face scratching (7, 8)
Meconium staining of amniotic fluid
Elevated serum magnesium levels when withdrawal signs are present (up to
twice normal)
Increased perinatal mortality; rates up to 37% in some series (13)

Random chromosome damage was significantly higher when Apgar scores were 6 or less (12, 17). However, only one case relating chromosome abnormalities to congenital anomalies has appeared (12). The lower incidence of hyaline membrane disease may be due to elevated prolactin blood levels in fetuses of addicted mothers (18).

Long-term effects on growth and behavior have been reported (19). As compared to controls, children aged 3–6 years delivered from addicted mothers were found to have lower weights, lower heights, and impaired behavior, perceptual, and organizational abilities.

[* Risk Factor D if used for prolonged periods or in high doses at term.]

Breast Feeding Summary

Heroin crosses into breast milk in sufficient quantities to cause addiction in the infant (20). A milk:plasma ratio has not been reported. Previous investigators have considered nursing as one method for treating the addicted newborn (21). The American Academy of Pediatrics considers heroin compatible with breast-feeding (22).

References

1. Anonymous. Diagnosis and management of reactions to drug abuse. Med Lett Drugs Ther 1980;22:74.
2. Thomas L. Notes of a biology-watcher. N Engl J Med 1972;286:531–3.
3. Chappel JN. Treatment of morphine-type dependence. JAMA 1972;221:1516.
4. Rementeria JL, Nunag NN. Narcotic withdrawal in pregnancy: stillbirth incidence with a case report. Am J Obstet Gynecol 1973;116:1152–6.
5. Gluck L, Kulovich MV. Lecithin/sphingomyelin ratios in amniotic fluid in normal and abnormal pregnancy. Am J Obstet Gynecol 1973;115:539–46.
6. Reddy AM, Harper RG, Stern G. Observations on heroin and methadone withdrawal in the newborn. Pediatrics 1971;48:353–8.
7. Stone ML, Salerno LJ, Green M, Zelson C. Narcotic addiction in pregnancy. Am J Obstet Gynecol 1971;109:716–23.
8. Zelson C, Rubio E, Wasserman E. Neonatal narcotic addiction: 10 year observation. Pediatrics 1971;48:178–89.

9. Ostrea EM, Chavez CJ. Perinatal problems (excluding neonatal withdrawal) in maternal drug addiction: a study of 830 cases. J Pediatr 1979;94:292–5.
10. Perlmutter JF. Drug addiction in pregnant women. Am J Obstet Gynecol 1967;99:569–72.
11. Krause SO, Murray PM, Holmes JB, Burch RE. Heroin addiction among pregnant women and their newborn babies. Am J Obstet Gynecol 1958;75:754–8.
12. Kushnick T, Robinson M, Tsao C. 45, X chromosome abnormality in the offspring of a narcotic addict. Am J Dis Child 1972;124:772–3.
13. Naeye RL, Blanc W, Leblanc W, Khatamee MA. Fetal complications of maternal heroin addiction: abnormal growth, infections and episodes of stress. J Pediatr 1973;83:1055–61.
14. Perlmutter JF. Heroin addiction and pregnancy. Obstet Gynecol Surv 1974;29:439–46.
15. Nathenson G, Cohen MI, Liff IF, McNamara H. The effect of maternal heroin addiction on neonatal jaundice. J Pediatr 1972;81:899–903.
16. Glass L, Rajegowda BK, Evans HE. Absence of respiratory distress syndrome in premature infants of heroin-addicted mothers. Lancet 1971;2:685–6.
17. Amarose AP, Norusis MJ. Cytogenetics of methadone-managed and heroin-addicted pregnant women and their newborn infants. Am J Obstet Gynecol 1976;124:635–40.
18. Parekh A, Mukherjee TK, Jhaveri R, Rosenfeld W, Glass L. Intrauterine exposure to narcotics and cord blood prolactin concentrations. Obstet Gynecol 1981;57:447–9.
19. Wilson GS, McCreary R, Kean J, Baxter JC. The development of preschool children of heroin-addicted mothers: a controlled study. Pediatrics 1979;63:135–41.
20. Lichlenstein PM. Infant drug addiction. NY Med J 1915;102:905. As reported by Cobrinik et al (21).
21. Cobrinik RW, Hood RT Jr, Chusid E. The effect of maternal narcotic addiction on the newborn infant. Pediatrics 1959;24:288–304.
22. Committee on Drugs, American Academy of Pediatrics. The transfer of drugs and other chemicals into human breast milk. Pediatrics 1983;72:375–83.

Name: **HETACILLIN**

Class: **Antibiotic**   Risk Factor: **B**

Fetal Risk Summary

Hetacillin, a penicillin antibiotic, breaks down in aqueous solution to ampicillin and acetone (see Ampicillin).

Breast Feeding Summary

See Ampicillin.

Name: **HEXAMETHONIUM**

Class: **Antihypertensive**   Risk Factor: **C**

Fetal Risk Summary

No reports linking the use of hexamethonium with congenital defects have been located. Hexamethonium crosses the placenta and accumulates in the amniotic fluid. The drug has been used in the treatment of pre-eclampsia and essential hypertension. Its use in these conditions is no longer recommended. Three cases of paralytic ileus and one case of delayed passage of meconium have been reported (1, 2).

Breast Feeding Summary

No data available.

References

1. Morris N. Hexamethonium in the treatment of pre-eclampsia and essential hypertension during pregnancy. Lancet 1953;1:322–4.
2. Hallum JL, Hatchuel WLF. Congenital paralytic ileus in a premature baby as a complication of hexamethonium bromide therapy for toxemia of pregnancy. Arch Dis Child 1954;29:354–6.

Name: **HEXOCYCLIUM**

Class: **Parasympatholytic (Anticholinergic)**   Risk Factor: **C**

Fetal Risk Summary

Hexocyclium is an anticholinergic agent. No reports of its use in pregnancy have been located (see also Atropine).

Breast Feeding Summary

No data available (see also Atropine).

Name: **HOMATROPINE**

Class: **Parasympatholytic (Anticholinergic)**   Risk Factor: **C**

Fetal Risk Summary

Homatropine is an anticholinergic agent. The Collaborative Perinatal Project monitored 50,282 mother-child pairs, 26 of which used homatropine in the 1st trimester (1). For use anytime during pregnancy, 86 exposures were recorded (2). Only for anytime use was a possible association with congenital defects discovered. In addition, when the group of parasympatholytics were taken as a whole (2,323 exposures), a possible association with minor malformations was found (1).

Breast Feeding Summary

See Atropine.

References

1. Heinonen OP, Slone D, Shapiro S. *Birth Defects and Drugs in Pregnancy*. Littleton:Publishing Sciences Group, 1977:346–53.
2. *Ibid*, 439.

Name: **HORMONAL PREGNANCY TEST TABLETS**

Class: **Estrogenic/Progestogenic Hormones**   Risk Factor: **X**

Fetal Risk Summary

See Oral Contraceptives.

Breast Feeding Summary

See Oral Contraceptives.

Name: **HYDRALAZINE**

Class: **Antihypertensive**   Risk Factor: **C**

Fetal Risk Summary

No reports linking the use of hydralazine with congenital defects have been located. Neonatal thrombocytopenia and bleeding secondary to maternal ingested hydralazine has been reported in three infants (1). In each case, the mother had consumed the drug daily throughout the 3rd trimester. This complication has also been reported in series examining severe maternal hypertension and may be related to the disease rather than to the drug (2).

Hydralazine readily crosses the placenta to the fetus (3). Serum concentrations in the fetus are equal to or greater than those in the mother.

The Collaborative Perinatal Project monitored 50,282 mother-child pairs, 8 of which had 1st trimester exposure to hydralazine (4). For use anytime during pregnancy, 136 cases were recorded (5). No defects were observed with 1st trimester use. There were eight infants born with defects who were exposed in the 2nd or 3rd trimesters. This incidence (5.8%) is greater than the expected frequency of occurrence.

Patients with pre-eclampsia are at risk for having a marked increase in fetal mortality (6–9). Use of hydralazine in 194 pre-eclamptic or eclamptic women was not associated with drug-induced fetal effects (6–9). Fatal maternal hypotension has been reported in one patient after combined therapy with hydralazine and diazoxide (10).

Breast Feeding Summary

Hydralazine is excreted into breast milk (3). In one patient treated with 50 mg three times daily, the milk:plasma ratio 2 hours after a dose was 1.4. This value is in close agreement with the predicted ratio calculated from the pK_a (11). The available dose of hydralazine in 75 ml of milk was estimated to be 13 μg (3). No adverse effects were noted in the nursing infant from this small concentration. The American Academy of Pediatrics considers hydralazine compatible with breast-feeding (12).

References

1. Widerlov E, Karlman I. Storsater J. Hydralazine-induced neonatal thrombocytopenia. N Engl J Med 1980;303:1235.

2. Brazy JE, Grimm JK, Little VA. Neonatal manifestations of severe maternal hypertension occurring before the thirty-sixth week of pregnancy. J Pediatr 1982;100:265–71.
3. Liedholm H, Wahlin-Boll E, Ingemarsson I, Melander A. Transplacental passage and breast milk concentrations of hydralazine. Eur J Clin Pharmacol 1982;21:417–9.
4. Heinonen OP, Slone D, Shapiro S. *Birth Defects and Drugs in Pregnancy*. Littleton:Publishing Sciences Group, 1977:372.
5. *Ibid*, 441.
6. Bott-Kanner G, Schweitzer A, Schoenfeld A, Joel-Cohen J, Rosenfeld JB. Treatment with propranolol and hydralazine throughout pregnancy in a hypertensive patient. Isr J Med Sci 1978;14:466–8.
7. Pritchard JA, Pritchard SA. Standardized treatment of 154 consecutive cases of eclampsia. Am J Obstet Gynecol 1975;123:543–52.
8. Chapman ER, Strozier WE, Magee RA. The clinical use of Apresoline in the toxemias of pregnancy. Am J Obstet Gynecol 1954;68:1109–17.
9. Johnson GT, Thompson RB. A clinical trial of intravenous Apresoline in the management of toxemia of late pregnancy. J Obstet Gynecol 1958;65:360–6.
10. Henrich WL, Cronin R, Miller PD, Anderson RJ. Hypotensive sequelae of diazoxide and hydralazine therapy. JAMA 1977;237:264–5.
11. Daily JW. Anticoagulant and cardiovascular drugs. In Wilson JT, ed. *Drugs in Breast Milk*. Balgowlah, Australia: ADIS Press, 1981:61–4.
12. Committee on Drugs, American Academy of Pediatrics. The transfer of drugs and other chemicals into human breast milk. Pediatrics 1983;72:375–83.

Name: **HYDRIODIC ACID**

Class: **Expectorant**   Risk Factor: **D**

Fetal Risk Summary

The active ingredient of hydriodic acid is iodide (see Potassium Iodide).

Breast Feeding Summary

See Potassium Iodide.

Name: **HYDROCHLOROTHIAZIDE**

Class: **Diuretic**   Risk Factor: **D**

Fetal Risk Summary

See Chlorothiazide.

Breast Feeding Summary

See Chlorothiazide.

Name: **HYDROCODONE**

Class: **Narcotic Analgesic/Antitussive**   Risk Factor: **B***

Fetal Risk Summary

No reports linking the use of hydrocodone with congenital defects have been located. Due to its narcotic properties, withdrawal could theoretically occur in infants exposed *in utero* to prolonged maternal ingestion of hydrocodone.

[* Risk Factor D if used for prolonged periods or in high doses at term.]

Breast Feeding Summary

No data available.

Name: **HYDROFLUMETHIAZIDE**

Class: **Diuretic**   Risk Factor: **D**

Fetal Risk Summary

See Chlorothiazide.

Breast Feeding Summary

See Chlorothiazide.

Name: **HYDROMORPHONE**

Class: **Narcotic Analgesic**   Risk Factor: **B***

Fetal Risk Summary

No reports linking the use of hydromorphone with congenital defects have been located. Withdrawal could occur in infants exposed *in utero* to prolonged maternal ingestion of hydromorphone. Use of the drug in pregnancy is primarily confined to labor. Respiratory depression in the neonate similar to that produced by meperidine or morphine should be expected (1).

[* Risk Factor D if used for prolonged periods or in high doses at term.]

Breast Feeding Summary

No data available.

References

1. Bonica J. *Principles and Practice of Obstetric Analgesia and Anesthesia.* Philadelphia:FA Davis Co, 1967:251.

Name: **HYDROXYPROGESTERONE**

Class: **Progestogenic Hormone**   Risk Factor: **D**

Fetal Risk Summary

The Food and Drug Administration mandated deletion of pregnancy-related indications from all progestins because of a possible association with congenital
anomalies. Ambiguous genitalia of both male and female fetuses have been
reported with hydroxyprogesterone (see also Norethindrone, Norethynodrel) (1–3).
The Collaborative Perinatal Project monitored 866 mother-child pairs with 1st
trimester exposure to progestational agents (including 162 with exposure to
hydroxyprogesterone) (4). An increase in the expected frequency of cardiovascular
defects and hypospadias was observed for both estrogens and progestogens (5,
6). Re-evaluation of these data in terms of timing of exposure, vaginal bleeding in
early pregnancy, and previous maternal obstetrical history, however, failed to
support an association between female sex hormones and cardiac malformations
(7).

Dillion (8, 9) reported six infants with malformations who had been exposed to
hydroxyprogesterone during various stages of gestation. The congenital defects
included spina bifida, anencephalus, hydrocephalus, Fallot's tetralogy, common
truncus arteriosus, cataract, and ventricular septal defect. Complete absence of
both thumbs and dislocated head of the right radius in a child have been associated
with hydroxyprogesterone (9). Use of diazepam in early pregnancy and the lack of
similar reports makes an association doubtful.

A 1985 study described 2,754 offspring born to mothers who had vaginal
bleeding during the 1st trimester (10). Of the total group, 1,608 of the newborns
were delivered from mothers treated during the 1st trimester with either oral
medroxyprogesterone (20–30 mg/day), 17-hydroxyprogesterone (500 mg/week
by injection), or a combination of the two. Medroxyprogesterone was used exclusively in 1,274 (79.2%) of the study group. The control group consisted of 1,146
infants delivered from mothers who bled during the 1st trimester but who were not
treated. There were no differences between the study and control groups in the
overall rate of malformations (120 vs 123.9/1,000, respectively) or in the rate of
major malformations (63.4 vs 71.5/1,000, respectively). Another 1985 study compared 988 infants, exposed *in utero* to various progesterones, to a matched cohort
of 1,976 unexposed controls (11). No association between the use of progestins,
primarily progesterone and 17-hydroxyprogesterone, and fetal malformations was
discovered.

Developmental changes in the psychosexual performance of boys has been
attributed to *in utero* exposure to hydroxyprogesterone (12). The mothers received
an estrogen/progestogen regimen for their diabetes. Hormone-exposed males
demonstrated a trend to have less heterosexual experience and fewer masculine
interests than controls.

The use of high-dose hydroxprogesterone during the 2nd and 3rd trimesters has
been advocated for the prevention of premature labor (13, 14). However, the use
of the steroid was not effective in twin pregnancies (15). Fetal adverse effects
were not observed.

Breast Feeding Summary

No data available.

References

1. Dayan E, Rosa FW. Fetal ambiguous genitalia associated with sex hormone use early in pregnancy. Food and Drug Administration, Division of Drug Experience, ADR Highlights 1981:1–14.
2. Wilkins L. Masculinization of female fetus due to use of orally given progestins. JAMA 1960;172;1028–32.
3. Wilkins L, Jones HW, Holman GH, Stempfel RS Jr. Masculinization of the female fetus associated with administration of oral and intramuscular progestins during gestation: non-adrenal female pseudohermaphrodism. J Clin Endocrinol Metab 1958;68:559–85
4. Heinonen OP, Slone D, Shapiro S. Birth Defects and Drugs in Pregnancy. Littleton:Publishing Sciences Group, 1977:389,391.
5. Ibid, 394.
6. Heinonen OP, Slone D, Monson RR, Hook EB, Shapiro S. Cardiovascular birth defects and antenatal exposure to female sex hormones. N Engl J Med 1977;296:67–70.
7. Wiseman RA, Dodds-Smith IC. Cardiovascular birth defects and antenatal exposure to female sex hormones: a reevaluation of some base data. Teratology 1984;30:359–70.
8. Dillion S. Congenital malformations and hormones in pregnancy. Br Med J 1976;2:1446.
9. Dillon S. Progestogen therapy in early pregnancy and associated congenital defects. Practitioner 1970;205:80–4.
10. Katz Z, Lancet M, Skornik J, Chemke J, Mogilner BM, Klinberg M. Teratogenicity of progestogens given during the first trimester of pregnancy. Obstet Gynecol 1985;65:775–80.
11. Resseguie LJ, Hick JF, Bruen JA, Noller KL, O'Fallon WM, Kurland LT. Congenital malformations among offspring exposed in utero to progestins, Olmsted County, Minnesota, 1936–1974. Fertil Steril 1985;43:514–9.
12. Yalom ID, Green R, Fisk N. Prenatal exposure to female hormones. Effect on psychosexual development in boys. Arch Gen Psychiatry 1973;28:554–61.
13. Johnson JWC, Austin KL, Jones GS, Davis GH, King TM. Efficacy of 17-hydroxyprogesterone caproate in the prevention of premature labor. N Engl J Med 1975;293:675–80.
14. Johnson JWC, Lee PA, Zachary AS, Calhoun S, Migeon CJ. High-risk prematurity—progestin treatment and steroid studies. Obstet Gynecol 1979;54:412–18.
15. Hartikainen-Sorri AL, Kauppila A, Tuimala R. Inefficacy of 17-hydroxyprogesterone caproate in the prevention of prematurity in twin pregnancy. Obstet Gynecol 1980;56:692–5.

Name: **HYDROXYZINE**

Class: **Tranquilizer**   Risk Factor: **C**

Fetal Risk Summary

Hydroxyzine belongs to the same class of compounds as buclizine, cyclizine, and meclizine. Although the drug is an animal teratogen in high doses, human teratogenicity has not been proven. In 100 patients treated in the 1st trimester with oral hydroxyzine (50 mg daily) for nausea and vomiting, no significant difference from nontreated controls was found in fetal wastage or anomalies (1). The Collaborative Perinatal Project monitored 50,282 mother-child pairs, 50 of which had 1st trimester exposure to hydroxyzine (2). For use anytime during pregnancy, 187 exposures were recorded (3). Based on five malformed children, a possible relationship was found between 1st trimester use and congenital defects, but the numbers were too small to determine statistical significance. The manufacturer considers the drug contraindicated in early pregnancy (4). During labor, hydroxyzine has been shown to be safe and effective for the relief of anxiety (5). No effect on the progress of labor or on neonatal Apgar scores was observed.

Breast Feeding Summary

No data available.

References

1. Erez S, Schifrin BS, Dirim O. Double-blind evaluation of hydroxyzine as an antiemetic in pregnancy. J Reprod Med 1971;7:57–9.
2. Heinonen OP, Slone D, Shapiro S. *Birth Defects and Drugs in Pregnancy*. Littleton:Publishing Sciences Group, 1977:335–7,341.
3. *Ibid*, 438.
4. Product information. Vistaril. Pfizer Laboratories, 1985.
5. Zsigmond EK, Patterson RL. Double-blind evaluation of hydroxyzine hydrochloride in obstetric anesthesia. Anesth Analg 1967;46:275.

Name: *l*-HYOSCYAMINE

Class: **Parasympatholytic (Anticholinergic)**   Risk Factor: **C**

Fetal Risk Summary

l-Hyoscyamine is an anticholinergic agent. No reports of its use in pregnancy have been located (see also Belladonna or Atropine).

Breast Feeding Summary

See Atropine.

Name: HYPERALIMENTATION, PARENTERAL

Class: **Nutrient**   Risk Factor: **C**

Fetal Risk Summary

Parenteral hyperalimentation (TPN) is the administration of an intravenous solution designed to provide complete nutritional support for a patient unable to maintain adequate nutritional intake. The solution is normally composed of dextrose (5–35%), amino acids (3.5–5%), vitamins, electrolytes, and trace elements. Lipids (intravenous fat emulsions) are often given with TPN to supply essential fatty acids and calories (see Lipids). Seventeen studies describing the use of TPN in 35 pregnant patients with delivery of 37 newborns have been located (1–17). Maternal indications for TPN were varied, with duration of therapy ranging from a few days to the entire pregnancy. Only two patients were treated during the 1st trimester with TPN (1–3). No fetal complications attributable to TPN, including newborn hypoglycemia, were identified in any of the reports. Intrauterine growth retardation occurred in five infants and one of these died, but the retarded growth and neonatal death were thought to be due to the underlying maternal disease (2–7).

Obstetrical complications included the worsening of one mother's renal hypertensive status after TPN was initiated, but the relationship between the effect and the therapy is not known (6). In a second case, resistance to oxytocin-induced labor was observed, but again, the relationship to TPN is not clear (7).

In summary, the use of total parenteral hyperalimentation does not seem to pose a risk to the fetus or newborn, provided that normal procedures, as with nonpregnant patients, are followed to prevent maternal complications.

Breast Feeding Summary

No problems should be expected in nursing infants whose mothers are receiving total parenteral hyperalimentation.

References

1. Hew LR, Deitel M. Total parenteral nutrition in gynecology and obstetrics. Obstet Gynecol 1980;55:464–8.
2. Tresadern JC, Falconer GF, Turnberg LA, Irving MH. Successful completed pregnancy in a patient maintained on home parenteral nutrition. Br Med J 1983;286:602–3.
3. Tresadern JC, Falconer GF, Turnberg LA, Irving MH. Maintenance of pregnancy in a home parenteral nutrition patient. JPEN 1984;8:199–202.
4. Gineston JL, Capron JP, Delcenserie R, Delamarre J, Blot M, Boulanger JC. Prolonged total parenteral nutrition in a pregnant woman with acute pancreatitis. J Clin Gastroenterol 1984;6:249–52.
5. Lakoff KM, Feldman JD. Anorexia nervosa associated with pregnancy. Obstet Gynecol 1972;39:699–701.
6. Lavin JP Jr, Gimmon Z, Miodovnik M, von Meyenfeldt M, Fischer JE. Total parenteral nutrition in a pregnant insulin-requiring diabetic. Obstet Gynecol 1982;59:660–4.
7. Weinberg RB, Sitrin MD, Adkins GM, Lin CC. Treatment of hyperlipidemic pancreatitis in pregnancy with total parenteral nutrition. Gastroenterology 1982;83:1300–5.
8. Di Costanzo J, Martin J, Cano N, Mas JC, Noirclerc M. Total parenteral nutrition with fat emulsions during pregnancy—nutritional requirements: a case report. JPEN 1982;6:534–8.
9. Young KR. Acute pancreatitis in pregnancy: two case reports. Obstet Gynecol 1982;60:653–7.
10. Rivera-Alsina ME, Saldana LR, Stringer CA. Fetal growth sustained by parenteral nutrition in pregnancy. Obstet Gynecol 1984;64:138–41.
11. Seifer DB, Silberman H, Catanzarite VA, Conteas CN, Wood R, Ueland K. Total parenteral nutrition in obstetrics. JAMA 1985;253:2073–5.
12. Benny PS, Legge M, Aickin DR. The biochemical effects of maternal hyperalimentation during pregnancy. NZ Med J 1978;88:283–5.
13. Cox KL, Byrne WJ, Ament ME. Home total parenteral nutrition during pregnancy: a case report. JPEN 1981;5:246–9.
14. Gamberdella FR. Pancreatic carcinoma in pregnancy: a case report. Am J Obstet Gynecol 1984;149:15–7.
15. Loludice TA, Chandrakaar C. Pregnancy and jejunoileal bypass: treatment complications with total parenteral nutrition. South Med J 1980;73:256–8.
16. Main ANH, Shenkin A, Black WP, Russell RI. Intravenous feeding to sustain pregnancy in patient with Crohn's disease. Br Med J 1981;283:1221–2.
17. Webb GA. The use of hyperalimentation and chemotherapy in pregnancy: a case report. Am J Obstet Gynecol 1980;137:263–6.

i

Name: **IBUPROFEN**

Class: **Nonsteroidal Anti-inflammatory**   Risk Factor: **B***

Fetal Risk Summary

No published reports linking the use of ibuprofen with congenital defects have been located. The manufacturer has nearly a dozen reports of ibuprofen use during pregnancy, all but one resulting in normal term infants (1). The one malformation involved an anencephalic infant exposed during the 1st trimester to ibuprofen and Bendectin (doxylamine succinate and pyridoxine hydrochloride). No cause and effect relationship could be established.

Theoretically, ibuprofen, a prostaglandin synthetase inhibitor, could cause constriction of the ductus arteriosus *in utero* (2). Persistent pulmonary hypertension of the newborn should also be considered (2). Drugs in this class have been shown to inhibit labor and prolong pregnancy (3). The manufacturer recommends that the drug not be used during pregnancy (4).

[* Risk Factor D if used in the 3rd trimester.]

Breast Feeding Summary

Ibuprofen apparently does not enter human milk in significant quantities. In 12 patients taking 400 mg every 6 hours for 24 hours, an assay capable of detecting 1 μg/ml failed to demonstrate ibuprofen in the milk (5, 6). In another case report, a woman was treated with 400 mg twice daily for 3 weeks (7). Milk levels shortly before and up to 8 hours after drug administration were all less than 0.5 μg/ml. The American Academy of Pediatrics considers ibuprofen compatible with breastfeeding (8).

References

1. Westland MM, The Upjohn Co, 1981. Personal communication.
2. Levin DL. Effects of inhibition of prostaglandin synthesis on fetal development, oxygenation, and the fetal circulation. Semin Perinatol 1980;4:35–44.
3. Fuchs F. Prevention of prematurity. Am J Obstet Gynecol 1976;126:809–20.
4. Product information. Motrin. The Upjohn Co, 1985.
5. Townsend RJ, Benedetti T, Erickson S, Gillespie WR, Albert KS. A study to evaluate the passage of ibuprofen into breast milk. Drug Intell Clin Pharm 1982;16:482–3 (Abstr).
6. Townsend RJ, Benedetti TJ, Erickson S, Cengiz C, Gillespie WR, Gschwend J, Albert KS. Excretion of ibuprofen into breast milk. Am J Obstet Gynecol 1984;149:184–6.
7. Weibert RT, Townsend RJ, Kaiser DG, Naylor AJ. Lack of ibuprofen secretion into human milk. Clin Pharm 1982;1:457–8.
8. Committee on Drugs, American Academy of Pediatrics. The transfer of drugs and other chemicals into human breast milk. Pediatrics 1983;72:375–83.

Name: **IDOXURIDINE**

Class: **Antiviral**   Risk Factor: **C**

Fetal Risk Summary

Idoxuridine has not been studied in human pregnancy. The drug is teratogenic in some species of animals after injection and ophthalmic use (1, 2).

Breast Feeding Summary

No data available.

References

1. Nishimura H, Tanimura T. *Clinical Aspects of the Teratogenicity of Drugs*. Amsterdam:Excerpta Medica, 1976:148, 258–9.
2. Itoi M, Gefter JW, Kaneko N, Ishii Y, Ramer RM, Gasset AR. Teratogenicities of ophthalmic drugs. I. Antiviral ophthalmic drugs. Arch Ophthalmol 1975;93:46–51.

Name: **IMIPRAMINE**

Class: **Antidepressant**   Risk Factor: **D**

Fetal Risk Summary

Bilateral amelia was reported in one child whose mother had ingested imipramine during pregnancy (1). An analysis of 546,505 births, 161 with 1st trimester exposure to imipramine, however, failed to find an association with limb reduction defects (2–14). Reported malformations other than limb reduction include (3–5):

Defective abdominal muscles (1 case)
Diaphragmatic hernia (2 cases)
Exencephaly, cleft palate, adrenal hypoplasia (1 case)
Cleft palate (2 cases)
Renal cystic degeneration (1 case)

These reports indicate that imipramine is not a major cause of congenital limb deformities.

Neonatal withdrawal symptoms have been reported with the use of imipramine during pregnancy (15–17). Symptoms observed in the infants during the first month of age were colic, cyanosis, rapid breathing, and irritability (15–17). Urinary retention in the neonate has been associated with maternal use of nortriptyline (chemically related to imipramine) (18).

Breast Feeding Summary

Imipramine and its metabolite, desipramine, enter breast milk in low concentrations (19, 20). A milk:plasma ratio of 1 has been suggested (19). Assuming a therapeutic serum level of 200 ng/ml, an infant consuming 1,000 ml of breast milk would ingest a daily dose of about 0.2 mg. The clinical significance of this amount is not known.

The American Academy of Pediatrics considers imipramine compatible with breast-feeding (21).

References

1. McBride WG. Limb deformities associated with iminodibenzyl hydrochloride. Med J Aust 1972; 1:492.
2. Heinonen OP, Slone D, Shapiro S. *Birth Defects and Drugs in Pregnancy*. Littleton:Publishing Sciences Group, 1977:336–7.
3. Kuenssberg EV, Knox JDE. Imipramine in pregnancy. Br Med J 1972;2:29.
4. Barson AJ. Malformed infant. Br Med J 1972; 2:45.
5. Idanpaan-Heikkila J, Saxen L. Possible teratogenicity of imipramine/chloropyramine. Lancet 1973;2:282–3.
6. Crombie DL, Pinsent R, Fleming D. Imipramine in pregnancy. Br Med J 1972; 1:745.
7. Sim M. Imipramine and pregnancy. Br Med J 1972; 2:45.
8. Scanlon FJ. Use of antidepressant drugs during the first trimester. Med J Aust 1969;2:1077.
9. Rachelefsky GS, Flynt JW, Eggin AJ, Wilson MG. Possible teratogenicity of tricyclic antidepressants. Lancet 1972;1:838.
10. Banister P, Dafoe C, Smith ESO, Miller J. Possible teratogenicity of tricyclic antidepressants. Lancet 1972; 1:838–9.
11. Jacobs D. Imipramine (Tofranil). S Afr Med J 1972;46:1023.
12. Australian Drug Evaluation Committee. Tricyclic antidepressant and limb reduction deformities. Med J Aust 1973;1:766–9.
13. Morrow AW. Imipramine and congenital abnormalities. NZ Med J 1972;75:228–9.
14. Wilson JG. Present status of drugs as teratogens in man. Teratology 1973;7:3–15.
15. Hill RM. Will this drug harm the unborn infant? South Med J 1977;67:1476–80.
16. Eggermont E. Withdrawal symptoms in neonate associated with maternal imipramine therapy. Lancet 1973;2:680.
17. Shrand H. Agoraphobia and imipramine withdrawal? Pediatrics 1982;70:825.
18. Shearer WT, Schreiner RL, Marshall RE. Urinary retention in a neonate secondary to maternal ingestion of nortriptyline. J Pediatr 1972;81:570–2.
19. Sovner R, Orsulak PJ. Excretion of imipramine and desipramine in human breast milk. Am J Psychiatry 1979;136:451–2.
20. Erickson SH, Smith GH, Heidrich F. Tricyclics and breast feeding. Am J Psychiatry 1979;136:1483.
21. Committee on Drugs, American Academy of Pediatrics. The transfer of drugs and other chemicals into human breast milk. Pediatrics 1983;72:375–83.

Name: # IMMUNE GLOBULIN, HEPATITIS B

Class: **Serum**   Risk Factor: **B**

Fetal Risk Summary

Hepatitis B immune globulin is used to provide passive immunity following exposure to hepatitis B. When hepatitis B occurs during pregnancy, an increased rate of abortion and prematurity may be observed (1). No risk to the fetus from the immune globulin has been reported (1, 2). The American College of Obstetricians and Gynecologists Technical Bulletin No. 64 recommends use of hepatitis B immune globulin in pregnancy for postexposure prophylaxis (1).

Breast Feeding Summary

No data available.

References

1. ACOG Technical Bulletin, No. 64, May 1982.
2. Amstey MS. Vaccination in pregnancy. Clin Obstet Gynaecol 1983;10:13–22.

Name: **IMMUNE GLOBULIN, RABIES**

Class: **Serum**   Risk Factor: **B**

Fetal Risk Summary

Rabies immune globulin is used to provide passive immunity following exposure to rabies combined with active immunization with rabies vaccine (1). Since rabies is nearly 100% fatal if contracted, both the immune globulin and the vaccine should be given for postexposure prophylaxis (1). No risk to the fetus from the immune globulin has been reported (see also Vaccine, Rabies Human) (1, 2).

Breast Feeding Summary

No data available.

References

1. ACOG Technical Bulletin, No. 64, May 1982.
2. Amstey MS. Vaccination in pregnancy. Clin Obstet Gynaecol 1983;10:13–22.

Name: **IMMUNE GLOBULIN, TETANUS**

Class: **Serum**   Risk Factor: **B**

Fetal Risk Summary

Tetanus immune globulin is used to provide passive immunity following exposure to tetanus combined with active immunization with tetanus toxoid (1). Tetanus produces severe morbidity and mortality in both the mother and newborn. No risk to the fetus from the immune globulin has been reported (1, 2).

Breast Feeding Summary

No data available.

References

1. ACOG Technical Bulletin, No. 64, May 1982.
2. Amstey MS. Vaccination in pregnancy. Clin Obstet Gynaecol 1983;10:13–22.

Name: **INDIGO CARMINE**

Class: **Dye**   Risk Factor: **B**

Fetal Risk Summary

Indigo carmine is used as a diagnostic dye. No reports linking its use with congenital defects have been located. Intra-amniotic injection has been conducted without apparent effect on the fetus (1, 2). Due to its known toxicities after intravenous administration, however, the dye should not be considered totally safe (3).

Breast Feeding Summary

No data available.

References

1. Elias S, Gerbie AB, Simpson JL, Nadler HL, Sabbagha RE, Shkolnik A. Genetic amniocentesis in twin gestations. Am J Obstet Gynecol 1980;138:169–74.
2. Horger EO III, Moody LO. Use of indigo carmine for twin amniocentesis and its effect on bilirubin analysis. Am J Obstet Gynecol 1984;150:858–60.
3. Fribourg S. Safety of intraamniotic injection of indigo carmine. Am J Obstet Gynecol 1981;140:350–1.

Name: **INDOMETHACIN**

Class: **Nonsteroidal Anti-inflammatory Analgesic**   Risk Factor: **B***

Fetal Risk Summary

A number of studies have described the use of indomethacin in the treatment of premature labor (1–26). The drug acts as a prostaglandin synthetase inhibitor and is apparently effective as a tocolytic agent, including in those cases resistant to β-mimetics. Niebyl (26) reviewed this topic in 1981. Daily doses ranged from 100 to 200 mg usually by the oral route, but rectal administration was often used. In most cases, indomethacin, either alone or in combination with other tocolytics, was successful in postponing delivery until fetal lung maturation had occurred.

Complications associated with the use of indomethacin during pregnancy may include premature closure of the ductus arteriosus, resulting in primary pulmonary hypertension of the newborn and in severe cases, neonatal death (1–5, 27–31). However, constriction of the ductus is apparently gestational age-dependent, occurring primarily after the 34th or 35th week of pregnancy (26). The fetus is relatively resistent to premature closure of the ductus before this time, when therapy for premature labor is most appropriate (26).

Other reported complications with indomethacin use in pregnancy are shown below. The relationship between the drug and these effects was not always known.

Phocomelia, agenesis of the penis (32) (1 case)
Stillborn (2)/neonatal death (1), meconium-stained severe oligohydramnion (33) (3 cases)

Hydrops fetalis in 1 twin, cardiac failure in the second, premature closure of the ductus (34) (twins)

Renal nonfunction but normal kidneys at autopsy, Potter's facies (35) (1 case)

[* Risk Factor D if used in the 3rd trimester.]

Breast Feeding Summary

Indomethacin is excreted in human breast milk, but a milk:plasma ratio has not been reported. It is known that milk levels are similar to those of maternal plasma (36). There is one case report of possible indomethacin-induced seizures in a breast-fed infant, although the causal link between the two events has been questioned (36, 37). The mother was taking 200 mg/day (3 mg/kg/day).

References

1. Atad J, David A, Moise J, Abramovici H. Classification of threatened premature labor related to treatment with a prostaglandin inhibitor: indomethacin. Biol Neonate 1980;37:291–6.
2. Gonzalez CHL, Jimenez PG, Pezzotti y R MA, Favela EL. Hipertension pulmonar persistente en el recien nacido por uso prenatal de inhibidores de las prostaglandinas (indometacina). Informe de un caso. Ginecol Obstet Mex 1980;48:103–10.
3. Sureau C, Piovani P. Clinical study of indomethacin for prevention of prematurity. Eur J Obstet Gynecol Reprod Biol 1983;46:400–2.
4. Van Kets H, Thiery M, Derom R, Van Egmond H, Baele G. Perinatal hazards of chronic antenatal tocolysis with indomethacin. Prostaglandins 1979;18:893–907.
5. Van Kets H, Thiery M, Derom R, Van Egmond H, Baele G. Prostaglandin synthase inhibitors in preterm labor. Lancet 1980;2:693.
6. Blake DA, Niebyl JR, White RD, Kumor KM, Dubin NH, Robinson JC, Egner PG. Treatment of premature labor with indomethacin. Adv Prostaglandin Thromboxane Res 1980;8:1465–7.
7. Grella P, Zanor P. Premature labor and indomethacin. Prostaglandins 1978;16:1007–17.
8. Karim SMM. On the use of blockers of prostaglandin synthesis in the control of labor. Adv Prostaglandin Thromboxane Res 1978;4:301–6.
9. Katz Z, Lancet M, Yemini M, Mogilner BM, Feigl A, Ben.Hur H. Treatment of premature labor contractions with combined ritodrine and indomethacin. Int J Gynaecol Obstet 1983;21:337–42.
10. Niebyl JR, Blake DA, White RD, Kumor KM, Dubin NH, Robinson JC, Egner PG. The inhibition of premature labor with indomethacin. Am J Obstet Gynecol 1980;136:1014–9.
11. Peteja J. Indometacyna w zapobieganiu porodom przedwczesnym. Ginekol Pol 1980;51:347–53.
12. Reiss U, Atad J, Rubinstein I, Zuckerman H. The effect of indomethacin in labour at term. Int J Gynaecol Obstet 1976;14:369–74.
13. Souka AR, Osman N, Sibaie F, Einen MA. Therapeutic value of indomethacin in threatened abortion. Prostaglandins 1980;19:457–60.
14. Spearing G. Alcohol, indomethacin, and salbutamol. Obstet Gynecol 1979;53:171–4.
15. Chimura T. The treatment of threatened premature labor by drugs. Acta Obstet Gynaecol Jpn 1980;32:1620–4.
16. Suzanne F, Fresne JJ, Portal B, Baudon J. Essai therapeutique de l'indometacine dans les menaces d'accouchement premature: a propos de 30 observations. Therapie 1980;35:751–60.
17. Tinga DJ, Aranoudse JG. Post-partum pulmonary oedema associated with preventive therapy for premature labor. Lancet 1979;1:1026.
18. Dudley DKL, Hardie MJ. Fetal and neonatal effects of indomethacin used as a tocolytic agent. Am J Obstet Gynecol 1985;151:181–4.
19. Gamissans O, Canas E, Cararach V, Ribas J, Puerto B, Edo A. A study of indomethacin combined with ritodrine in threatened preterm labor. Eur J Obstet Reprod Biol 1978;8:123–8.
20. Wiqvist N, Lundstrom V, Green K. Premature labor and indomethacin. Prostaglandins 1975;10:515–26.
21. Wiqvist N, Kjellmer I, Thiringer K, Ivarsson E, Karlsson K. Treatment of premature labor by prostaglandin synthetase inhibitors. Acta Biol Med Ger 1978;37:923–30.
22. Zuckerman H, Reiss U, Rubinstein I. Inhibition of human premature labor by indomethacin. Obstet Gynecol 1974;44:787–92.

23. Zuckerman H, Reiss U, Atad J, Lampert I, Ben Ezra S, Sklan D. The effect of indomethacin on plasma levels of prostaglandin F_{2a} in women in labour. Br J Obstet Gynaecol 1977;84:339–43.
24. Zuckerman H, Shalev E, Gilad G, Katzuni E. Further study of the inhibition of premature labor by indomethacin. Part I. J Perinat Med 1984;12:19–23.
25. Ibid. Part II, 25–9.
26. Niebyl JR. Prostaglandin synthetase inhibitors. Semin Perinatol 1981;5:274–87.
27. Levin DL. Effects of inhibition of prostaglandin synthesis on fetal development, oxygenation, and the fetal circulation. Semin Perinatol 1980;4:35–44.
28. Csaba IF, Sulyok E, Ertl T. Relationship of maternal treatment with indomethacin to persistence of fetal circulation syndrome. J Pediatr 1978;92:484.
29. Levin DL, Fixler DE, Morriss FC, Tyson J. Morphologic analysis of the pulmonary vascular bed in infants exposed in utero to prostaglandin synthetase inhibitors. J Pediatr 1978;92:478–83.
30. Rubaltelli FF, Chiozza ML, Zanardo V, Cantarutti F. Effect on neonate of maternal treatment with indomethacin. J Pediatr 1979;94:161.
31. Manchester D, Margolis HS, Sheldon RE. Possible association between maternal indomethacin therapy and primary pulmonary hypertension of the newborn. Am J Obstet Gynecol 1976;126:467–9.
32. Di Battista C, Landizi L, Tamborino G. Focomelia ed agenesia del pene in neonato. Minerva Pediatr 1975;27:675. As cited in Dukes MNG, ed. Side Effects of Drugs Annual 1. Amsterdam: Excerpta Medica, 1977:89.
33. Itskovitz J, Abramovici H, Brandes JM. Oligohydramnion, meconium and perinatal death concurrent with indomethacin treatment in human pregnancy. J Reprod Med 1980;24:137–40.
34. Mogilner BM, Ashkenazy M, Borenstein R, Lancet M. Hydrops fetalis caused by maternal indomethacin treatment. Acta Obstet Gynecol Scand 1982;61:183–5.
35. Veersema D, de Jong PA, van Wijck JAM. Indomethacin and the fetal renal nonfunction syndrome. Eur J Obstet Gynecol Reprod Biol 1983;16:113–21.
36. Eeg-Olofsson O, Malmros I, Elwin CE, Steen B. Convulsions in a breast-fed infant after maternal indomethacin. Lancet 1978;2:215.
37. Fairhead FW. Convulsions in a breast-fed infant after maternal indomethacin. Lancet 1978;2:576.

Name: **INSULIN**

Class: **Antidiabetic**　　　　　　　　　　　　　Risk Factor: **B**

Fetal Risk Summary

Insulin, a natural occurring hormone, is the drug of choice for the control of diabetes mellitus in pregnancy. Infants of diabetic mothers are at risk for an increased incidence of congenital anomalies, up to 2–4 times that of normal controls (1–4). The rate of malformations seems to be related to the severity of the maternal disease. The exact mechanisms causing this increase are unknown. Human insulin does not cross the placenta, at least when administered in the 2nd trimester (5). Studies prior to this time have not been conducted. This distinction is of interest since most major malformations observed in infants of diabetic mothers were induced sometime prior to the 7th week of gestation (1). Several mechanisms have been offered as a cause of the malformations, including exogenous insulin itself and insulin-induced hypoglycemia. However, a recent study using hemoglobin A_{1c}, a normal minor hemoglobin whose levels are indicative of diabetic control, found a significantly higher percentage of major congenital anomalies in the offspring of mothers with elevated levels of this hemoglobin (3). The authors concluded that poorly controlled diabetes (i.e., hyperglycemia) was associated with an increased risk of defects. Congenital malformations are now the most common cause of perinatal death in infants of diabetic mothers (1, 2). Not only is the frequency of major defects increased, but also the frequency of multiple malformations (affecting more than one organ system) (1). Malformations observed in infants of diabetic mothers usually involve one or more of five systems (1):

Most common
  Skeletal: vertebrae and limbs
  Cardiovascular: transposition of great vessels; ventricular septal defects; coarctation of the aorta
  Central nervous system: neural tube defects
Less common
  Genitourinary: varied
  Gastrointestinal: tracheoesophageal fistula; bowel atresias; imperforate anus; narrowed colon

Infants of diabetic mothers may have significant perinatal morbidity, even when the mothers have been under close diabetic control (6). Perinatal morbidity in one series affected 65% (169 of 260) of the infants and included hypoglycemia, hyperbilirubinemia, hypocalcemia, and polycythemia (6).

Breast Feeding Summary

Insulin is a naturally occurring constituent of the blood. It does not pass into breast milk.

References

1. Dignan PSJ. Teratogenic risk and counseling in diabetes. Clin Obstet Gynecol 1981;24:149–59.
2. Friend JR. Diabetes. Clin Obstet Gynaecol 1981;8:353–82.
3. Miller E, Hare JW, Cloherty JP, et al. Elevated maternal hemoglobin A_{1c} in early pregnancy and major congenital anomalies in infants in diabetic mothers. N Engl J Med 1981;304:1331–4.
4. Soler NG, Walsh CH, Malins JM. Congenital malformations in infants of diabetic mothers. Q J Med 1976;45:303–13.
5. Adam PAJ, Teramo K, Raiha N, Gitlin D, Schwartz R. Human fetal insulin metabolism early in gestation. Diabetes 1969;18:409–16.
6. Gabbe SG, Mestman JH, Freeman RK, et al. Management and outcome of pregnancy in diabetes mellitus, classes B to R. Am J Obstet Gynecol 1977;129:723–32.

Name: **IOCETAMIC ACID**

Class: **Diagnostic**   Risk Factor: **D**

Fetal Risk Summary

Iocetamic acid contains a high concentration of organically bound iodine. See Diatrizoate for possible effects on the fetus and neonate.

Breast Feeding Summary

See Potassium Iodide.

Name: **IODAMIDE**

Class: **Diagnostic**   Risk Factor: **D**

Fetal Risk Summary

The various preparations of iodamide contain a high concentration of organically bound iodine. See Diatrizoate for possible effects on the fetus and newborn.

Breast Feeding Summary

See Potassium Iodide.

Name: **IODINATED GLYCEROL**

Class: **Expectorant**   Risk Factor: X_M

Fetal Risk Summary

Iodinated glycerol is a stable complex containing 50% organically bound iodine (see Potassium Iodide). The manufacturer considers the drug to be contraindicated in pregnancy (1).

Breast Feeding Summary

See Potassium Iodide. The manufacturer considers iodinated glycerol to be contraindicated in nursing mothers (1).

References

1. Product information. Organidin. Wallace Laboratories. Physician's Desk Reference. Oradell:Medical Economics Co, 1984:2076.

Name: **IODINE**

Class: **Anti-infective**   Risk Factor: **D**

Fetal Risk Summary

See Potassium Iodide.

Breast Feeding Summary

See Potassium Iodide.

Name: **IODIPAMIDE**

Class: **Diagnostic**   Risk Factor: **D**

Fetal Risk Summary

The various preparations of iodipamide contain a high concentration of organically bound iodine. See Diatrizoate for possible effects on the fetus and newborn.

Breast Feeding Summary

See Potassium Iodide.

Name: **IODOQUINOL**

Class: **Amebicide**   Risk Factor: **C**

Fetal Risk Summary

No data available.

Breast Feeding Summary

No data available.

Name: **IODOTHYRIN**

Class: **Thyroid**   Risk Factor: **A**

Fetal Risk Summary

Iodothyrin is a combination product containing thyroid, iodized calcium, and peptone. See Thyroid.

Breast Feeding Summary

See Levothyroxine and Liothyronine.

Name: **IODOXAMATE**

Class: **Diagnostic**   Risk Factor: **D**

Fetal Risk Summary

The various preparations of iodoxamate contain a high concentration of organically bound iodine. See Diatrizoate for possible effects on the fetus and newborn.

Breast Feeding Summary

See Potassium Iodide.

Name: **IOPANOIC ACID**

Class: **Diagnostic**   Risk Factor: **D**

Fetal Risk Summary

Iopanoic acid contains a high concentration of organically bound iodine. See Diatrizoate for possible effects on the fetus and newborn.

Breast Feeding Summary

Iopanoic acid is excreted in breast milk. Cholecystography was performed with iopanoic acid in 11 lactating patients (1). The mean amount of iodine administered to five patients was 2.77 g (range 1.98–3.96 g) and the mean amount excreted in breast milk during the next 19–29 hours was 20.8 mg (0.08%) (range 6.72–29.9 mg). The nursing infants showed no reaction to the contrast media.

References

1. Holmdahl KH. Cholecystography during lactation. Acta Radiol 1956;45: 305–7.

Name: **IOTHALAMATE**

Class: **Diagnostic**   Risk Factor: **D**

Fetal Risk Summary

Iothalamate has been used for diagnostic procedures during pregnancy. Amniography was performed in one patient to diagnose monoamniotic twinning shortly before an elective cesarean section (1). No effect on the two newborns was mentioned. In a second study, 17 women were given either iothalamate or metrizoate for ascending phlebography during various stages of pregnancy (2). Two patients, one exposed in the 1st trimester and one in the 2nd trimester, were found to have deep vein thrombosis and were treated with heparin. While the baby from the 2nd trimester patient was normal, the other newborn had hyperbilirubinemia and undescended testis. The relationship between the diagnostic agents (or other drugs) and the defects is not known.

   Use of other organically bound iodine preparations near term has resulted in hypothyroidism in some newborns (see Diatrizoate). Thus, appropriate measures should be taken to treat neonatal hypothyroidism if diagnostic tests with iothalamate are required close to delivery.

Breast Feeding Summary

See Potassium Iodide.

References

1. Dunnihoo DR, Harris RE. The diagnosis of monoamniotic twinning by amniography. Am J Obstet Gynecol 1966;96:894–5.
2. Kierkegaard A. Incidence and diagnosis of deep vein thrombosis associated with pregnancy. Acta Obstet Gynecol Scand 1983;62:239–43.

Name: **IPODATE**

Class: **Diagnostic**   Risk Factor: **D**

Fetal Risk Summary

Ipodate contains a high concentration of organically bound iodine. See Diatrizoate for possible effects on the fetus and newborn.

Breast Feeding Summary

See Potassium Iodide.

Name: **IPRINDOLE**

Class: **Antidepressant**   Risk Factor: **D**

Fetal Risk Summary

No data available (see Imipramine).

Breast Feeding Summary

No data available (see Imipramine).

Name: **IPRONIAZID**

Class: **Antidepressant**   Risk Factor: **C**

Fetal Risk Summary

No data available (see Phenelzine).

Breast Feeding Summary

No data available (see Phenelzine).

Name: **ISOCARBOXAZID**

Class: **Antidepressant**   Risk Factor: **C**

Fetal Risk Summary

Isocarboxazid is a monoamine oxidase inhibitor. The Collaborative Perinatal Project monitored 21 mother-child pairs exposed to these drugs during the 1st trimester, 1 of which was exposed to isocarboxazid (1). An increased risk of malformations was found. Details of the single case with exposure to isocarboxazid were not given.

Breast Feeding Summary

No data available.

References

1. Heinonen OP, Slone D, Shapiro S. *Birth Defects and Drugs in Pregnancy*. Littleton:Publishing Sciences Group, 1977:336–7.

Name: **ISOETHARINE**

Class: **Sympathomimetic (Adrenergic)**   Risk Factor: **C**

Fetal Risk Summary

No reports linking the use of isoetharine with congenital defects have been located. Isoetharine-like drugs are teratogenic in some animal species, but human teratogenicity has not been suspected (1, 2). Recent data may require a reappraisal of this opinion. The Collaborative Perinatal Project monitored 50,282 mother-child pairs, 3,082 of which had 1st trimester exposure to sympathomimetic drugs (3). For use anytime during pregnancy, 9,719 exposures were recorded (4). An association in the 1st trimester was found between the sympathomimetic class of drugs as a whole and minor malformations (not life-threatening or major cosmetic defects), inguinal hernia, and clubfoot (3). Sympathomimetics are often administered in combination with other drugs to alleviate the symptoms of upper respiratory infections. Thus, the fetal effects of sympathomimetics, other drugs, and viruses cannot be totally separated. However, indiscriminate use of this class of drugs, especially in the 1st trimester, is not without risk.

Breast Feeding Summary

No data available.

References

1. Nishimura H, Tanimura T. *Clinical Aspects of the Teratogenicity of Drugs*. Amsterdam:Excerpta Medica, 1976:231.
2. Shepard TH. *Catalog of Teratogenic Agents*, ed 3. Baltimore:The Johns Hopkins University Press, 1980:134–5.
3. Heinonen OP, Slone D, Shapiro S. *Birth Defects and Drugs in Pregnancy*. Littleton:Publishing Sciences Group, 1977:345–56.
4. *Ibid*, 439.

Name: **ISOFLUROPHATE**

Class: **Parasympathomimetic (Cholinergic)**   Risk Factor: **C**

Fetal Risk Summary

Isoflurophate is used in the eye. No reports of its use in pregnancy have been located. As a quaternary ammonium compound, it is ionized at physiologic pH and transplacental passage in significant amounts would not be expected (see also Neostigmine).

Breast Feeding Summary

No data available.

Name: **ISONIAZID**

Class: **Antituberculosis Agent**   Risk Factor: **C**

Fetal Risk Summary

Reports discussing fetal effects of isoniazid during pregnancy may reflect multiple drug therapies. These reports have identified retarded psychomotor activity, psychic retardation, convulsions, myoclonia, myelomeningocele with spina bifida and talipes, and hypospadias as possible effects related to isoniazid therapy during pregnancy (1, 2). The Collaborative Perinatal Project monitored 85 patients who received isoniazid during the 1st trimester (3). They reported 10 malformations, an incidence almost twice the expected rate. The above observations have not been confirmed by other studies (4–8). Retrospective analysis of over 4,900 pregnancies in which isoniazid was administered demonstrated rates of malformations similar to control populations (0.7%–2.3%). A 1980 review found no association between isoniazid and fetal anomalies (9).

A case report of a malignant mesothelioma in a 9-year-old child who was exposed to isoniazid *in utero* has been published (10). The authors suggested a possible carcinogenic effect because of the rarity of malignant mesotheliomas during the 1st decade and supportive animal data. Hammond and co-workers (11) reported an earlier study which followed 660 children up to 16 years of age. No carcinogenic effects were observed in this study.

An association between isoniazid and hemorrhagic disease of the newborn has been suspected in two infants (12). The mothers were also treated with rifampicin and ethambutol and in a third case, only with these latter two drugs. Although other reports of this potentially serious reaction have not been found, prophylactic vitamin K is recommended at birth (see Phytonadione).

The bulk of clinical experience supports the use of isoniazid during gestation for the treatment and prophylaxis of tuberculosis.

Breast Feeding Summary

No reports of isoniazid-induced effects in the nursing infant have been located. A milk:plasma ratio of 1.0 has been reported (13). Milk levels 3 hours after a maternal

5 mg/kg dose were 6 μg/ml (14). Doubling the maternal dose doubled the milk concentration. Timing of single-dose isoniazid regimens may limit the total amount of drug available to the infant. Patients who choose to breast-feed should be counselled that experimental studies have suggested carcinogenic effects. The American Academy of Pediatrics considers isoniazid compatible with breast-feeding (15).

References

1. Weinstein L, Dalton AC. Host determinants of response to antimicrobial agents. N Engl J Med 1968;279:524–31.
2. Lowe CR. Congenital defects among children born to women under supervision or treatment for pulmonary tuberculosis. Br J Prev Soc Med 1964;18:14–6.
3. Heinonen OP, Slone D, Shapiro S. *Birth Defects and Drugs in Pregnancy.* Littleton:Publishing Sciences Group, 1977:299, 313.
4. Marynowski A, Sianozecka E. Comparison of the incidence of congenital malformations in neonates from healthy mothers and from patients treated because of tuberculosis. Ginekol Pol 1972;43:713.
5. Jentgens H. Antituberkulose chimotherapie und schwangerschaft sabbruch. Prax Klin Pneumol 1973;27:479.
6. Ludford J, Doster B, Woolpert SF. Effect of isoniazid on reproduction. Am Rev Respir Dis 1973;108:1170–4.
7. Scheinhorn DJ, Angelillo VA. Antituberculosis therapy in pregnancy; risks to the fetus. West J Med 1977;127:195–8.
8. Good JT, Iseman MD, Davidson PT, Lakshminarayan S, Sahn SA. Tuberculosis in association with pregnancy. Am J Obstet Gynecol 1981;140:492–8.
9. Snider DE Jr, Layde PM, Johnson MW, Lyle MA. Treatment of tuberculosis during pregnancy. Am Rev Respir Dis 1980;122:65–79.
10. Tuman KJ, Chilcote RR, Gerkow RI, Moohr JW. Mesothelioma in child with prenatal exposure to isoniazid. Lancet 1980;2:362.
11. Hammond DC, Silidoff IJ, Robitzek EH. Isoniazid therapy in relation to later occurrence of cancer in adults and in infants. Br Med J 1967;2:792–5.
12. Eggermont E, Logghe N, Van De Casseye W, Casteels-Van Daele M, Jaeken J, Cosemans J, Verstraete M, Renaer M. Haemorrhagic disease of the newborn in the offspring of rifampicin and isoniazid treated mothers. Acta Paediatr Belg 1976;29:87–90.
13. Vorherr H. Drugs excretion in breast milk. Postgrad Med 1974;56:97–104.
14. Ricci G, Copaitich T. Modalta di eliminazione dili'isoniazide somministrata per via orale attraverso il latte di donna. Rass Clin Ter 1954–5;209:53–4.
15. Committee on Drugs, American Academy of Pediatrics. The transfer of drugs and other chemicals into human breast milk. Pediatrics 1983;72:375–83.

Name: **ISOPROPAMIDE**

Class: **Parasympatholytic**   Risk Factor: **C**

Fetal Risk Summary

Isopropamide is an anticholinergic quaternary ammonium iodide. The Collaborative Perinatal Project monitored 50,282 mother-child pairs, 180 of which used isopropamide in the 1st trimester (1). For use anytime during pregnancy, 1,071 exposures were recorded (2). In neither case was evidence found for an association with malformations. However, when the group of parasympatholytics were taken as a whole (2,323 exposures), a possible association with minor malformations was found (1).

Breast Feeding Summary

No data available (see also Atropine).

References

1. Heinonen OP, Slone D, Shapiro S. *Birth Defects and Drugs in Pregnancy*. Littleton:Publishing Sciences Group, 1977:346–53.
2. *Ibid*, 439.

Name: **ISOPROTERENOL**

Class: **Sympathomimetic (Adrenergic)**   Risk Factor: **C**

Fetal Risk Summary

No reports linking the use of isoproterenol with congenital defects have been located. Isoproterenol is teratogenic in some animal species, but human teratogenicity has not been suspected (1, 2). Recent data may require a reappraisal of this opinion. The Collaborative Perinatal Project monitored 50,282 mother-child pairs, 31 of which had 1st trimester exposure to isoproterenol (3). No evidence was found to suggest a relationship with large categories of major or minor malformations or to individual defects. However, an association in the 1st trimester was found between the sympathomimetic class of drugs as a whole and minor malformations (not life-threatening or major cosmetic defects), inguinal hernia, and clubfoot (4). Sympathomimetics are often administered in combination with other drugs to alleviate the symptoms of upper respiratory infections. Thus, the fetal effects of sympathomimetics, other drugs, and viruses cannot be totally separated. However, indiscriminate use of this class of drugs, especially in the 1st trimester, is not without risk.

Breast Feeding Summary

No data available.

References

1. Nishimura H, Tanimura T. *Clinical Aspects of the Teratogenicity of Drugs*. Amsterdam:Excerpta Medica, 1976;231–2.
2. Shepard TH. *Catalog of Teratogenic Agents*, ed 3. Baltimore:The Johns Hopkins University Press, 1980;191.
3. Heinonen OP, Slone D, Shapiro S. *Birth Defects and Drugs in Pregnancy*. Littleton:Publishing Sciences Group, 1977:346–7.
4. *Ibid*, 345–56.

Name: **ISOSORBIDE**

Class: **Diuretic**   Risk Factor: **C**

Fetal Risk Summary

No data available.

Breast Feeding Summary

No data available.

Name: **ISOSORBIDE DINITRATE**

Class: **Vasodilator**   Risk Factor: **C**

Fetal Risk Summary

See Nitroglycerin or Amyl Nitrite.

Breast Feeding Summary

No data available.

Name: **ISOTRETINOIN**

Class: **Vitamin**   Risk Factor: **X**

Fetal Risk Summary

Isotretinoin is a vitamin A isomer used for the treatment of severe, recalcitrant cystic acne. The animal teratogenicity of this drug was well documented prior to its approval for human use in 1982 (1, 2). In the 22 months following its introduction (September 1982–July 1, 1984), the United States Food and Drug Administration (FDA) received reports on pregnancies in 69 isotretinoin-exposed women, which resulted in 24 spontaneous abortions, 21 major birth defects, and 24 apparently normal children (3). In 25 of these pregnancies in women known to have been exposed during the critical time of 4–10 weeks following the onset of the last menstrual period, 11 ended in spontaneous abortion. Of the remaining 14 pregnancies, 4 babies were born with defects and 1 apparently normal infant died unexplainably at 7 weeks of age, a 36% incidence of adverse outcome in those pregnancies going to term. Some of the 24 normal infants in the total group may not have been exposed *in utero* to isotretinoin during the critical period (3). Of further concern, major defects may not be apparent at birth. Thus, until sufficient time has elapsed for adequate follow-up studies, the exact number of affected children will not be known.

Several reports have appeared describing the syndrome of defects produced by isotretinoin (4–15). This syndrome may consist of all or part of the following:

Central Nervous System:	Hydrocephalus
	Microcephaly
	Dandy-Walker cyst (posterior fossa)
Facial Dysmorphia:	Small mouth and lower jaw
	Malformed skull
	Depressed nasal bridge
	Microtia or absent external ears
	Cleft palate
	Microphthalmia
Cardiovascular:	Transposition of great vessels
	Anomalies of aortic arch
	Ventricular septal defect
	Atrial septal defect
	Tetralogy of Fallot
	Hypoplastic adrenal cortex

In summary, isotretinoin has proven to be one of the most potent human teratogens known to man. Critically important to prescribers is the fact that a high percentage of the recipients of this drug are women in their child-bearing years. Estimates have appeared indicating that 38% of isotretinoin users are women aged 13–19 years (5). Pregnancy must be excluded and prevented in these and other female patients before isotretinoin is prescribed. Therapy should be stopped at least 1 month prior to conception (5). Fortunately, in one study the drug did not interfere with the action of oral contraceptive steroids (16). If conception does occur during therapy, strong consideration should be given to terminating the pregnancy.

Breast Feeding Summary

No data available. The manufacturer recommends that isotretinoin not be used in nursing mothers (17).

References

1. Voorhees JJ, Orfanos CE. Oral retinoids. Arch Dermatol 1981;117:418–21.
2. Kamm JJ. Toxicology, carcinogenicity, and teratogenicity of some orally administered retinoids. J Am Acad Dermatol 1982;6:652–9.
3. FDA Drug Bulletin. Update on birth defects with isotretinoin. 1984;14:15–6.
4. Rosa FW. Teratogenicity of isotretinoin. Lancet 1983;2:513.
5. FDA Drug Bulletin. Adverse effects with isotretinoin. 1983;13:21–3.
6. Braun JT, Franciosi RA, Mastri AR, Drake RM, O'Neil BL. Isotretinoin dysmorphic syndrome. Lancet 1984;1:506–7.
7. Stern RS, Rosa F, Baum C. Isotretinoin and pregnancy. J Am Acad Dermatol 1984;10:851–4.
8. Benke PJ. The isotretinoin teratogen syndrome. JAMA 1984;251:3267–9.
9. Marwick C. More cautionary labeling appears on isotretinoin. JAMA 1984;251:3208–9
10. Zarowny DP. Accutane Roche: risk of teratogenic effects. Can Med Assoc J 1984;131:273.
11. Lott IT, Bocian M, Pribram HW, Leitner M. Fetal hydrocephalus and ear anomalies associated with maternal use of isotretinoin. J Pediatr 1984;105:597–600.
12. Fernhoff PM, Lammer EJ. Craniofacial features of isotretinoin embryopathy. J Pediatr 1984;105:595–7.
13. Hall JG. Vitamin A: A newly recognized human teratogen. Harbinger of things to come? J Pediatr 1984;105:583–4.
14. De La Cruz E, Sun S, Vangvanichyakorn K, Desposito F. Multiple congenital malformations associated with maternal isotretinoin therapy. Pediatrics 1984;74:428–30.
15. Hersh JH, Danhauer DE, Hand ME, Weisskopf B. Retinoic acid embryopathy: timing of exposure and effects on fetal development. JAMA 1985;254:909–10.
16. Orme M, Back DJ, Shaw MA, Allen WL, Tjia J, Cunliffe WJ, Jones DH. Isotretinoin and contraception. Lancet 1984;2:752–3.
17. Product information. Accutane. Hoffmann-La Roche, 1985.

Name: **ISOXSUPRINE**

Class: **Sympathomimetic (Adrenergic)**   Risk Factor: **C**

Fetal Risk Summary

No reports linking the use of isoxsuprine with congenital defects have been located. Isoxsuprine, a β-sympathomimetic, is indicated for vasodilation, but it has been used to prevent premature labor (1–6). Uterine inhibitory effects usually require high intravenous doses which increase the risk for serious adverse effects (7, 8).

Maternal heart rate increases and blood pressure decreases are usually mild at lower doses (2, 4, 6). A decrease in the incidence of neonatal respiratory distress syndrome has been observed (9). However, in one study, neonatal respiratory depression was increased if cord serum levels exceeded 10 ng/ml (10). The depression was always associated with hypotension, so the mechanism of the defect may have been related to pulmonary hypoperfusion. Neonatal toxicity is generally rare if cord levels of isoxsuprine are less than 2 ng/ml (corresponding to a drug-free interval of more than 5 hours), but levels greater than 10 ng/ml (drug-free interval of 2 hours of less) were associated with severe neonatal problems (10). These problems include hypocalcemia, hypoglycemia, ileus, hypotension, and death (10–12). Hypotension and neonatal death occurred primarily in infants of 26–31 weeks gestation, especially if cord levels exceeded 10 ng/ml, and in infants whose mothers developed hypotension or tachycardia during isoxsuprine infusion (10, 11). Neonatal ileus, up to 33% in some series, was not related to cord isoxsuprine concentrations, but hypotension and hypocalcemia were directly related, reaching 89 and 100%, respectively, when cord levels exceeded 10 ng/ml (10, 12). Fetal tachycardia is a common side effect. As compared to controls, no increase in late or variable decelerations was seen (10). In contrast to the above, infusion of isoxsuprine 30 minutes prior to cesarean section under general anesthesia was not observed to produce adverse effects in the mother, fetus or newborn (13). Cord concentrations were not measured. Long term evaluation of infants exposed to β-mimetics *in utero* has been reported, but not specifically for isoxsuprine (14). No harmful effects in the infants resulting from this exposure were observed.

Breast Feeding Summary

No data available.

References

1. Bishop EH, Woutersz TB. Isoxsuprine, a myometrial relaxant. A preliminary report. Obstet Gynecol 1961;17:442–6.
2. Hendricks CH, Cibils LA, Pose SV, Eskes TKAB. The pharmacological control of excessive uterine activity with isoxsuprine. Am J Obstet Gynecol 1961;82:1064–78.
3. Bishop EH, Woutersz TB. Arrest of premature labor. JAMA 1961;178:812–4.
4. Stander RW, Barden TP, Thompson JF, Pugh WR, Werts CE. Fetal cardiac effects of maternal isoxsuprine infusion. Am J Obstet Gynecol 1964;89:792–800.
5. Hendricks CH. The use of isoxsuprine for the arrest of premature labor. Clin Obstet Gynecol 1964;7:687–94.
6. Allen HH, Short H, Fraleigh DM. The use of isoxsuprine in the management of premature labor. Appl Ther 1965;7:544–7.
7. Anonymous. Drugs acting on the uterus. Br Med J 1964;1:1234–6.
8. Briscoe CC. Failure of oral isoxsuprine to prevent prematurity. Am J Obstet Gynecol 1966;95:885–6.
9. Kero P, Hirvonen T, Valimaki I. Perinatal isoxsuprine and respiratory distress syndrome. Lancet 1973;2:198.
10. Brazy JE, Little V, Grimm J, Pupkin M. Risk:benefit considerations for the use of isoxsuprine in the treatment of premature labor. Obstet Gynecol 1981;58:297–303.
11. Brazy JE, Pupkin MJ. Effects of maternal isoxsuprine administration on preterm infants. J Pediatr 1979;94:444–8.
12. Brazy JE, Little V, Grimm J. Isoxsuprine in the perinatal period. II. Relationships between neonatal symptoms, drug exposure, and drug concentration at the time of birth. J Pediatr 1981;98:146–51.
13. Jouppila R, Kauppila A, Tuimala R, Pakarinen A, Moilanen K. Maternal, fetal and neonatal effects

of beta-adrenergic stimulation in connection with cesarean section. Acta Obstet Gynecol Scand 1980;59:489–93.

14. Freysz H, Willard D, Lehr A, Messer J. Boog G. A long term evaluation of infants who received a beta-mimetic drug while in utero. J Perinat Med 1977;5:94–9.

15. Heinonen OP, Slone D, Shapiro S. *Birth Defects and Drugs in Pregnancy*. Littleton:Publishing Sciences Group, 1977:345–56.

16. *Ibid*, 439.

Name: **KANAMYCIN**

Class: **Antibiotic**   Risk Factor: **D**

Fetal Risk Summary

Kanamycin is an aminoglycoside antibiotic. At term, the drug is detectable in cord serum 15 minutes after a 500-mg intramuscular maternal dose (1). Mean cord serum levels at 3–6 hours were 6 μg/ml. Amniotic fluid levels were undetectable during the first hours, then rose during the next 6 hours to a mean value of 5.5 μg/ml. No effects on the infants were mentioned.

Eighth cranial nerve damage has been reported following *in utero* exposure to kanamycin (2, 3). In a retrospective survey of 391 mothers who had received kanamycin, 50 mg/kg, for prolonged periods during pregnancy, 9 children were found to have hearing loss (2.3% incidence) (2). Complete hearing loss in a mother and her infant was reported after the mother had been treated during pregnancy with kanamycin, 1 g/day intramuscularly for 4.5 days (3). Ethacrynic acid, an ototoxic diuretic, was also given to the mother during pregnancy.

Except for ototoxicity, no reports of congenital defects due to kanamycin have been located. Embryos were examined from five patients who aborted during the 11th–12th week of pregnancy and who had been treated with kanamycin during the 6th and 8th week (2). No abnormalities in the embryos were found.

Breast Feeding Summary

Kanamycin is excreted in breast milk. Milk:plasma ratios of 0.05–0.40 have been reported (4). A 1-g intramuscular dose produced peak milk levels of 18.4 μg/ml (5). No effects were reported in the nursing infants. Since oral absorption of kanamycin is poor, ototoxicity would not be expected. However, three potential problems exist for the nursing infant: modification of bowel flora, direct effects on the infant, and interference with the interpretation of culture results if a fever work-up is required.

References

1. Good R, Johnson G. The placental transfer of kanamycin during late pregnancy. Obstet Gynecol 1971;38:60-2.
2. Nishimura H, Tanimura T. *Clinical Aspects of the Teratogenicity of Drugs*. Amsterdam:Excerpta Medica, 1976:131.
3. Jones HC. Intrauterine ototoxicity. A case report and review of literature. J Natl Med Assoc 1973;65:201-3.
4. Wilson JT. Milk/plasma ratios and contraindicated drugs. In Wilson JT, ed. *Drugs in Breast Milk*. Balgowlah, Australia:ADIS Press, 1981:79.
5. O'Brien T. Excretion of drugs in human milk. Am J Hosp Pharm 1974;31:844-54.

Name: **LABETALOL**

Class: **Sympatholytic**

Risk Factor: **C$_M$**

Fetal Risk Summary

Labetalol, a combined α/β-adrenergic blocking agent, has been used for the treatment of hypertension occurring during pregnancy (1–19). The drug crosses the placenta to produce cord serum concentrations averaging 40–80% of peak maternal levels (1–5). Maternal serum and amniotic fluid concentrations are approximately equivalent 1–3 hours after a single intravenous dose (4). The pharmacokinetics of labetalol in pregnant patients have been reported (6, 7).

No fetal malformations attributable to labetalol have been reported, but experience during the 1st trimester is lacking. Similarly, no adverse effects on birth weight, head circumference, Apgar scores, or blood glucose control have been observed. One case of neonatal hypoglycemia has been mentioned, but the mother was also taking a thiazide diuretic (2). Offspring of mothers treated with labetalol had a significantly higher birth weight than infants of atenolol-treated mothers, 3,280 g vs 2,750 g ($p < 0.001$), respectively (8).

Fetal heart rate is apparently unaffected by labetalol treatment of hypertensive pregnant women. However, two studies have observed newborn bradycardia in a total of five infants (9, 10). In one of these infants, bradycardia was marked (<100) and persistent (10). All five infants survived. Hypotension was noted in another infant delivered by cesarean section at 28 weeks gestation (1).

Several investigations have shown a lack of effect of labetalol treatment on uterine contractions (1–3, 9, 11, 12). One study did report a higher incidence of spontaneous labor in labetalol-treated mothers (6 of 10) than in a similar group treated with methyldopa (2 of 9) (13). In another report, 3 of 31 patients treated with labetalol experienced spontaneous labor, one of whom delivered prematurely (14). The authors attributed the uterine activity to the drug as no other causes were found. However, since most trials with labetalol in hypertensive women have not shown this effect, it is questionable whether the drug has any direct effect on uterine contractility.

Labetalol does not change uteroplacental blood flow despite a drop in blood pressure (2, 4, 5, 15). The lack of effect on blood flow was probably due to reduced peripheral resistance. As a result, fetal growth retardation has not been reported as a complication of labetalol therapy.

Labetalol apparently reduces the incidence of hyaline membrane disease in premature infants by increasing the production of pulmonary surfactant (1, 2, 4, 9, 16). This effect may be mediated through β-2-adrenoceptor agonist activity, which the drug partially possesses (1, 2, 4, 9, 16).

Follow-up studies have been completed at 6 months of age on 10 infants exposed *in utero* to labetalol (17). All infants demonstrated normal growth and development. In addition, no ocular toxicity has been observed in newborns, even though labetalol has an affinity for ocular melanin (1, 2, 16).

In summary, the use of labetalol for the treatment of maternal hypertension does not seem to pose a risk to the fetus and may offer advantages over the use of agents with only β-blocker activity . Although the majority of newborns have shown no adverse clinical signs after exposure, they should be closely observed during the first 24–48 hours for bradycardia, hypotension, and other symptoms of α/β blockade. Long-term effects (>6 months) of *in utero* exposure to labetalol have not been studied but warrant evaluation.

Breast Feeding Summary

Labetalol is excreted into breast milk (1). In 24 lactating women, 3 days postpartum, administration of 330–800 mg/day produced a mean milk level of 33 ng/ml. No adverse effects were observed in the nursing infants. One patient, consuming 1,200 mg/day, had a mean milk concentration of 600 ng/ml; however, this women did not breast-feed. Although no adverse effects have been reported, nursing infants should be closely observed for bradycardia, hypotension, and other symptoms of α/β-blockade. Long-term effects of exposure to labetalol from milk have not been studied but warrant evaluation.

References

1. Michael CA. Use of labetalol in the treatment of severe hypertension during pregnancy. Br J Clin Pharmacol 1979;8(Suppl 2):211S–5S.
2. Riley AJ. Clinical pharmacology of labetalol in pregnancy. J Cardiovasc Pharmacol 1981;3(Suppl 1):S53–S9.
3. Andrejak M, Coevoet B, Fievet P, Gheerbrant JD, Comoy E, Leuillet P, Verhoest P, Boulanger JC, Vitse M, Fournier A. Effect of labetalol on hypertension and the renin-angiotensin-aldosterone and adrenergic systems in pregnancy. In Riley A, Symonds EM, eds. *The Investigation of Labetalol in the Management of Hypertension in Pregnancy*. Amsterdam:Excerpta Medica, 1982:77–87.
4. Lunel NO, Hjemdahl P, Fredholm BB, Lewander R, Nisell H, Nylund L, Persson B, Sarby J, Wager J, Thornstrom S. Acute effects of labetalol on maternal metabolism and uteroplacental circulation in hypertension of pregnancy. *Ibid*, 34–45.
5. Nylund L, Lunell NO, Lewander R, Sarby B, Thornstrom S. Labetalol for the treatment of hypertension in pregnancy. Acta Obstet Gynecol Scand 1984;118(Suppl):71–3.
6. Rubin PC. Drugs in pregnancy. In Riley A, Symonds EM, eds. *The Investigation of Labetalol in the Management of Hypertension in Pregnancy*. Amsterdam:Excerpta Medica, 1982:28–33.
7. Rubin PC, Butters L, Kelman AW, Fitzsimons C, Reid JL. Labetalol disposition and concentration-effect relationships during pregnancy. Br J Clin Pharmacol 1983;15:465–70.
8. Lardoux H, Gerard J, Blazquez G, Chouty F, Flouvat B. Hypertension in pregnancy: evaluation of two beta blockers atenolol and labetalol. Eur Heart J 1983;4(Suppl G):35–40.
9. Michael CA, Potter JM. A comparison of labetalol with other antihypertensive drugs in the treatment of hypertensive disease of pregnancy. In Riley A, Symonds EM, eds. *The Investigation of Labetalol in the Management of Hypertension in Pregnancy*. Amsterdam:Excerpta Medica, 1982:111–22.
10. Davey DA, Dommisse J, Garden A. Intravenous labetalol and intravenous dihydralazine in severe hypertension in pregnancy. *Ibid*, 52–61.
11. Redman CWG. A controlled trial of the treatment of hypertension in pregnancy: labetalol compared with methyldopa. *Ibid*, 101–10.
12. Walker JJ, Crooks A, Erwin L, Calder AA. Labetalol in pregnancy-induced hypertension: fetal and maternal effects. *Ibid*, 148–60.
13. Lamming GD, Symonds EM. Use of labetalol and methyldopa in pregnancy-induced hypertension. Br J Clin Pharmacol 1979;8(Suppl 2):217S–22S.
14. Jorge CS, Fernandes L, Cunha S. Labetalol in the hypertensive states of pregnancy. In Riley A,

Symonds EM, eds. *The Investigation of Labetalol in the Management of Hypertension in Pregnancy*. Amsterdam:Excerpta Medica, 1982:124–30.

15. Lunell NO, Nylund L, Lewander R, Sarby B. Acute effect of an antihypertensive drug, labetalol, on uteroplacental blood flow. Br J Obstet Gynaecol 1982;89:640–4.

16. Michael CA. The evaluation of labetalol in the treatment of hypertension complicating pregnancy. Br J Clin Pharmacol 1982;13(Suppl):127S–31S.

17. Symonds EM, Lamming GD, Jadoul F, Broughton Pipkin F. Clinical and biochemical aspects of the use of labetalol in the treatment of hypertension in pregnancy: comparison with methyldopa. In Riley A, Symonds EM, eds. *The Investigation of Labetalol in the Management of Hypertension in Pregnancy*. Amsterdam:Excerpta Medica, 1982:62–76.

18. Smith AM. Beta-blockers for pregnancy hypertension. Lancet 1983;1:708–9.

19. Walker JJ, Bonduelle M, Greer I, Calder AA. Antihypertensive therapy in pregnancy. Lancet 1983;1:932–3.

Name: **LACTULOSE**

Class: **Laxative/Ammonia Detoxicant**   Risk Factor: **C**

Fetal Risk Summary

No data available.

Breast Feeding Summary

No data available.

Name: **LAETRILE**

Class: **Unclassified/Antineoplastic**   Risk Factor: **C**

Fetal Risk Summary

Laetrile is a nonapproved agent used for the treatment of cancer. There are no studies of laetrile in pregnancy. A concern for possible gestational cyanide poisoning has been reported (1). Due to an increased amount of β-glycosidase present in the intestinal flora, the oral route would theoretically be more toxic than the parenteral route in liberation of hydrogen cyanide, which is present in various sources of laetrile (1). Long-term follow-up has been recommended, as neurologic evidence of chronic cyanide exposure may not be recognizable in the infant.

Breast Feeding Summary

No data available.

References

1. Peterson RG, Ruman BH. Laetrile and pregnancy. Clin Toxicol 1979;15:181–4.

Name: **LANATOSIDE C**

Class: **Cardiac Glycoside**   Risk Factor: **C**

Fetal Risk Summary

See Digitalis.

Breast Feeding Summary

See Digitalis.

Name: **LEUCOVORIN**

Class: **Vitamin**   Risk Factor: **C$_M$**

Fetal Risk Summary

Leucovorin (folinic acid) is an active metabolite of folic acid (1). It has been used for the treatment of megaloblastic anemia during pregnancy (2). See Folic Acid.

Breast Feeding Summary

Leucovorin (folinic acid) is an active metabolite of folic acid (1). See Folic Acid.

References

1. American Hospital Formulary Service. *Drug Information 1985*. Bethesda:American Society of Hospital Pharmacists, 1985:1745–7.
2. Scott JM. Folinic acid in megaloblastic anaemia of pregnancy. Br Med J 1957:2:270–2.

Name: **LEVALLORPHAN**

Class: **Narcotic Antagonist**   Risk Factor: **D**

Fetal Risk Summary

Levallorphan is a narcotic antagonist that is used to reverse respiratory depression from narcotic overdose. It has been used in combination with alphaprodine or meperidine during labor to reduce neonatal depression (1–6). Although some benefits were initially claimed, caution in the use of levallorphan during labor has been advised for the following reasons (7):

A statistically significant reduction in neonatal depression has not been demonstrated.

The antagonist also reduces analgesia.

The antagonist may increase neonatal depression if an improper narcotic-narcotic antagonist ratio is used.

As indicated above, levallorphan may cause respiratory depression in the absence of narcotics or if a critical ratio is exceeded (7). Because of these considerations, the use of levallorphan either alone or in combination therapy in pregnancy should be discouraged. If a narcotic antagonist is indicated, other agents that do not cause respiratory depression, such as naloxone, are preferred.

Breast Feeding Summary

No data available.

References

1. Backner DD, Foldes FF, Gordon EH. The combined use of alphaprodine (Nisentil) hydrochloride and levallorphan tartrate for analgesia in obstetrics. Am J Obstet Gynecol 1957;74:271–82.
2. Roberts H, Kuck MAC. Use of alphaprodine and levallorphan during labour. Can Med Assoc J 1960;83:1088–93.
3. Roberts H, Kane KM, Percival N, Snow P, Please NW. Effects of some analgesic drugs used in childbirth. Lancet 1957;1:128–32.
4. Bullough J. Use of premixed pethidine and antagonists in obstetrical analgesia with special reference to cases in which levallorphan was used. Br Med J 1959;2:859–62.
5. Posner AC. Combined pethidine and antagonists in obstetrics. Br Med J 1960;1:124–5.
6. Bullough J. Combined pethidine and antagonists in obstetrics. Br Med J 1960;1:125.
7. Bonica JJ. *Principles and Practice of Obstetric Analgesia and Anesthesia.* Philadelphia:FA Davis Co, 1967:254–9.

Name: **LEVARTERENOL**

Class: **Sympathomimetic (Adrenergic)**   Risk Factor: **D**

Fetal Risk Summary

Levarterenol is a sympathomimetic used in emergency situations to treat hypotension. Because of the nature of its indication, experience in pregnancy is limited. Levarterenol readily crosses the placenta (1). Uterine vessels are normally maximally dilated, and they have only α-adrenergic receptors (2). Use of the α- and β-adrenergic stimulant, levarterenol, could cause constriction of these vessels and reduce uterine blood flow, thereby producing fetal hypoxia (bradycardia). Levarterenol may also interact with oxytocics or ergot derivatives to produce severe persistent maternal hypertension (2). Rupture of a cerebral vessel is possible. If a pressor agent is indicated, other drugs such as ephedrine should be considered.

Breast Feeding Summary

No data available.

References

1. Morgan CD, Sandler M, Panigel M. Placental transfer of catecholamines in vitro and in vivo. Am J Obstet Gynecol 1972;112:1068–75.
2. Smith NT, Corbascio AN. The use and misuse of pressor agents. Anesthesiology 1970;33:58–101.

Name: **LEVORPHANOL**

Class: **Narcotic Analgesic**   Risk Factor: **B***

Fetal Risk Summary

No reports linking the use of levorphanol with congenital defects have been located. Use of the drug during labor should be expected to produce neonatal depression to the same degree as other narcotic analgesics (1).

[* Risk Factor D if used for prolonged periods or in high doses at term.]

Breast Feeding Summary

No data available.

References

1. Bonica JJ. *Principles and Practice of Obstetric Analgesia and Anesthesia*. Philadelphia:FA Davis Co, 1967:251.

Name: **LEVOTHYROXINE**

Class: **Thyroid**   Risk Factor: **A$_M$**

Fetal Risk Summary

Levothyroxine (T$_4$) is a naturally occurring thyroid hormone produced by the mother and the fetus. It is used during pregnancy for the treatment of hypothyroidism (see also Liothyronine and Thyroid). There is little or no transplacental passage of the drug at physiologic serum concentrations (1–5).

Several reports have described the direct administration of T$_4$ to the fetus and amniotic fluid (5–10). In almost identical cases, two fetuses were treated in the 3rd trimester with intramuscular injections of T$_4$, 120 μg, every 2 weeks for four doses in an attempt to prevent congenital hypothyroidism (5, 6). Their mothers had been treated with radioactive iodine (^{131}I) at 13 and 13 ½ weeks gestation, respectively. Both newborns were hypothyroid at birth and developed respiratory stridor, but neither had physical signs of cretinism. At the time of the reports, one infant had mild developmental retardation at 3 years of age (5). The second infant was stable with a tracheostomy tube in place at 6 months of age (6). In a third mother who inadvertently received ^{131}I at 10–11 weeks gestation, intra-amniotic T$_4$, 500 μg, was given weekly during the last 7 weeks of pregnancy (7). Evidence was found that the T$_4$ was absorbed by the fetus. A male infant was delivered who developed normally. In a study to determine the metabolic fate of T$_4$ *in utero*, 700 μg of T$_4$ was injected intra-amniotically 24 hours prior to delivery in five full-term healthy patients (8). Serum T$_4$ levels were increased in all infants. Intra-amniotic T$_4$, 200 μg, was given to eight women in whom premature delivery was inevitable or indicated to enhance fetal lung maturity (9). The patients ranged in gestational age between 29 and 32 weeks. No respiratory distress syndrome was found in the eight newborn infants. Delivery occurred 1–49 days after the injection. The dimensions of a large fetal goiter, secondary to propylthiouracil, were decreased but not eliminated within 5 days of an intra-amniotic 200-μg dose of T_4 administered at 34.5 weeks gestation (10). Serial lecithin/sphingomyelin ratios before and after the injection demonstrated no effect of T_4 on fetal lung maturity.

In a large prospective study, 537 mother-child pairs were exposed to levothyroxine and thyroid during the 1st trimester (11). For use anytime during pregnancy, 780 exposures were reported (12). After 1st trimester exposure, possible associations were found with cardiovascular anomalies (nine cases), Down's syndrome (three cases), and polydactyly in blacks (three cases). Due to the small numbers involved, the statistical significance of these findings is unknown and independent confirmation is required. Maternal hypothyroidism itself has been reported to be responsible for poor pregnancy outcome (13–15). Others have not found this association, claiming that fetal development is not directly affected by maternal thyroid function (16).

Combination therapy with thyroid-antithyroid drugs was advocated at one time for the treatment of hyperthyroidism but is now considered inappropriate (see Propylthiouracil).

Breast Feeding Summary

T_4 is excreted into breast milk in low concentrations. The effect of this hormone on the nursing infant is controversial (see also Liothyronine and Thyrotropin). Two reports have claimed that sufficient quantities are present to partially treat neonatal hypothyroidism (17, 18). A third study measured high T_4/ levels in breast-fed infants but was unsure of its significance (19). In contrast, four competing studies have found that breast-feeding does not alter either T_4 levels or thyroid function in the infant (20–23). Although all of the investigators, on both sides of the issue, used sophisticated available methods to arrive at their conclusions, the balance of evidence weighs in on the side of those claiming lack of effect since they have relied on increasingly refined means to measure the hormone (24–26). The reports are briefly summarized below.

In 19 healthy euthyroid mothers not taking thyroid replacement therapy, mean milk T_4 concentrations in the first postpartum week were 3.8 ng/ml (17). Between 8 and 48 days, the levels rose to 42.7 ng/ml and then decreased to 11.1 ng/ml after 50 days postpartum. The daily excretion of T_4 at the higher levels is about the recommended daily dose for hypothyroid infants. An infant was diagnosed as athyrotic shortly after breast-feeding was stopped at age 10 months (18). Growth was at the 97th percentile during breast-feeding, but the bone age remained that of a newborn. In this study, mean levels of T_4 in breast milk during the last trimester (12 patients) and within 48 hours of delivery (22 patients) were 14 and 7 ng/ml, respectively. A 1983 report measured significantly greater serum levels of T_4 in 22 breast-fed infants than in 25 formula-fed babies, 131.1 ng/ml vs 118.4 ng/ml, respectively (19). The overlap between the two groups, however, cast doubt on the physiologic significance of the differences.

In 77 euthyroid mothers, measurable amounts of T_4 were found in only 5 of 88 milk specimens collected over 43 months of lactation with 4 of the positive samples occurring within 4 days of delivery (20). Concentrations ranged from 8 to 13 ng/ml. A 1980 report described four exclusively breast-fed infants with congenital hypothyroidism that was diagnosed between the ages of 2 and 79 days (21).

Breast-feeding did not hinder making the diagnosis. Another 1980 research report evaluated clinical and biochemical thyroid parameters in 45 hypothyroid infants, 12 of whom were breast-fed (22). No difference was detected between the breast-fed and bottle-fed babies, leading to the conclusion that breast milk did not offer protection against the effects of congenital hypothyroidism. In a 1985 study, serum concentrations of T_4 were similar in breast-fed and bottle-fed infants at 5, 10, and 15 days postpartum (23).

The discrepancies described above can be partially explained by the various techniques used to measure milk T_4 concentrations. Japanese researchers failed to detect milk T_4 using four different methods of radioimmunoassay (RIA) (24). Using three competitive protein-binding assays, highly variable T_4 levels were recovered from milk and a standard solution. Although the RIA methods were not completely reliable since recovery from a standardized solution exceeded 100% with one method, they concluded that milk T_4 concentrations must be very low and had no influence on the pituitary-thyroid axis of normal babies. No difficulty was encountered with measuring serum T_4 levels which were not significantly different between breast-fed and bottle-fed infants (24). Swedish investigators using RIA methods also failed to find T_4 in milk (25). A second group of Swedish researchers utilized a gas chromatography-mass spectrometry technique to determine that the concentration of T_4 in milk was less than 4 ng/ml (26).

In summary, levothyroxine breast milk levels, as determined by modern laboratory techniques, are apparently too low to completely protect a hypothyroid infant from the effects of the disease. The levels are also too low to interfere with neonatal thyroid screening programs (23). Breast-feeding, however, probably offers better protection to infants with congenital hypothyroidism than does formula feeding.

References

1. Grumbach MM, Werner SC. Transfer of thyroid hormone across the human placenta at term. J Clin Endocrinol Metab 1956;16:1392–5.
2. Kearns JE, Hutson W. Tagged isomers and analogues of thyroxine (their transmission across the human placenta and other studies). J Nucl Med 1963;4:453–61.
3. Fisher DA, Lehman H, Lackey C. Placental transport of thyroxine. J Clin Endocrinol Metab 1964;24:393–400.
4. Fisher DA, Klein AH. Thyroid development and disorders of thyroid function in the newborn. N Engl J Med 1981;304:702–12.
5. Van Herle AJ, Young RT, Fisher DA, Uller RP, Brinkman CR III. Intrauterine treatment of a hypothyroid fetus. J Clin Endocrinol Metab 1975;40:474–7.
6. Jafek BW, Small R, Lillian DL. Congenital radioactive-iodine induced stridor and hypothyroidism. Arch Otolaryngol 1974;99:369–71.
7. Lightner ES, Fisher DA, Giles H, Woolfenden J. Intra-amniotic injection of thyroxine (T_4) to a human fetus. Am J Obstet Gynecol 1977;127:487–90.
8. Klein AH, Hobel CJ, Sack J, Fisher DA. Effect of intraamniotic fluid thyroxine injection on fetal serum and amniotic fluid iodothyronine concentrations. J Clin Endocrinol Metab 1978;47:1034–7.
9. Mashiach S, Barkai G, Sach J, Stern E, Goldman B, Brish M, Serr DM. Enhancement of fetal lung maturity by intra-amniotic administration of thyroid hormone. Am J Obstet Gynecol 1978;130:289–93.
10. Weiner S, Scharf JI, Bolognese RJ, Librizzi RJ. Antenatal diagnosis and treatment of fetal goiter. J Reprod Med 1980;24:39–42.
11. Heinonen OP, Slone D, Shapiro S. *Birth Defects and Drugs in Pregnancy*. Littleton:Publishing Sciences Group, 1977:388–400.
12. *Ibid*, 443.
13. Potter JD. Hypothyroidism and reproductive failure. Surg Gynecol Obstet 1980;150:251–5.
14. Pekonen F, Teramo K, Ikonen E, Osterlund K, Makinen T, Lamberg BA. Women on thyroid hormone

therapy: pregnancy course, fetal outcome, and amniotic fluid thyroid hormone level. Obstet Gynecol 1984;63: 635–8.

15. Man EB, Shaver BA Jr, Cooke RE. Studies of children born to women with thyroid disease. Am J Obstet Gynecol 1958;75:728–41.
16. Montoro M, Collea JV, Frasier SD, Mestman JH. Successful outcome of pregnancy in women with hypothyroidism. Ann Intern Med 1981;94:31–4.
17. Sack J, Amado O, Lunenfeld. Thyroxine concentration in human milk. J Clin Endocrinol Metab 1977;45:171–3.
18. Bode HH, Vanjonack WJ, Crawford JD. Mitigation of cretinism by breast-feeding. Pediatrics 1978;62:13–6.
19. Hahn HB Jr, Spiekerman AM, Otto WR, Hossalla DE. Thyroid function tests in neonates fed human milk. Am J Dis Child 1983;137:220–2.
20. Varma SK, Collins M, Row A, Haller WS, Varma K. Thyroxine, triiodothyronine, and reverse triiodothyronine concentrations in human milk. J Pediatr 1978;93:803–6.
21. Abbassi V, Steinour TA. Successful diagnosis of congenital hypothyroidism in four breast-fed neonates. J Pediatr 1980;97:259–61.
22. Letarte J, Guyda H, Dussault JH, Glorieux J. Lack of protective effect of breast-feeding in congenital hypothyroidism: report of 12 cases. Pediatrics 1980;65:703–5.
23. Franklin R, O'Grady C, Carpenter L. Neonatal thyroid function: comparison between breast-fed and bottle-fed infants. J Pediatr 1985;106:124–6.
24. Mizuta H, Amino N, Ichihara K, Harada T, Nose O, Tanizawa O, Miyai K. Thyroid hormones in human milk and their influence on thyroid function of breast-fed babies. Pediatr Res 1983;17:468–71.
25. Jansson L, Ivarsson S, Larsson I, Ekman R. Tri-iodothyronine and thyroxine in human milk. Acta Paediatr Scand 1983;72:703–5.
26. Moller B, Bjorkhem I, Falk O, Lantto O, Larsson A. Identification of thyroxine in human breast milk by gas chromatography-mass spectrometry. J Clin Endocrinol Metab 1983;56:30–4.

Name: **LINCOMYCIN**

Class: **Antibiotic**   Risk Factor: **B**

Fetal Risk Summary

No reports linking the use of lincomycin with congenital defects have been located. The antibiotic crosses the placenta, achieving cord serum levels about 25% of the maternal serum (1, 2). Multiple intramuscular injections of 600 mg did not result in accumulation in the amniotic fluid (2). No effects on the newborn were observed.

The progeny of 302 patients treated at various stages of pregnancy with oral lincomycin, 2 g/day for 7 days, were evaluated at various intervals up to 7 years after birth (3). As compared to a control group, no increases in malformations or delayed developmental defects were observed.

Breast Feeding Summary

Lincomycin is excreted into breast milk. Six hours following oral dosing of 500 mg every 6 hours for 3 days, serum and milk levels in nine patients averaged 1.37 and 1.28 μg/ml, respectively, a milk:plasma ratio of 0.9 (1). Much lower milk:plasma ratios of 0.13–0.17 have also been reported (4). Although no adverse effects have been reported, three potential problems exist for the nursing infant: modification of bowel flora, direct effects on the infant, and interference with the interpretation of culture results if a fever work-up is required.

References

1. Medina A, Fiske N, Hjelt-Harvey I, Brown CD, Prigot A. Absorption, diffusion, and excretion of a new antibiotic, lincomycin. Antimicrob Agents Chemother 1963;189–96.
2. Duignan NM, Andrews J, Williams JD. Pharmacological studies with lincomycin in late pregnancy. Br Med J 1973;3:75–8.
3. Mickal A, Panzer JD. The safety of lincomycin in pregnancy. Am J Obstet Gynecol 1975;121:1071–4.
4. Wilson JT. Milk/plasma ratios and contraindicated drugs. In Wilson JT, ed. *Drugs in Breast Milk*. Balgowlah, Australia: ADIS Press, 1981:78–9.

Name: **LINDANE**

Class: **Scabicide/Pediculicide**   Risk Factor: **C**

Fetal Risk Summary

Lindane (γ-benzene hexachloride) is used topically for the treatment of lice and scabies. Small amounts are absorbed through the intact skin and mucous membranes (1). No reports linking the use of this drug with toxic or congenital defects have been located, but one reference suggested it should be used with caution due to its potential to produce neurotoxicity, convulsions, and aplastic anemia (2). Limited animal studies have not shown a teratogenic effect (3, 4). In one animal study, lindane seemed to have a protective effect when given with known teratogens (5). The manufacturer recommends using lindane with caution during pregnancy (6). Because of the potential serious toxicity, pyrethrins with piperonyl butoxide is recommended for the treatment of lice infestations occurring during pregnancy (see Pyrethrins with Piperonyl Butoxide).

Breast Feeding Summary

No reports describing the use of lindane in lactating women have been located. Based on theoretical considerations, the manufacturer estimates the upper limit of lindane levels in breast milk to be approximately 30 ng/ml after maternal application (7). A nursing infant taking 1 liter of milk per day would thus ingest about 30 μg/day of lindane. This is in the same general range that the infant would absorb after direct topical application (7). These amounts are probably clinically insignificant.

References

1. American Hospital Formulary Service. *Drug Information 1985*. Bethesda:American Society of Hospital Pharmacists, 1985:1600–1601.
2. Sanmiguel GS, Ferrer AP, Alberich MT, Genaoui BM. Consideraciones sobre el tratamiento de la infancia y en el embarazo. Actas Dermosifilogr 1980;71:105–8.
3. Palmer AK, Cozens DD, Spicer EJF, Worden AN. Effects of lindane upon reproduction function in a 3-generation study of rats. Toxicology 1978;10:45–54.
4. Palmer AK, Bottomley AM, Worden AN, Frohberg H, Bauer A. Effect of lindane on pregnancy in the rabbit and rat. Toxicology 1978;10:239–47.
5. Shtenberg AI, Torchinski I. Adaptation to the action of several teratogens as a consequence of preliminary administration of pesticides to females. Biul Eksp Biol Med 1977;83:227–8.
6. Product information. Kwell. Reed & Carnrick, 1985.
7. Rickard ED, Clinical Research Associate, Reed & Carnrick, May 13,1983. Personal communication.

Name: **LIOTHYRONINE**

Class: **Thyroid**   Risk Factor: **A**

Fetal Risk Summary

Liothyronine (T_3) is a naturally occurring thyroid hormone produced by the mother and the fetus. It is used during pregnancy for the treatment of hypothyroidism (see also Levothyroxine and Thyroid). There is little or no transplacental passage of the hormone at physiologic serum concentrations (1–3). Limited placental passage of T_3 to the fetus has been demonstrated following very large doses (4, 5).

In a large prospective study, 34 mother-child pairs were exposed to liothyronine during the 1st trimester (6). No association between the drug and fetal defects was found. Maternal hypothyroidism itself has been reported to be responsible for poor pregnancy outcome (7). Others have not found this association, claiming that fetal development is not directly affected by maternal thyroid function (8).

Combination therapy with thyroid-antithyroid drugs was advocated at one time for the treatment of hyperthyroidism but is now considered inappropriate (see Propylthiouracil).

Breast Feeding Summary

T_3 is excreted into breast milk in low concentrations. The effect on the nursing infant is not thought to be physiologically significant although at least one report concluded otherwise (9). An infant was diagnosed as athyrotic shortly after breast-feeding was stopped at age 10 months (9). Growth was at the 97th percentile during breast-feeding, but the bone age remained that of a newborn. Mean levels of T_3 in breast milk during the last trimester (12 patients) and within 48 hours of delivery (22 patients) were 1.36 and 2.86 ng/ml, respectively. A 1978 study reported milk concentrations varying between 0.4 and 2.38 ng/ml (range 0.1–5 ng/ml) from the day of delivery to 148 days postpartum (10). No liothyronine was detected in a number of the samples. Levels in three instances, collected 16, 20, and 43 months postpartum, ranged from 0.68 to 4.5 ng/ml with the highest concentration measured at 20 months. From the first week through 148 days postdelivery, the calculated maximum amount of T_3 that a nursing infant would have ingested was 2.1–2.6 μg/day, far less than the dose required to treat congenital hypothyroidism (10). However, the authors concluded this was enough to mask the symptoms of the disease without halting its progression. In a study comparing serum T_3 levels between 22 breast-fed and 29 formula-fed infants, significantly higher levels were found in the breast-feeding group (11). The levels, 2.24 and 1.79 ng/ml, were comparable to previous reports and probably were of doubtful clinical significance. A 1980 report described four exclusively breast-fed infants with congenital hypothyroidism that was diagnosed between the ages of 2 and 79 days (12). Breast-feeding did not hinder making the diagnosis. Another 1980 research report evaluated clinical and biochemical thyroid parameters in 45 hypothyroid infants, 12 of whom were breast-fed (13). No difference was detected between the breast-fed and bottle-fed babies, leading to the conclusion that breast milk does not offer protection against the effects of congenital hypothyroidism. In a 1985 paper, serum concentrations of T_3 were similar in breast-fed and bottle-fed infants at 5, 10, and 15 days postpartum (14).

Japanese researchers found a T_3 milk:plasma ratio of 0.36 (15). No correlation was discovered between serum T_3 and milk T_3 or total daily T_3 excretion, nor was there a correlation between milk T_3 levels and milk protein concentration or daily volume of milk. They concluded that breast-feeding has no influence on the pituitary-thyroid axis of normal babies. A Swedish investigation measured higher levels of T_3 in milk 1–3 months after delivery as compared to early colostrum (16). The concentrations were comparable to those in the studies cited above.

In summary, liothyronine breast milk concentrations are too low to completely protect a hypothyroid infant from the effects of the disease. The levels are also too low to interfere with neonatal thyroid screening programs (14).

References

1. Grumbach MM, Werner SC. Transfer of thyroid hormone across the human placenta at term. J Clin Endocrinol Metab 1956;16:1392–5.
2. Kearns JE, Hutson W. Tagged isomers and analogues of thyroxine (their transmission across the human placenta and other studies). J Nucl Med 1963;4:453–61.
3. Fisher DA, Lehman H, Lackey C. Placental transport of thyroxine. J Clin Endocrinol Metab 1964;24:393–400.
4. Raiti S, Holzman GB, Scott RI, Blizzard RM. Evidence for the placental transfer of tri-iodothyronine in human beings. N Engl J Med 1967;277: 456–9.
5. Dussault J, Row VV, Lickrish G, Volpe R. Studies of serum triiodothyronine concentration in maternal and cord blood: transfer of triiodothyronine across the human placenta. J Clin Endocrinol Metab 1969; 29:595–606.
6. Heinonen OP, Slone D, Shapiro S. *Birth Defects and Drugs in Pregnancy*. Littleton:Publishing Sciences Group, 1977:388–400.
7. Potter JD. Hypothyroidism and reproductive failure. Surg Gynecol Obstet 1980;150:251–5.
8. Montoro M, Collea JV, Frasier SD, Mestman JH. Successful outcome of pregnancy in women with hypothyroidism. Ann Intern Med 1981;94:31–4.
9. Bode HH, Vanjonack WJ, Crawford JD. Mitigation of cretinism by breast-feeding. Pediatrics 1978;62:13–6.
10. Varma SK, Collins M, Row A, Haller WS, Varma K. Thyroxine, triiodothyronine, and reverse triiodothyronine concentrations in human milk. J Pediatr 1978;93:803–6.
11. Hahn HB Jr, Spiekerman AM, Otto WR, Hossalla DE. Thyroid function tests in neonates fed human milk. Am J Dis Child 1983;137:220–2.
12. Abbassi V, Steinour TA. Successful diagnosis of congenital hypothyroidism in four breast-fed neonates. J Pediatr 1980;97:259–61.
13. Letarte J, Guyda H, Dussault JH, Glorieux J. Lack of protective effect of breast-feeding in congenital hypothyroidism: report of 12 cases. Pediatrics 1980;65:703–5.
14. Franklin R, O'Grady C, Carpenter L. Neonatal thyroid function: comparison between breast-fed and bottle-fed infants. J Pediatr 1985;106:124–6.
15. Mizuta H, Amino N, Ichihara K, Harade T, Nose O, Tanizawa O, Miyai K. Thyroid hormones in human milk and influence on thyroid function of breast-fed babies. Pediatr Res 1983;17:468–71.
16. Jansson L, Ivarsson S, Larsson I, Ekman R. Tri-iodothyronine and thyroxine in human milk. Acta Paediatr Scand 1983;72:703–5.

Name: LIOTRIX

Class: **Thyroid**   Risk Factor: **A**

Fetal Risk Summary

Liotrix is a synthetic combination of levothyroxine and liothyronine (see Levothyroxine and Liothyronine).

Breast Feeding Summary

See Levothyroxine and Liothyronine.

Name: **LIPIDS**

Class: **Nutrient**   Risk Factor: **C**

Fetal Risk Summary

Lipids (intravenous fat emulsions) are a mixture of neutral triglycerides, primarily unsaturated fatty acids, prepared from either soybean or safflower oil. Egg yolk phospholipids are used as an emulsifier. The triglyceride fatty acids readily cross the placenta to the fetus (1).

Reports have described the use of lipids during pregnancy in conjunction with dextrose/amino acid solutions (see Hyperalimentation, Parenteral) in 19 patients (2–9). Heller, in 1976 (10), wrote that lipid infusions were contraindicated during pregnancy for several reasons: 1) an excessive increase in serum triglycerides, often with ketonemia, would result because of the physiologic hyperlipemia present during pregnancy, 2) premature labor would occur, and 3) placental infarctions would occur from fat deposits and cause placental insufficiency. Fortunately, none of these complications has been observed in the mothers and fetuses treated with lipids.

Based on limited clinical experience, intravenous lipids apparently do not pose a risk to the mother or fetus. Standard precautions, as taken with nonpregnant patients, should be followed when these solutions are administered during pregnancy.

Breast Feeding Summary

No data available.

References

1. Elphick MC, Filshie GM, Hull D. The passage of fat emulsion across the human placenta. Br J Obstet Gynaecol 1978;85:610–8.
2. Hew LR, Deitel M. Total parenteral nutrition in gynecology and obstetrics. Obstet Gynecol 1980;55:464–8.
3. Tresadern JC, Falconer GF, Turnberg LA, Irving MH. Successful completed pregnancy in a patient maintained on home parenteral nutrition. Br Med J 1983;286:602–3.
4. Tresadern JC, Falconer GF, Turnberg LA, Irving MH. Maintenance of pregnancy in a home parenteral nutrition patient. JPEN 1984;8:199–202.
5. Seifer DB, Silberman H, Catanzarite VA, Conteas CN, Wood R, Ueland K. Total parenteral nutrition in obstetrics. JAMA 1985;253;2073–5.
6. Lavin JP Jr, Gimmon Z, Miodovnik M, von Meyenfeldt M, Fischer JE. Total parenteral nutrition in a pregnant insulin-requiring diabetic. Obstet Gynecol 1982;59:660–4.
7. Rivera-Alsina ME, Saldana LR, Stringer CA. Fetal growth sustained by parenteral nutrition in pregnancy. Obstet Gynecol 1984;64:138–41.
8. Di Costanzo J, Martin J, Cano N, Mas JC, Noirclerc M. Total parenteral nutrition with fat emulsions during pregnancy—nutritional requirements: a case report. JPEN 1982;6:534–8.
9. Young KR. Acute pancreatitis in pregnancy: two case reports. Obstet Gynecol 1982;60:653–7.
10. Heller L. Parenteral nutrition in obstetrics and gynecology. In Greep JM, Soeters PB, Wesdorp RIC, et al, eds. *Current Concepts in Parenteral Nutrition*. The Hague:Martinus Nijhoff Medical Division, 1977:179–86.

Name: **LITHIUM**

Class: **Tranquilizer**   Risk Factor: **D**

Fetal Risk Summary

The use of lithium during the 1st trimester may be related to an increased incidence of congenital defects, particularly of the cardiovascular system. The drug freely crosses the placenta, equilibrating between maternal and cord serum (1–5). Amniotic fluid concentrations exceed cord serum levels (2). Frequent reports have described the fetal effects of lithium, the majority from data accumulated by the Lithium Baby Register (1, 6–14). The Register, founded in Denmark in 1968 and later expanded internationally, collects data on known cases of 1st trimester exposure to lithium. By 1977, the Register included 183 infants, 20 (11%) with major congenital anomalies (12). Of the 20 malformed infants, there were 15 instances of cardiovascular defects, including 5 with the rare Ebstein's anomaly. Others have also noted the increased incidence of Ebstein's anomaly in lithium-exposed babies (15). Two new case reports bring the total number of infants with cardiovascular defects to 17, or 77% (17 of 22) of the known malformed children (16, 17). Ebstein's anomaly has been diagnosed in the fetus during the 2nd trimester by echocardiography (18). Details on 16 of the malformed infants are shown below.

In 60 of the children born without malformations, follow-up comparisons with nonexposed siblings did not show an increased frequency of physical or mental anomalies (19).

Author	Case No.	Defect
Weinstein (11)	1	Coarctation of aorta
	2	High intraventricular septal defect
	3	Stenosis of aqueduct with hydrocephalus, spina bifida with sacral meningomyelocele, bilateral talipes equivovarus with paralysis; atonic bladder, patulous rectal sphincter and rectal prolapse (see also Ref. 7)
	4	Unilateral microtia
	5	Mitral atresia, rudimentary left ventricle without inlet or outlet, aorta and pulmonary artery arising from right ventricle, patent ductus arteriosus, left superior vena cava
	6	Mitral atresia
	7	Ebstein's anomaly
	8	Single umbilical artery, bilateral hypoplasia of maxilla
	9	Ebstein's anomaly
	10	Atresia of tricuspid valve
	11	Ebstein's anomaly
	12	Patent ductus arteriosus, ventricular septal defect
	13	Ebstein's anomaly
Rane (14)	14	Detrocardia and situs colitus, patent ductus arteriosus, juxta-ductal aortic coarctation
Weinstein (12)	15	Ebstein's anomaly
Arnon (17)	16	Massive tricuspid regurgitation, atrial flutter, congestive heart failure

Lithium toxicity in the newborn has been reported frequently:

Cyanosis (2, 16, 20–23, 29)
Hypotonia (2, 10, 20–26, 29)

Bradycardia (16, 21, 25, 27, 29)
Thyroid depression with goiter (2, 10, 26)
Atrial flutter (28)
Hepatomegaly (29)
Electrocardiogram abnormalities (T wave inversion) (21, 27)
Cardiomegaly (22, 28, 29)
Gastrointestinal bleeding (27)
Diabetes insipidus (2, 29)
Shock (29)

Most of these toxic effects are self-limiting, returning to normal in 1–2 weeks. This corresponds with the renal elimination of lithium from the infant. The serum half-life of lithium in newborns is prolonged, averaging 68–96 hours, as compared to the adult value of 10–20 hours (3, 16). The two reported cases of nephrogenic diabetes insipidus persisted for 2 months or longer (2, 29).

Fetal red blood cell choline levels are elevated during maternal therapy with lithium (30). The clinical significance of this effect on choline, the metabolic precursor to acetycholine, is unknown but may be related to the teratogenicity of lithium due to its effect on cellular lithium transport (30). In an *in vitro* study, lithium had no effect on human sperm motility (31).

In the mother, renal lithium clearance rises during pregnancy, returning to prepregnancy levels shortly after delivery (32). In four patients, the mean clearance before delivery was 29 ml/min, declining to 15 ml/min 6–7 weeks after delivery, a statistically significant difference ($p < 0.01$). These data emphasize the need to closely monitor lithium levels before and after pregnancy.

In summary, lithium should be avoided during pregnancy if possible, especially during the 1st trimester. Use of the drug near term may produce severe toxicity in the newborn, which is usually reversible.

Breast Feeding Summary

Lithium is excreted into breast milk (5, 21, 33, 34). Milk levels average 40% of the maternal serum concentration (21, 34). Infant serum and milk levels are approximately equal. Although no toxic effects in the nursing infant have been reported, long-term effects from this exposure have not been studied. The American Academy of Pediatrics considers lithium compatible with breast-feeding (35).

References

1. Weinstein MR, Goldfield M. Lithium carbonate treatment during pregnancy: report of a case. Dis Nerv Syst 1969;30:828–32.
2. Mizrahi EM, Hobbs JF, Goldsmith DI. Nephrogenic diabetes insipidus in transplacental lithium intoxication. J Pediatr 1979;94:493–5.
3. Mackay AVP, Loose R, Glen AIM. Labour on lithium. Br Med J 1976;1:878.
4. Schou M, Amdisen A. Lithium and placenta. Am J Obstet Gynecol 1975;122:541.
5. Sykes PA, Quarrie J, Alexander FW. Lithium carbonate and breast-feeding. Br Med J 1976;2:1299.
6. Schou M, Amdisen A. Lithium in pregnancy. Lancet 1970;1:1391.
7. Aoki FY, Ruedy J. Severe lithium intoxication: management without dialysis and report of a possible teratogenic effect of lithium. Can Med Assoc J 1971;105:847–8.
8. Goldfield M, Weinstein MR. Lithium in pregnancy: a review with recommendations. Am J Psychiatry 1971;127:888–93.
9. Goldfield MD, Weinstein MR. Lithium carbonate in obstetrics: guidelines for clinical use. Am J Obstet Gynecol 1973;116:15–22.
10. Schou M, Goldfield MD, Weinstein MR, Villeneuve A. Lithium and pregnancy. I. Report from the register of lithium babies. Br Med J 1973;2:135–6.

11. Weinstein MR, Goldfield MD. Cardiovascular malformations with lithium use during pregnancy. Am J Psychiatry 1975;132:529–31.
12. Weinstein MR. Recent advances in clinical psychopharmacology. I. Lithium carbonate. Hosp Formul 1977;12:759–62.
13. Linden S, Rich CL. The use of lithium during pregnancy and lactation. J Clin Psychiatry 1983; 44:358–61.
14. Pitts FN. Editorial. Lithium and pregnancy. J Clin Psychiatry 1983;44:357.
15. Nora JJ, Nora AH, Toews WH. Lithium, Ebstein's anomaly, and other congenital heart defects. Lancet 1974;2:594–5.
16. Rane A, Tomson G, Bjarke B. Effects of maternal lithium therapy in a newborn infant. J Pediatr 1978;93:296–7.
17. Arnon RG, Marin-Garcia J, Peeden JN. Tricuspid valve regurgitation and lithium carbonate toxicity in a newborn infant. Am J Dis Child 1981;135:941–3.
18. Allan LD, Desai G, Tynan MJ. Prenatal echocardiographic screening for Ebstein's anomaly for mothers on lithium therapy. Lancet 1982;2:875–6.
19. Schou M. What happened later to the lithium babies? A follow-up study of children born without malformations. Acta Psychiatr Scand 1976;54:193–7.
20. Woody JN, London WL, Wilbanks GD Jr. Lithium toxicity in a newborn. Pediatrics 1971;47:94–6.
21. Tunnessen WW Jr, Hertz CG. Toxic effects of lithium in newborn infants: a commentary. J Pediatr 1972;81:804–7.
22. Piton M, Barthe ML, Laloum D, Davy J, Poilpre E, Venezia R. Acute lithium intoxication. Report of two cases: mother and her newborn. Therapie 1973;28:1123–44.
23. Wilbanks GD, Bressler B, Peete CH Jr, Cherny WB, London WL. Toxic effects of lithium carbonate in a mother and newborn infant. JAMA 1970;213:865–7.
24. Silverman JA, Winters RW, Strande C. Lithium carbonate therapy during pregnancy: apparent lack of effect upon the fetus. Am J Obstet Gynecol 1971;109:934–6.
25. Strothers JK, Wilson DW, Royston N. Lithium toxicity in the newborn. Br Med J 1973;3:233–4.
26. Karlsson K, Lindstedt G, Lundberg PA, Selstam U. Transplacental lithium poisoning: reversible inhibition of fetal thyroid. Lancet 1975;1:1295.
27. Stevens D, Burman D, Midwinter A. Transplacental lithium poisoning. Lancet 1974;2:595.
28. Wilson N, Forfar JC, Godman MJ. Atrial flutter in the newborn resulting from maternal lithium ingestion. Arch Dis Child 1983;58:538–9.
29. Morrell P, Sutherland GR, Buamah PK, Oo M, Bain HH. Lithium toxicity in a neonate. Arch Dis Child 1983;58:539–41.
30. Mallinger AG, Hanin I, Stumpf RL, Mallinger J, Kopp U, Erstling C. Lithium treatment during pregnancy: a case study of erythrocyte choline content and lithium transport. J Clin Psychiatry 1983;44:381–4.
31. Levin RM, Amsterdam JD, Winokur A, Wein AJ. Effects of psychotropic drugs on human sperm motility. Fertil Steril 1981;36:503–6.
32. Schou M, Amdisen A, Steenstrup OR. Lithium and pregnancy. II. Hazards to women given lithium during pregnancy and delivery. Br Med J 1973;2:137–8.
33. Fries H. Lithium in pregnancy. Lancet 1970;1:1233.
34. Schou M, Amdisen A. Lithium and pregnancy. III. Lithium ingestion by children breast-fed by women on lithium treatment. Br Med J 1973;2:138.
35. Committee on Drugs, American Academy of Pediatrics. The transfer of drugs and other chemicals into human breast milk. Pediatrics 1983;72:375–83.

Name: **LOPERAMIDE**

Class: **Antidiarrheal**   Risk Factor: **B$_M$**

Fetal Risk Summary

No reports linking the use of loperamide with congenital defects have been located. Animal studies have not indicated a teratogenic effect (1).

Breast Feeding Summary

Data relating to the excretion of loperamide into breast milk are lacking. One source recommends that the drug should not be used in the lactating mother (2).

References

1. Product information. Imodium. Janssen Pharmaceutica, 1985.
2. Stewart JJ. Gastrointestinal drugs. In Wilson JT, ed. *Drugs in Breast Milk*. Balgowlah, Australia:ADIS Press, 1981:71.

Name: **LORAZEPAM**

Class: **Sedative**   Risk Factor: **C**

Fetal Risk Summary

Lorazepam is a benzodiazepine. No reports linking the use of lorazepam with congenital defects have been located. Other drugs in this group have been suspected of causing fetal malformations (see also Diazepam or Chlordiazepoxide). Lorazepam crosses the placenta, achieving cord levels similar to maternal serum concentrations (1–4). Placental transfer is slower than diazepam, but high intravenous doses may produce the "floppy infant" syndrome (2).

Lorazepam has been used in labor to potentiate the effects of narcotic analgesics (5). Although not statistical significant, a higher incidence of respiratory depression occurred in the exposed newborn infants.

Breast Feeding Summary

Lorazepam is excreted into breast milk in low concentrations (6). No effects on the nursing infant were reported, but the slight delay in establishing feeding was a cause of concern (7). In a subsequent study, 5 mg of oral lorazepam was given 1 hour before labor induction and the effects on feeding behavior were measured in the newborn infants (8). During the first 48 hours, no significant effect was observed on volume of milk consumed or duration of feeding.

References

1. de Groot G, Maes RAA, Defoort P, Thiery M. Placental transfer of lorazepam. IRCS Med Sci 1975;3:290.
2. McBride RJ, Dundee JW, Moore J, Toner W, Howard PJ. A study of the plasma concentrations of lorazepam in mother and neonate. Br J Anaesth 1979;51:971–8.
3. Kanto J, Aaltonen L, Liukko P, Maenpaa K. Transfer of lorazepam and its conjugate across the human placenta. Acta Pharmacol Toxicol (Copenh) 1980;47:130–4.
4. Kanto JH. Use of benzodiazepines during pregnancy, labour and lactation, with particular reference to pharmacokinetic considerations. Drugs 1982;23:354–80.
5. McAuley DM, O'Neill MP, Moore J, Dundee JW. Lorazepam premedication for labour. Br J Obstet Gynaecol 1982;89:149–54.
6. Whitelaw AGL, Cummings AJ, McFadyen IR. Effect of maternal lorazepam on the neonate. Br Med J 1981;282:1106–8.
7. Johnstone M. Effect of maternal lorazepam on the neonate. Br Med J 1981;282:1973.
8. Johnstone MJ. The effect of lorazepam on neonatal feeding behaviour at term. Pharmatherapeutica 1982;3:259–62.

Name: **LOXAPINE**

Class: **Tranquilizer**   Risk Factor: **C**

Fetal Risk Summary

No data available.

Breast Feeding Summary

No data available.

Name: **LYNESTRENOL**

Class: **Progestogenic Hormone**   Risk Factor: **D**

Fetal Risk Summary

The Food and Drug Administration mandated deletion of pregnancy-related indications from all progestins because of a possible association with congenital anomalies. No reports linking the use of lynestrenol with congenital defects have been located (see Hydroxyprogesterone, Norethynodrel, Norethindrone, Medroxyprogesterone, Ethisterone). Ravn (1) observed 16 women who had used lynestrenol for contraception and gave birth to normal infants following cessation of treatment. No conclusions can be made from this report. Use of progestogens during pregnancy is not recommended.

Breast Feeding Summary

See Oral Contraceptives.

References

1. Ravn J. Pregnancy and progeny after long-term contraceptive treatment with low-dose progestogens. Curr Med Res Opin 1975;2:616–9.

Name: **LYPRESSIN**

Class: **Pituitary Hormone, Synthetic**   Risk Factor: **B**

Fetal Risk Summary

Lypressin is a synthetic polypeptide structurally identical to the major active component of vasopressin. See Vasopressin.

Breast Feeding Summary

See Vasopressin.

Name: **MAGNESIUM SULFATE**

Class: **Anticonvulsant/Cathartic**   Risk Factor: **B**

Fetal Risk Summary

Magnesium sulfate ($MgSO_4$) is commonly used as an anticonvulsant for toxemia and as a tocolytic agent for premature labor during the last half of pregnancy. Concentrations of magnesium, a natural constituent of human serum, are readily increased in both the mother and fetus following maternal therapy with cord serum levels ranging from 70 to 100% of maternal concentrations (1–5). Elevated levels in the newborn may persist for up to 7 days with an elimination half-life of 43.2 hours (2). The elimination rate is the same in premature and full-term infants (2).

No reports linking the use of magnesium sulfate with congenital defects have been located. The Collaborative Perinatal Project monitored 50,282 mother-child pairs, 141 of which had exposure to magnesium sulfate during pregnancy (6). No evidence was found to suggest a relationship to congenital malformations.

Most studies have been unable to find a correlation between cord serum magnesium levels and newborn condition (2, 5, 7–11). In a study of 7,000 offspring of mothers treated with $MgSO_4$ for toxemia, no adverse effects from the therapy were noted in fetuses or newborns (5). Other studies have also observed a lack of toxicity (12, 13). A 1983 investigation of women with pregnancy-induced hypertension at term compared newborns of magnesium-treated mothers with newborns of untreated mothers (11). No differences in neurologic behavior were observed between the two groups except that exposed infants had decreased active tone of the neck extensors on the 1st day after birth.

Newborn depression and hypotonia have been reported as an effect of maternal magnesium therapy in some series, but intrauterine hypoxia could not be eliminated as a potential cause or contributing factor (2, 7, 8). A 1971 report described two infants with magnesium levels above 8 mg/100 ml who were severely depressed at birth (9). Spontaneous remission of toxic symptoms occurred after 12 hours in one infant, but the second had residual effects of anoxic encephalopathy. In a 1982 study, activities requiring sustained muscle contraction, such as head lag, ventral suspension, suck reflex, and cry response, were impaired up to 48 hours after birth in infants exposed *in utero* to magnesium (10). A hypertensive woman, treated with 11 g of magnesium sulfate within 3.5 hours of delivery, gave birth to a depressed infant without spontaneous respirations, movement, or reflexes (14). An exchange transfusion at 24 hours reversed the condition. In another study, decreased gastrointestinal motility, ileus, hypotonia, and patent ductus arteriosus occurring in the offspring of mothers with severe hypertension were thought to be due to maternal drug therapy, including magnesium sulfate (15). However, the authors could not relate their findings to any particular drug or drugs and could not completely eliminate the possibility that the effects were due to the severe maternal disease.

A mild decrease in cord calcium concentrations has been reported in mothers treated with magnesium (3, 9, 11). In contrast, a 1970 study reported elevated calcium levels in cord blood following magnesium therapy (4). No newborn symptoms were associated with either change in serum calcium concentrations.

An interaction between *in utero* acquired magnesium and gentamicin has been reported in a newborn 24 hours after birth (16). The mother had received 24 g of MgSO$_4$ during the 32 hours preceding birth of a neurologically depressed female infant. Gentamicin, 2.5 mg/kg intramuscularly every 12 hours, was begun at 12 hours of age for presumed sepsis. The infant developed respiratory arrest following the second dose of gentamicin which resolved after administration of the antibiotic was stopped. Animal experiments confirmed the interaction.

In summary, the administration of magnesium sulfate to the mother for anticonvulsant or tocolytic effects does not usually pose a risk to the fetus or newborn. Neonatal neurologic depression may occur, however, with respiratory depression, muscle weakness, and loss of reflexes. The toxicity is not usually correlated with cord serum magnesium levels. Offspring of mothers treated with this drug close to delivery should be closely observed for signs of toxicity during the first 24–48 hours after birth. Caution is advocated with the use of aminoglycoside antibiotics during this period.

Breast Feeding Summary

Magnesium salts may be encountered by nursing mothers using over-the-counter laxatives. A study in which 50 mothers received an emulsion of magnesium and liquid petrolatum or mineral oil found no evidence of changes or frequency of stools in nursing infants (17). In 10 preeclamptic patients receiving magnesium sulfate, 1 g/hr intravenously during the first 24 hours after delivery, magnesium levels in breast milk were 64 μg/ml as compared to 48 μg/ml in nontreated controls (18). Twenty-four hours after the drug was stopped, milk levels in treated and nontreated patients were 38 and 32 μg/ml, respectively. By 48 hours, the levels were identical in the two groups. Milk:plasma ratios were 1.9 and 2.1 in treated and nontreated patients, respectively. The American Academy of Pediatrics considers magnesium sulfate compatible with breast-feeding (19).

References

1. Chesley LC, Tepper I. Plasma levels of magnesium attained in magnesium sulfate therapy for preeclampsia and eclampsia. Surg Clin N Am 1957;37:353–67.
2. Dangman BC, Rosen TS. Magnesium levels in infants of mothers treated with MgSO$_4$. Pediatr Res 1977;11:415 (Abstr 262).
3. Cruikshank DP, Pitkin RM, Reynolds WA, Williams GA, Hargis GK. Effects of magnesium sulfate treatment on perinatal calcium metabolism. I. Maternal and fetal responses. Am J Obstet Gynecol 1979;134:243–9.
4. Donovan EF, Tsang RC, Steichen JJ, Strub RJ, Chen IW, Chen M. Neonatal hypermagnesemia: effect on parathyroid hormone and calcium homeostasis. J Pediatr 1980;96:305–10.
5. Stone SR, Pritchard JA. Effect of maternally administered magnesium sulfate on the neonate. Obstet Gynecol 1970;35:574–7.
6. Heinonen OP, Slone D, Shapiro S. *Birth Defects and Drugs in Pregnancy*. Littleton:Publishing Sciences Group, 1977:440.
7. Lipsitz PJ, English IC. Hypermagnesemia in the newborn infant. Pediatrics 1967;40:856–62.
8. Lipsitz PJ. The clinical and biochemical effects of excess magnesium in the newborn. Pediatrics 1971;47:501–9.

9. Savory J, Monif GRG. Serum calcium levels in cord sera of the progeny of mothers treated with magnesium sulfate for toxemia of pregnancy. Am J Obstet Gynecol 1971;110:556–9.
10. Rasch DK, Huber PA, Richardson CJ, L'Hommedieu CS, Nelson TE, Reddi R. Neurobehavioral effects of neonatal hypermagnesemia. J Pediatr 1982;100:272–6.
11. Green KW, Key TC, Coen R, Resnik R. The effects of maternally administered magnesium sulfate on the neonate. Am J Obstet Gynecol 1983;146:29–33.
12. Sibai BM, Lipshitz J, Anderson GD, Dilts PV Jr. Reassessment of intravenous MgSO₄ therapy in preeclampsia-eclampsia. Obstet Gynecol 1981;57:199–202.
13. Hutchinson HT, Nichols MM, Kuhn CR, Vasicka A. Effects of magnesium sulfate on uterine contractility, intrauterine fetus, and infant. Am J Obstet Gynecol 1964;88:747–58.
14. Brady JP, Williams HC. Magnesium intoxication in a premature infant. Pediatrics 1967;40:100–3.
15. Brazy JE, Grimm JK, Little VA. Neonatal manifestations of severe maternal hypertension occurring before the thirty-sixth week of pregnancy. J Pediatr 1982;100:265–71.
16. L'Hommedieu CS, Nicholas D, Armes DA, Jones P, Nelson T, Pickering LK. Potentiation of magnesium sulfate-induced neuromuscular weakness by gentamicin, tobramycin, and amikacin. J Pediatr 1983;102:629–31.
17. Baldwin WF. Clinical study of senna administration to nursing mothers: assessment of effects on infant bowel habits. Can Med Assoc J 1963;89:566–8.
18. Cruikshank DP, Varner MW, Pitkin RM. Breast milk magnesium and calcium concentrations following magnesium sulfate treatment. Am J Obstet Gynecol 1982;143:685–8.
19. Committee on Drugs, American Academy of Pediatrics. The transfer of drugs and other chemicals into human breast milk. Pediatrics 1983;72:375–83.

Name: **MANDELIC ACID**

Class: **Urinary Germicide**   Risk Factor: **C**

Fetal Risk Summary

Mandelic acid is available as a single agent and in combination with methenamine (see also Methenamine). The Collaborative Perinatal Project reported 30 1st trimester exposures for this drug (1). For use anytime in pregnancy, 224 exposures were recorded (2). Only in the latter group was a possible association with malformations found. The statistical significance of this association is not known. Independent confirmation is required.

Breast Feeding Summary

Mandelic acid is excreted into breast milk. In six mothers given 12 g/day, milk levels averaged 550 μg/ml (3). The drug was found in the urine of all infants. It was estimated that an infant would receive an average dose of 86 mg/kg/day by this route. The significance of this amount is not known.

References

1. Heinonen OP, Slone D, Shapiro S. *Birth Defects and Drugs in Pregnancy*. Littleton:Publishing Sciences Group, 1977:299, 302.
2. *Ibid*, 435.
3. Berger H. Excretion of mandelic acid in breast milk. Am J Dis Child 1941;61:256–61.

Name: **MANNITOL**

Class: **Diuretic**   Risk Factor: **C**

Fetal Risk Summary

Mannitol is an osmotic diuretic. No reports of its use in pregnancy following intravenous administration have been located. Mannitol, given by intra-amniotic injection, has been used for the induction of abortion (1).

Breast Feeding Summary

No data available.

References

1. Craft IL, Mus BD. Hypertonic solutions to induce abortions. Br Med J 1971;2:49.

Name: **MAPROTILINE**

Class: **Antidepressant**   Risk Factor: **B$_M$**

Fetal Risk Summary

No reports linking the use of maprotiline with congenital defects have been located. Animal studies have failed to demonstrate teratogenicity, carcinogenicity, mutagenicity, or impairment of fertility (1).

Breast Feeding Summary

Maprotiline is excreted into breast milk (2). Milk:plasma ratios of 1.5 and 1.3 have been reported following a 100-mg single dose and 150 mg in divided doses for 120 hours. Multiple dosing resulted in milk concentrations of unchanged maprotiline of 0.2 μg/ml. Although this amount is low, the significance to the nursing infant is not known.

References

1. Product information. Ludiomil. CIBA Pharmaceutical Co, 1985.
2. Reiss W. The relevance of blood level determinations during the evaluation of maprotiline in man. In *Research and Clinical Investigation in Depression*. Northampton, England: Cambridge Medical Publications, 1980:19–38.

Name: **MAZINDOL**

Class: **Central Stimulant/Anorectant**   Risk Factor: **C**

Fetal Risk Summary

No data available.

Breast Feeding Summary

No data available.

Name: **MEBANAZINE**

Class: **Antidepressant**   Risk Factor: **C**

Fetal Risk Summary

No data available (see Phenelzine).

Breast Feeding Summary

No data available (see Phenelzine).

Name: **MECHLORETHAMINE**

Class: **Antineoplastic**   Risk Factor: **D**

Fetal Risk Summary

Mechlorethamine is an alkylating antineoplastic agent. The drug has been used in pregnancy, usually in combination with other antineoplastic drugs. Most reports have not shown an adverse effect in the fetus even when mechlorethamine was given during the 1st trimester (1–4). Two malformed infants have resulted following 1st trimester use of mechlorethamine (5, 6):

> Oligodactyly of both feet with webbing of third and fourth toes, four metatarsals on left, three on right, bowing of right tibia, cerebral hemorrhage (5) (1 case)
> Malformed kidneys—markedly reduced size and malpositioned (6) (1 case)

Data from one review indicated that 40% of the infants exposed to anticancer drugs were of low birth weight (3). Long-term studies of growth and mental development in offspring exposed to mechlorethamine during the 2nd trimester, the period of neuroblast multiplication, have not been conducted (7).

Ovarian function has been evaluated in 27 women previously treated with mechlorethamine and other antineoplastic drugs (8). Excluding three patients who received pelvic radiation, 13 (54%) maintained regular cyclic menses and overall, 13 normal children were born after therapy. Other successful pregnancies have been reported following combination chemotherapy with mechlorethamine (9–14). Ovarian failure is apparently often gradual in onset and is age-related (8). Mechlorethamine therapy in men has been observed to produce testicular germinal cell depletion and azoospermia (13–16).

Breast Feeding Summary

No data available.

References

1. Hennessy JP, Rottino A. Hodgkin's disease in pregnancy with a report of twelve cases. Am J Obstet Gynecol 1952;63:756–64.
2. Riva HL, Andreson PS, O'Grady JW. Pregnancy and Hodgkin's disease: a report of eight cases. Am J Obstet Gynecol 1953;66:866–70.
3. Nicholson HO. Cytotoxic drugs in pregnancy: review of reported cases. J Obstet Gynaecol Br Commonw 1968;75:307–12.

4. Jones RT, Weinerman ER. MOPP (nitrogen mustard, vincristine, procarbazine, and prednisone) given during pregnancy. Obstet Gynecol 1979;54:477–8.
5. Garrett MJ. Teratogenic effects of combination chemotherapy. Ann Intern Med 1974;80:667.
6. Mennuti MT, Shepard TH, Mellman WJ. Fetal renal malformation following treatment of Hodgkin's disease during pregnancy. Obstet Gynecol 1975;46:194–6.
7. Dobbing J. Pregnancy and leukaemia. Lancet 1977;1:1155.
8. Schilsky RL, Sherins RJ, Hubbard SM, Wesley MN, Young RC, DeVita VT Jr. Long-term follow-up of ovarian function in women treated with MOPP chemotherapy for Hodgkin's disease. Am J Med 1981;71:552–6.
9. Ross GT. Congenital anomalies among children born of mothers receiving chemotherapy for gestational trophoblastic neoplasms. Cancer 1976;37:1043–7.
10. Johnson SA, Goldman JM, Hawkins DF. Pregnancy after chemotherapy for Hodgkin's disease. Lancet 1979;2:93.
11. Whitehead E, Shalet SM, Blackledge G, Todd I, Crowther D, Beardwell CG. The effect of combination chemotherapy on ovarian function in women treated for Hodgkin's disease. Cancer 1983;52:988–993.
12. Andrieu JM, Ochoa-Molina ME. Menstrual cycle, pregnancies and offspring before and after MOPP therapy for Hodgkin's disease. Cancer 1983;52:435–8.
13. Dein RA, Mennuti MT, Kovach P, Gabbe SG. The reproductive potential of young men and women with Hodgkin's disease. Obstet Gynecol Surv 1984;39:474–82.
14. Schilsky RL, Lewis BJ, Sherins RJ, Young RC. Gonadal dysfunction in patients receiving chemotherapy for cancer. Ann Intern Med 1980;93:109–14.
15. Sherins RJ, Olweny CLM, Ziegler JL. Gynecomastia and gonadal dysfunction in adolescent boys treated with combination chemotherapy for Hodgkin's disease. N Engl J Med 1978;299:12–6.
16. Sherins RJ, DeVita VT Jr. Effect of drug treatment for lymphoma on male reproductive capacity: studies of men in remission after therapy. Ann Intern Med 1973;79:216–20.

Name: **MECLIZINE**

Class: **Antihistamine/Antiemetic**   Risk Factor: **B$_M$**

Fetal Risk Summary

Meclizine is a piperazine antihistamine which is frequently used as an antiemetic (see also Buclizine and Cyclizine). The drug is teratogenic in animals but apparently not in humans. Since late 1962, the question of the effect of meclizine on the fetus has been argued in numerous citations, the bulk of which are case reports and letters (1–27). Three studies involving large numbers of patients have concluded that meclizine is not a human teratogen (28–32).

The Collaborative Perinatal Project (CPP) monitored 50,282 mother-child pairs, 1,014 of which had exposure to meclizine in the 1st trimester (28). For use anytime during pregnancy, 1,463 exposures were recorded (29). In neither case was evidence found to suggest a relationship to large categories of major or minor malformations. Several possible associations with individual malformations were found, but the statistical significance of these are unknown (28–30). Independent confirmation is required to determine the actual risk.

Respiratory defects (7 cases)
Eye and ear defects (7 cases)
Inguinal hernia (18 cases)
Hypoplasia cordis (3 cases)
Hypoplastic left heart syndrome (3 cases)

The CPP study indicated a possible relationship to ocular malformations, but the authors warned that the results must be interpreted with extreme caution (33). The FDA's OTC Laxative Panel, acting on the data from the CPP study, concluded that meclizine was not teratogenic (34).

A second large prospective study covering 613 1st trimester exposures supported these negative findings (31). No harmful effects were found in the exposed offspring as compared to the total sample.

Finally, in a 1971 report, significantly fewer infants with malformations were exposed to antiemetics in the 1st trimester as compared to controls (32). Meclizine was the third most commonly used antiemetic.

Breast Feeding Summary

No data available.

References

1. Watson GI. Meclozine ("Ancoloxin") and foetal abnormalities. Br Med J 1962;2:1446.
2. Smithells RW. "Ancloxin" and foetal abnormalities. Br Med J 1962;2:1539.
3. Diggorg PLC, Tomkinson JS. Meclozine and foetal abnormalities. Lancet 1962;2:1222.
4. Carter MP, Wilson FW. "Ancoloxin'' and foetal abnormalities. Br Med J 1962;2:1609.
5. Macleod M, Ibid.
6. Lask S, Ibid.
7. Leck IM, Ibid, 1610.
8. McBride WG. Drugs and foetal abnormalities. Br Med J 1962;2:1681.
9. Fagg CG, Ibid.
10. Barwell TE, Ibid.
11. Woodall J. Ibid, 1682.
12. McBride WG. Drugs and congenital abnormalities. Lancet 1962;2:1332.
13. Lenz W. Ibid.
14. David A. Goodspeed AH. "Ancoloxin" and foetal abnormalities. Br Med J 1963;1:121.
15. Gallagher C, Ibid, 121–2.
16. Watson GI, Ibid, 122.
17. Mellin GW, Katzenstein M. Meclozine and foetal abnormalities. Lancet 1963;1:222–3.
18. Salzmann KD. "Ancloxin" and foetal abnormalities. Br Med J 1963;1:471.
19. Burry AF. Meclozine and foetal abnormalities. Br Med J 1963;1:1476.
20. Smithells RW, Chinn ER. Meclozine and feotal abnormalities. Br Med J 1963;1:1678.
21. O'Leary JL, O'Leary JA. Nonthalidomide ectromelia. Report of a case. Obstet Gynecol 1964;23:17–20.
22. Smithells RW, Chinn ER. Meclozine and foetal malformations: a prospective study. Br Med J 1964;1:217–8.
23. Pettersson F. Meclozine and congenital malformations. Lancet 1964;1:675.
24. Yerushalmy J, Milkovich L. Evaluation of the teratogenic effect of meclizine in man. Am J Obstet Gynecol 1965;93:553–62.
25. Sadusk JF Jr, Palmisano PA. Teratogenic effect of meclizine, cyclizine, and chlorcyclizine. JAMA 1965;194:987–9.
26. Lenz W. Malformations caused by drugs in pregnancy. Am J Dis Child 1966;112:99–106.
27. Lenz W. How can the teratogenic action of a factor be established in man? South Med J 1971;64(Suppl 1):41–7.
28. Heinonen OP, Slone D, Shapiro S, Birth Defects and Drugs in Pregnancy. Littleton:Publishing Sciences Group, 1977:328.
29. Ibid, 437.
30. Ibid, 475.
31. Milkovich L, Van den Berg BJ. An evaluation of the teratogenicity of certain antinauseant drugs. Am J Obstet Gynecol 1976;125:244–8.
32. Nelson MM, Forfar JO. Associations between drugs administered during pregnancy and congenital abnormalities of the fetus. Br Med J 1971;1:523–7.

33. Shapiro S, Kaufman DW, Rosenberg L, Slone D, Monson RR, Siskind V, Heinonen OP. Meclizine in pregnancy in relation to congenital malformations. Br Med J 1978;1:483.
34. Anonymous. Pink Sheets. Meclizine, cyclizine not teratogenic. FDC Reports 1974;2.

Name: **MECLOFENAMATE**

Class: **Nonsteroidal Anti-inflammatory** Risk Factor: **B***

Fetal Risk Summary

No reports linking the use of meclofenamate with congenital defects have been located. Theoretically, meclofenamate, a prostaglandin synthetase inhibitor, could cause constriction of the ductus arteriosus *in utero* (1). Persistent pulmonary hypertension of the newborn should also be considered (2). Drugs in this class have been shown to inhibit labor and prolong pregnancy (2). The manufacturer recommends that the drug not be used during pregnancy (3).

[* Risk Factor D if used in the 3rd trimester.]

Breast Feeding Summary

No data available. The manufacturer recommends that the drug not be used when breast-feeding (3).

References

1. Levin DL. Effects of inhibition of prostaglandin synthesis on fetal development, oxygenation, and the fetal circulation. Semin Perinatol 1980;4:35–44.
2. Fuchs F. Prevention of prematurity. Am J Obstet Gynecol 1976;126:809–20.
3. Product information. Meclomen. Parke-Davis, 1985.

Name: **MEDROXYPROGESTERONE**

Class: **Progestogenic Hormone** Risk Factor: **D**

Fetal Risk Summary

The Food and Drug Administration mandated deletion of pregnancy-related indications from all progestins because of a possible association with congenital anomalies. Fourteen cases of ambiguous genitalia of the fetus have been reported to the FDA, although the literature is more supportive of the 19-nortestosterone derivatives (see Norethindrone, Norethynodrel) (1). The Collaborative Perinatal Project monitored 866 mother-child pairs with 1st trimester exposure to progestational agents, including 130 with exposure to medroxyprogesterone (2). An increase in the expected frequency of cardiovascular defects and hypospadias was observed for the progestational agents as a group (3). The cardiovascular defects included a ventricular septal defect and tricuspid atresia (4). Re-evaluation of these data in terms of timing of exposure, vaginal bleeding in early pregnancy, and previous maternal obstetrical history, however, failed to support an association between female sex hormones and cardiac malformations (5). Other studies have also failed to find any relationship with nongenital malformations (6, 7).

A 1985 study described 2,754 infants born to mothers who had vaginal bleeding during the 1st trimester (8). Of the total group, 1,608 of the newborns were delivered from mothers treated during the 1st trimester with either oral medroxy-progesterone (20–30 mg/day), 17-hydroxyprogesterone (500 mg/week by injection), or a combination of the two. Medroxyprogesterone was used exclusively in 1,274 (79.2%) of the study group. The control group consisted of 1,146 infants delivered from mothers who bled during the 1st trimester, but who were not treated. There were no differences between the study and control groups in the overall rate of malformations (120 vs 123.9/1,000, respectively) or in the rate of major malformations (63.4 vs 71.5/1,000, respectively). Another 1985 study compared 988 infants exposed *in utero* to various progesterones to a matched cohort of 1,976 unexposed controls (9). Only 60 infants were exposed to medroxypro-gesterone. No association between progestins, primarily progesterone and 17-hydroxyprogesterone, and fetal malformations was discovered.

Breast Feeding Summary

Medroxyprogesterone has not been shown to adversely affect lactation (10, 11). A 1981 review concluded that use of the drug by the mother would not have a significant effect on the nursing infant (12). Milk production and duration of lactation may be increased if the drug is given in the puerperium. If breast-feeding is desired, medroxyprogesterone may be used safely.

References

1. Dayan E, Rosa FW. Fetal ambiguous genitalia associated with sex hormones use early in pregnancy. Food and Drug Administration, Division of Drug Experience. ADR Highlights 1981:1–14.
2. Heinonen OP, Slone D, Shapiro S. *Birth Defects and Drugs in Pregnancy*. Littleton:Publishing Sciences Group, 1977:389.
3. *Ibid*, 394.
4. Heinonen OP, Slone D, Monson RR, Hook EB, Shapiro S. Cardiovascular birth defects and antenatal exposure to female sex hormones. N Engl J Med 1977;296:67–70.
5. Wiseman RA, Dodds-Smith IC. Cardiovascular birth defects and antenatal exposure to female sex hormones: a reevaluation of some base data. Teratology 1984;30:359–70.
6. Wilson JG, Brent RL. Are female sex hormones teratogenic? Am J Obstet Gynecol 1981;141:567–80.
7. Dahlberg K. Some effects of depo-medroxyprogesterone acetate (DMPA): observations in the nursing infant and in the long-term user. Int J Gynaecol Obstet 1982;20:43–8.
8. Katz Z, Lancet M, Skornik J, Chemke J, Mogilner BM, Klinberg M. Teratogenicity of progestogens given during the first trimester of pregnancy. Obstet Gynecol 1985;65:775–80.
9. Resseguie LJ, Hick JF, Bruen JA, Noller KL, O'Fallon WM, Kurland LT. Congenital malformations among offspring exposed in utero to progestins, Olmsted County, Minnesota, 1936–74. Fertil Steril 1985;43:514–9.
10. Guiloff E, Ibarra-Polo A, Zanartu J, Toscanini C, Mischler TW, Gomez-Rogers C. Effect of contraception on lactation. Am J Obstet Gynecol 1974;118:42–5.
11. Karim M, Ammar R, El Mahgoub S, El Ganzoury B, Fikri F, Abdou Z. Injected progesterone and lactation. Br Med J 1971;1:200–3.
12. Schwallie PC. The effect of depot-medroxyprogesterone acetate on the fetus and nursing infant: a review. Contraception 1981;23:375–86.

Name: **MELPHALAN**

Class: **Antineoplastic**   Risk Factor: **D$_M$**

Fetal Risk Summary

No reports linking the use of melphalan with congenital defects have been located. Melphalan is mutagenic as well as carcinogenic (1–8). These effects have not been described in infants following *in utero* exposure. Data from one review indicated that 40% of the infants exposed to anticancer drugs were of low birth weight (9). Long-term studies of growth and mental development in offspring exposed to melphalan and other antineoplastic drugs during the 2nd trimester, the period of neuroblast multiplication, have not been conducted (10).

Melphalan has caused suppression of ovarian function resulting in amenorrhea (10–13). These effects should be considered prior to administering the drug to patients in their reproductive years. Although there are no supportive data to suggest a teratogenic effect, melphalan is structurally similar to other alkylating agents which have produced defects (see Chlorambucil, Mechlorethamine, Cyclophosphamide).

Breast Feeding Summary

No data available.

References

1. Sharpe HB. Observations on the effect of therapy with nitrogen mustard or a derivative on chromosomes of human peripheral blood lymphocytes. Cell Tissue Kinet 1971;4:501–4.
2. Kyle RA, Pierre RV, Bayrd ED. Multiple myeloma and acute myelomonocytic leukemia. N Engl J Med 1970;283:1121–5.
3. Kyle RA. Primary amyloidosis in acute leukemia associated with melphalan. Blood 1974;44:333–7.
4. Burton IE, Abbott CR, Roberts BE, Antonis AH. Acute leukemia after four years of melphalan treatment for melanoma. Br Med J 1976;1:20.
5. Peterson HS. Erythroleukemia in a melphalan treated patient with primary macroglobulinaemia. Scand J Haematol 1973;10:5–11.
6. Stavem P, Harboe M. Acute erythroleukaemia in a patient treated with melphalan for the cold agglutinin syndrome. Scand J Haematol 1971;8:375–9.
7. Einhorn N. Acute leukemia after chemotherapy (melphalan). Cancer 1978;41:444–7.
8. Reimer RR, Hover R, Fraumen JF, Young RC. Acute leukemia after alkylating agent therapy of ovarian cancer. N Engl J Med 1977;297:177–81.
9. Nicholson HO. Cytotoxic drugs in pregnancy: review of reported cases. J Obstet Gynaecol Br Commonw 1968;75:307–12.
10. Dobbing J. Pregnancy and leukaemia. Lancet 1977;1:11–15.
11. Rose DP, David PE. Ovarian function in patients receiving adjuvant chemotherapy for breast cancer. Lancet 1977;1:1174–6.
12. Ahmann DL. Repeated adjuvant chemotherapy with phenylalanine mustard or 5-fluorouracil, cyclophosphamide and prednisone with or without radiation. Lancet 1978;1:893–6.
13. Schilsky RL, Lewis BJ, Sherins RJ, Young RC. Gonadal dysfunction in patients receiving chemotherapy for cancer. Ann Intern Med 1980;93:109–14.

Name: **MENADIONE**

Class: **Vitamin**   Risk Factor: **C***

Fetal Risk Summary

Menadione (vitamin K_3) is a synthetic, fat-soluble form of vitamin K used to prevent hypoprothrombinemia due to vitamin K deficiency (1). The water-soluble derivative of menadione, menadiol sodium phosphate, also known as vitamin K_3, is available for parenteral use.

Vitamin K_1 occurs naturally in a variety of foods and is synthesized by the normal intestinal flora (see Phytonadione) (1). Administration of vitamin K during pregnancy is usually not required unless the mother develops hypoprothrombinemia or is taking certain drugs that may produce severe vitamin K deficiency in the fetus, resulting in hemorrhagic disease of the newborn (e.g., anticonvulsants, warfarin, rifampin, isoniazid). Early attempts to prevent maternal-induced hemorrhagic disease of the newborn by administering vitamin K_3 to the mother shortly before delivery often resulted in marked hyperbilirubinemia and kernicterus in the newborn, especially in premature infants (2–5). Several large reviews have described the relationship between vitamin K and bilirubin and have discussed the toxicity of the vitamin K analogues (2–5). Because menadione and menadiol may produce newborn toxicity, phytonadione is considered the drug of choice for administration during pregnancy or to the newborn (6, 7).

[* Risk Factor X if used in 3rd trimester or close to delivery.]

Breast Feeding Summary

See Phytonadione.

References

1. American Hospital Formulary Service. *Drug Information 1985*. Bethesda:American Society of Hospital Pharmacists, 1985:1707–8.
2. Lane PA, Hathaway WE. Vitamin K in infancy. J Pediatr 1985;106:351–9.
3. Payne NR, Hasegawa DK. Vitamin K deficiency in newborns: a case report in α-1-antitrypsin deficiency and a review of factors predisposing to hemorrhage. Pediatrics 1984;73:712–6.
4. Wynn RM. The obstetric significance of factors affecting the metabolism of bilirubin, with particular reference to the role of vitamin K. Obstet Gynecol Surv 1963;18:333–54.
5. Finkel MJ. Vitamin K_1 and the vitamin K analogues. J Clin Pharmacol Ther 1961;2:795–814.
6. Committee on Nutrition, American Academy of Pediatrics. Vitamin K compounds and the water-soluble analogues. Pediatrics 1961;28:501–7.
7. Committee on Nutrition, American Academy of Pediatrics. Vitamin and mineral supplement needs in normal children in the United States. Pediatrics 1980;66:1015–21.

Name: **MEPENZOLATE**

Class: **Parasympatholytic (Anticholinergic)**   Risk Factor: **C**

Fetal Risk Summary

Mepenzolate is an anticholinergic quaternary ammonium bromide. In a large prospective study, 2,323 patients were exposed to this class of drugs during the

1st trimester, 1 of whom took mepenzolate (1). A possible association was found between the total group and minor malformations.

Breast Feeding Summary

No data available (see also Atropine).

References

1. Heinonen OP, Slone D, Shapiro S. *Birth Defects and Drugs in Pregnancy*. Littleton:Publishing Sciences Group, 1977:346–53.

Name: **MEPERIDINE**

Class: **Narcotic Analgesic**   Risk Factor: **B***

Fetal Risk Summary

Fetal problems have not been reported from the therapeutic use of meperidine in pregnancy except when it has been given during labor. Like all narcotics, maternal and neonatal addiction are possible from inappropriate use. Neonatal depression, at times fatal, has historically been the primary concern following obstetrical meperidine analgesia. Controversy has now risen over the potential long-term adverse effects resulting from this use.

The placental transfer of meperidine is very rapid, appearing in cord blood within 2 minutes following intravenous administration (1). It is detectable in amniotic fluid 30 minutes after intramuscular injection (2). Cord blood concentrations average 70–77% (range 45–106%) of maternal plasma levels (3, 4). The drug has been detected in the saliva of newborns for 48 hours following maternal administration during labor (5). Concentrations in pharyngeal aspirates were higher than either arterial or venous cord blood.

Respiratory depression in the newborn following use of the drug in labor is time- and dose-dependent. The incidence of depression increases markedly if delivery occurs 60 minutes or longer after injection, reaching a peak around 2–3 hours (6, 7). Whether this depression is due to metabolites of meperidine (e.g., normeperidine) or the drug itself is currently not known (2, 8–10). However, recent work by Belfrage and co-workers (7) suggests that these effects are related to unmetabolized meperidine and not to normeperidine.

Impaired behavioral response and electroencephalogram changes persisting for several days have been observed (11, 12). These persistent effects may be partially explained by the slow elimination of meperidine and normeperidine from the neonate over several days (13, 14). Belsey and co-workers (15) related depressed attention and social responsiveness during the first 6 weeks of life to high cord blood levels of meperidine. An earlier study reported long-term follow-up of 70 healthy neonates born to mothers who had received meperidine within 2 hours of birth (16, 17). Psychological and physical parameters at age 5 years were similar in both exposed and control groups. Academic progress and behavior during the 3rd and 4th year in school were also similar.

The Collaborative Perinatal Project monitored 50,282 mother-child pairs, 268 of which had 1st trimester exposure to meperidine (18). For use anytime during pregnancy, 1,100 exposures were recorded (19). No evidence was found to suggest a relationship to large categories of major or minor malformations. A possible association between the use of meperidine in the 1st trimester and inguinal hernia was found based on six cases (20). The statistical significance of this association is unknown, and independent confirmation is required.

[* Risk Factor D if used for prolonged periods or in high doses at term.]

Breast Feeding Summary

Meperidine is excreted into breast milk (21, 22). In a group of mothers who had received meperidine during labor, the breast-fed infants had higher saliva levels of the drug for up to 48 hours after birth than a similar group that was bottle-fed (5). In nine nursing mothers, a single 50-mg intramuscular dose produced peak levels of 0.13 µg/ml at 2 hours (22). After 24 hours, the concentrations decreased to 0.02 µg/ml. Average milk:plasma ratios for the nine patients were greater than 1.0. No adverse effects in nursing infants were reported in any of the above studies. The American Academy of Pediatrics considers meperidine compatible with breast-feeding (23).

References

1. Crawford JS, Rudofsky S. The placental transmission of pethidine. Br J Anaesth 1965;37:929–33.
2. Szeto HH, Zervoudakis IA, Cederquist LL, Inturrise CE. Amniotic fluid transfer of meperidine from maternal plasma in early pregnancy. Obstet Gynecol 1978;52:59–62.
3. Apgar V, Burns JJ, Brodie BB, Papper EM. The transmission of meperidine across the human placenta. Am J Obstet Gynecol 1952;64:1368–70.
4. Shnider SM, Way EL, Lord MJ. Rate of appearance and disappearance of meperidine in fetal blood after administration of narcotic to the mother. Anesthesiology 1966;27:227–8.
5. Freeborn SF, Calvert RT, Black P, MacFarlane T, D'Souza SW. Saliva and blood pethidine concentrations in the mother and the newborn baby. Br J Obstet Gynaecol 1980;87:966–9.
6. Morrison JC, Wiser WL, Rosser SI, et al. Metabolites of meperidine related to fetal depression. Am J Obstet Gynecol 1973;115:1132–7.
7. Belfrage P, Boreus LO, Hartvig P, Irestedt L, Raabe N. Neonatal depression after obstetrical analgesia with pethidine. The role of the injection-delivery time interval and the plasma concentrations of pethidine and norpethidine. Acta Obstet Gynecol Scand 1981;60:43–9.
8. Morrison JC, Whybrew WD, Rosser SI, Bucovaz ET, Wiser WL, Fish SA. Metabolites of meperidine in the fetal and maternal serum. Am J Obstet Gynecol 1976;126:97–1002.
9. Clark RB, Lattin DL. Metabolites of meperidine in serum. Am J Obstet Gynecol 1978;130:113–5.
10. Morrison JC. Reply to Drs. Clark and Lattin. Am J Obstet Gynecol 1978;130:115–7.
11. Borgstedt AD, Rosen MG. Medication during labor correlated with behavior and EEG of the newborn. Am J Dis Child 1968;115:21–4.
12. Hodgkinson R, Bhatt M, Wang CN. Double-blind comparison of the neurobehaviour of neonates following the administration of different doses of meperidine to the mother. Can Anaesth Soc J 1978;25:405–11.
13. Cooper LV, Stephen GW, Aggett PJA. Elimination of pethidine and bupivacaine in the newborn. Arch Dis Child 1977;52:638–41.
14. Kuhnert BR, Kuhnert PM, Prochaska AL, Sokol RJ. Meperidine disposition in mother, neonate and nonpregnant females. Clin Pharmacol Ther 1980;27:486–91.
15. Belsey EM, Rosenblatt DB, Lieberman BA, et al. The influence of maternal analgesia on neonatal behaviour. I. Pethidine. Br J Obstet Gynaecol 1981;88:398–406.
16. Buck C, Gregg R, Stavraky K, Subrahmaniam K, Brown J. The effect of single prenatal and natal complications upon the development of children of mature birthweight. Pediatrics 1969;43:942–55.

17. Buck C. Drugs in pregnancy. Can Med Assoc J 1975;112:1285.
18. Heinonen O, Slone D, Shapiro S. *Birth Defects and Drugs in Pregnancy*. Littleton:Publishing Sciences Group, 1977:287–95.
19. *Ibid*, 434.
20. *Ibid*, 471.
21. Vorherr H. Drug excretion in breast milk. Postgrad Med 1974;56:97–104.
22. Peiker G, Muller B, Ihn W, Noschel H. Excretion of pethidine in mother's milk. Zentralbl Gynaekol 1980;102:537–41.
23. Committee on Drugs, American Academy of Pediatrics. The transfer of drugs and other chemicals into human breast milk. Pediatrics 1983;72:375–83.

Name: **MEPHENTERMINE**

Class: **Sympathomimetic (Adrenergic)**   Risk Factor: **C**

Fetal Risk Summary

Mephentermine is a sympathomimetic used in emergency situations to treat hypotension. Because of the nature of its indication, experience in pregnancy with mephentermine is limited. The primary action of mephentermine is to increase cardiac output due to enhanced cardiac contraction and, to a lesser extent, from peripheral vasoconstriction (1). Its effect on uterine blood flow should be minimal (1).

Breast Feeding Summary

No data available.

References

1. Smith NT, Corbascio AN. The use and misuse of pressor agents. Anesthesiology 1970;33:58–101.

Name: **MEPHENYTOIN**

Class: **Anticonvulsant**   Risk Factor: **C**

Fetal Risk Summary

Mephenytoin is a hydantoin anticonvulsant similar to phenytoin (see Phenytoin). The drug is infrequently prescribed because of the greater incidence of serious side effects as compared with phenytoin (1). There have been reports of 12 infants with 1st trimester exposure to mephenytoin (2–5). No evidence of adverse fetal effects were found.

Breast Feeding Summary

No data available.

References

1. Rall TW, Shleifer LS. Drugs effective in the treatment of the epilepsies. In Goodman AG, Goodman LS, Gilman A, eds. *The Pharmacological Basis of Therapeutics*, ed 6. New York:Macmillan Publishing Co, 1980:456.

2. Fedrick J. Epilepsy and pregnancy: a report from the Oxford Linkage Study. Br Med J 1973;2:442–8.
3. Heinonen O, Slone D, Shapiro S. *Birth Defects and Drugs in Pregnancy*. Littleton:Publishing Sciences Group, 1977:358–9.
4. Annegers JF, Elveback LR, Hauser WA, Kurland LT. Do anticonvulsants have a teratogenic effect? Arch Neurol 1974;31:364–73.
5. Speidel BD, Meadow SR. Maternal epilepsy and abnormalities of the fetus and newborn. Lancet 1972;2:839–43.

Name: **MEPHOBARBITAL**

Class: **Anticonvulsant/Sedative**   Risk Factor: **D**

Fetal Risk Summary

No reports linking the use of mephobarbital with congenital defects have been located. The drug is demethylated by the liver to phenobarbital (see Phenobarbital). The Collaborative Perinatal Project monitored 50,282 mother-child pairs, 8 of which had 1st trimester exposure to mephobarbital (1). No evidence was found to suggest a relationship to large categories of major or minor malformations or to individual defects. Hemorrhagic disease and barbiturate withdrawal in the newborn are theoretically possible, although this has not been reported with mephobarbital.

Breast Feeding Summary

See Phenobarbital.

References

1. Heinonen O, Slone D, Shapiro S. *Birth Defects and Drugs in Pregnancy*. Littleton:Publishing Sciences Group, 1977:336.

Name: **MEPINDOLOL**

Class: **Sympatholytic (β-Adrenergic Blocker)**   Risk Factor: **C**

Fetal Risk Summary

Mepindolol is a nonselective β-adrenergic blocking agent. No reports of its use in pregnancy have been located. The use near delivery of some agents in this class has resulted in persistent β-blockade in the newborn (see Acebutolol, Atenolol, and Nadolol). Thus, newborns exposed *in utero* to mepindolol should be closely observed during the first 24–48 hours after birth for bradycardia and other symptoms. The long-term effects of *in utero* exposure to β-blockers have not been studied but warrant evaluation.

Breast Feeding Summary

Mepindolol is excreted into breast milk (1). Following a 20-mg dose, mean milk concentrations in five mothers at 2 and 6 hours were 18 and 16 ng/ml, respectively, with a milk:plasma ratio at 2 hours of 0.35. Continuous dosing of 20 mg daily for

5 days produced milk levels at 2 and 6 hours of 22 and 33 ng/ml. The milk:plasma ratio at 6 hours was 0.61. At a detection limit of 1 ng/ml, mepindolol could only be found in the serum of one of the five breast-fed infants. Although no adverse effects were observed, nursing infants should be closely watched for bradycardia and other signs and symptoms of β-blockade. Long-term effects of exposure to β-blockers from milk have not been studied but warrant evaluation.

References

1. Krause W, Stoppelli I, Milia S, Rainer E. Transfer of mepindolol to newborns by breast-feeding mothers after single and repeated daily doses. Eur J Clin Pharmacol 1982;22:53–5.

Name: **MEPROBAMATE**

Class: **Sedative**   Risk Factor: **D**

Fetal Risk Summary

Meprobamate use in pregnancy has been associated with an increased risk of congenital anomalies (1.9–12.1%) (1, 2). In 395 patients, Milkovich and van den Berg (1) observed eight defects:

Congenital heart disease (2 with multiple other defects) (5 cases)
Down's syndrome (1 case)
Deafness (partial) (1 case)
Deformed elbows and joints (1 case)

One other report described congenital heart defects in a newborn exposed to meprobamate (3). The mother of this patient was treated very early in the 1st trimester with meprobamate and propoxyphene:

Omphalocele, defective anterior abdominal wall, defect in diaphragm, congenital heart disease with partial ectopic cordis secondary to sternal cleft, dysplastic hips

Multiple defects of the eye and central nervous system were observed in a newborn exposed to multiple drugs, including meprobamate and LSD (4).

The Collaborative Perinatal Project monitored 50,282 mother-child pairs, 356 of which were exposed in the 1st trimester to meprobamate (5, 6). No association of meprobamate with large classes of malformations or to individual defects was found. Others have also failed to find a relationship between the use of meprobamate and congenital malformations (7).

Since few indications exist for this drug in the pregnant woman, it should be used with extreme caution, if at all, during pregnancy. Use during the first 6 weeks of pregnancy may be correlated with an increased risk for fetal malformations.

Breast Feeding Summary

Meprobamate is excreted into breast milk (8). Milk concentrations are 2–4 times that of maternal plasma (8, 9). The effect on the nursing infant is not known. The American Academy of Pediatrics considers meprobamate compatible with breast-feeding (10).

References

1. Milkovich L, van den Berg BJ. Effects of prenatal meprobamate and chlordiazepoxide hydrochloride on human embryonic and fetal development. N Engl J Med 1974;291:1268-71.
2. Crombie DL, Pinsent RJ, Fleming DM, Rumeau-Rouguette C, Goujard J, Huel G. Fetal effects of tranquilizers in pregnancy. N Engl J Med 1975;293:198-9.
3, Ringrose CAD. The hazard of neurotropic drugs in the fertile years. Can Med Assoc J 1972;106:1058.
4. Bogdanoff B, Rorke LB, Yanoff M, Warren WS. Brain and eye abnormalities: possible sequelae to prenatal use of multiple drugs including LSD. Am J Dis Child 1972;123:145-8.
5. Heinonen OP, Slone D, Shapiro S. *Birth Defects and Drugs in Pregnancy*. Littleton:Publishing Sciences Group, 1977:336-7.
6. Hartz SC, Heinonen OP, Shapiro S, Siskind V, Slone D. Antenatal exposure to meprobamate and chlordiazepoxide in relation to malformations, mental development, and childhood mortality. N Engl J Med 1975;292:726-8.
7. Belafsky HA, Breslow S, Hirsch LM, Shangold JE, Stahl MB. Meprobamate during pregnancy. Obstet Gynecol 1969;34:378-86.
8. Product information. Miltown. Wallace Laboratories, 1985.
9. Wilson JT, Brown RD, Cherek DR, Dailey JW, Hilman B, Jobe PC, Manno BR, Manno JE, Redetzki HM, Stewart JJ. Drug excretion in human breast milk: principles, pharmacokinetics and projected consequences. Clin Pharmacokinet 1980;5:1-66.
10. Committee on Drugs, American Academy of Pediatrics. The transfer of drugs and other chemicals into human breast milk. Pediatrics 1983;72:375-83.

Name: **MERCAPTOPURINE**

Class: **Antineoplastic**   Risk Factor: **D**

Fetal Risk Summary

Mercaptopurine is an antimetabolite antineoplastic agent. Experience with mercaptopurine in pregnancy has been reviewed by Moloney in 1964 (1), Nicholson in 1968 (2), and Gililland and Weinstein in 1983 (3). A total of 62 exposed pregnancies have been described, including 29 in the 1st trimester (1–10). Excluding those pregnancies that ended in abortion or stillbirths, abnormalities or toxicity were found in six infants:

Pancytopenia (infant exposed to six antineoplastic agents in 3rd trimester) (6)
Microangiopathic hemolytic anemia (9)
Cleft palate, microphthalmia, hypoplasia of the ovaries and thyroid gland, corneal opacity, cytomegaly and intrauterine growth retardation (also exposed to busulfan and radiation) (10).
Pulmonary atelectasis (3) (2 cases)
Cushingoid appearance (3)

Data from one review indicated that 40% of the infants exposed to anticancer drugs were of low birth weight (2). This finding was not related to the timing of exposure. In addition, long-term studies of growth and mental development in infants exposed to mercaptopurine during the 2nd trimester, the period of neuroblast multiplication, have not been conducted (11).

Severe oligospermia has been described in a 22-year-old man receiving sequential chemotherapy of cyclophosphamide, methotrexate, and mercaptopurine for leukemia (12). After treatment was stopped, the sperm count returned to normal, and the patient fathered a healthy female child. Others have also observed reversible testicular dysfunction (13). Ovarian function in females exposed to mercaptopurine does not seem to be adversely affected (14–18). However, long-term analysis of human reproduction following mercaptopurine therapy has not been reported (19).

Breast Feeding Summary

No data available.

References

1. Moloney WC. Management of leukemia in pregnancy. Ann NY Acad Sci 1964;114:857–67.
2. Nicholson HO. Cytotoxic drugs in pregnancy: review of reported cases. J Obstet Gynaecol Br Commonw 1968;75:307–12.
3. Gililland J, Weinstein L. The effects of cancer chemotherapeutic agents on the developing fetus. Obstet Gynecol Survey 1983;38:6–13.
4. Wegelius R. Successful pregnancy in acute leukaemia. Lancet 1975;2:1301.
5. Nicholson HO. Leukaemia and pregnancy: a report of five cases and discussion of management. J Obstet Gynaecol Br Commonw 1968;75:517–20.
6. Pizzuto J, Aviles A, Noriega L, Niz J, Morales M, Romero F. Treatment of acute leukemia during pregnancy: presentation of nine cases. Cancer Treat Rep 1980;64:679–83.
7. Burnier AM. Discussion. In Plows CW. Acute myelomonocytic leukemia in pregnancy: report of a case. Am J Obstet Gynecol 1982;143:41–3.
8. Dara P, Slater LM, Armentrout SA. Successful pregnancy during chemotherapy for acute leukemia. Cancer 1981;47:845–6.
9. McConnell JF, Bhoola R. A neonatal complication of maternal leukemia treated with 6-mercapto-purine. Postgrad Med J 1973;49:211–3.
10. Diamond J, Anderson MM, McCreadie SR. Transplacental transmission of busulfan (Myleran) in a mother with leukemia: production of fetal malformation and cytomegaly. Pediatrics 1960;25:85–90.
11. Dobbing J. Pregnancy and leukaemia. Lancet 1977;1:1155.
12. Hinkes E, Plotkin D. Reversible drug-induced sterility in a patient with acute leukemia. JAMA 1973;223:1490–1.
13. Lendon M, Palmer MK, Hann IM, Shalet SM, Jones PHM. Testicular histology after combination chemotherapy in childhood for acute lymphoblastic leukaemia. Lancet 1978;2:439–41.
14. Schilsky RL, Lewis BJ, Sherins RJ, Young RC. Gonadal dysfunction in patients receiving chemo-therapy for cancer. Ann Intern Med 1980;93:109–14.
15. Gasser C. Long-term survival (cures) in childhood acute leukemia. Paediatrician 1980;9:344–57.
16. Bacon C, Kernahan J. Successful pregnancy in acute leukaemia. Lancet 1975;2:515.
17. Walden PAM, Bagshawe KD. Pregnancies after chemotherapy for gestational trophoblastic tu-mours. Lancet 1979;2:1241.
18. Sanz MH, Rafecas FJ. Successful pregnancy during chemotherapy for acute promyelocytic leuke-mia. N Engl J Med 1982;306:939.
19. Steckman ML. Treatment of Crohn's disease with 6-mercaptopurine: what effects on fertility? N Engl J Med 1980;303:817.

Name: **MESORIDAZINE**

Class: **Tranquilizer**   Risk Factor: **C**

Fetal Risk Summary

Mesoridazine is a piperidyl phenothiazine. Phenothiazines readily cross the placenta (1). No specific information on its use in pregnancy has been located. Although occasional reports have attempted to link various phenothiazine compounds with congenital malformations, the bulk of the evidence indicates that these drugs are safe for the mother and fetus (see Chlorpromazine).

Breast Feeding Summary

No reports describing the excretion of mesoridazine into breast milk have been located. The American Academy of Pediatrics considers the drug compatible with breast-feeding (2).

References

1. Moya F, Thorndike V. Passage of drugs across the placenta. Am J Obstet Gynecol 1962;84:1778–98.
2. Committee on Drugs, American Academy of Pediatrics. The transfer of drugs and other chemicals into human breast milk. Pediatrics 1983;72:375–83.

Name: **MESTRANOL**

Class: **Estrogenic Hormone**   Risk Factor: **X**

Fetal Risk Summary

Mestranol is the 3-methyl ester of ethinyl estradiol. Mestranol is used frequently in combination with progestins for oral contraception (see Oral Contraceptives). Congenital malformations attributed to the use of mestranol alone have not been reported. The Collaborative Perinatal Project monitored 614 mother-child pairs with 1st trimester exposure to estrogenic agents, including 179 with exposure to mestranol (1). An increase in the expected frequency of cardiovascular defects, eye and ear anomalies, and Down's syndrome was found for estrogens as a group but not for mestranol (1, 2). Re-evaluation of these data in terms of timing of exposure, vaginal bleeding in early pregnancy, and previous maternal obstetrical history, however, failed to support an association between estrogens and cardiac malformations (3). An earlier study also failed to find any relationship with nongenital malformations (4). The use of estrogenic hormones during pregnancy is contraindicated.

Breast Feeding Summary

Estrogens are frequently used for suppression of postpartum lactation (5). Doses of 100–150 μg of ethinyl estradiol (equivalent to 160–240 μg of mestranol) for 5–7 days are used (5). Mestranol, when used in oral contraceptives with doses of 30–80 μg, has been associated with decreased milk production, lower infant weight gain, and decreased composition of nitrogen and protein content of human milk (6–8). The magnitude of these changes is low. However, the changes in milk production and composition may be of nutritional importance in malnourished mothers. If breast-feeding is desired, the lowest dose of oral contraceptives should be chosen. Monitoring of infant weight gain and the possible need for nutritional supplementation should be considered (see Oral Contraceptives).

References

1. Heinonen OP, Slone D, Shapiro S. *Birth Defects and Drugs in Pregnancy*. Littleton:Publishing Sciences Group, 1977:389, 391.
2. *Ibid*, 395.

3. Wiseman RA, Dodds-Smith IC. Cardiovascular birth defects and antenatal exposure to female sex hormones: a reevaluation of some base data. Teratology 1984;30:359–70.
4. Wilson JG, Brent RL. Are female sex hormones teratogenic? Am J Obstet Gynecol 1981;141:567–80.
5. Gilman AG, Goodman LS, Gilman A, eds. *The Pharmacological Basis of Therapeutics*, ed 6. New York:Macmillan Publishing Co, 1980:1431.
6. Kora SJ. Effect of oral contraceptives on lactation. Fertil Steril 1969;20:419–23.
7. Miller GH, Hughs LR. Lactation and genital involution effects of a new low-dose oral contraceptive on breast-feeding mothers and their infants. Obstet Gynecol 1970;35:44–50.
8. Lonnerdal B, Forsum E, Hambraeus L. Effect of oral contraceptives on composition and volume of breast milk. Am J Clin Nutr 1980;33:816–24.

Name: **METAPROTERENOL**

Class: **Sympathomimetic (Adrenergic)**   Risk Factor: C_M

Fetal Risk Summary

No reports linking the use of metaproterenol with congenital defects have been located. Metaproterenol, a β-sympathomimetic, has been used to prevent premature labor (1–3). Its use for this purpose has been largely assumed by ritodrine, albuterol, or terbutaline. Like all β-mimetics, metaproterenol causes maternal, and to a lesser degree, fetal tachycardia. Maternal hypotension, hyperglycemia, and neonatal hypoglycemia should be expected (see also Ritodrine, Albuterol, or Terbutaline). Long-term evaluation of infants exposed to *in utero* β-mimetics has been reported but not specifically for metaproterenol (4). No harmful effects in the infants were observed.

Breast Feeding Summary

No data available.

References

1. Baillie P, Meehan FP, Tyack AJ. Treatment of premature labour with orciprenaline. Br Med J 1970;4:154–5.
2. Tyack AJ, Baillier P, Meehan FP. In-vivo response of the human uterus to orciprenaline in early labour. Br Med J 1971;2:741–3.
3. Zilianti M, Aller J. Action of orciprenaline on uterine contractility during labor, maternal cardiovascular system, fetal heart rate, and acid-base balance. Am J Obstet Gynecol 1971;109:1073–9.
4. Freysz H, Willard D, Lehr A, Messer J, Boog G. A long term evaluation of infants who received a beta-mimetic drug while in utero. J Perinat Med 1977;5:94–9.

Name: **METARAMINOL**

Class: **Sympathomimetic (Adrenergic)**   Risk Factor: **D**

Fetal Risk Summary

Metaraminol is a sympathomimetic used in emergency situations to treat hypotension. Because of the nature of its indications, experience in pregnancy with metaraminol is limited. Uterine vessels are normally maximally dilated, and they have only α-adrenergic receptors (1). Use of the predominantly α-adrenergic stimulant, metaraminol, could cause constriction of these vessels and reduce uterine blood flow, thereby producing fetal hypoxia (bradycardia). Metaraminol may also interact with oxytocics or ergot derivatives to produce severe persistent maternal hypertension (1). Rupture of a cerebral vessel is possible. If a pressor agent is indicated, other drugs such as ephedrine should be considered.

Breast Feeding Summary

No data available.

References

1. Smith NT, Corbascio AN. The use and misuse of pressor agents. Anesthesiology 1970;33:58–101.

Name: **METHACYCLINE**

Class: **Antibiotic**   Risk Factor: **D**

Fetal Risk Summary

See Tetracycline.

Breast Feeding Summary

See Tetracycline.

Name: **METHADONE**

Class: **Narcotic Analgesic**   Risk Factor: **B***

Fetal Risk Summary

Methadone use in pregnancy is almost exclusively related to the treatment of heroin addiction. No increase in congenital defects has been observed. However, since these patients normally consume a wide variety of drugs, it is not possible to completely separate the effects of methadone from the effects of other agents. Neonatal narcotic withdrawal and low birth weight seem to be the primary problems.

Withdrawal symptoms occur in approximately 60–90% of the infants (1–6). One study concluded that the intensity of withdrawal was increased if the daily maternal dosage exceeded 20 mg (5). When withdrawal symptoms do occur, they normally start within 48 hours after delivery, but a small percentage may be delayed up to 7–14 days (1). One report observed initial withdrawal symptoms appearing up to 28 days after birth, but the authors do not mention if mothers of these infants were breast-feeding (6). Methadone concentrations in breast milk are reported to be sufficient to prevent withdrawal in addicted infants (See Breast Feeding Summary below). Some authors believe methadone withdrawal is more intense than that occurring with heroin (1). Less than one third of symptomatic infants require therapy (1–5). A lower incidence of hyaline membrane disease is seen in infants exposed *in utero* to chronic methadone and may be due to elevated blood levels of prolactin (7).

Infants of drug-addicted mothers are often small for gestational age. In some series, one third or more of the infants weigh less than 2,500 g (1, 2, 4). The newborn of methadone addicts may have a higher birth weight than comparable offspring of heroin addicts for reasons that remain unclear (4).

Other problems occurring in the offspring of methadone addicts are increased mortality, sudden infant death syndrome (SIDS), jaundice, and thrombocytosis. A correlation between drug addiction and SIDS has been suggested with 20 cases (2.8%) in a group of 702 infants, but the data could not attribute the increase to a single drug (8, 9). Another study of 313 infants of methadone-addicted mothers reported 2 cases (0.6%) of SIDS, an incidence similar to the overall experience of that location (4). In one study, a positive correlation was found between severity of neonatal withdrawal and the incidence of SIDS (9). Maternal withdrawal during pregnancy has been observed to produce a marked response of the fetal adrenal glands and sympathetic nervous system (10). An increased stillborn and neonatal mortality rate has also been reported (11). Both reports recommend against detoxification of the mother during gestation. Jaundice is comparatively infrequent in both heroin- and methadone-exposed newborns. However, a higher rate of severe hyperbilirubinemia in methadone-exposed infants than in a comparable group of heroin-exposed infants has been observed (1). Thrombocytosis developing in the 2nd week of life, with some platelet counts exceeding $1,000,000/mm^3$ and persisting for over 16 weeks, has been reported (12). The condition was not related to withdrawal symptoms or neonatal treatment. Some of these infants also had increased circulating platelet aggregates.

Respiratory depression is not a significant problem, as Apgar scores are comparable to those of a nonaddicted population (1–5). Long-term effects on the behavior and gross motor development skills are not known.

[* Risk Factor D if used for prolonged periods or in high doses at term.]

Breast Feeding Summary

Methadone enters breast milk in concentrations approaching plasma levels and may prevent withdrawal symptoms in addicted infants. One study reported an average milk concentration in 10 patients of 0.27 μg/ml, representing an average milk:plasma ratio of 0.83 (13). The same investigators earlier reported levels ranging from 0.17 to 5.6 μg/ml in the milk of mothers on methadone maintenance (2). At least one infant death has been attributed to methadone obtained through breast milk (14). However, a recent report claimed that methadone enters breast milk in very low quantities which are clinically insignificant (15). The American Academy of Pediatrics considers methadone compatible with breast-feeding (16).

References

1. Zelson C, Lee SJ, Casalino M. Neonatal narcotic addiction. N Engl J Med 1973;289:1216–20.
2. Blinick G, Jerez E, Wallach RC. Methadone maintenance, pregnancy and progeny. JAMA 1973;225:477–9.
3. Strauss ME, Andresko M, Stryker JC, Wardell JN, Dunkel LD. Methadone maintenance during pregnancy: pregnancy, birth and neonate characteristics. Am J Obstet Gynecol 1974;120:895–900.
4. Newman RG, Bashkow S, Calko D. Results of 313 consecutive live births of infants delivered to

patients in the New York City methadone maintenance program. Am J Obstet Gynecol 1975;121:233–7.

5. Ostrea EM, Chavez CJ, Strauss ME. A study of factors that influence the severity of neonatal narcotic withdrawal. J Pediatr 1976;88:642–5.

6. Kandall SR, Gartner LM. Delayed presentation of neonatal methadone withdrawal. Pediatr Res 1973;7:320.

7. Parekh A, Mukherjee TK, Jhaveri R, Rosenfeld W, Glass L. Intrauterine exposure to narcotics and cord blood prolactin concentrations. Obstet Gynecol 1981;57:447–9.

8. Pierson PS, Howard P, Kleber HD. Sudden deaths in infants born to methadone-maintained addicts. JAMA 1972;220:1733–4.

9. Chavez CJ, Ostrea EM, Stryker JC, Smialek Z. Sudden infant death syndrome among infants of drug-dependent mothers. J Pediatr 1979;95:407–9.

10. Zuspan FP, Gumpel JA, Mejia-Zelaya A, Madden J, David R. Fetal stress from methadone withdrawal. Am J Obstet Gynecol 1975;122:43–6.

11. Rementeria JL, Nunag NN. Narcotic withdrawal in pregnancy: stillbirth incidence with a case report. Am J Obstet Gynecol 1973;116:1152–6.

12. Burstein Y, Giardina PJV, Rausen AR, Kandall SR, Siljestrom K, Peterson CM. Thrombocytosis and increased circulating platelet aggregates in newborn infants of polydrug users. J Pediatr 1979;94:895–9.

13. Blinick G, Inturrisi CE, Jerez E, Wallach RC. Methadone assays in pregnant women and progeny. Am J Obstet Gynecol 1975;121:617–21.

14. Smialek JE, Monforte JR, Aronow R, Spitz WU. Methadone deaths in children—a continuing problem. JAMA 1977;238:2516–7.

15. Anonymous. Methadone in breast milk. Med Lett Drugs Ther 1979;21:52.

16. Committee on Drugs, American Academy of Pediatrics. The transfer of drugs and other chemicals into human breast milk. Pediatrics 1983;72:375–83.

Name: **METHANTHELINE**

Class: **Parasympatholytic (Anticholinergic)**   Risk Factor: **C**

Fetal Risk Summary

Methantheline is an anticholinergic quaternary ammonium bromide. In a large prospective study, 2,323 patients were exposed to this class of drugs during the 1st trimester, 2 of whom took methantheline (1). A possible association was found between the total group and minor malformations.

Breast Feeding Summary

No data available (see also Atropine).

References

1. Heinonen OP, Slone D, Shapiro S. *Birth Defects and Drugs in Pregnancy*. Littleton:Publishing Sciences Group, 1977:346–53.

Name: **METHAQUALONE**

Class: **Hypnotic**   Risk Factor: **D**

Fetal Risk Summary

No reports linking the use of methaqualone with congenital defects have been located. One manufacturer was not aware of any adverse effects following 1st trimester use (1). The autopsy of a 6-day-old infant found a congenital hypothalamic hamartoblastoma and multiple malformations (2). The baby had been exposed to methaqualone, marijuana, and cocaine early in gestation, but the correlation to any of these agents is unknown. Methaqualone is often used as an illicit abuse drug. Separating fetal effects from adulterants or other drugs is not possible. Due to the abuse potential, methaqualone is not recommended during pregnancy.

Breast Feeding Summary

No data available.

References

1. Smith RR. William H. Rorer, Inc, 1972. Personal communication.
2. Huff DS, Fernandes M. Two cases of congenital hypothalamic hamartoblastoma, polydactyly, and other congenital anomalies (Pallister-Hall syndrome). N Engl J Med 1982;306:430–1.

Name: **METHARBITAL**

Class: **Anticonvulsant/Sedative**   Risk Factor: **D**

Fetal Risk Summary

No reports linking the use of metharbital with congenital defects have been located. Metharbital is demethylated to barbital by the liver (see also Phenobarbital).

Breast Feeding Summary

The metabolite of metharbital metabolite, barbital, has been demonstrated in breast milk in trace amounts (1). No reports linking the use of metharbital with adverse effects in the nursing infant have been located.

References

1. Kwit NT, Hatcher RA. Excretion of drugs in milk. Am J Dis Child 1935;40:900–4.

Name: **METHDILAZINE**

Class: **Antihistamine**   Risk Factor: **C**

Fetal Risk Summary

No data available. See Promethazine for representative agent in this class.

Breast Feeding Summary

No data available.

Name: **METHENAMINE**

Class: **Urinary Germicide**   Risk Factor: **C$_M$**

Fetal Risk Summary

Methenamine, in either the mandelate or hippurate salt form, is used for chronic suppressive treatment of bacteriuria. In two studies, the mandelate form was given to 120 patients and the hippurate to 70 patients (1, 2). No increase in congenital defects or other problems as compared to controls were observed. The Collaborative Perinatal Project reported 49 1st trimester exposures to methenamine (3). For use anytime in pregnancy, 299 exposures were recorded (4). Only in the latter group was a possible association with malformations found. The statistical significance of this is not known. Independent confirmation is required.

Methenamine interferes with the determination of urinary estrogen (5). Urinary estrogen was formerly used to assess the condition of the fetoplacental unit, depressed levels being associated with fetal distress. This assessment is now made by measuring unconjugated estriol, which is not affected by methenamine.

Breast Feeding Summary

Methenamine is excreted into breast milk. Peak levels occur at 1 hour (6). No adverse effects on the nursing infant have been reported.

References

1. Gordon SF. Asymptomatic bacteriuria of pregnancy. Clin Med 1972;79:22–4.
2. Furness ET, McDonald PJ, Beasley NV. Urinary antiseptics in asymptomatic bacteriuria of pregnancy. NZ Med J 1975;81:417–9.
3. Heinonen OP, Slone D, Shapiro S. *Birth Defects and Drugs in Pregnancy*. Littleton:Publishing Sciences Group, 1977:299, 302.
4. *Ibid*, 435.
5. Kivinen S, Tuimala R. Decreased urinary oestriol concentrations in pregnant women during hexamine hippurate treatment. Br Med J 1977;2:682.
6. Sapeika N. The excretion of drugs in human milk—a review. J Obstet Gynaecol Br Emp 1947;54:426–31.

Name: **METHICILLIN**

Class: **Antibiotic**   Risk Factor: **B$_M$**

Fetal Risk Summary

Methicillin is a penicillin antibiotic (see also Penicillin G). The drug rapidly crosses the placenta into the fetal circulation and amniotic fluid (1, 2). Following a 500-mg intravenous dose over 10–15 minutes, peak levels of 13.0 and 10.5 μg/ml were measured in maternal and fetal serums, respectively, at 30 minutes (1). Equilibration occurred between the two serums within 1 hour. No effects were reported in the infants.

No reports linking the use of methicillin with congenital defects have been located. The Collaborative Perinatal Project monitored 50,282 mother-child pairs, 3,546 of which had 1st trimester exposure to penicillin derivatives (3). For use anytime during pregnancy, 7,171 exposures were recorded (4). In neither case was evidence found to suggest a relationship to large categories of major or minor malformations or to individual defects.

Breast Feeding Summary

No data available (see Penicillin G).

References

1. Depp R, Kind A, Kirby W, Johnson W. Transplacental passage of methicillin and dicloxacillin into the fetus and amniotic fluid. Am J Obstet Gynecol 1970;107:1054–7.
2. MacAulay M, Molloy W, Charles D. Placental transfer of methicillin. Am J Obstet Gynecol 1973;115:58–65.
3. Heinonen OP, Slone D, Shapiro S. *Birth Defects and Drugs in Pregnancy*. Littleton:Publishing Sciences Group, 1977:297–313.
4. *Ibid*, 435.

Name: **METHIMAZOLE**

Class: **Antithyroid**   Risk Factor: **D**

Fetal Risk Summary

Five cases of scalp defects (aplasia cutis) in newborns exposed *in utero* to methimazole have been reported (1, 2). In one of these newborns, an imperforate anus was also present (2). A 1980 study included one patient, whose condition was well controlled with carbimazole (converted *in vivo* to methimazole), giving birth to an infant who died at 3 days of age secondary to transposition of the great arteries (3). In a large prospective study, 25 patients were exposed to one or more noniodide thyroid suppressants during the 1st trimester, nine of whom took methimazole (4). From the total group, four children with nonspecified malformations were found, suggesting that the group may be teratogenic. However, since 18 of the group took other antithyroid drugs, the relationship between methimazole and the anomalies cannot be determined. Finally, two infants (of 25) from Ireland exposed to carbimazole were found to have defects: bilateral congenital cataracts (one case) and partial adactyly of the the right foot (one case) (5). Other reports have described the use of methimazole and carbimazole during pregnancy without fetal anomalies (6–18).

Methimazole readily crosses the placenta to the fetus. Two patients undergoing 2nd trimester therapeutic abortions were given a single 10-mg ^{35}S-labeled oral dose 2 hours before pregnancy termination (19). Fetal:maternal serum ratios were 0.72 and 0.81, representing 0.22 and 0.24% of the administered dose. In the same study, three patients at 14, 14, and 20 weeks gestation were given an equimolar dose of carbimazole (16.6 mg). Fetal:maternal serum ratios were 0.80–1.09 with 0.17–0.87% of the total radioactivity in the fetus. The highest serum and tissue levels were found in the 20-week-old fetus. In separate pregnancies in a mother with Graves' disease, fetal thyrotoxicosis was treated with 20–40 mg/day of carbimazole with successful resolution of fetal tachycardia in both cases and disappearance of fetal goiter in the first infant (17).

Treatment of maternal hyperthyroidism may result in mild fetal hypothyroidism due to increased levels of fetal pituitary thyrotropin (11, 14, 20). This usually resolves within a few days without treatment (14). An exception to this occurred in one newborn exposed to 30 mg of carbimazole daily to term who appeared normal at birth but who developed hypothyroidism evident at 2 months of age with subsequent mental retardation (6). Small, usually nonobstructing, goiters in the newborn have been reported frequently with propylthiouracil (see Propylthiouracil). Only two goiters have been reported in carbimazole-exposed newborns and none with methimazole (3). Long-term follow-up of 25 children exposed *in utero* to carbimazole has shown normal growth and development (5).

Combination therapy with thyroid-antithyroid drugs was advocated at one time but is now considered inappropriate (see also Propylthiouracil) (12, 16, 20, 21). Two reasons contributed to this change: 1) use of thyroid hormones may require higher doses of the antithyroid drug to be used, and 2) placental transfer of levothroxine and liothyronine are minimal and not sufficient to reverse fetal hypothyroidism (see also Levothyroxine and Liothyronine) (14).

Due to the possible association with aplasia cutis and passage of methimazole into breast milk, many experts consider propylthiouracil to be the drug of choice for the medical treatment of hyperthyroidism during pregnancy. If methimazole or carbimazole is used, the smallest possible dose to control the maternal disease should be given (3, 20).

Breast Feeding Summary

Methimazole is excreted into breast milk (22–25). In a patient given 10 mg of radiolabeled carbimazole (hydrolyzed *in vivo* to methimazole), the milk:plasma (M:P) ratio was a fairly constant 1.05 over 24 hours (22). This represented about 0.47% of the given radioactive dose. In a second study, a patient was administered 2.5 mg of methimazole every 12 hours (23). The mean M:P ratio was 1.16, representing 16–39 μg of methimazole in the daily milk supply. Extrapolation of these results to a daily dose of 20 mg indicated that approximately 3 mg/day would be excreted into the milk (23). Five lactating women were given 40 mg of carbimazole, producing a mean M:P ratio at 1 hour of 0.72 (24). For the 8-hour period after dosing, the M:P ratio was 0.98. A new radioimmunoassay was used to measure methimazole milk levels after a single 40-mg oral dose in four lactating women (25). The mean M:P ratio during the first 8 hours was 0.97, with 70 μg excreted in the milk. Because the amounts found in the above studies may cause thyroid dysfunction in the nursing infant, methimazole and carbimazole should be avoided during lactation (26). If antithyroid drug therapy is required, propylthiouracil should be considered (see Propylthiouracil).

References

1. Milham S Jr, Elledge W. Maternal methimazole and congenital defects in children. Teratology 1972;5:125.
2. Mujtaba Q, Burrow GN. Treatment of hyperthyroidism in pregnancy with propylthiouracil and methimazole. Obstet Gynecol 1975;46:282–6.
3. Sugrue D, Drury MI. Hyperthyroidism complicating pregnancy: results of treatment by antithyroid drugs in 77 pregnancies. Br J Obstet Gynaecol 1980;87:970–5.
4. Heinonen OP, Slone D, Shapiro S. *Birth Defects and Drugs in Pregnancy*. Littleton:Publishing Sciences Group, 1977:388–400.

5. McCarroll AM, Hutchinson M, McAuley R, Montgomery DAD. Long-term assessment of children exposed in utero to carbimazole. Arch Dis Child 1976;51:532–6.
6. Hawe P, Francis HH. Pregnancy and thyrotoxicosis. Br Med J 1962;2:817–22.
7. Herbst AL. Selenkow HA. Combined antithyroid-thyroid therapy of hyperthyroidism in pregnancy. Obstet Gynecol 1963;21:543–50.
8. Reveno WS, Rosenbaum H. Observation on the use of antithyroid drugs. Ann Intern Med 1964;60:982–9.
9. Herbst AL, Selenkow HA. Hyperthyroidism during pregnancy. N Engl J Med 1965;273:627–33.
10. Talbert LM, Thomas CG Jr, Holt WA, Rankin P. Hyperthyroidism during pregnancy. Obstet Gynecol 1970;36:779–85.
11. Refetoff S, Ochi Y, Selenkow HA, Rosenfield RL. Neonatal hypothyroidism and goiter in one infant of each of two sets of twins due to maternal therapy with antithyroid drugs. J Pediatr 1974;85:240–4.
12. Mestman JH, Manning PR, Hodgman J. Hyperthyroidism and pregnancy. Ann Intern Med 1974;134:434–9.
13. Ramsay I. Attempted prevention of neonatal thyrotoxicosis. Br Med J 1976;2:1110.
14. Low L, Ratcliffe W, Alexander W. Intrauterine hypothyroidism due to antithyroid-drug therapy for thyrotoxicosis during pregnancy. Lancet 1978;2:370–1.
15. Robinson PL, O'Mullane NH, Alderman B. Prenatal treatment of fetal thyrotoxicosis. Br Med J 1979;1:383–4.
16. Kock HCLV, Merkus JMWM. Graves' disease during pregnancy. Eur J Obstet Gynecol Reprod Biol 1983;14:323–30.
17. Pekonen F, Teramo K, Makinen T, Ikonen E, Osterlund K, Lamberg BA. Prenatal diagnosis and treatment of fetal thyrotoxicosis. Am J Obstet Gynecol 1984;150:893–4.
18. Jeffcoate WJ, Bain C. Recurrent pregnancy-induced thyrotoxicosis presenting as hyperemesis gravidarum. Case report. Br J Obstet Gynaecol 1985;92:413–5.
19. Marchant B, Brownlie EW, Hart DM, Horton PW, Alexander WD. The placental transfer of propylthiouracil, methimazole and carbimazole. J Clin Endocrinol Metab 1977;45:1187–93.
20. Burr WA. Thyroid disease. Clin Obstet Gynecol 1981;8:341–51.
21. Anonymous. Transplacental passage of thyroid hormones. N Engl J Med 1967;277:486–7.
22. Low LCK, Lang J, Alexander WD. Excretion of carbimazole and propylthiouracil in breast milk. Lancet 1979;2:1011.
23. Tegler L, Lindstrom B. Antithyroid drugs in milk. Lancet 1980;2:591.
24. Johansen K, Andersen AN, Kampmann JP, Hansen JM, Mortensen HB. Excretion of methimazole in human milk. Eur J Clin Pharmacol 1982;23:339–41.
25. Cooper DS, Bode HH, Nath B, Saxe V, Malcof F, Ridgway EC. Methimazole in man: studies using a newly developed radioimmunoassay for methimazole. J Clin Endocrinol Metab 1984;58:473–9.
26. Committee on Drugs, American Academy of Pediatrics. The transfer of drugs and other chemicals into human breast milk. Pediatrics 1983;72:375–83.

Name: **METHIXENE**

Class: **Parasympatholytic**   Risk Factor: **C**

Fetal Risk Summary

Methixene is an anticholinergic agent. No reports of its use in pregnancy have been located (see also Atropine).

Breast Feeding Summary

No data available (see also Atropine).

Name: **METHOTREXATE**

Class: **Antineoplastic**   Risk Factor: **D**

Fetal Risk Summary

Methotrexate is a folic acid antagonist. References describing the use of this antineoplastic agent in 15 pregnancies, eight in the 1st trimester, have been located (1–7). Three of the eight 1st trimester exposures resulted in malformed infants (2, 3, 6). Methotrexate-induced congenital defects are similar to those produced by another folic acid antagonist, aminopterin (see also Aminopterin) (6). Two such infants are described below:

> Absence of lambdoid and coronal sutures, oxycephaly, absence of frontal bone, low set ears, hypertelorism, dextroposition of heart, absence of digits on feet, growth retardation, very wide posterior fontanel, hypoplastic mandible, multiple anomalous ribs (2)
>
> Oxycephaly due to absent coronal sutures, large anterior fontanel, depressed/ wide nasal bridge, low set ears, long webbed fingers, wide set eyes (3)

Possible retention of methotrexate in maternal tissues prior to conception was suggested as the cause of desquamating fibrosing alveolitis in a newborn (8). Previous studies have shown that methotrexate may persist for prolonged periods in human tissues (9). The only other apparent adverse effect observed following methotrexate use in pregnancy was in a 1,000-g male infant born with pancytopenia after exposure to six different antineoplastic agents in the 3rd trimester (4). However, data from one review indicated that 40% of the infants exposed to cytotoxic drugs were of low birth weight (1). This finding was not related to the timing of the exposure. Long-term studies of growth and mental development in offspring exposed to antineoplastic agents during the 2nd trimester, the period of neuroblast multiplication, have not been conducted (10, 11).

Successful pregnancies have followed the use of methotrexate prior to conception (8, 12–19). Apparently, ovarian and testicular dysfunction are reversible (11, 20–23).

Breast Feeding Summary

Methotrexate is excreted into breast milk in low concentrations (24). After a dose of 22.5 mg/day, milk concentrations of 6×10^9 M (0.26 μg/dl) have been measured with a milk:plasma ratio of 0.08. The significance of this small amount is not known. However, since the drug may accumulate in neonatal tissues, breast-feeding is not recommended.

References

1. Nicholson HO. Cytotoxic drugs in pregnancy: review of reported cases. J Obstet Gynaecol Br Commonw 1968;75:307–12.
2. Milunsky A, Graef JW, Gaynor MF. Methotrexate-induced congenital malformations. J Pediatr 1968;72:790–5.
3. Powell HR, Ekert H. Methotrexate-induced congenital malformations. Med J Aust 1971;2:1076–7.
4. Pizzuto J, Aviles A, Noriega L, Niz J, Morales M, Romero F. Treatment of acute leukemia during pregnancy: presentation of nine cases. Cancer Treat Rep 1980;64:679–83.
5. Dara P, Slater LM, Armentrout SA. Successful pregnancy during chemotherapy for acute leukemia. Cancer 1981;47:845–6.

6. Warkany J. Teratogenicity of folic acid antagonists. Cancer Bull 1981;33:76–7.
7. Burnier AM. Discussion. In Plows CW. Acute myelomonocytic leukemia in pregnancy: report of a case. Am J Obstet Gynecol 1982;143:41–3.
8. Walden PAM, Bagshawe KD. Pregnancies after chemotherapy for gestational trophoblastic tumours. Lancet 1979;2:1241.
9. Charache S, Condit PT, Humphreys SR. Studies on the folic acid vitamins. IV. The persistance of amethopterin in mammalian tissues. Cancer 1960;13:236–40.
10. Dobbing J. Pregnancy and leukaemia. Lancet 1977;1:1155.
11. Schilsky RL, Lewis BJ, Sherins RJ, Young RC. Gonadal dysfunction in patients receiving chemotherapy for cancer. Ann Intern Med 1980;93:109–14.
12. Bacon C, Kernahan J. Successful pregnancy in acute leukaemia. Lancet 1975;2:515.
13. Wegelius R. Successful pregnancy in acute leukaemia. Lancet 1975;2:1301.
14. Ross GT. Congenital anomalies among children born of mothers receiving chemotherapy for gestational trophoblastic neoplasms. Cancer 1976;37:1043–7.
15. Gasser C. Long-term survival (cures) in childhood acute leukemia. Paediatrician 1980;9:344–57.
16. Sanz MA, Rafecas FJ. Successful pregnancy during chemotherapy for acute promyelocytic leukemia. N Engl J Med 1982;306:939.
17. Barnes AB, Link DA. Childhood dermatomyositis and pregnancy. Am J Obstet Gynecol 1983;146:335–6.
18. Deeg HJ, Kennedy MS, Sanders JE, Thomas ED, Storb R. Successful pregnancy after marrow transplantation for severe aplastic anemia and immunosuppression with cyclosporine. JAMA 1983;250:647.
19. Rustin GJS, Booth M, Dent J, Salt S, Rustin F, Bagshawe KD. Pregnancy after cytotoxic chemotherapy for gestational trophoblastic tumours. Br Med J 1984;288:103–6.
20. Hinkes E, Plotkin D. Reversible drug-induced sterility in a patient with acute leukemia. JAMA 1973;223:1490–1.
21. Sherins RJ, DeVita VT Jr. Effect of drug treatment for lymphoma on male reproductive capacity. Ann Intern Med 1973;79:216–20.
22. Lendon M, Palmer MK, Hann IM, Shalet SM, Jones PHM. Testicular histology after combination chemotherapy in childhood for acute lymphoblastic leukaemia. Lancet 1978;2:439–41.
23. Evenson DP, Arlin Z, Welt S, Claps ML, Melamed MR. Male reproductive capacity may recover following drug treatment with the L-10 protocol for acute lymphocytic leukemia. Cancer 1984;53:30–6.
24. Johns DG, Rutherford LD, Keighton PC, Vogel CL. Secretion of methotrexate into human milk. Am J Obstet Gynecol 1972;112:978–80.

Name: **METHOXAMINE**

Class: **Sympathomimetic (Adrenergic)**   Risk Factor: **D**

Fetal Risk Summary

Methoxamine is a sympathomimetic used in emergency situations to treat hypotension. It has been recently discontinued by the manufacturer. Because of the nature of its indications, experience in pregnancy with methoxamine is limited. Uterine vessels are normally maximally dilated, and they have only α-adrenergic receptors (1). Use of the predominantly α-adrenergic stimulant, methoxamine, could cause constriction of these vessels and reduce uterine blood flow, thereby producing fetal hypoxia (bradycardia). Methoxamine may also interact with oxytocics or ergot derivatives to produce severe persistent maternal hypertension (1). Rupture of a cerebral vessel is possible. If a pressor agent is indicated, other drugs such as ephedrine should be considered.

Breast Feeding Summary

No data available.

References

1. Smith NT, Corbascio AN. The use and misuse of pressor agents. Anesthesiology 1970;33:58–101.

Name: **METHSCOPOLAMINE**

Class: **Parasympatholytic (Anticholinergic)**   Risk Factor: **C**

Fetal Risk Summary

Methscopolamine is an anticholinergic quaternary ammonium bromide derivative of scopolamine (see also Scopolamine). In a large prospective study, 2,323 patients were exposed to this class of drugs during the 1st trimester, two of whom took methscopolamine (1). A possible association was found between the total group and minor malformations.

Breast Feeding Summary

No data available (see also Atropine).

References

1. Heinonen OP, Slone D, Shapiro S. *Birth Defects and Drugs in Pregnancy*. Littleton:Publishing Sciences Group, 1977:346–53.

Name: **METHSUXIMIDE**

Class: **Anticonvulsant**   Risk Factor: **C**

Fetal Risk Summary

Methsuximide is a succinimide anticonvulsant used in the treatment of petit mal epilepsy. The use of methsuximide during the 1st trimester has been reported in only five pregnancies (1, 2). No evidence of adverse fetal effects was found. Methsuximide has a much lower teratogenic potential than the oxazolidinedione class of anticonvulsants (see Trimethadione) (3, 4). The succinimide anticonvulsants should be considered the anticonvulsants of choice for the treatment of petit mal epilepsy during the 1st trimester (see Ethosuximide).

Breast Feeding Summary

No data available.

References

1. Annegers JF, Elveback LR, Hauser WA, Kurland LT. Do anticonvulsants have a teratogenic effect? Arch Neurol 1974;31:364–73.

2. Heinonen OP, Slone D, Shapiro S. *Birth Defects and Drugs in Pregnancy*. Littleton:Publishing Sciences Group, 1977:358–9.
3. Fabro S, Brown NA. Teratogenic potential of anticonvulsants. N Engl J Med 1979;300:1280–1.
4. The National Institutes of Health. Anticonvulsants found to have teratogenic potential. JAMA 1981;241:36.

Name: **METHYCLOTHIAZIDE**

Class: **Diuretic**   Risk Factor: **D**

Fetal Risk Summary

See Chlorothiazide.

Breast Feeding Summary

See Chlorothiazide.

Name: **METHYLDOPA**

Class: **Antihypertensive**   Risk Factor: **C**

Fetal Risk Summary

Methyldopa crosses the placenta and achieves fetal concentrations similar to those of the maternal serum (1–3). The Collaborative Perinatal Project monitored only one mother-child pair in which 1st trimester exposure to methyldopa was recorded (4). No abnormalities were found. A decrease in intracranial volume has been reported after 1st trimester exposure to methyldopa (5, 6). Infants evaluated at 4 years of age showed no association between small head size and retarded mental development (7). Review of 1,157 hypertensive pregnancies demonstrated no adverse effects from methyldopa administration (8–20). A reduced systolic blood pressure of 4–5 mm Hg in 24 infants for the first 2 days after delivery has been reported (21). This mild reduction in blood pressure was not considered significant. An infant born with esophageal atresia with fistula, congenital heart disease, absent left kidney, and hypospadias was exposed to methyldopa throughout gestation (22). The mother also took clomiphene early in the 1st trimester.

Breast Feeding Summary

Methyldopa is excreted into breast milk in small amounts. In four lactating women taking 750–2,000 mg/day, milk levels of free and conjugated methyldopa ranged from 0.1 to 0.9 μg/ml (1). A milk:plasma ratio could not be determined since simultaneous plasma levels were not obtained. The American Academy of Pediatrics considers methyldopa compatible with breast-feeding (23).

References

1. Jones HMR, Cummings AJ. A study of the transfer of α-methyldopa to the human foetus and newborn infant. Br J Clin Pharmacol 1978;6:432–4.

2. Jones HMR, Cummings AJ, Setchell KDR, Lawson AM. Pharmacokinetics of methyldopa in neonates. Br J Clin Pharmacol 1979;8:433–40.

3. Cummings AJ, Whitelaw AGL. A study of conjugation and drug elimination in the human neonate. Br J Clin Pharmacol 1981;12:511–5.

4. Heinonen OP, Slone D, Shapiro S. *Birth Defects and Drugs in Pregnancy*. Littleton:Publishing Sciences Group, 1977:372.

5. Myerscough PR. Infant growth and development after treatment of maternal hypertension. Lancet 1980;1:883.

6. Moar VA, Jefferies MA, Mutch LMM, Dunsted MK, Redman CWG. Neonatal head circumference and the treatment of maternal hypertension. Br J Obstet Gynaecol 1978;85:933–7.

7. Dunsted M, Moar VA, Redman CWG. Infant growth and development following treatment of maternal hypertension. Lancet 1980;1:705.

8. Redman CWG, Beilin LJ, Bonnar J, Ounsted MK. Fetal outcome in trial of antihypertensive treatment in pregnancy. Lancet 1976;2:753–6.

9. Hamilton M, Kopelman H. Treatment of severe hypertension with methyldopa. Br Med J 1963;1:151–5.

10. Abramowsky CR, Vegas ME, Swinehart G, Gyves MT. Decidual vasculopathy of the placenta in lupus erythematosus. N Engl J Med 1980;303:668–72.

11. Gallery EDM, Sounders DM, Hunyor SN, Gyory AZ. Randomised comparison of methyldopa and oxprenolol for treatment of hypertension in pregnancy. Br Med J 1979;1:1591–4.

12. Gyory AZ, Gallery ED, Hunyor SN. Effect of treatment of maternal hypertension with oxprenolol and α-methyldopa on plasma volume, placental and birth weights. Presented at the Eighth World Congress of Cardiology, Tokyo, 1978, Abstr. 1098.

13. Arias F, Zamora J. Antihypertensive treatment and pregnancy outcome in patients with mild chronic hypertension. Obstet Gynecol 1979;53:489–94.

14. Redman CWG, Beilin LJ, Bonnar J. A trial of hypotensive treatment in pregnancy. Clin Sci Mol Med 1975;49:3–4.

15. Tcherdakoff P, Milliez P. Traitement de l'hypertension arterielle par alphamethyldopa au cours de lo grossesse. In Proceedings Premier Symposium National, Hypertension Arterielle, Cannes, 1970:207–9.

16. Lselve A, Berger R, Vial JY, Gaillard MF. Alpha-methyldopa/Aldomet and reserpine/Serpasil: treatment of pregnancy hypertensions. J Med Lyon 1968;1369–75.

17. Leather HM, Humphreys DM, Baker P, Chadd MA. A controlled trial of hypotensive agents in hypertension in pregnancy. Lancet 1968;2:488–90.

18. Hamilton H. Some aspects of the long-term treatment of severe hypertension with methyldopa. Postgrad Med J 1968;44:66–9.

19. Skacel K, Sklendvsky A, Gazarek F, Matlocha Z, Mohapl M. Therapeutic use of alpha-methyldopa in cases of late toxemia of pregnancy. Cesk Gynekol 1967;32:78–80.

20. Kincaid-Smith P, Bullen M. Prolonged use of methyldopa in severe hypertension in pregnancy. Br Med J 1966;1:274–6.

21. Whitelaw A. Maternal methyldopa treatment and neonatal blood pressure. Br Med J 1981;283:471.

22. Ylikorkala O. Congenital anomalies and clomiphene. Lancet 1975;2:1262–3.

23. Committee on Drugs, American Academy of Pediatrics. The transfer of drugs and other chemicals into human breast milk. Pediatrics 1983;72:375–83.

Name: **METHYLENE BLUE**

Class: **Urinary Germicide/Diagnostic Dye**   Risk Factor: **C*$_M$**

Fetal Risk Summary

Methylene blue may be administered orally for its weak urinary germicide properties or injected into the amniotic fluid to diagnose premature rupture of the membranes. For oral dosing, nine exposures in the 1st trimester have been reported (1). No congenital abnormalities were observed. For use anytime during pregnancy, 46 exposures were reported (2). A possible association with malformations was found, but the statistical significance is not known.

Diagnostic intra-amniotic injection of methylene blue has resulted in hemolytic anemia, hyperbilirubinemia, and methemoglobinemia in the newborn (3–7). Doses of the dye ranged from 10 to 70 mg. One author suggested that smaller doses, such as 1.6 mg, would be adequate to confirm the presence of ruptured membranes without causing hemolysis (3). Inadvertent intrauterine injection in the 1st trimester has been reported (8). No adverse effects were reported in the full-term neonate.

[* Risk Factor D if injected intra-amniotically.]

Breast Feeding Summary

No data available.

References

1. Heinonen OP, Slone D, Shapiro S. *Birth Defects and Drugs in Pregnancy*. Littleton:Publishing Sciences Group, 1977:299.
2. *Ibid*, 434–5.
3. Plunkett GD. Neonatal complications. Obstet Gynecol 1973;41:476–7.
4. Cowett RM, Hakanson DO, Kocon RW, Oh W. Untoward neonatal effect of intraamniotic adminis- tration of methylene blue. Obstet Gynecol 1976;48:74s–5s.
5. Kirsch IR, Cohen HJ. Heinz body hemolytic anemia from the use of methylene blue in neonates. J Pediatr 1980;96:276–8.
6. Crooks J. Haemolytic jaundice in a neonate after intra-amniotic injection of methylene blue. Arch Dis Child 1982;57:872–3.
7. McEnerney JK. McEnerney LN. Unfavorable neonatal outcome after intraamniotic injection of methylene blue. Obstet Gynecol 1983;61:35S–6S.
8. Katz Z, Lancet M. Inadvertent intrauterine injection of methylene blue in early pregnancy. N Engl J Med 1981;304:1427.

Name: **METHYLPHENIDATE**

Class: **Central Stimulant**   Risk Factor: **C**

Fetal Risk Summary

No reports linking the use of methylphenidate with congenital defects have been located. The Collaborative Perinatal Project monitored 3,082 mother-child pairs with exposure to sympathomimetic drugs, 11 of which were exposed to methyl- phenidate (1). No evidence for an increased malformation rate was found.

Breast Feeding Summary

No data available.

References

1. Heinonen OP, Slone D, Shapiro S. *Birth Defects and Drugs in Pregnancy*. Littleton:Publishing Sciences Group, 1977:346–7.

Name: **METOLAZONE**

Class: **Diuretic**   Risk Factor: **D**

Fetal Risk Summary

Metolazone is structurally related to the thiazide diuretics. See Chlorothiazide.

Breast Feeding Summary

See Chlorothiazide.

Name: **METOPROLOL**

Class: **Sympatholytic (β-Adrenergic Blocker)**   Risk Factor: **B$_M$**

Fetal Risk Summary

Metoprolol, a cardioselective β-adrenergic blocking agent, has been used during pregnancy for the treatment of maternal hypertension and tachycardia (1–6). The drug readily crosses the placenta, producing approximately equal concentrations of metoprolol in maternal and fetal serum at delivery (1–3). The serum half-lives of metoprolol determined in five women during the 3rd trimester and repeated 3–5 months after delivery were similar, 1.3 vs 1.7 hours, respectively, but peak levels during pregnancy were only 20–40% of those measured later (4). Neonatal serum levels of metoprolol increase up to 4-fold in the first 2–5 hours after birth then decline rapidly over the next 15 hours (2, 3).

No fetal malformations attributable to metoprolol have been reported, but experience during the 1st trimester is lacking. In a 1978 study, 101 hypertensive pregnant patients treated with metoprolol alone (57 patients) or combined with hydralazine (44 patients) were compared to 97 patients treated with hydralazine alone (1). The duration of pregnancy at the start of antihypertensive treatment was 34.1 weeks (range 13–41) for the metoprolol group and 32.5 weeks (range 12–40) for the hydralazine group. The metoprolol group experienced a lower rate of perinatal mortality (2% vs 8%) and a lower incidence of intrauterine growth retardation (11.7% vs 16.3%). No signs or symptoms of β-blockade were noted in the fetuses or newborns in this or other studies (1, 2, 5).

The use of metoprolol in a pregnant patient with pheochromocytoma has been reported (5). High blood pressure had been controlled with prazosin, an α-adrenergic blocking agent, but the onset of maternal tachycardia required the addition of metoprolol during the last few weeks of pregnancy. No adverse effects were observed in the newborn.

Although the use of metoprolol for maternal disease does not seem to pose a risk to the fetus, the long-term effects of *in utero* exposure to β-blockers have not been studied. Persistent β-blockade has been observed in newborns exposed near delivery to other members of this class (see Acebutolol, Atenolol, and Nadolol). Thus, newborns exposed *in utero* to metoprolol should be closely observed during the first 24–48 hours after birth for bradycardia and other symptoms.

Breast Feeding Summary

Metoprolol is excreted into breast milk (1, 3, 7–9). Milk concentrations are approximately three times those found simultaneously in the maternal serum (reported range 2.0–3.7). No adverse effects have been observed in nursing infants exposed to metoprolol in milk. Based on calculations from a 1984 study, a mother ingesting 200 mg/day of metoprolol would only provide about 225 μg in a liter of her milk (3). To minimize this exposure even further, one reference suggested waiting 3–4 hours after a dose to breast-feed (9). Although these levels are probably clinically insignificant, nursing infants should be closely observed for signs or symptoms of β-blockade. The long-term effects of exposure to β-blockers from milk have not been studied but warrant evaluation. The American Academy of Pediatrics considers the drug compatible with breast-feeding (10).

References

1. Sandstrom B. Antihypertensive treatment with the adrenergic beta-receptor blocker metoprolol during pregnancy. Gynecol Invest 1978;9:195–204.
2. Lundborg P, Agren G, Ervik M, Lindeberg S, Sandstrom B. Disposition of metoprolol in the newborn. Br J Clin Pharmacol 1981;12:598–600.
3. Lindeberg S, Sandstrom B, Lundborg P, Regardh CG. Disposition of the adrenergic blocker metoprolol in the late-pregnant woman, the amniotic fluid, the cord blood and the neonate. Acta Obstet Gynecol Scand 1984;118(Suppl):61–4.
4. Hogstedt S, Lindberg B, Rane A. Increased oral clearance of metoprolol in pregnancy. Eur J Clin Pharmacol 1983;24:217–20.
5. Venuto R, Burstein P, Schneider R. Pheochromocytoma: antepartum diagnosis and management with tumor resection in the puerperium. Am J Obstet Gynecol 1984;150:431–2.
6. Robson DJ, Jeeva Ray MV, Storey GAC, Holt DW. Use of amiodarone during pregnancy. Postgrad Med J 1985;61:75–7.
7. Sandstrom B, Regardh CG. Metoprolol excretion into breast milk. Br J Clin Pharmacol 1980;9:518–9.
8. Liedholm H, Melander A, Bitzen PO, Helm G, Lonnerholm G, Mattiasson I, Nilsson B. Accumulation of atenolol and metoprolol in human breast milk. Eur J Clin Pharmacol 1981;20:229–31.
9. Kulas J, Lunell NO, Rosing U, Steen B, Rane A. Atenolol and metoprolol. A comparison of their excretion into human breast milk. Acta Obstet Scand 1984;118(Suppl):65–9.
10. Committee on Drugs, American Academy of Pediatrics. The transfer of drugs and other chemicals into human breast milk. Pediatrics 1983;72:375–83.

Name: **METRIZAMIDE**

Class: **Diagnostic**   Risk Factor: **D**

Fetal Risk Summary

Metrizamide contains a high concentration of organically bound iodine. See Diatrizoate for possible effects on the fetus and newborn.

Breast Feeding Summary

Metrizamide is excreted into milk in small quantities (1). A woman was injected with 5.06 g of metrizamide into the subarachnoid space. Milk levels increased linearly with time but only 1.1 mg (0.02%) of the dose was recovered in 44.3 hours. This amount of contrast media probably does not pose a risk to the nursing infant.

The American Academy of Pediatrics considers metrizamide compatible with breast-feeding (2).

References

1. Ilett KF, Hackett LP, Paterson JW, McCormick CC. Excretion of metrizamide in milk. Br J Radiol 1981;54:537–8.
2. Committee on Drugs, American Academy of Pediatrics. The transfer of drugs and other chemicals into human breast milk. Pediatrics 1983;72:375–83.

Name: **METRONIDAZOLE**

Class: **Antiprotozoal/Antibacterial**   Risk Factor: **B$_M$**

Fetal Risk Summary

Metronidazole possesses trichomonacidal and amebacidal activity as well as effectiveness against certain bacteria. The drug crosses the placenta to the fetus throughout gestation with a cord:maternal plasma ratio at term of approximately 1.0 (1–3). The pharmacokinetics of metronidazole in pregnant women have been reported (4).

The use of metronidazole in pregnancy is controversial. The drug is mutagenic in bacteria and carcinogenic in rodents, and although these properties have never been shown in humans, concern for these toxicities have led some to advise against the use of metronidazole in pregnancy (5, 6). To date, no association with human cancer has been proven (6, 7).

Several studies, individual case reports, and reviews have described the safe use of metronidazole during pregnancy (8–21). Included among these is a 1972 review summarizing 20 years of experience with the drug and involving 1,469 pregnant women, 206 of whom were treated during the 1st trimester (21). No association with congenital malformations, abortions, or stillbirths was found. Some investigations, however, have found an increased risk when the agent was used early in pregnancy (7, 22, 23).

The Collaborative Perinatal Project monitored 50,282 mother-child pairs, 31 of which had 1st trimester exposure to metronidazole (22). A possible association with malformations was found (relative risk 2.02) based on defects in four children. The statistical significance of this finding is unknown. Independent confirmation is required to determine the actual risk. In a 1979 report, metronidazole was used in 57 pregnancies, including 23 during the 1st trimester (7). Three of the 1st trimester exposures ended in spontaneous abortion (a normal incidence) and in the remaining 20 births, there were five congenital anomalies: hydrocele (2), congenital dislocated hip (female twin), metatarsus varus, and mental retardation (both parents mentally retarded). Analysis of the data is not possible because of the small numbers and possible involvement of genetic factors (7).

Two mothers, treated with metronidazole during the 5th–7th weeks of gestation for amebiasis, gave birth to infants with midline facial defects (23). Diiodohydroxyquinoline was also used in one of the pregnancies. One of the infants had holotelencephaly and one had unilateral cleft lip and palate. The relationship between the drug and the defects is unknown.

In summary, the available reports have arrived at conflicting conclusions on the safety of metronidazole in pregnancy. It is not possible to assess the risk to the fetus until additional data have been collected. The long-term risks from exposure to this drug, including the potential for cancer, have not been completely evaluated. The manufacturer and the Center for Disease Control consider metronidazole contraindicated during the 1st trimester in patients with trichomoniasis (24, 25). Use for trichomoniasis during the 2nd and 3rd trimesters may be acceptable if alternate therapies have failed (24, 25). Single-dose therapy should be avoided (25). For other indications, the risk:benefit ratio must be carefully weighed prior to the use of metronidazole, especially in the 1st trimester.

Breast Feeding Summary

Metronidazole is excreted into breast milk. Following a single 2-g oral dose in three patients, peak milk concentrations in the 50–60 μg/ml range were measured at 2–4 hours (26). With normal breast-feeding, infants would have received about 25 mg of metronidazole over the next 48 hours. By interrupting feedings for either 12 or 24 hours, infant exposure to the drug would have been reduced to 9.8 or 3.5 mg, respectively (26).

In women treated with divided oral doses of either 600 or 1200 mg/day, the mean milk levels were 5.7 and 14.4 μg/ml, respectively (27). The milk:plasma ratios in both groups were approximately 1.0. The mean plasma concentrations in the exposed infants were about 20% of the maternal plasma drug level. Eight women treated with metronidazole rectal suppositories, 1 g every 8 hours, produced a mean milk drug level of 10 μg/ml with maximum concentrations of 25 μg/ml (28).

One report described diarrhea and secondary lactose intolerance in a breast-fed infant whose mother was receiving metronidazole (29). The relationship between the drug and the events is unknown. Except for this one case, no reports of adverse effects in metronidazole-exposed nursing infants have been located. However, since the drug is mutagenic and carcinogenic in some test species (see Fetal Risk Summary), unnecessary exposure to metronidazole should be avoided. A single, 2-g oral dose has been recommended by the Center for Disease Control if metronidazole is used for trichomoniasis during lactation (24). If this dose is given, the American Academy of Pediatrics recommends discontinuing breast-feeding for 12–24 hours to allow excretion of the drug (30).

References

1. Amon K, Amon I, Huller H. Maternal-fetal passage of metronidazole. In *Advances in Antimicrobial and Antineoplastic Chemotherapy*. Proceedings of the VII International Congress of Chemotherapy, Prague, 1971:113–5.
2. Heisterberg L. Placental transfer of metronidazole in the first trimester of pregnancy. J Perinat Med 1984;12:43–5.
3. Karhunen M. Placental transfer of metronidazole and tinidazole in early human pregnancy after a single infusion. Br J Clin Pharmacol 1984;18:254–7.
4. Amon I, Amon K, Franke G, Mohr C. Pharmacokinetics of metronidazole in pregnant women. Chemotherapy 1981;27:73–9.
5. Anonymous. Is Flagyl dangerous? Med Lett Drugs Ther 1975;17:53–4.
6. Finegold SM. Metronidazole. Ann Intern Med 1980;93:585–7.
7. Beard CM, Noller KL, O'Fallon WM, Kurland LT, Dockerty MB. Lack of evidence for cancer due to use of metronidazole. N Engl J Med 1979;301:519–22.
8. Gray MS. Trichomonas vaginalis in pregnancy: the results of metronidazole therapy on the mother and child. J Obstet Gynaecol Br Commonw 1961;68:723–9.

9. Robinson SC, Johnston DW. Observations on vaginal trichomoniasis. II. Treatment with metroni-dazole. Can Med Assoc J 1961;85:1094–6.
10. Luthra R, Boyd JR. The treatment of trichomoniasis with metronidazole. Am J Obstet Gynecol 1962;83:1288–93.
11. Schram M, Kleinman H. Use of metronidazole in the treatment of trichomoniasis. Am J Obstet Gynecol 1962;83:1284–7.
12. Andrews MC, Andrews WC. Systemic treatment of trichomonas vaginitis. South Med J 1963;56:1214–8.
13. Zacharias LF, Salzer RB, Gunn JC, Dierksheide EB. Trichomoniasis and metronidazole. Am J Obstet Gynecol 1963;86:748–52.
14. Kotcher E, Frick CA, Giesel LO, Jr. The effect of metronidazole on vaginal microbiology and maternal and neonatal hematology. Am J Obstet Gynecol 1964;88:184–9.
15. Scott-Gray M. Metronidazole in obstetric practice. J Obstet Gynaecol Br Commonw 1964;71:82–5.
16. Perl G. Metronidazole treatment of trichomoniasis in pregnancy. Obstet Gynecol 1965;25:273–6.
17. Peterson WF, Stauch JE, Ryder CD. Metronidazole in pregnancy. Am J Obstet Gynecol 1966;94:343–9.
18. Robinson SC, Mirchandani G. Trichomonas vaginalis. V. Further observations on metronidazole (Flagyl) (including infant follow-up). Am J Obstet Gynecol 1965;93:502–5.
19. Mitchell RW, Teare AJ. Amoebic liver abscess in pregnancy. Case reports. Br J Obstet Gynaecol 1984;91:393–5.
20. Morgan I. Metronidazole treatment in pregnancy. Int J Gynaecol Obstet 1978;15:501–2.
21. Berget A, Weber T. Metronidazole and pregnancy. Ugeskr Laeg 1972;134:2085–9. As cited in Shepard TH. Catalog of Teratogenic Agents, ed 3. Baltimore:The Johns Hopkins University Press, 1980:228.
22. Heinonen OP, Slone D, Shapiro S. Birth Defects and Drugs in Pregnancy. Littleton:Publishing Sciences Group, 1977:298, 299, 302.
23. Cantu JM, Garcia-Cruz D. Midline facial defect as a teratogenic effect of metronidazole. Birth Defects 1982;18:85–8.
24. American Hospital Formulary Service. Drug Information 1985. Bethesda:American Society of Hospital Pharmacists, 1985:322–6.
25. Product information. Flagyl. Searle & Company, 1985.
26. Erickson SH, Oppenheim GL, Smith GH. Metronidazole in breast milk. Obstet Gynecol 1981;57:48–50.
27. Heisterberg L, Branebjerg PE. Blood and milk concentrations of metronidazole in mothers and infants. J Perinat Med 1983;11:114–20.
28. Moore B, Collier J. Drugs and breast-feeding. Br Med J 1979;2:211.
29. Clements CJ. Metronidazole and breast feeding. NZ Med J 1980;92:329.
30. Committee on Drugs, American Academy of Pediatrics. The transfer of drugs and other chemicals into human breast milk. Pediatrics 1983;72:375–83.

Name: **MICONAZOLE**

Class: **Antifungal Antibiotic**   Risk Factor: **B**

Fetal Risk Summary

Miconazole is normally used as a topical antifungal agent. Small amounts are absorbed from the vagina (1). Use in pregnant patients with vulvovaginal candidiasis (moniliasis) has not been associated with an increase in congenital malformations (1–5). Effects following intravenous use are not known.

Breast Feeding Summary

No data available.

References

1. Product information. Monistat. Ortho Pharmaceutical Corp, 1985.
2. Culbertson C. Monistat: a new fungicide for treatment of vulvovaginal candidiasis. Am J Obstet Gynecol 1974;120:973–6.
3. Wade A, ed. *Martindale. The Extra Pharmacopoeia*, ed 27. London:Pharmaceutical Press, 1977:648.
4. Davis JE, Frudenfeld JH, Goddard JL. Comparative evaluation of Monistat and Mycostatin in the treatment of vulvovaginal candidiasis. Obstet Gynecol 1974;44:403–6.
5. Wallenburg HCS, Wladimiroff JW. Recurrence of vulvovaginal candidosis during pregnancy. Comparison of miconazole vs nystatin treatment. Obstet Gynecol 1976;48:491–4.

Name: **MINERAL OIL**

Class: **Laxative**   Risk Factor: **C**

Fetal Risk Summary

Mineral oil is an emollient laxative. The drug is generally considered nonabsorbable. Chronic use may lead to decreased absorption of fat-soluble vitamins.

Breast Feeding Summary

No data available.

Name: **MINOCYCLINE**

Class: **Antibiotic**   Risk Factor: **D**

Fetal Risk Summary

See Tetracycline.

Breast Feeding Summary

See Tetracycline.

Name: **MINOXIDIL**

Class: **Antihypertensive**   Risk Factor: **C**

Fetal Risk Summary

Minoxidil has been used throughout gestation in one woman (1). No effects of this exposure were seen in the healthy newborn.

Breast Feeding Summary

Minoxidil is excreted into breast milk (1). Levels in the milk ranged from 41.7 ng/ml (1 hour) to 0.3 ng/ml (12 hours), with milk:plasma ratios during this interval varying from 0.67 to 1.0. No adverse effects were observed in the infant.

References

1. Valdivieso A, Valdes G, Spiro TE, Westerman RL. Minoxidil in breast milk. Ann Intern Med 1985;102:135.

Name: **MITHRAMYCIN**

Class: **Antineoplastic**   Risk Factor: **D**

Fetal Risk Summary

No data available.

Breast Feeding Summary

No data available.

Name: **MOLINDONE**

Class: **Tranquilizer**   Risk Factor: **C**

Fetal Risk Summary

Molindone is an antipsychotic drug. The only reported use of it in pregnancy was in a woman who gave birth at term to normal twin boys (1). The mother had ingested 9,800 mg of molindone during her 9-month pregnancy. No abnormalities in physical or mental development were noted in their first 20 years of life.

Breast Feeding Summary

No data available.

References

1. Ayd FJ Jr. Moban: the first of a new class of neuroleptics. In Ayd FJ Jr., ed. *Rational Psychopharmacotherapy and the Right to Treatment*. Baltimore:Ayd Medical Communications, 1975:91–106.

Name: **MORPHINE**

Class: **Narcotic Analgesic**   Risk Factor: **B***

Fetal Risk Summary

No reports linking the therapeutic use of morphine with major congenital defects have been located. Bilateral horizontal nystagmus persisting for 1 year was reported in one addicted newborn (1). Like all narcotics, placental transfer of morphine is very rapid (2, 3). Maternal addiction with subsequent neonatal withdrawal is well known following illicit use (see also Heroin) (1, 4, 5). Morphine was widely used in labor until the 1940's when it was largely displaced by meperidine.

Clinical impressions that meperidine caused less respiratory depression in the newborn were apparently confirmed (6, 7). Other clinicians reported no difference between narcotics in the degree of neonatal depression when equianalgesic intravenous doses were used (3). Epidural use of morphine has been reported in women in labor but with unsatisfactory analgesic effects (8). The intrathecal route, however, has provided safe and effective analgesia without fetal or newborn toxicity (9–11).

The Collaborative Perinatal Project monitored 50,282 mother-child pairs, 70 of which had 1st trimester exposure to morphine (12). For use anytime during pregnancy, 448 exposures were recorded (13). No evidence was found to suggest a relationship to large categories of major or minor malformations. A possible association with inguinal hernia (10 cases) after anytime use was observed (14). The statistical significance of this association is unknown and independent confirmation is required.

[* Risk Factor D if used for prolonged periods or in high doses at term.]

Breast Feeding Summary

Only trace amounts of morphine enter breast milk. The significance is unknown (15–17). The American Academy of Pediatrics considers morphine compatible with breast-feeding (18).

References

1. Perlstein MA. Congenital morphinism. A rare cause of convulsions in the newborn. JAMA 1947;135:633.
2. Fisher DE, Paton JB. The effect of maternal anesthetic and analgesic drugs on the fetus and newborn. Clin Obstet Gynaecol 1974;17:275–87.
3. Bonica JJ. *Principles and Practice of Obstetric Analgesia and Anesthesia*. Philadelphia:FA Davis Co, 1967:247.
4. McMullin GP, Mobarak AN. Congenital narcotic addiction. Arch Dis Child 1970;45:140–1.
5. Cobrinik RW, Hodd RT Jr, Chusid E. The effect of maternal narcotic addiction on the newborn infant. Pediatrics 1959;24:288–304.
6. Gilbert G, Dixon AB. Observations on Demerol as an obstetric analgesic. Am J Obstet Gynecol 1943;45:320–6.
7. Way WL, Costley EC, Way EL. Respiratory sensitivity of the newborn infant to meperidine and morphine. Clin Pharmacol Ther 1965;6:454–61.
8. Nybell-Lindahl G, Carlsson C, Ingemarsson I, Westgren M, Paalzow L. Maternal and fetal concentrations of morphine after epidural administration during labor. Am J Obstet Gynecol 1981;139:20–1.
9. Baraka A, Noueihid R, Hajj S. Intrathecal injection of morphine for obstetric analgesia. Anesthesiology 1981;54:136–40.
10. Bonnardot JP, Maillet M, Colau JC, Millot F, Deligne P. Maternal and fetal concentration of morphine after intrathecal administration during labour. Br J Anaesth 1982;54:487–9.
11. Brizgys RV, Shnider SM. Hyperbaric intrathecal morphine analgesia during labor in a patient with Wolff-Parkinson-White syndrome. Obstet Gynecol 1984;64:44S–6S.
12. Heinonen OP, Slone D, Shapiro S. *Birth Defects and Drugs in Pregnancy*. Littleton:Publishing Sciences Group, 1977:287–95.
13. *Ibid*, 434.
14. *Ibid*, 484.
15. Terwilliger WG, Hatcher RA. The elimination of morphine and quinine in human milk. Surg Gynecol Obstet 1934;58:823–6.
16. Kwit NT, Hatcher RA. Excretion of drugs in milk. Am J Dis Child 1935;49:900–4.
17. Anonymous. Drugs in breast milk. Med Lett Drugs Ther 1979;21:21–4.
18. Committee on Drugs, American Academy of Pediatrics. The transfer of drugs and other chemicals into human breast milk. Pediatrics 1983;72:375–83.

Name: **MOXALACTAM**

Class: **Antibiotic**   Risk Factor: **C$_M$**

Fetal Risk Summary

Moxalactam is a cephalosporin antibiotic. No controlled studies on its use in pregnancy have been located. The drug crosses the placenta to the fetus, producing a mean peak level at 1 hour in the cord blood of 38.4 μg/ml following a 1-g intravenous dose (1). Peak amniotic fluid levels of 10.3 μg/ml occurred at 7.5 hours.

Breast Feeding Summary

Moxalactam is excreted into breast milk (2). In eight women receiving 2 g every 8 hours, mean daily concentrations of the antibiotic varied from 1.56 to 3.66 mg/ml, representing a daily dose of 0.86–2.01 mg. Since moxalactam is acid-stable, the authors cautioned that colonization of the infant's bowel with gram-positive organisms could occur, resulting in a risk for enterocolitis (2). Due to this theoretical risk, they advised against breast-feeding if the mother was being treated with moxalactam.

References

1. Cho N, et al. Fundamental and clinical studies on 6059-S in the field of obstetrics and gynecology. J Chemother 1980;2(suppl):109.
2. Miller RD, Keegan KA, Thrupp LD, Brann J. Human breast milk concentration of moxalactam. Am J Obstet Gynecol 1984;148:348–9.

Name: **NADOLOL**

Class: **Sympatholytic (β-Adrenergic Blocker)**   Risk Factor: **C$_M$**

Fetal Risk Summary

Nadolol is a nonselective β-adrenergic blocking agent used for hypertension and angina pectoris. Only one reported case of its use in pregnancy has been located (1). A mother with IgA nephropathy and hypertension was treated throughout pregnancy with nadolol, 20 mg/day, plus a diuretic (triamterene/hydrochlorothiazide) and thyroid. The infant, delivered by emergency cesarean section at 35 weeks gestation, was growth-retarded and exhibited tachypnea (68 breaths/min) and mild hypoglycemia (20 mg/100 ml). Depressed respirations (23 breaths/min), slowed heart rate (112 beats/min), and hypothermia (96.5°F) occurred at 4.5 hours of age. The lowered body temperature responded to warming, but the cardiorespiratory depression, with brief episodes of bradycardia, persisted for 72 hours. Nadolol serum concentrations in cord blood and in the infant at 12 and 38 hours after delivery were 43, 145, and 80 ng/ml, respectively.

The etiology of some or all of the effects observed in this infant may have been β-blockade (1). However, maternal disease could not be excluded as the sole or contributing factor behind the intrauterine growth retardation and hypoglycemia (1). In addition, hydrochlorothiazide may have contributed to the low blood glucose level (see Chlorothiazide).

The authors identified several characteristics of nadolol in the adult that could potentially increase its toxicity in the fetus and newborn, including a long serum half-life (17–24 hours), lack of metabolism (excreted unchanged by the kidneys), and low protein binding (30%) (1). Because of these factors, other β-blockers may be safer for use during pregnancy although persistent β-blockade has also been observed with acebutolol and atenolol. As with other agents in this class, long-term effects of in utero β-blockade have not been studied but warrant evaluation.

Breast Feeding Summary

Nadolol is excreted into breast milk (1, 2). A mother taking 20 mg of nadolol per day had a concentration in her milk of 146 ng/ml 38 hours after delivery (1). In 12 lactating women ingesting 80 mg/day for 5 days, mean steady levels of nadolol were approximately 357 ng/ml, 4.6 times higher than maternal serum levels (2). By calculation, a 5-kg infant would have received 2–7% of the adult therapeutic dose, but the infants were not allowed to breast-feed (2).

Because experience is lacking, nursing infants of mothers consuming nadolol should be closely observed for symptoms of β-blockade. Long-term effects of exposure to β-blockers from milk have not been studied but warrant evaluation.

The American Academy of Pediatrics considers nadolol compatible with breast-feeding (3).

References

1. Fox RE, Marx C, Stark AR. Neonatal effects of maternal nadolol therapy. Am J Obstet Gynecol 1985;152:1045–6.
2. Devlin RG, Duchin KL, Fleiss PM. Nadolol in human serum and breast milk. Br J Clin Pharmacol 1981;12:393–6.
3. Committee on Drugs, American Academy of Pediatrics. The transfer of drugs and other chemicals into human breast milk. Pediatrics 1983;72:375–83.

Name: **NAFCILLIN**

Class: **Antibiotic**   Risk Factor: **B**

Fetal Risk Summary

Nafcillin is a pencillin antibiotic (see also Pencillin G). No reports linking its use with congenital defects have been located. The Collaborative Perinatal Project monitored 50,282 mother-child pairs, 3,546 of which had 1st trimester exposure to pencillin derivatives (1). For use anytime during pregnancy, 7,171 exposures were recorded (2). In neither case was evidence found to suggest a relationship to large categories of major or minor malformations or to individual defects.

Breast Feeding Summary

No data available (see Pencillin G).

References

1. Heinonen OP, Slone D, Shapiro S. Birth Defects and Drugs in Pregnancy. Littleton:Publishing Sciences Group, 1977:297–313.
2. Ibid, 435.

Name: **NALBUPHINE**

Class: **Analgesic**   Risk Factor: **B***

Fetal Risk Summary

No congenital defects have been reported in humans or in experimental animals (1). Nalbuphine has both narcotic agonist and antagonist effects. Prolonged use during pregnancy could theoretically result in fetal addiction with subsequent withdrawal in the newborn (see also Pentazocine). Use of the drug in labor produces neonatal respiratory depression comparable to meperidine (1).

[* Risk Factor D if used for prolonged periods or in high doses at term.]

Breast Feeding Summary

No data available.

References

1. Miller RR. Evaluation of nalbuphine hydrochloride. Am J Hosp Pharm 1980;37:942–9.

Name: **NALIDIXIC ACID**

Class: **Urinary Germicide**   Risk Factor: **B**

Fetal Risk Summary

No reports linking the use of nalidixic acid with congenital defects have been located. Chromosome damage was not observed in human leukocytes cultured with varying concentrations of the drug (1). One author cautioned that the drug should be avoided in late pregnancy since it may produce hydrocephalus (2). However, a subsequent report examined the newborns of 63 patients treated with nalidixic acid at various stages of gestation (3). No defects attributable to the drug or intracranial hypertension were observed.

Breast Feeding Summary

Nalidixic acid is excreted into breast milk in low concentrations. Hemolytic anemia was reported in one infant with glucose-6-phosphate dehydrogenase deficiency whose mother was taking 1 g four times a day (4). Milk levels were not measured in this case, but the author noted data from the manufacturer in which milk levels from four women taking a similar dose were found to be 4 μg/ml. The milk:plasma ratio has been reported as 0.08–0.13 (5). These quantities are normally considered insignificant (6).

References

1. Stenchever MA, Powell W, Jarvis JA. Effect of nalidixic acid on human chromosome integrity. Am J Obstet Gynecol 1970;107:329–30.
2. Asscher AW. Diseases of the urinary system. Urinary tract infections. Br Med J 1977;1:1332.
3. Murray EDS. Nalidixic acid in pregnancy. Br Med J 1981;282:224.
4. Belton EM, Jones RV. Hemolytic anemia due to nalidixic acid. Lancet 1965;2:691.
5. Wilson JT. Milk/plasma ratios and contraindicated drugs. In Wilson JT, ed. *Drugs in Breast Milk.* Balgowlah, Australia: ADIS Press, 1981:78–9.
6. Takyi BE. Excretion of drugs in human milk. J Hosp Pharm 1970;28:317–25.

Name: **NALORPHINE**

Class: **Narcotic Antagonist**   Risk Factor: **D**

Fetal Risk Summary

Nalorphine is a narcotic antagonist that is used to reverse respiratory depression from narcotic overdose. It has been used either alone or in combination with meperidine or morphine during labor to reduce neonatal depression (1–6). Nalorphine has also been given to the newborn to prevent neonatal asphyxia (3, 7).

Although some benefits were initially claimed, caution in the use of nalorphine during labor has been advised for the following reasons (8):

A statistically significant reduction in neonatal depression has not been demonstrated.

The antagonist reduces analgesia.

The antagonist may increase neonatal depression if an improper narcotic-narcotic antagonist ratio is used.

An adverse effect on fetal cord blood pH, pCO_2 and base deficit was shown when nalorphine was given in combination with meperidine during labor (9). As indicated above, nalorphine may cause respiratory depression in the absence of narcotics or if the critical ratio is exceeded (8). Because of these considerations, the use of nalorphine either alone or in combination therapy in pregnancy should be discouraged. If a narcotic antagonist is indicated, other agents that do not cause respiratory depression, such as naloxone, are preferred.

Breast Feeding Summary

No data available.

References

1. Cappe BE, Himel SZ, Grossman F. Use of a mixture of morphine and N-allynormorphine as an analgesic. Am J Obstet Gynecol 1953;66:1231–4.
2. Echenhoff JE, Hoffman GL, Funderburg LW. N-allynormorphine: an antagonist to neonatal narcosis produced by sedation of the parturient. Am J Obstet Gynecol 1953;65:1269–75.
3. Echenhoff JE, Funderburg LW. Observations in the use of the opiate antagonists nalorphine and levallorphan. Am J Med Sci 1954;228:546–53.
4. Baker FJ. Pethidine and nalorphine in labor. Anaesthesia 1957;12:282–92.
5. Gordon DWS, Pinker GD. Increased pethidine dosage in obstetrics associated with the use of nalorphine. J Obstet Gynaecol Br Commonw 1958;65:606–11.
6. Bullough J. Use of premixed pethidine and antagonists in obstetrical analgesia with special reference to cases in which levallorphan was used. Br Med J 1959;2:859–62.
7. Paterson S, Prescott F. Nalorphine in prevention of neonatal asphyxia due to maternal sedation with pethidine. Lancet 1954;1:490–3.
8. Bonica JJ. *Principles and Practice of Obstetric Analgesia and Anesthesia*. Philadelphia:FA Davis Co, 1967:254–9.
9. Hounslow D, Wood C, Humphrey M, Chang A. Intrapartum drugs and fetal blood pH and gas status. J Obstet Gynaecol Br Commonw 1973;80:1007–12.

Name: **NALOXONE**

Class: **Narcotic Antagonist**   Risk Factor: **B$_M$**

Fetal Risk Summary

Naloxone is a narcotic antagonist that is used to reverse the effects of narcotic overdose. The drug has no intrinsic respiratory depressive actions or other narcotic effects of its own (1). Naloxone has been shown to cross the placenta, appearing in fetal blood 2 minutes after a maternal dose and gradually increasing over 10–30 minutes (2).

In three reports, naloxone was given to mothers in labor after the administration of meperidine (3–5). Clark and co-workers (4) found that 18–40 μg/kg (maternal weight) intravenously provided the best results in comparison with controls that did not receive meperidine or naloxone. In measurements of newborn neurobehavior, groups treated in labor with either meperidine or meperidine plus naloxone (0.4 mg) were compared with a nontreated control group (5). The control group scored better in the first 24 hours than either of the treated groups and, after 2 hours, no difference was found between meperidine or meperidine plus naloxone-treated patients. Women in active labor received 1.0 mg of morphine intrathecally followed in 1 hour by a 0.4-mg intravenous bolus of naloxone plus 0.6 mg/hr or placebo as constant infusion for 23 hours (6). A reduction in some morphine-induced maternal side effects was seen with naloxone, but no significant differences with placebo were found for fetal heart rate or variability, Apgar scores, umbilical venous and arterial gasses, neonatal respirations, or neurobehavioral examination scores. Cord:maternal serum ratio for naloxone was 0.50. Naloxone has also been safely given to newborns within a few minutes of delivery (7–12).

Naloxone has been used at term to treat fetal heart rate baselines with low beat-to-beat variability not due to maternally administered narcotics (13). This use was based on the assumption that the heart rate patterns were due to elevated fetal endorphins. In one case, however, naloxone may have enhanced fetal asphyxia, leading to fatal respiratory failure in the newborn (13). Based on the above data, naloxone should not be given to the mother just prior to delivery to reverse the effects of narcotics in the fetus or newborn unless narcotic toxicity is evident. Information on its fetal effects during pregnancy, other than labor, are not available.

Breast Feeding Summary

No data available.

References

1. Jaffe JH, Martin WR. Opioid analgesics and antagonists. In Gilman AG, Goodman LS, Gilman A, eds. *The Pharmacological Basis of Therapeutics*, ed 6. New York:Macmillan Publishing Co, 1980:522–5.
2. Finster M, Gibbs C, Dawes GS, et al. Placental transfer of meperidine (Demerol) and naloxone (Narcan). Presented at the Annual Meeting of the American Society of Anesthesiologists, Boston, October 4, 1972. In Clark RB, Beard AG, Greifenstein FE, Barclay DL. South Med J 1976;69:570–5.
3. Clark RB. Transplacental reversal of meperidine depression in the fetus by naloxone. J Arkansas Med Soc 1971;68:128–30.
4. Clark RB, Beard AG, Greifenstein FE, Barclay DL. Naloxone in the parturient and her infant. South Med J 1976;69:570–5.
5. Hodgkinson R, Bhatt M, Grewal G, Marx GF. Neonatal neurobehavior in the first 48 hours of life: effect of the administration of meperidine with and without naloxone in the mother. Pediatrics 1978;62:294–8.
6. Brookshire GL, Shnider SM, Abboud TK, Kotelko DM, Nouiehed R, Thigpen JW, Khoo SS, Raya JA, Foutz SE, Brizgys RV. Effects of naloxone on the mother and neonate after intrathecal morphine for labor analgesia. Anesthesiology 1983;59:A417.
7. Evans JM, Hogg MIJ, Rosen M. Reversal of narcotic depression in the neonate by naloxone. Br Med J 1976;2:1098–1100.
8. Wiener PC, Hogg MIJ, Rosen M. Effects of naloxone on pethidine-induced neonatal depression. II. Intramuscular naloxone. Br Med J 1977;2:229–31.
9. Wiener PC, Hogg MIJ, Rosen M. Effects of naloxone on pethidine-induced neonatal depression. I. Intravenous naloxone. Br Med J 1977;2:228–9.

10. Gerhardt T, Bancalari E, Cohen H, Rocha LF. Use of naloxone to reverse narcotic respiratory depression in the newborn infant. J Pediatr 1977;90:1009–12.
11. Bonta BW, Gagliardi JV, Williams V, Warshaw JB. Naloxone reversal of mild neurobehavioral depression in normal newborn infants after routine obstetric analgesia. J Pediatr 1979;94:102–5.
12. Welles B, Belfrage P, de Chateau P. Effects of naloxone on newborn infant behavior after maternal analgesia with pethidine during labor. Acta Obstet Gynecol Scand 1984;63:617–9.
13. Goodlin RC. Naloxone and its possible relationship to fetal endorphin levels and fetal distress. Am J Obstet Gynecol 1981;139:16–9.

Name: **NAPROXEN**

Class: **Nonsteroidal Anti-inflammatory**   Risk Factor: **B*$_M$**

Fetal Risk Summary

Naproxen is a potent inhibitor of prostaglandin synthetase. Drugs in this class have been shown to inhibit labor and to prolong the length of pregnancy (1). Naproxen readily crosses the placenta to the fetal circulation (2, 3). In a mother treated with 250 mg of naproxen every 8 hours for four doses, cord blood levels in twins 5 hours after the last dose were 59.5 and 68 μg/ml, respectively (3). Prostaglandin synthetase inhibitors may cause constriction of the ductus arteriosus *in utero*, which may result in primary pulmonary hypertension of the newborn (4, 5). The dose, duration, and period of gestation are important determinants of these effects. Most studies of nonsteroidal anti-inflammatory agents used as tocolytics have indicated that the fetus is relatively resistant to premature closure of the ductus before the 34th or 35th week of gestation (see Indomethacin). However, three fetuses (one set of twins) exposed to naproxen at 30 weeks for 2–6 days in an unsuccessful attempt to halt premature labor had markedly decreased plasma concentrations of prostaglandin E (3, 6). Primary pulmonary hypertension of the newborn with severe hypoxemia, increased blood clotting times, hyperbilirubinemia, and impaired renal function were observed in the newborns. One infant died 4 days after birth, probably due to subarachnoid hemorrhage. Autopsy revealed a short and constricted ductus arteriosus. Use in other patients for premature labor at 34 weeks or earlier did not result in neonatal problems (7, 8). Because of the potential newborn toxicity, naproxen should not be used late in the 3rd trimester (2, 3, 9).

[* Risk Factor D if used in 3rd trimester or near delivery.]

Breast Feeding Summary

Naproxen passes into breast milk in very small quantities. The milk:plasma ratio is approximately 0.01 (2). Following 250 or 375 mg twice daily, maximum milk levels were found 4 hours after a dose and ranged from 0.7 to 1.25 μg/ml and from 1.76 to 2.37 μg/ml, respectively (10). The total amount of naproxen excreted in the infant's urine was 0.26% of the mother's dose. The effect on the infant from these amounts is not known. The American Academy of Pediatrics considers naproxen compatible with breast-feeding (11).

References

1. Fuchs F. Prevention of prematurity. Am J Obstet Gynecol 1976;126:809–20.
2. Product information. Naprosyn. Syntex, 1985.

3. Wilkinson AR. Naproxen levels in preterm infants after maternal treatment. Lancet 1980;2:591–2.
4. Levin DL. Effects of inhibition of prostaglandin synthesis on fetal development, oxygenation, and the fetal circulation. Semin Perinatol 1980;4:35–44.
5. Rudolph AM. The effects of nonsteroidal antiinflammatory compounds on fetal circulation and pulmonary function. Obstet Gynecol 1981;58(Suppl): 63s–7s.
6. Wilkinson AR, Aynsley-Green A, Mitchell MD. Persistent pulmonary hypertension and abnormal prostaglandin E levels in preterm infants after maternal treatment with naproxen. Arch Dis Child 1979;54:942–5.
7. Gerris J, Jonckheer M, Sacre-Smits L. Acute hyperthyroidism during pregnancy: a case report and critical analysis. Eur J Obstet Gynecol Reprod Biol 1981;12:271–80.
8. Wiqvist N, Kjellmer I, Thiringer K, Ivarsson E, Karlsson K. Treatment of premature labor by prostaglandin synthetase inhibitors. Acta Biol Med Germ 1978;37:923–30.
9. Anonymous. PG-synthetase inhibitors in obstetrics and after. Lancet 1980;2:185–6.
10. Jamali F, Tam YK, Stevens RD. Naproxen excretion in breast milk and its uptake by suckling infant. Drug Intell Clin Pharm 1982;16:475 (Abstr).
11. Committee on Drugs, American Academy of Pediatrics. The transfer of drugs and other chemicals into human breast milk. Pediatrics 1983;72:375–83.

Name: **NEOMYCIN**

Class: **Antibiotic**   Risk Factor: **C**

Fetal Risk Summary

Neomycin is an aminoglycoside antibiotic. No reports describing its passage across the placenta to the fetus have been located, but this should be expected (see other aminoglycosides: Amikacin, Gentamicin, Kanamycin, Streptomycin, and Tobramycin).

Ototoxicity, which is known to occur after oral, topical, and parenteral neomycin therapy, has not been reported as an effect of *in utero* exposure. However, eighth cranial nerve toxicity in the fetus is well known following exposure to kanamycin and streptomycin and may potentially occur with neomycin.

Oral neomycin therapy, 2 g daily, depresses urinary estrogen excretion apparently by inhibiting steroid conjugate hydrolysis in the gut (1). The fall in estrogen excretion resembles the effect produced by ampicillin but occurs about 2 days later. Urinary estriol was formerly used to assess the condition of the fetoplacental unit, depressed levels being associated with fetal distress. This assessment is now made by measuring plasma conjugated estriol, which is not usually affected by neomycin.

No reports linking the use of neomycin to congenital defects have been located. The Collaborative Perinatal Project monitored 50,282 mother-child pairs, 30 of which had 1st trimester exposure to neomycin (2). No evidence was found to suggest a relationship to large categories of major or minor malformations or to individual defects.

Breast Feeding Summary

No data available.

References

1. Pulkkinen M, Willman K. Reduction of maternal estrogen excretion by neomycin. Am J Obstet Gynecol 1973;115:1153.

2. Heinonen OP, Slone D, Shapiro S. *Birth Defects and Drugs in Pregnancy*. Littleton:Publishing Sciences Group, 1977:297–301.

Name: **NEOSTIGMINE**

Class: **Parasympathomimetic (Cholinergic)**   Risk Factor: C_M

Fetal Risk Summary

Neostigmine is a quaternary ammonium compound with anticholinesterase activity used in the diagnosis and treatment of myasthenia gravis. Because it is ionized at physiologic pH, it would not be expected to cross the placenta in significant amounts. Use of the drug during pregnancy, including the 1st trimester, has been reported for the treatment of maternal myasthenia gravis (1–10). One study reported 22 exposures to neostigmine in the 1st trimester (1). No relationship to congenital defects was found. A 1973 study described the use of 0.5 mg orally per day for 3 days in 27 pregnant patients (5–14 weeks) (2). One patient aborted and 26 went to term without complications. McNall and Jafarnia (3) consider neostigmine to be one of the drugs of choice for pregnant patients with myasthenia gravis. They also cautioned that intravenous anticholinesterases should not be used in pregnancy for fear of inducing premature labor and suggest that intramuscular neostigmine be used in place of intravenous edrophonium for diagnostic purposes. Other investigators have reported the safe use of neostigmine for myasthenia gravis in pregnancy (4–6).

Transient muscular weakness has been observed in about 20% of newborns of mothers with myasthenia gravis (9). The neonatal myasthenia is due to transplacental passage of anti-acetylcholine receptor immunoglobulin G antibodies (9).

Breast Feeding Summary

Because it is ionized at physiologic pH, neostigmine is apparently not excreted into breast milk (10, 11). However, pyridostigmine, another quaternary ammonium compound, is found in breast milk as determined by modern analytical techniques (see Pyridostigmine). Thus, the passage of neostigmine from maternal plasma to milk cannot be totally excluded at the present time.

References

1. Heinonen OP, Slone D, Shapiro S. *Birth Defects and Drugs in Pregnancy*. Littleton:Publishing Sciences Group, 1977:345–56.
2. Brunclik V, Hauser GA. Short-term therapy in secondary amenorrhea. Ther Umsch 1973;30:496–502.
3. McNall PG, Jafarnia MR. Management of myasthenia gravis in the obstetrical patient. Am J Obstet Gynecol 1965;92:518–25.
4. Foldes FF, McNall PG. Myasthenia gravis: a guide for anesthesiologists. Anesthesiology 1962;23:837–72.
5. Chambers DC, Hall JE, Boyce J. Myasthenia gravis and pregnancy. Obstet Gynecol 1967;29:597–603.
6. Hay DM. Myasthenia gravis and pregnancy. J Obstet Gynaecol Br Commonw 1969;76:323–9.
7. Blackhall MI, Buckley GA, Roberts DV, Roberts JB, Thomas BH, Wilson A. Drug-induced neonatal myasthenia. J Obstet Gynaecol Br Commonw 1969;76:157–62.
8. Eden RD, Gall SA. Myasthenia gravis and pregnancy: a reappraisal of thymectomy. Obstet Gynecol 1983;62:328–33.

9. Plauche WC. Myasthenia gravis in pregnancy: an update. Am J Obstet Gynecol 1979;135:691–7.
10. Fraser D, Turner JWA. Myastenia gravis and pregnancy. Proc R Soc Med 1963;56:379–81.
11. Wilson JT. Pharmacokinetics of drug excretion. In Wilson JT, ed. *Drugs in Breast Milk*. Balgowlah, Australia: ADIS Press, 1981:17.

Name: **NIACIN**

Class: **Vitamin**   Risk Factor: **A***

Fetal Risk Summary

Niacin, a B complex vitamin, is converted in humans to niacinamide, the active form of vitamin B_3. See Niacinamide.

[* Risk Factor C if used in doses above the RDA.]

Breast Feeding Summary

See Niacinamide.

Name: **NIACINAMIDE**

Class: **Vitamin**   Risk Factor: **A***

Fetal Risk Summary

Niacinamide, a water-soluble B complex vitamin, is an essential nutrient required for lipid metabolism, tissue respiration, and glycogenolysis (1). Both niacin, which is converted to niacinamide *in vivo*, and niacinamide are available commercially and are collectively known as vitamin B_3. The American RDA for niacinamide in pregnancy is 15–17 mg (2).

Only two reports have been located that link niacinamide with maternal or fetal complications. A 1948 study observed an association between niacinamide deficiency and pregnancy-induced hypertension (PIH, toxemia, etc.) (3). Other B complex vitamins have also been associated with this disease, but any relationship between vitamins and pregnancy-induced hypertension is controversial (see other B complex vitamins). One patient with hyperemesis gravidarum was seen with neuritis, reddened tongue, and psychosis (4). She was treated with 100 mg of niacin plus other B complex vitamins, resulting in rapid disappearance of her symptoms. The authors attributed her response to the niacin.

Niacinamide is actively transported to the fetus (5, 6). Higher concentrations are found in the fetus and newborn than in the mother (6–9). Deficiency of niacinamide in pregnancy is uncommon except in women with poor nutrition (7, 8). At term, mean niacinamide values in 174 mothers were 3.9 μg/ml (range 2.0–7.2) and in their newborns 5.8 μg/ml (range 3.0–10.5) (7). Conversion of the amino acid, tryptophan, to niacin and then to niacinamide is enhanced in pregnancy (10).

[* Risk Factor C if used in doses above the RDA.]

Breast Feeding Summary

Niacin, the precursor to niacinamide, is actively exceted in human breast milk (11). Reports on the excretion of niacinamide in milk have not been located, but it is probable that it also is actively transferred. In a study of lactating women with low nutritional status, supplementation with niacin in doses of 2.0–60.0 mg/day resulted in mean milk concentrations of 1.17–2.75 μg/ml (11). Milk concentrations were directly proportional to dietary intake. A 1983 English study measured niacin levels in pooled human milk obtained from preterm (26 mothers: 29–34 weeks) and term (35 mothers: 39 weeks or longer) patients (12). Preterm milk level rose from 0.65 μg/ml (colostrum) to 2.05 μg/ml (16–196 days) while term milk level increased over the same period from 0.50 to 1.82 μg/ml.

The American RDA for niacinamide during lactation is 18–20 mg (2). If the diet of the lactating woman adequately supplies this amount, supplementation with niacinamide is not needed. Maternal supplementation with the RDA for niacinamide is recommended for those patients with inadequate nutritional intake.

References

1. American Hospital Formulary Service. *Drug Information 1985*. Bethesda:American Society of Hospital Pharmacists, 1985:1685–7.
2. *Recommended Dietary Allowances*, ed 9. Washington, DC:National Academy of Sciences, 1980.
3. Hobson W. A dietary and clinical survey of pregnant women with particular reference to toxaemia of pregnancy. J Hyg 1948;46:198–216.
4. Hart BF, McConnell WT. Vitamin B factors in toxic psychosis of pregnancy and the puerperium. Am J Obstet Gynecol 1943;46:283.
5. Hill EP, Longo LD. Dynamics of maternal-fetal nutrient transfer. Fed Proc 1980;39:239–44.
6. Kaminetzky HA, Baker H, Frank O, Langer A. The effects of intravenously administered water-soluble vitamins during labor in normovitaminemic and hypovitaminemic gravidas on maternal and neonatal blood vitamin levels at delivery. Am J Obstet Gynecol 1974;120:697–703.
7. Baker H, Frank O, Thomson AD, Langer A, Munves ED, De Angelis B, Kaminetzky HA. Vitamin profile of 174 mothers and newborns at parturition. Am J Clin Nutr 1975;28:59–65.
8. Baker H, Frank O, Deangelis B, Feingold S, Kaminetzky HA. Role of placenta in maternal-fetal vitamin transfer in humans. Am J Obstet Gynecol 1981;141:792–6.
9. Baker H, Thind IS, Frank O, DeAngelis B, Caterini H, Lquria DB. Vitamin levels in low-birth-weight newborn infants and their mothers. Am J Obstet Gynecol 1977;129:521–4.
10. Wertz AW, Lojkin ME, Bouchard BS, Derby MB. Tryptophan-niacin relationships in pregnancy. Am J Nutr 1958;64:339–53.
11. Deodhar AD, Rajalakshmi R, Ramakrishnan CV. Studies on human lactation. Part III. Effect of dietary vitamin supplementation on vitamin contents of breast milk. Acta Paediatr Scand 1964;53:42–8.
12. Ford JE, Zechalko A, Murphy J, Brooke OG. Comparison of the B vitamin composition of milk from mothers of preterm and term babies. Arch Dis Child 1983;58:367–72.

Name: **NIALAMIDE**

Class: **Antidepressant**   Risk Factor: **C**

Fetal Risk Summary

No data available (see Phenelzine).

Breast Feeding Summary

No data available (see Phenelzine).

Name: **NICOTINYL ALCOHOL**

Class: **Vasodilator**

Risk Factor: **C**

Fetal Risk Summary

Nicotinyl alcohol is converted in the body to niacin, the active form. Only one report of its use in pregnancy has been located. The Collaborative Perinatal Project recorded one 1st trimester exposure to nicotinyl alcohol plus 14 other patients exposed to other vasodilators (1). From this small group of 15 patients, 4 malformed children were produced, a statistically significant incidence ($p < 0.02$). It was not stated if nicotinyl alcohol was taken by a mother of one of the affected infants. Although the data serve as a warning, the number of patients is so small that conclusions as to the relative safety of this drug in pregnancy cannot be made.

Breast Feeding Summary

No data available.

References

1. Heinonen OP, Slone D, Shapiro S. *Birth Defects and Drugs in Pregnancy*. Littleton:Publishing Sciences Group, 1977:371–3.

Name: **NICOUMALONE**

Class: **Anticoagulant**

Risk Factor: **D**

Fetal Risk Summary

See Coumarin Derivatives.

Breast Feeding Summary

See Coumarin Derivatives.

Name: **NIFEDIPINE**

Class: **Cardiac Drug**

Risk Factor: **C$_M$**

Fetal Risk Summary

Nifedipine, a calcium channel-blocking agent, has been used during the 2nd and 3rd trimesters for the treatment of severe hypertension (1). No fetal heart rate changes after reduction of maternal blood pressure or other adverse effects in the fetus or newborn were observed. Its use as a tocolytic agent has been described in two human studies totaling 11 patients (2, 3). In one patient, nifedipine, 20 mg three times daily, was given for a total of 55 days (3). Terbutaline was used concurrently for most of that time. No complications of the therapy were found in

310/nNifedipine–Nitrofurantoin

any of the infants. In follow-up examinations at 5–12 months of age, all were alive and well.

Although limited use in humans has not demonstrated toxicity, intravenous nifedipine in pregnant rhesus monkeys has been associated with fetal hypoxemia and acidosis (4). As a consequence, nifedipine should be used with caution until this toxicity has been more carefully studied.

Breast Feeding Summary

No data available.

References

1. Walters BNJ, Redman CWG. Treatment of severe pregnancy-associated hypertension with the calcium antagonist nifedipine. Br J Obstet Gynaecol 1984;91:330–6.
2. Ulmsten U, Andersson K-E, Wingerup L. Treatment of premature labor with the calcium antagonist nifedipine. Arch Gynecol 1980;229:1–5.
3. Kaul AF, Osathanondh R, Safon LE, Frigoletto FD Jr, Friedman PA. The management of preterm labor with the calcium channel-blocking agent nifedipine combined with the β-memetic terbutaline. Drug Intell Clin Pharm 1985;19:369–71.
4. Ducsay CA, Cook MJ, Veille JC, Novy MJ. Nifedipine tocolysis in pregnant rhesus monkeys: maternal and fetal cardiorespiratory effects. Abstract No. 79, Society of Perinatal Obstetricians Annual Meeting, Las Vegas, February, 1985.

Name: **NITROFURANTOIN**

Class: **Urinary Germicide**   Risk Factor: **B**

Fetal Risk Summary

No reports linking the use of nitrofurantoin with congenital defects have been located. One manufacturer (Norwich Eaton Pharmaceuticals) has collected over 1,700 case histories describing the use of this drug during various stages of pregnancy (95 references) (1). None of the reports observed deleterious effects on the fetus. In a published study, a retrospective analysis of 91 pregnancies in which nitrofurantoin was used yielded no evidence of fetal toxicity (2). Other studies have also supported the safety of this drug in pregnancy (3).

Nitrofurantoin is capable of inducing hemolytic anemia in glucose-6-phosphate dehydrogenase-deficient patients and in patients whose red blood cells are deficient in reduced glutathione (4). Since the red blood cells of newborns are deficient in reduced glutathione, the manufacturer's package insert (Norwich Eaton) carries a warning against use of the drug at term. However, hemolytic anemia in the newborn as a result of *in utero* exposure to nitrofurantoin has not been reported.

Nitrofurantoin has been reported to cause discoloration of the primary teeth when given to an infant, and by implication, this could occur from *in utero* exposure (5). However, the fact that the baby was also given a 14-day course of tetracycline and the lack of other confirming reports makes the likelihood for a causal relationship remote (6).

When given orally in high doses of 10 mg/kg/day to young males, nitrofurantoin may produce slight to moderate transient spermatogenic arrest (7). The lower doses used clinically do not seem to have this effect.

Breast Feeding Summary

Nitrofurantoin is excreted into breast milk in very low concentrations. The drug could not be detected in 20 samples from mothers receiving 100 mg four times daily (8). In a second study, nine mothers were given 100 mg every 6 hours for 1 day, then either 100 or 200 mg the next morning (9). Only two of the four patients receiving the 200-mg dose excreted measurable amounts of nitrofurantoin, 0.3–0.5 μg/ml. Although these amounts are negligible, the authors cautioned that infants with glucose-6-phosphate dehydrogenase deficiency may develop hemolytic anemia from this exposure.

References

1. Norwich Eaton Pharmaceuticals, 1981. Personal communication.
2. Hailey FJ, Fort H, Williams JC, Hammers B. Foetal safety of nitrofurantoin macrocrystals therapy during pregnancy: a retrospective analysis. J Int Med Res 1983;11:364–9.
3. Lenke RR, VanDorsten JP, Schifrin BS. Pyelonephritis in pregnancy: a prospective randomized trial to prevent recurrent disease evaluating suppressive therapy with nitrofurantoin and close surveillance. Am J Obstet Gynecol 1983;146:953–7.
4. Powell RD, DeGowin RL, Alving AS. Nitrofurantoin-induced hemolysis. J Lab Clin Med 1963;62:1002–3.
5. Ball JS, Ferguson AN. Permanent discoloration of primary dentition by nitrofurantoin. Br Med J 1962;2:1103.
6. Duckworth R, Swallow JN. Nitrofurantoin and teeth. Br Med J 1962;2:1617.
7. Nelson WO, Bunge RG. The effect of therapeutic dosages of nitrofurantoin (Furadantin) upon spermatogenesis in man. J Urol 1957;77:275–81.
8. Hosbach RE, Foster RB. Absence of nitrofurantoin from human milk. JAMA 1967;202:1057.
9. Varsano I, Fischl J, Shochet SB. The excretion of orally ingested nitrofurantoin in human milk. J Pediatr 1973;82:886–7.

Name: **NITROGLYCERIN**

Class: **Vasodilator**   Risk Factor: C_M

Fetal Risk Summary

Nitroglycerin is a rapid acting, short duration vasodilator used primarily for the treatment or prevention of angina pectoris. Due to the nature of its indication, experience in pregnancy is limited. The drug has been used to control severe hypertension during cesarean section (1, 2). No hypotension or other effects of the drug were observed in the newborn infants. Use of nitroglycerin sublingually for angina during pregnancy without fetal harm has also been reported (3). The Collaborative Perinatal Project recorded 7 1st trimester exposures to nitroglycerin and amyl nitrite plus 8 other patients exposed to other vasodilators (4). From this small group of 15 patients, 4 malformed children were produced, a statistically significant incidence ($p < 0.02$). The data did not indicate if nitroglycerin was taken by any of the mothers of the affected infants. Although the data serve as a warning, the number of patients is so small that conclusions as to the relative safety of nitroglycerin in pregnancy cannot be made.

Breast Feeding Summary

No data available.

References

1. Snyder SW, Wheeler AS, James FM III. The use of nitroglycerin to control severe hypertension of pregnancy during cesarean section. Anesthesiology 1979;51:563–4.
2. Hood DD, Dewan DM, James FM III, Bogard TD, Floyd HM. The use of nitroglycerin in preventing the hypertensive response to tracheal intubation in severe preeclamptics. Anesthesiology 1983;59:A423.
3. Diro M, Beydown SN, Jaramillo B, O'Sullivan MJ, Kieval J. Successful pregnancy in a woman with a left ventricular cardiac aneurysm: a case report. J Reprod Med 1983;28:559–63.
4. Heinonen OP, Slone D, Shapiro S. *Birth Defects and Drugs in Pregnancy*. Littleton:Publishing Sciences Group, 1977:371–3.

Name: **NORETHINDRONE**

Class: **Progestogenic Hormone**   Risk Factor: **D**

Fetal Risk Summary

Norethindrone is a progestogen derived from 19-nortestosterone. It is used in oral contraceptives and as a hormonal pregnancy test (no longer available in the United States). Masculinization of the female fetus has been associated with norethindrone (1–3). Jacobson (2) observed an 18% incidence of masculinization of female infants born to mothers given norethindrone. A more conservative estimate for the incidence of masculinization due to synthetic progestogens has been reported as 0.3% (4). The Collaborative Perinatal Project monitored 866 mother-child pairs with 1st trimester exposure to progestational agents (including 132 with exposure to norethindrone) (5). Evidence of an increased risk of malformation was found for norethindrone. An increase in the expected frequency of cardiovascular defects and hypospadias was also observed for progestational agents as a group (6, 7). Re-evaluation of these data in terms of timing of exposure, vaginal bleeding in early pregnancy, and previous maternal obstetrical history, however, failed to support an association between female sex hormones and cardiac malformations (8). An earlier study also failed to find any relationship with nongenital malformations (3). Dillion (9) observed two infants with malformations who had been exposed to norethindrone. The congenital defects included spina bifida and hydrocephalus.

Breast Feeding Summary

Norethindrone exhibits a dose-dependent suppression of lactation (10). Lower infant weight gain, decreased milk production, and decreased composition of nitrogen and protein content of human milk have been associated with norethindrone and estrogenic agents (11–14). The magnitude of these changes is low. However, the changes in milk production and composition may be of nutritional importance in malnourished mothers. If breast-feeding is desired, the lowest dose of oral contraceptives should be chosen. Monitoring of infant weight gain and the possible need for nutritional supplementation should be considered.

References

1. Hagler S, Schultz A, Hankin H, Kunstadter RN. Fetal effects of steroid therapy during pregnancy. Am J Dis Child 1963;106:586–90.
2. Jacobson BD. Hazards of norethindrone therapy during pregnancy. Am J Obstet Gynecol 1962;84:962–8.

3. Wilson JG, Brent RL. Are female sex hormones teratogenic? Am J Obstet Gynecol 1981;141:567–80.
4. Bongiovanni AM, McFadden AJ. Steroids during pregnancy and possible fetal consequences. Fertil Steril 1960;11:181–4.
5. Heinonen OP, Slone D, Shapiro S. *Birth Defects and Drugs in Pregnancy*. Littleton:Publishing Sciences Group, 1977:389, 391.
6. *Ibid*, 394.
7. Heinonen OP, Slone D, Monson RR, Hook EB, Shapiro S. Cardiovascular birth defects and antenatal exposure to female sex hormones. N Engl J Med 1977;296:67–70.
8. Wiseman RA, Dodds-Smith IC. Cardiovascular birth defects and antenatal exposure to female sex hormones: a reevaluation of some base data. Teratology 1984;30:359–70.
9. Dillon S. Congenital malformations and hormones in pregnancy. Br Med J 1976;2:1446.
10. Guiloff E, Ibarra-Polo A, Zanartu J, Toscanini C, Mischler TW, Gomez-Rogers C. Effect of contraception on lactation. Am J Obstet Gynecol 1974;118:42–5.
11. Karim M, Ammarr R, El-Mahgoubh S, El-Ganzoury B, Fikri F, Abdou I. Injected progestogen and lactation. Br Med J 1971;1:200–3.
12. Kora SJ. Effect of oral contraceptives on lactation. Fertil Steril 1969;20:419–23.
13. Miller GH, Hughes LR. Lactation and genital involution effects of a new low-dose oral contraceptive on breast-feeding mothers and their infants. Obstet Gynecol 1970;35:44–50.
14. Lonnerdal B, Forsum E, Hambraeus L. Effect of oral contraceptives on composition and volume of breast milk. Am J Clin Nutr 1980;33:816–24.

Name: **NORETHYNODREL**

Class: **Progestogenic Hormone**   Risk Factor: **D**

Fetal Risk Summary

Norethynodrel is a progestogen derived from 19-nortestosterone. It is used in oral contraceptive agents and as a hormonal pregnancy test (no longer available in the United States). Masculinization of the female infant has been associated with norethynodrel (1, 2). The Collaborative Perinatal Project monitored 866 mother-child pairs with 1st trimester exposure to progestational agents (including 154 with exposure to norethynodrel) (3). Fetuses exposed to norethynodrel were not at an increased risk for malformation. However, an increase in the expected frequency of cardiovascular defects and hypospadias was observed for progestational agents as a group (4, 5). Re-evaluation of these data in terms of timing of exposure, vaginal bleeding in early pregnancy, and previous maternal obstetrical history, however, failed to support an association between female sex hormones and cardiac malformations (6). An earlier study also failed to find any relationship with nongenital malformations (1). Dillion (7) observed three infants who were exposed to norethynodrel and mestranol during the 1st trimester. The congenital defects reported included atrial and ventricular septal defects (one infant), hypospadias (one infant), and inguinal hernias (two infants).

Breast Feeding Summary

Norethynodrel exhibits a dose-dependent suppression of lactation (8). Lower infant weight gain, decreased milk production, and decreased composition of nitrogen and protein content of human milk have been associated with similar synthetic progestogens and estrogen products (see Norethindrone, Mestranol, Ethinyl Estradiol, Oral Contraceptives) (9–11). The magnitude of these changes is low. However, the changes in milk production and composition may be of nutritional importance in malnourished mothers. If breast-feeding is desired, the lowest dose of oral contraceptives should be chosen. Monitoring of infant weight gain and the possible need for nutritional supplementation should be considered.

References

1. Wilson JG, Brent RL. Are female sex hormones teratogenic? Am J Obstet Gynecol 1981;141:567–80.
2. Hagler S. Schultz A, Hankin H, Kunstadter RN. Fetal effects of steroid therapy during pregnancy. Am J Dis Child 1963;106:586–90.
3. Heinonen OP, Slone D, Shapiro S. *Birth Defects and Drugs in Pregnancy*. Littleton:Publishing Sciences Group, 1977:389, 391.
4. *Ibid*, 394.
5. Heinonen OP, Slone D, Monson RR, Hook EB, Shapiro S. Cardiovascular birth defects and antenatal exposure to female hormones. N Engl J Med 1977;296:67–70.
6. Wiseman RA, Dodds-Smith IC. Cardiovascular birth defects and antenatal exposure to female sex hormones: a reevaluation of some base data. Teratology 1984;30:359–70.
7. Dillion S. Congenital malformations and hormones in pregnancy. Br Med J 1976;2:1446.
8. Guiloff E, Ibarra-Polo A, Zanartu J, Toscanini C, Mischler TW, Gomez-Rogers C. Effect of contraception on lactation. Am J Obstet Gynecol 1974;118:42–5.
9. Kora SJ. Effect of oral contraceptives on lactation. Fertil Steril 1969;20:419–23.
10. Miller GH, Hughes LR. Lactation and genital involution effects of a new low-dose oral contraceptive on breast-feeding mothers and their infants. Obstet Gynecol 1970;35:44–50.
11. Lonnerdal B, Forsum E, Hambraeus L. Effect of oral contraceptives on composition and volume of breast milk. Am J Clin Nutr 1980;33:816–24.

Name: **NORGESTREL**
Class: **Progestogenic Hormone** Risk Factor: **D**

Fetal Risk Summary

Norgestrel is commonly used as an oral contraceptive either alone or in combination with estrogens (see Oral Contraceptives).

Breast Feeding Summary

No data available (see Oral Contraceptives).

Name: **NORTRIPTYLINE**
Class: **Antidepressant** Risk Factor: **D**

Fetal Risk Summary

Limb reduction anomalies have been reported with nortriptyline (1, 2). However, one of these children was not exposed until after the critical period for limb development (3). The second infant was also exposed to sulfamethizole and heavy cigarette smoking (1). Evaluation of data from 86 patients with 1st trimester exposure to amitriptyline, the active precursor of nortriptyline, does not support the drug as a major cause of congenital limb deformities (see Amitriptyline). Urinary retention in the neonate has been associated with maternal use of nortriptyline (4).

Breast Feeding Summary

Nortriptyline is excreted into breast milk in low concentrations (5–7). A milk level in one patient was 59 ng/ml, representing a milk:serum ratio of 0.7 (6). Nortriptyline was not been detected in the serum of breast-fed infants when their mothers were taking the drug (6, 7). The significance of chronic exposure is not known (see also Amitriptyline).

References

1. Bourke GM. Antidepressant teratogenicity? Lancet 1974;1:98.
2. McBride WG. Limb deformities associated with iminobenzyl hydrochloride. Med J Aust 1972;1:492.
3. Australian Drug Evaluation Committee. Tricyclic antidepressants and limb reduction deformities. Med J Aust 1973;1:768–9.
4. Shearer WT, Schreiner RL, Marshall RE. Urinary retention in a neonate secondary to maternal ingestion of nortriptyline. J Pediatr 1972;81:570–2.
5. Bader TF, Newman K. Amitriptyline in human breast milk and the nursing infant's serum. Am J Psychiatry 1980;137:855–6.
6. Erickson SH, Smith GH, Heidrich F. Tricyclics and breast feeding. Am J Psychiatry 1979;136:1483.
7. Brixen-Rasmussen L, Halgrener J, Jorgensen A. Amitriptyline and nortriptyline excretion in human breast milk. Psychopharmacology (Berlin) 1982;76:94–5.

Name: **NOVOBIOCIN**

Class: **Antibiotic** Risk Factor: **C**

Fetal Risk Summary

No reports linking the use of novobiocin with congenital defects have been located. One study listed 21 patients exposed to the drug in the 1st trimester (1). No association with malformations was found. Since novobiocin may cause jaundice due to inhibition of glucuronyl transferase, its use near term is not recommended (2).

Breast Feeding Summary

Novobiocin is excreted into breast milk. Concentrations up to 7 μg/ml have been reported with milk:plasma ratios of 0.1–0.25 (3, 4). While adverse effects have not been reported, three potential problems exist for the nursing infant: modification of bowel flora, direct effects on the infant, and interference with the interpretation of culture results if a fever work-up is required.

References

1. Heinonen OP, Slone D, Shapiro S. *Birth Defects and Drugs in Pregnancy*. Littleton:Publishing Sciences Group, 1977:297, 301.
2. Weistein L. Antibiotics. IV. Miscellaneous antimicrobial, antifungal, and antiviral agents. In Goodman LS, Gilman A, eds. *The Pharmacological Basis of Therapeutics*, ed 4. New York:Macmillan Publishing Co, 1970:1292.
3. Knowles JA. Excretion of drugs in milk—a review. J Pediatr 1965;66:1068–82.
4. Anderson PO. Drugs and breast feeding—a review. Drug Intell Clin Pharm 1977;11:208–23.

Name: **NYLIDRIN**

Class: **Vasodilator**   Risk Factor: **C$_M$**

Fetal Risk Summary

Nylidrin is a β-adrenergic receptor stimulant used as a vasodilator in the United States. The drug has been studied in Europe as a tocolytic agent for premature labor and for the treatment of hypertension in pregnancy (1–7). Systolic blood pressure is usually unchanged, with a fall in total peripheral resistance greater than the decrease in diastolic pressure (8, 9). Although maternal hyperglycemia has been observed, especially in diabetic patients, this or other serious adverse effects were not reported in the above studies in mothers or in newborns.

Breast Feeding Summary

No data available.

References

1. Neubuser D. Comparative investigation of two inhibitors of labour (TV 399 and buphenin). Geburtshilfe Fraunheilkd 1972;32:781–6.
2. Castren O, Gummerus M, Saarikoski S. Treatment of imminent premature labour. Acta Obstet Gynecol Scand 1975;54:95–100.
3. Gummerus M. Prevention of premature birth with nylidrin and verapamil. Z Geburtshilfe Perinatol 1975;179:261–6.
4. Wolff F, Bolte A, Berg R. Does an additional administration of acetylsalicylic acid reduce the requirement of betamimetics in tocolytic treatment? Geburtshilfe Fraunheilkd 1981;41:293–6.
5. Hofer U, Ammann K. The oral tocolytic longtime therapy and its effects on the child. Ther Umsch 1978;35:417–21.
6. Retzke VU, Schwarz R, Lanckner W, During R. Dilatol for hypertension therapy in pregnancy. Zentralbl Gynaekol 1979;101:1034–8.
7. During VR, Mauch I. Effects of nylidrin (Dilatol) on blood pressure of hypertensive patients in advanced pregnancy. Zentralbl Gynaekol 1980;102:193–8.
8. Retzke VU, Schwarz R, Barten G. Cardiovascular effects of nylidrin (Dilatol) in pregnancy. Zentralbl Gynaekol 1976;98:1059–65.
9. During VR, Reincke R. Action of nylidrin (Dilatol) on utero-placental blood supply. Zentralbl Gynaekol 1981;103:214–9.

Name: **NYSTATIN**

Class: **Antifungal Antibiotic**   Risk Factor: **B**

Fetal Risk Summary

Nystatin is poorly absorbed after oral administration and from intact skin and mucous membranes. The Collaborative Perinatal Project found a possible association with congenital malformations after 142 1st trimester exposures, but this was probably due to its use as an adjunct to tetracycline therapy (1). No association was found following 230 exposures anytime in pregnancy (2). Other investigators have reported its safe use in pregnancy (3–5).

Breast Feeding Summary

Since nystatin is poorly absorbed, if at all, serum and milk levels would not occur.

References

1. Heinonen OP, Slone D, Shapiro S. *Birth Defects and Drugs in Pregnancy*. Littleton:Publishing Sciences Group, 1977:313.
2. *Ibid*, 435.
3. Culbertson C. Monistat: a new fungicide for treatment of vulvovaginal candidiasis. Am J Obstet Gynecol 1974;120:973–6.
4. David JE, Frudenfeld JH, Goddard JL. Comparative evaluation of Monistat and Mycostatin in the treatment of vulvovaginal candidiasis. Obstet Gynecol 1974;44:403–6.
5. Wallenburg HCS, Wladimiroff JW. Recurrence of vulvovaginal candidosis during pregnancy. Comparison of miconazole vs nystatin treatment. Obstet Gynecol 1976;48:491–4.

Name: **OLEANDOMYCIN**

Class: **Antibiotic**   Risk Factor: **C**

Fetal Risk Summary

No reports linking the use of oleandomycin or its triacetyl ester, troleandomycin, with congenital defects have been located. One study listed nine patients exposed to the drugs in the 1st trimester (1). No association with malformations was found.

Breast Feeding Summary

No data available.

References

1. Heinonen OP, Slone D, Shapiro S. *Birth Defects and Drugs in Pregnancy*. Littleton:Publishing Sciences Group, 1977:297, 301.

Name: **OPIPRAMOL**

Class: **Antidepressant**   Risk Factor: **D**

Fetal Risk Summary

No data available (see Imipramine).

Breast Feeding Summary

No data available (see Imipramine).

Name: **OPIUM**

Class: **Narcotic Antidiarrheal**   Risk Factor: **B***

Fetal Risk Summary

The effects of opium are due to morphine (see Morphine). The Collaborative Perinatal Project monitored 50,282 mother-child pairs, 36 of which had 1st trimester exposure to opium (1). For use anytime during pregnancy, 181 exposures were recorded (2). Although these numbers are small, a possible relationship may exist between the use of this drug and major and minor malformations. Further, a possible association with inguinal hernia (seven cases) after anytime use was observed (3). The statistical significance of these associations is unknown, and independent confirmation is required.

Narcotic withdrawal was observed in a newborn whose mother was treated for regional ileitis with deodorized tincture of opium during the 2nd and 3rd trimesters (4). Symptoms of withdrawal in the infant began at 48 hours of age.

[* Risk Factor D if used for prolonged periods or in high doses at term.]

Breast Feeding Summary

See Morphine.

References

1. Heinonen OP, Slone D, Shapiro S. *Birth Defects and Drugs in Pregnancy*. Littleton:Publishing Sciences Group, 1977:287–295.
2. *Ibid*, 424.
3. *Ibid*, 485.
4. Fisch GR, Henley WL. Symptoms of narcotic withdrawal in a newborn infant secondary to medical therapy of the mother. Pediatrics 1961;28:852–3.

Name: **ORAL CONTRACEPTIVES**

Class: **Estrogenic/Progestogenic Hormones**   Risk Factor: **X**

Fetal Risk Summary

Oral contraceptives contain a 19-nortestosterone progestin and a synthetic estrogen (see Mestranol, Norethindrone, Norethynodrel, Ethinyl Estradiol, Progesterone, Hydroxyprogesterone, Ethisterone). Because oral contraceptives are primarily combination products, it is difficult to separate entirely the fetal effects of progestogens and estrogens. Ambani and co-workers in 1977 (1) and Wilson and Brent in 1981 (2) reviewed the effects of these hormones on the fetus (133 references). Several potential problems were discussed: congenital heart defects, central nervous system defects, limb reduction malformations, general malformations, and modified development of sexual organs. Except for the latter category, no firm evidence has appeared that establishes a causal relationship between oral contraceptives and various congenital anomalies. The acronym VACTERL (vertebral, anal, cardiac, tracheal, esophageal, renal or radial, and limb) has been used to describe the fetal malformations produced by oral contraceptives or the related hormonal pregnancy test preparations (no longer available in the United States) (2, 3). The use of this acronym should probably be abandoned in favor of more conventional terminology as a large variety of malformations have been reported with estrogen/progestogen-containing products (1–11). The Population Council estimates that even if the study findings for VACTERL malformations are accurate, such abnormalities would occur in only 0.07% of the pregnancies exposed to oral contraceptives (12). Finally, Wilson and Brent (2) concluded from their review that the risk to the fetus for nongenital malformations after *in utero* exposure to these agents is small, if indeed it exists at all.

In contrast to the above, the effect of estrogens and some synthetic progestogens on the development of the sexual organs is well established (2). Masculinization of the female infant has been associated with norethindrone, norethynodrel, hydroxyprogesterone, medroxyprogesterone, and diethylstilbestrol (2, 13, 14). Bongiovanni and McFadden (15) reported that the incidence of masculinization of female infants exposed to synthetic progestogens is 0.3%. Pseudohermaphroditism in the male infant is not a problem, due to the low doses of estrogen employed in oral contraceptives (14).

McConnell and co-workers (16) reported increased serum bilirubin in neonates of mothers taking oral contraceptives or progestogens before and after conception. Icterus occasionally reached clinically significant levels in infants whose mothers were exposed to the progestogens.

Concern that oral contraceptives may act as a risk factor for preeclampsia has been suggested on the basis of the known effects of oral contraceptives on blood pressure (16 references) (17). In a retrospective controlled review of 341 patients, no association was found between this effect and oral contraceptives.

Possible interactions between oral contraceptives and tetracycline, rifampin, ampicillin, or chloramphenicol, resulting in pregnancy have been reported (18–25). The mechanism for this interaction may involve the interruption of the enterhepatic circulation of contraceptive steroids by inhibition of gut hydrolysis of steroid conjugates, resulting in lower concentrations of circulating steroids.

Breast Feeding Summary

Use of oral contraceptives during lactation has been associated with shortened duration of lactation, decreased infant weight gain, decreased milk production, and decreased composition of nitrogen and protein content of milk (26–29). The American Academy of Pediatrics has reviewed this subject (30) (37 references). Although the magnitude of these changes is low, the changes in milk production and composition may be of nutritional importance in malnourished mothers.

In general, progestin-only contraceptives demonstrate no consistent alteration of breast milk composition, volume, or duration of lactation (30). The composition and volume of breast milk will vary considerably even in the absence of steroidal contraceptives (29). Both estrogens and progestins cross into milk. An infant consuming 600 ml of breast milk daily from a mother using contraceptives containing 50 μg of ethinyl estradiol will probably receive a daily dose in the range of 10 ng (30). This is in the same range as the amount of natural estradiol received by infants of mothers not using oral contraceptives. Progestins also pass into breast milk, although naturally occurring progestins have not been identified. One study estimated 0.03, 0.15, and 0.3 μg of d-norgestrel per 600 ml of milk from mothers receiving 30, 150, and 250 μg of the drug, respectively (31). A milk:plasma ratio of 0.15 for norgestrel was calculated by the authors (31). A ratio of 0.16 has been calculated for lynestrol (31, 32).

Reports of adverse effects are lacking except for one child with mild breast tenderness and hypertrophy who was exposed to large doses of estrogen (30). If breast-feeding is desired, the lowest effective dose of oral contraceptives should be chosen. Infant weight gain should be monitored and the possible need for nutritional supplements should be considered.

References

1. Ambani LM, Joshi NJ, Vaidya RA, Devi PK. Are hormonal contraceptives teratogenic? Fertil Steril 1977;28:791–7.

2. Wilson JG, Brent RL. Are female sex hormones teratogenic? Am J Obstet Gynecol 1981;141:567–80.
3. Corcoran R, Entwistle GC. VACTERL congenital malformations and the male fetus. Lancet 1975;2:981–2.
4. Nora JJ, Nora AH. Can the pill cause birth defects. N Engl J Med 1974;294:731–2.
5. Kasan PN, Andrews J. Oral contraceptives and congenital abnormalities. Br J Obstet Gynaecol 1980;87:545–51.
6. Kullander S, Kallen B. A prospective study of drugs and pregnancy. Acta Obstet Gynecol Scand 1976;55:221–4.
7. Oakley GP, Flynt JW. Hormonal pregnancy test and congenital malformations. Lancet 1973; 2:256–7.
8. Savolainen E, Saksela E, Saxen L. Teratogenic hazards of oral contraceptives analyzed in a national malformation register. Am J Obstet Gynecol 1981;140:521–4.
9. Frost O. Tracheo-oesophageal fistula associated with hormonal contraception during pregnancy. Br Med J 1976;3:978.
10. Redline RW, Abramowsky CR. Transposition of the great vessels in an infant exposed to massive doses of oral contraceptives. Am J Obstet Gynecol 1981;141:468–9.
11. Farb HF, Thomason J, Carandang FS, Sampson MB, Spellacy WH. Anencephaly twins and HLA-B27. J Reprod Med 1980;25:166–9.
12. Department of Medical and Public Affairs. Population Reports. The George Washington University Medical Center, Washington, DC, 1975;2:A 29–51.
13. Bongiovanni AM, DiGeorge AM, Grumbach MM. Masculinization of the female infant associated with estrogenic therapy alone during gestation: four cases. J Clin Endocrinol Metab 1959;19:1004–11.
14. Hagler S, Schultz A, Hankin H, Kunstadter RH. Fetal effects of steroid therapy during pregnancy. Am J Dis Child 1963;106:586–90.
15. Bongiovanni AM, McFadden AJ. Steroids during pregnancy and possible fetal consequences. Fertil Steril 1960;11:181–4.
16. McConnell JB, Glasgow JF, McNair R. Effect on neonatal jaundice of oestrogens and progestogens taken before and after conception. Br Med J 1973;3:605–7.
17. Bracken MB, Srisuphan W. Oral contraception as a risk factor for preeclampsia. Am J Obstet Gynecol 1982;142:191–6.
18. Bacon JF, Shenfield GM. Pregnancy attributable to interaction between tetracycline and oral contraceptives. Br Med J 1980;1:283.
19. Stockley I. Interactions with oral contraceptives. Pharm J 1976;216:140.
20. Reiners D, Nockefinck L, Breurer H. Rifampin and the "pill" do not go well together. JAMA 1974;227:608.
21. Dosseter EJ. Drug interactions with oral contraceptives. Br Med J 1975;1:1967.
22. Pullskinnen MO, Williams K. Reduced maternal plasma and urinary estriol during ampicillin treatment. Am J Obstet Gynecol 1971;109:895–6.
23. Friedman GI, Huneke AL, Kim MH, Powell J. The effect of ampicillin on oral contraceptive effectiveness. Obstet Gynecol 1980;55:33–7.
24. Back DJ, Breckenridge AM. Drug interactions with oral contraceptives. IPFF Med Bull 1978; 12:1–2.
25. Orme ML, Back DJ. Therapy with oral contraceptive steroids and antibiotics J Antimicrob Chemother 1979;5:124–6.
26. Miller GH, Hughes LR. Lactation and genital involution effects of a new low-dose oral contraceptive on breast-feeding mothers and their infants. Obstet Gynecol 1970;35:44–50.
27. Kora SJ. Effect of oral contraceptives on lactation. Fertil Steril 1969;20:419–23.
28. Guiloff E, Ibarra-Polo A, Zanartu J, Tuscanini C, Mischler TW, Gomez-Rodgers C. Effect of contraception on lactation. Am J Obstet Gynecol 1974;118:42–5.
29. Lonnerdal B, Forsum E. Hambraeus L. Effect of oral contraceptives on consumption and volume of breast milk. Am J Clin Nutr 1980;33:816–24.
30. Committee on Drugs, American Academy of Pediatrics. Breast-feeding and contraception. Pediatrics 1981;68:138–40.
31. Nilsson S, Nygren KC, Johansson EDB. d-Norgestrel concentrations in maternal plasma, milk, and child plasma during administration of oral contraceptives to nursing women. Am J Obstet Gynecol 1977;129:178–83.

32. van der Molen HJ, Hart PG, Wijmenga HG. Studies with 4-$_{14}$C-lynestrol in normal and lactating women. Acta Endocrinol (Copenh) 1969;61:255–74.

Name: **ORPHENADRINE**

Class: **Parasympatholytic**   Risk Factor: **C**

Fetal Risk Summary

Orphenadrine is an anticholinergic agent used in the treatment of parkinsonism. No reports of its use in pregnancy have been located (see also Atropine).

Breast Feeding Summary

No data available (see also Atropine).

Name: **OUABAIN**

Class: **Cardiac Glycoside**   Risk Factor: **B**

Fetal Risk Summary

See Digitalis.

Breast Feeding Summary

See Digitalis.

Name: **OXACILLIN**

Class: **Antibiotic**   Risk Factor: **B$_M$**

Fetal Risk Summary

Oxacillin is a penicillin antibiotic (see also Penicillin G). The drug crosses the placenta in low concentrations. Cord serum and amniotic fluid levels were less than 0.3 μg/ml in 15 of 18 patients given 500 mg orally 0.5–4 hours prior to cesarean section (1). No effects were seen in the infants.

No reports linking the use of oxacillin with congenital defects have been located. The Collaborative Perinatal Project monitored 50,282 mother-child pairs, 3,546 of which had 1st trimester exposure to penicillin derivatives (2). For use anytime during pregnancy, 7,171 exposures were recorded (3). In neither case was evidence found to suggest a relationship to large categories of major or minor malformations or to individual defects.

An interaction between oxacillin and oral contraceptives resulting in pregnancy has been reported (4). Other penicillins (e.g., see Ampicillin) have been suspected of this interaction, but not all investigators believe it occurs. Although controversial, an alternate means of contraception may be a practical solution if both drugs are consumed at the same time.

Breast Feeding Summary

Oxacillin is excreted in breast milk in low concentrations. Although no adverse effects have been reported, three potential problems exist for the nursing infant: modification of bowel flora, direct effects on the infant (e.g., allergic response), and interference with the interpretation of culture results if a fever work-up is required.

References

1. Prigot A, Froix C, Rubin E. Absorption, diffusion, and excretion of new penicillin, oxacillin. Antimicrob Agents Chemother 1962:402–10.
2. Heinonen OP, Slone D, Shapiro S. *Birth Defects and Drugs in Pregnancy*. Littleton:Publishing Sciences Group, 1977:297–313.
3. *Ibid*, 435.
4. Silber TJ. Apparent oral contraceptive failure associated with antibiotic administration. J Adolesc Health Care 1983;4:287–9.

Name: **OXAZEPAM**

Class: **Sedative**   Risk Factor: **C**

Fetal Risk Summary

Oxazepam is an active metabolite of diazepam (see also Diazepam). It is a member of the benzodiazepine group. The drug in both free and conjugated forms crosses the placenta, achieving average cord:maternal serum ratios during the 2nd trimester of 0.6 and at term of 1.1 (1). Large variations between patients for placental transfer have been observed (1–3). Passage of oxazepam is slower than that of diazepam, but the clinical significance of this is unknown (4). No reports linking the use of oxazepam with congenital defects have been located. Other drugs in this group have been suspected of causing fetal malformations (see also Diazepam or Chlordiazepoxide). Two reports have suggested that the use of oxazepam in preeclampsia would be safer for the newborn infant than diazepam (5, 6).

Breast Feeding Summary

Specific data relating to oxazepam usage in lactating women have not been located. Oxazepam has been detected in the urine of an infant exposed to high doses of diazepam during lactation (7). The infant was lethargic and demonstrated an electroencephalogram pattern compatible with sedative medication (see Diazepam).

References

1. Kangas L, Erkkola R, Kanto J, Eronen M. Transfer of free and conjugated oxazepam across the human placenta. Eur J Clin Pharmacol 1980;17:301–4.
2. Kanto J, Erkkola R, Sellman R. Perinatal metabolism of diazepam. Br Med J 1974;1:641–2.
3. Mandelli M, Morselli PL, Nordio S, et al. Placental transfer of diazepam and its disposition in the newborn. Clin Pharmacol Ther 1975;17:564–72.

4. Kanto JH. Use of benzodiazepines during pregnancy, labour and lactation, with particular reference to pharmacokinetic considerations. Drugs 1982;23:354–80.
5. Gillberg C. "Floppy infant syndrome" and maternal diazepam. Lancet 1977;2:612–3.
6. Drury KAD, Spalding E, Donaldson D, Rutherford D. Floppy-infant syndrome: is oxazepam the answer? Lancet 1977;2:1126–7.
7. Patrick MJ, Tilstone WJ, Reavey P. Diazepam and breast-feeding. Br Med J 1972; 1:542–3.

Name: **OXPRENOLOL**

Class: **Sympatholytic (β-Adrenergic Blocker)**   Risk Factor: **C**

Fetal Risk Summary

Oxprenolol, a nonselective β-adrenergic blocking agent, has been used for the treatment of hypertension occurring during pregnancy (1–4). The drug crosses the placenta, but mean fetal serum levels at term are only about 25–37% of maternal concentrations (4, 5).

No fetal malformations or other fetal adverse effects attributable to oxprenolol have been reported, but experience during the 1st trimester is lacking. The drug has been compared with methyldopa in two studies of pregnant hypertensive women (1, 2). In one of these studies, oxprenolol-exposed infants were significantly larger, 3,051 g vs 2,654 g, than offspring of methyldopa-treated mothers (1). The difference was thought to be due to the greater maternal plasma volume expansion and placental growth observed in the β-blocker group (1). A 1983 study, however, found no difference between oxprenolol- and methyldopa-treated groups in birth weight, placental weight, head circumference, and Apgar scores (2). In a third study, the combination of oxprenolol and prazosin (an α-adrenergic blocking agent) was effective for the control of severe essential hypertension in 25 pregnant women but not effective in 19 patients with pregnancy-induced hypertension (3).

Although β-blockade of the newborn has not been reported in the offspring of oxprenolol-treated mothers, this complication has occurred with other members of this class (see Acebutolol, Atenolol, and Nadolol). Thus, close observation of the newborn for bradycardia and other symptoms of β-blockade is recommended during the first 24–48 hours after birth. Long-term effects of *in utero* exposure to β-blockers have not been studied but warrant evaluation.

Breast Feeding Summary

Oxprenolol is excreted into breast milk (5, 6). In nine lactating women given 80 mg twice daily, the mean milk concentration of oxprenolol 105–135 minutes after a dose was 118 ng/ml (6). When a dose of 160 mg twice daily was given to three women, mean milk levels were 160 ng/ml. Finally, one woman was treated with 320 mg twice daily, producing a milk level of 470 ng/ml. The milk:plasma ratios for the three regimens were 0.14, 0.16, and 0.43, respectively. The mean milk:plasma ratio in another study was 0.45 (5). These low ratios, relative to other β-blockers, may be due to the high maternal serum protein binding (80%) which negates trapping of the weakly basic drug in the relative acidic milk (5). Based on calculations, a mother ingesting 240 mg/day would only provide a 3-kg infant with a dose of 0.07 mg/kg in 500 ml of milk (5). This amount is probably clinically insignificant.

Although no adverse reactions have been noted in nursing infants of mothers treated with oxprenolol, infants should be closely observed for bradycardia and other symptoms of β-blockade. Long-term effects of exposure to β-blockers from milk have not been studied but warrant evaluation.

References

1. Gallery EDM, Saunders DM, Hunyor SN, Gyory AZ. Randomized comparison of methyldopa and oxprenolol for treatment of hypertension in pregnancy. Br Med J 1979;1:1591–4.
2. Fidler J, Smith V, Fayers P, DeSwiet M. Randomized controlled comparative study of methyldopa and oxprenolol in treatment of hypertension in pregnancy. Br Med J 1983;286:1927–30.
3. Lubbe WF, Hodge JV. Combined α- and β-adrenoceptor antagonism with prazosin and oxprenolol in control of severe hypertension in pregnancy. NZ Med J 1981;94:169–72.
4. Lubbe WF. More on beta-blockers in pregnancy. N Engl J Med 1982;307:753.
5. Sioufi A, Hillion D, Lumbroso P, Wainer R, Olivier-Martin M, Schoeller JP, Colussi D, Leroux F, Mangoni P. Oxprenolol placental transfer, plasma concentrations in newborns and passage into breast milk. Br J Clin Pharmacol 1984;18:453–6.
6. Fidler J, Smith V, DeSwiet M. Excretion of oxprenolol and timolol in breast milk. Br J Obstet Gynaecol 1983;90:961–5.

Name: **OXTRIPHYLLINE**

Class: **Spasmolytic/Vasodilator**   Risk Factor: **C**

Fetal Risk Summary

Oxtriphylline is a methylxanthine which is metabolized to theophylline. Theophylline has been found in cord blood but not in the serum of an infant whose mother had taken oxtriphylline during pregnancy (1). No adverse effects in the infant were observed (see also Theophylline).

Breast Feeding Summary

No data available. See also Theophylline.

References

1. Labovitz E, Spector S. Placental theophylline transfer in pregnant asthmatics. JAMA 1982;247:786–8.

Name: **OXYCODONE**

Class: **Narcotic Analgesic**   Risk Factor: **B***

Fetal Risk Summary

No reports linking the use of oxycodone with congenital defects have been located. The drug is rarely used in pregnancy.

[* Risk Factor D if used for prolonged periods or in high doses at term.]

Breast Feeding Summary

No data available.

Name: **OXYMORPHONE**

Class: **Narcotic Analgesic**   Risk Factor: **B***

Fetal Risk Summary

No reports linking the use of oxymorphone with congenital defects have been located. Use of this drug during labor produces neonatal respiratory depression to the same degree as other narcotic analgesics (1–4).

[* Risk Factor D if used for prolonged periods or in high doses at term.]

Breast Feeding Summary

No data available.

References

1. Simeckova M, Shaw W, Pool E, Nichols EE. Numorphan in labor—a preliminary report. Obstet Gynecol 1960;16:119–23.
2. Sentnor MH, Solomons E, Kohl SG. An evaluation of oxymorphone in labor. Am J Obstet Gynecol 1962;84:956–61.
3. Eames GM, Pool KRS. Clinical trial of oxymorphone in labor. Br Med J 1964;2:353–5.
4. Ransom S. Oxymorphone as an obstetric analgesic—a clinical trial. Anesthesia 1966;21:464–71.

Name: **OXYPHENBUTAZONE**

Class: **Nonsteroidal Anti-Inflammatory**   Risk Factor: **D**

Fetal Risk Summary

See Phenylbutazone.

Breast Feeding Summary

See Phenylbutazone.

Name: **OXYPHENCYCLIMINE**

Class: **Parasympatholytic (Anticholinergic)**   Risk Factor: **C**

Fetal Risk Summary

Oxyphencyclimine is an anticholinergic agent. In a large prospective study, 2,323 patients were exposed to this class of drugs during the 1st trimester, 1 of whom took oxyphencyclimine (1). A possible association was found between the total group and minor malformations.

Breast Feeding Summary

No data available (see also Atropine).

References

1. Heinonen OP, Slone D, Shapiro S. *Birth Defects and Drugs in Pregnancy*. Littleton:Publishing Sciences Group, 1977:346–53.

Name: **OXYPHENONIUM**

Class: **Parasympatholytic (Anticholinergic)**   Risk Factor: **C**

Fetal Risk Summary

Oxyphenonium is an anticholinergic quaternary ammonium bromide. No reports of its use in pregnancy have been located (see also Atropine).

Breast Feeding Summary

No data available (see also Atropine).

Name: **OXYTETRACYCLINE**

Class: **Antibiotic**   Risk Factor: **D**

Fetal Risk Summary

See Tetracycline.

Breast Feeding Summary

See Tetracycline.

Name: **PANTOTHENIC ACID**

Class: **Vitamin**   Risk Factor: **A***

Fetal Risk Summary

Pantothenic acid, a water-soluble B complex vitamin, acts as a coenzyme in the metabolism or synthesis of a number of carbohydrates, proteins, lipids, and steroid hormones (1). The American RDA for pantothenic acid or its derivatives (dexpanthenol and calcium pantothenate) in pregnancy is 10.0 mg (2).

No reports of maternal or fetal complications associated with pantothenic acid have been located. Deficiency of this vitamin was not found in two studies evaluating maternal vitamin levels during pregnancy (3, 4). Like other B complex vitamins, newborn pantothenic acid levels are significantly greater than maternal levels (3–6). At term, mean pantothenate levels in 174 mothers were 430 ng/ml (range 250–710) and in their newborns 780 ng/ml (range 400–1,480) (3). Placental transfer of pantothenate to the fetus is by active transport but slower than other B complex vitamins (7, 8). In one report, low-birth-weight infants had significantly lower levels of pantothenic acid than normal-weight infants (6).

[* Risk Factor C in amounts above the RDA.]

Breast Feeding Summary

Pantothenic acid is excreted in human breast milk with concentrations directly proportional to intake (9, 10). With a dietary intake of 8–15 mg/day, mean milk concentrations average 1.93–2.35 μg/ml (9). In a group of mothers who had delivered premature babies (28–34 weeks gestational age), pantothenic acid milk levels were significantly greater than in a comparable group with term babies (39–41 weeks) (10). Milk levels in the preterm group averaged 3.91 μg/ml up to 40 weeks gestational age and then fell to 3.16 μg/ml. For the term group, levels at 2 and 12 weeks postpartum were 2.57 and 2.55 μg/ml, respectively. A 1983 English study measured pantothenic acid levels in pooled human milk obtained from preterm (26 mothers: 29–34 weeks) and term (35 mothers: 39 weeks or longer) patients (11). Preterm milk levels rose from 1.29 μg/ml (colostrum) to 2.27 μg/ml (16–196 days) while term milk levels increased over the same period from 1.26 to 2.61 μg/ml.

A RDA for pantothenic acid during lactation has not been established. However, since this vitamin is required for good health, amounts at least equal to the RDA for pregnancy are recommended. If the diet of the lactating woman adequately supplies this amount, maternal supplementation with pantothenic acid is probably not required. Supplementation with the pregnancy RDA for pantothenic acid is recommended for those women with inadequate nutritional intake.

References

1. American Hospital Formulary Service. *Drug Information 1985*. Bethesda:American Society of Hospital Pharmacists, 1985:1687–8.
2. *Recommended Dietary Allowances*, ed 9. Washington, DC:National Academy of Sciences, 1980:122–4.
3. Baker H, Frank O, Thomson AD, Langer A, Munves ED, De Angelis B, Kaminetzky HA. Vitamin profile of 174 mothers and newborns at parturition. Am J Clin Nutr 1975;28:59–65.
4. Baker H, Frank O, Deangelis B, Feingold S, Kaminetzky HA. Role of placenta in maternal-fetal vitamin transfer in humans. Am J Obstet Gynecol 1981;141:792–6.
5. Cohenour SH, Calloway DH. Blood, urine, and dietary pantothenic acid levels of pregnant teenagers. Am J Clin Nutr 1972;25:512–7.
6. Baker H, Thind IS, Frank O, DeAngelis B, Caterini H, Louria DB. Vitamin levels in low-birth-weight newborn infants and their mothers. Am J Obstet Gynecol 1977;129:521–4.
7. Hill EP, Longo LD. Dynamics of maternal-fetal nutrient transfer. Fed Proc 1980;39:239–44.
8. Kaminetsky HA, Baker H, Frank O, Langer A. The effects of intravenously administered water-soluble vitamins during labor in normovitaminemic and hypovitaminemic gravidas on maternal and neonatal blood vitamin levels at delivery. Am J Obstet Gynecol 1974;120:697–703.
9. Deodhar AD, Rajalakshmi R, Ramakrishnan CV. Studies on human lactation. Part III. Effect of dietary vitamin supplementation on vitamin contents of breast milk. Acta Paediatr (Stockholm) 1964;53:42–8.
10. Song WO, Chan GM, Wyse BW, Hansen RG. Effect of pantothenic acid status on the content of the vitamin in human milk. Am J Clin Nutr 1984;40:317–24.
11. Ford JE, Zechalko A, Murphy J, Brooke OG. Comparison of the B vitamin composition of milk from mothers of preterm and term babies. Arch Dis Child 1983;58:367–72.

Name: **PARAMETHADIONE**

Class: **Anticonvulsant**
Risk Factor: **D$_M$**

Fetal Risk Summary

Paramethadione is an oxazolidinedione anticonvulsant used in the treatment of petit mal epilepsy. There have been three families (10 pregnancies) in which an increase in spontaneous abortion or abnormalities have been reported (1, 2). Paramethadione is considered equivalent to trimethadione in regard to its fetal effects. In fact, one of the families described by German and co-workers (3) was included in the fetal trimethadione syndrome (see Trimethadione). This patient had one normal infant after anticonvulsant medications were withdrawn. Malformations reported in two additional families by Rutman (2) are consistent with the fetal paramethadione/trimethadione syndrome. The malformations included: tetralogy of Fallot, mental retardation, failure to thrive, and increased incidence of spontaneous abortions (2). Because paramethadione has demonstrated both clinical and experimental fetal risk greater than other anticonvulsants, its use should be abandoned in favor of other anticonvulsants for the treatment of petit mal epilepsy (see also Ethosuximide, Phensuximide, Methsuximide) (4–6).

Breast Feeding Summary

No data available.

References

1. German J, Ehlers KH, Kowal A, DeGeorge PU, Engle MA, Passarge E. Possible teratogenicity of trimethadione and paramethadione. Lancet 1970;2:261–2.

2. Rutman JT. Anticonvulsants and fetal damage. N Engl J Med 1973;189:696–7.
3. German J, Kowal A, Ehlers KH. Trimethadione and human teratogenesis. Teratology 1970;3:349–62.
4. National Institutes of Health. Anticonvulsants found to have teratogenic potential. JAMA 1981;245:36.
5. Fabro S, Brown NA. Teratogenic potential of anticonvulsants. N Engl J Med 1979;300:1280–1.
6. Hill RM. Managing the epileptic patient during pregnancy. Drug Ther 1976:204–5.

Name: **PAREGORIC**

Class: **Antidiarrheal**   Risk Factor: **B**

Fetal Risk Summary

Paregoric is a mixture of opium powder, anise oil, benzoic acid, camphor, glycerin, and ethanol. Its action is mainly due to morphine (see also Morphine). The Collaborative Perinatal Project monitored 50,282 mother-child pairs, 90 of which had 1st trimester exposure to paregoric (1). For use anytime during pregnancy, 562 exposures were recorded (2). No evidence was found to suggest a relationship to large categories of major or minor malformations or to individual defects.

[* Risk Factor D if used for prolonged periods or in high doses at term.]

Breast Feeding Summary

See Morphine.

References

1. Heinonen OP, Slone D, Shapiro S. *Birth Defects and Drugs in Pregnancy*. Littleton:Publishing Sciences Group, 1977:287–95.
2. *Ibid*, 434.

Name: **PARGYLINE**

Class: **Antihypertensive**   Risk Factor: **C$_M$**

Fetal Risk Summary

No data available.

Breast Feeding Summary

No data available.

Name: **PENICILLAMINE**
Class: **Heavy Metal Antagonist**   Risk Factor: **D**

Fetal Risk Summary

The use of penicillamine during pregnancy has been reported in less than 100 pregnancies (1–13). The mothers were treated for rheumatoid arthritis, cystinuria, or Wilson's disease. From these pregnancies, anomalies were observed in eight infants:

Cutis laxa, hypotonia, hyperflexion of hips and shoulders, pyloric stenosis, vein fragility, varicosities, impaired wound healing, death (2)
Cutis laxa, growth retardation, inguinal hernia, simian crease, perforated bowel, death (6)
Cutis laxa (3)
Cutis laxa, mild micrognathia, low-set ears, inguinal hernia (12)
Cutis laxa, inguinal hernia (13)
Congenital contractures, hydrocephalus, hypertonia, death (14)
Cerebral palsy, blindness, bilateral clubfeet, sudden infant death at 3 months (14)
Hydrocephalus (14)

The relationship of the last three cases listed above to penicillamine is controversial since they did not include connective tissue anomalies. The drug may be partially responsible but other factors, such as maternal infections and surgery, may have a stronger association with the defects (14). A small ventricular septal defect was observed in another newborn, but this was probably not related to penicillamine (8). Although the evidence is incomplete, maintaining the daily dose at 500 mg or less may reduce the incidence of penicillamine-induced toxicity in the newborn (5, 10).

Breast Feeding Summary

No data available.

References

1. Crawhall JC, Scowen EF, Thompson CJ, Watts RWE. Dissolution of cystine stones during d-penicillamine treatment of a pregnant patient with cystinuria. Br Med J 1967;2:216–8.
2. Mjolnerod OK, Rasmussen K, Dommerud SA, Gjeruldsen ST. Congenital connective-tissue defect probably due to d-penicillamine treatment in pregnancy. Lancet 1971;1:673–5.
3. Laver M, Fairley KF. D-penicillamine treatment in pregnancy. Lancet 1971;1:1019–20.
4. Scheinberg IH, Sternlieb I. Pregnancy in penicillamine-treated patients with Wilson's disease. N Engl J Med 1975; 293:1300–3.
5. Marecek Z, Graf M. Pregnancy in penicillamine-treated patients with Wilson's disease. N Engl J Med 1976;295:841–2.
6. Solomon L, Abrams G, Dinner M, Berman L. Neonatal abnormalities associated with d-penicillamine treatment during pregnancy. N Engl J Med 1977;296:54–5.
7. Walshe JM. Pregnancy in Wilson's disease. Q J Med 1977;46:73–83.
8. Lyle WH. Penicillamine in pregnancy. Lancet 1978;1:606–7.
9. Linares A, Zarranz JJ, Rodriguez-Alarcon J, Diaz-Perez JL. Reversible cutis laxa due to maternal d-penicillamine treatment. Lancet 1979;2:43.
10. Endres W. D-penicillamine in pregnancy—to ban or not to ban? Klin Wochenschr 1981;59:535–7.
11. Briggs GG. Unpublished data, 1982.

12. Harpey JP, Jaudon MC, Clavel JP, Galli A, Darbois Y. Cutis laxa and low serum zinc after antenatal exposure to penicillamine. Lancet 1983;2:858.

13. Beck RB, et al. Ultrastructural findings in the fetal penicillamine syndrome (Abstr). Read before the 13th Annual Birth Defects Conference, March of Dimes and University of California, San Diego, June, 1980. As cited in Gal P, Ravenel SD. Contractures and hydrocephalus with penicillamine and maternal hypotension. J Clin Dysmorphol 1984;2:9–12.

14. Gal P, Ravenel SD. Contractures and hydrocephalus with penicillamine and maternal hypotension. J Clin Dysmorphol 1984;2:9–12.

Name: **PENICILLIN G**

Class: **Antibiotic**   Risk Factor: **B**

Fetal Risk Summary

Penicillin G is used routinely for maternal infections during pregnancy. Several investigators have documented its rapid passage into the fetal circulation and amniotic fluid (1–5). Therapeutic levels are reached in both sites except for the amniotic fluid during the 1st trimester (5). At term, maternal serum and amniotic fluid concentrations are equal 60–90 minutes after intravenous (IV) administration (2). Continuous IV infusions (10,000 units/hr) produced equal concentrations of penicillin G at 20 hours in maternal serum, cord serum, and amniotic fluid (2).

The early use of penicillin G was linked to increased uterine activity and abortion (6–10). It is not known if this was due to impurities in the drug or to penicillin itself. No reports of this effect have appeared since a reference in 1950 (10). An anaphylactic reaction in a pregnant patient reportedly led to the death of her fetus *in utero* (11).

Only one reference has linked the use of penicillin G with congenital abnormalities (12). An examination of hospital records indicated that in three of four cases the administration of penicillin G had been followed by the birth of a malformed baby. A retrospective review of additional patients exposed to antibiotics in the 1st trimester indicated an increase in congenital defects. Unfortunately, the authors did not analyze their data for each antibiotic, so no causal relationship to penicillin G could be shown (12, 13). In another case, a patient was treated in early pregnancy with high doses of penicillin G procaine IV (?), cortisone, and sodium salicylate (14). A cyclopic male was delivered at term but died 5 minutes later. The defect was attributed to salicylates, cortisone, or maternal viremia. (Penicillin G procaine should not be given IV. The Editors are assuming the drug was either given intramuscularly or the procaine form was not used. We have not been able to contact the authors to clarify these assumptions.)

In a controlled study, 110 patients received one to three antibiotics during the 1st trimester for a total of 589 weeks (15). Penicillin G was given for a total of 107 weeks. The incidence of birth defects was no different from that in a nontreated control group.

The Collaborative Perinatal Project monitored 50,282 mother-child pairs, 3,546 of which had 1st trimester exposure to penicillin derivatives (16). For use anytime during pregnancy, 7,171 exposures were recorded (17). In neither case was evidence found to suggest a relationship to large categories of major or minor malformations or to individual defects. Based on these data, it is unlikely that penicillin G is teratogenic.

Breast Feeding Summary

Penicillin G is excreted into breast milk in low concentrations. Milk:plasma ratios following intramuscular doses of 100,000 units in 11 patients varied between 0.02 and 0.13 (18). The maximum concentration measured in milk was 0.6 unit/ml after this dose. Although no adverse effects were reported, three potential problems exist for the nursing infant: modification of bowel flora, direct effects on the infant (e.g., allergic response), and interference with the interpretation of culture results if a fever work-up is required.

References

1. Herrel W, Nichols D, Heilman D. Penicillin. Its usefulness, limitations, diffusion and detection, with analysis of 150 cases in which it was employed. JAMA 1944;125:1003–11.
2. Woltz J, Zintel H. The transmission of penicillin to amniotic fluid and fetal blood in the human. Am J Obstet Gynecol 1945;50:338–40.
3. Hutter A, Parks J. The transmission of penicillin through the placenta. A preliminary report. Am J Obstet Gynecol 1945;49:663–5.
4. Woltz J, Wiley M. The transmission of penicillin to the previable fetus. JAMA 1946;131:969–70.
5. Wasz-Hockert O, Nummi S, Vuopala S, Jarvinen P. Transplacental passage of azidocillin, ampicillin and penicillin G during early and late pregnancy. Acta Paediatr Scand 1970;206 (Suppl):109–10.
6. Lentz J, Ingraham N Jr, Beerman H, Stokes J. Penicillin in the prevention and treatment of congenital syphilis. JAMA 1944;126:408–13.
7. Leavitt H. Clinical action of penicillin on the uterus. J Vener Dis Inf 1945;26:150–3.
8. McLachlan A, Brown D. The effects of penicillin administration on menstrual and other sexual functions. Br J Vener Dis 1947;23:1–10.
9. Mazingarbe A. Le pencilline possede-t-elle une action abortive? Gynecol Obstet 1946;45:487.
10. Perin L, Sissmann R, Detre F, Chertier A. La pencilline a-t-elle une action abortive? Bull Soc Fr Dermatol 1950;57:534–8.
11. Kosim H. Intrauterine fetal death as a result of anaphylactic reaction to penicillin in a pregnant woman. Dapim Refuiim 1959;18:136–7.
12. Carter M, Wilson F. Antibiotics and congenital malformations. Lancet 1963;1:1267–8.
13. Carter M, Wilson F. Antibiotics in early pregnancy and congenital malformations. Dev Med Child Neurol 1965;7:353–9.
14. Khudr G, Olding L. Cyclopia. Am J Dis Child 1973;125:120–2.
15. Ravid R, Toaff R. On the possible teratogenicity of antibiotic drugs administered during pregnancy— a prospective study. In Klingberg M, Abramovici A, Chemki J, eds. Drugs and Fetal Development. New York:Plenum Press, 1972:505–10.
16. Heinonen OP, Slone D, Shapiro S. Birth Defects and Drugs in Pregnancy. Littleton:Publishing Sciences Group, 1977:297–313.
17. Ibid, 435.
18. Greene H, Burkhart B, Hobby G. Excretion of penicillin in human milk following parturition. Am J Obstet Gynecol 1946;51:732–3.

Name: **PENICILLIN G, BENZATHINE**

Class: **Antibiotic**   Risk Factor: **B**

Fetal Risk Summary

Benzathine penicillin G is a combination of an ammonium base and penicillin G suspended in water. See Penicillin G.

Breast Feeding Summary

See Penicillin G.

Name: **PENICILLIN G, PROCAINE**

Class: **Antibiotic**   Risk Factor: **B**

Fetal Risk Summary

Procaine penicillin G is an equimolar combination of procaine and penicillin G suspended in water (1). The combination is broken down *in vivo* into the two components. See also Penicillin G.

A case report described the use of high doses of penicillin G procaine intravenously (?), cortisone, and sodium salicylate in early pregnancy followed by the delivery at term of a cyclopic male infant (2). The lethal defect was attributed to salicylates, cortisone, or maternal viremia. (Note: Penicillin G procaine should not be given intravenously. The Editors are assuming the drug was either given intramuscularly or the procaine form was not used. We have been unable to contact the authors of the paper to clarify these assumptions.)

Breast Feeding Summary

See Penicillin G.

References

1. Mandel G, Sande M. Antimicrobial agents (continued). Penicillins and cephalosporins. In Gilman AG, Goodman LS, Gilman A, eds. *The Pharmacological Basis of Therapeutics*, ed 6. New York:Macmillan Publishing Co, 1980:1137.
2. Khudr G, Olding L. Cyclopia. Am J Dis Child 1973;125:120–2.

Name: **PENICILLIN V**

Class: **Antibiotic**   Risk Factor: **B**

Fetal Risk Summary

No reports linking the use of penicillin V with congenital defects have been located. The Collaborative Perinatal Project monitored 50,282 mother-child pairs, 3,546 of which had 1st trimester exposure to penicillin derivatives (1). For use anytime during pregnancy, 7,171 exposures were recorded (2). In neither case was evidence found to suggest a relationship to large categories of major or minor malformations or to individual defects.

Penicillin V depresses both plasma-bound and urinary-excreted estriol (3). Urinary estriol was formerly used to assess the condition of the fetoplacental unit, depressed levels being associated with fetal distress. This assessment is now made by measuring plasma-unconjugated estriol, which is not usually affected by penicillin V.

Breast Feeding Summary

No data available (see Penicillin G).

References

1. Heinonen OP, Slone D, Shapiro S. *Birth Defects and Drugs in Pregnancy*. Littleton:Publishing Sciences Group, 1977:297–313.

2. *Ibid*, 435.
3. Pulkkinen M, Willman K. Maternal oestrogen levels during penicillin treatment. Br Med J 1971;4:48.

Name: **PENTAERYTHRITOL TETRANITRATE**

Class: **Vasodilator**   Risk Factor: **C**

Fetal Risk Summary

Pentaerythritol tetranitrate is a long-acting agent used for the prevention of angina pectoris. Due to the nature of its indication, experience in pregnancy is limited. The Collaborative Perinatal Project recorded 3 1st trimester exposures to pentaerythritol tetranitrate plus 12 other patients exposed to other vasodilators (1). From this small sample, four malformed children were produced, a statistically significant incidence ($p < 0.02$). It was not reported if pentaerythritol tetranitrate was taken by any of the mothers of the affected infants. Although these data serve as a warning, the number of patients is so small that conclusions as to the relative safety of this drug cannot be made.

Breast Feeding Summary

No data available.

References

1. Heinonen OP, Slone D, Shapiro S. *Birth Defects and Drugs in Pregnancy*. Littleton:Publishing Sciences Group, 1977:371–3.

Name: **PENTAZOCINE**

Class: **Analgesic**   Risk Factor: **B***

Fetal Risk Summary

No reports linking the use of pentazocine with congenital defects have been located. The drug rapidly crosses the placenta, resulting in cord blood levels of 40–70% of maternal serum (1). Withdrawal has been reported in infants exposed *in utero* to chronic maternal ingestion of pentazocine (2–4). Symptoms, presenting within 24 hours of birth, consist of trembling and jitteriness, marked hyperirritability, hyperactivity with hypertonia, high-pitched cry, diaphoresis, diarrhea, vomiting and opisthotonic posturing.

During labor, increased overall uterine activity has been observed after pentazocine, but without changes in fetal heart rate (5). In equianalgesic doses, most studies report no significant differences between meperidine and pentazocine in pain relief, length of labor, or Apgar scores (6–11). However, meperidine in one study was observed to produce significantly lower Apgar scores than pentazocine, especially with repeated doses (12). Severe neonatal respiratory depression may also occur with pentazocine (6, 12).

A report from New Orleans described 24 infants born of mothers using the intravenous combination of pentazocine and tripelennamine ('T's and Blue's) (13). Doses were unknown but probably ranged from 200 to 600 mg of pentazocine and 100 to 250 mg of tripelennamine. Six of the newborns were exposed early in pregnancy. Birth weights for 11 of the infants were less than 2,500 g; nine of these were premature (less than 37 weeks) and two were small for gestational age. Daily or weekly exposure throughout pregnancy produced withdrawal symptoms, occurring within 7 days of birth, in 15 of 16 infants. Withdrawal was thought to be due to pentazocine, but antihistamine withdrawal has been reported (see Diphenhydramine). Thirteen of 15 infants became asymptomatic 3–11 days following onset of withdrawal, but in two symptoms persisted for up to 6 months.

[* Risk Factor D if used for prolonged periods or in high doses at term.]

Breast Feeding Summary

No data available.

References

1. Beckett AH, Taylor JF. Blood concentrations of pethidine and pentazocine in mother and infant at time of birth. J Pharm Pharmacol 1967;19(Suppl):50s–2s.
2. Goetz RL, Bain RV. Neonatal withdrawal symptoms associated with maternal use of pentazocine. J Pediatr 1974;84:887–8.
3. Scanlon JW. Pentazocine and neonatal withdrawal symptoms. J Pediatr 1974;85:735–6.
4. Kopelman AE. Fetal addiction to pentazocine. Pediatrics 1975;55:888–9.
5. Filler WW, Filler NW. Effect of a potent non-narcotic analgesic agent (pentazocine) on uterine contractility and fetal heart rate. Obstet Gynecol 1966;28:224–32.
6. Freedman H, Tafeen CH, Harris H. Parenteral Win 20,228 as analgesic in labor. NY State J Med 1967;67:2849–51.
7. Duncan SLB, Ginsburg J, Morris NF. Comparison of pentazocine and pethidine in normal labor. Am J Obstet Gynecol 1969;105:197–202.
8. Moore J, Hunter RJ. A comparison of the effects of pentazocine and pethidine administered during labor. J Obstet Gynaecol Br Commonw 1970;77:830–6.
9. Mowat J, Garrey MM. Comparison of pentazocine and pethidine in labour. Br Med J 1970;2:757–9.
10. Levy DL. Obstetric analgesia. Pentazocine and meperidine in normal primiparous labor. Obstet Gynecol 1971;38:907–11.
11. Moore J, Ball HG. A sequential study of intravenous analgesic treatment during labour. Br J Anaesth 1974;46:365–72.
12. Refstad SO, Lindbaek E. Ventilatory depression of the newborn of women receiving pethidine or pentazocine. Br J Aneasth 1980;52:265–70.
13. Dunn DW, Reynolds J. Neonatal withdrawal symptoms associated with 'T's and Blue's (pentazocine and tripelennamine). Am J Dis Child 1982;136:644–5.

Name: **PENTOBARBITAL**

Class: **Sedative/Hypnotic**   Risk Factor: D_M

Fetal Risk Summary

No reports linking the use of pentobarbital with congenital defects have been located. The Collaborative Perinatal Project monitored 50,282 mother-child pairs, 250 of which had 1st trimester exposure to pentobarbital (1). No evidence was found to suggest a relationship to large categories of major or minor malformations or to individual defects. Hemorrhagic disease and barbiturate withdrawal in the newborn are theoretical possibilities (see also Phenobarbital).

Breast Feeding Summary

Pentobarbital is excreted into breast milk (2). Breast milk levels of 0.17 μg/ml have been detected 19 hours after a dose of 100 mg daily for 32 days. The effect on the nursing infant is not known.

References

1. Heinonen OP, Slone D, Shapiro S. *Birth Defects and Drugs in Pregnancy*. Littleton:Publishing Sciences Group, 1977:336–7.
2. Wilson JT, Brown RD, Cherek DR, Dailey JW, Hilman B, Jobe PC, Manno BR, Manno JE, Redetzki HM, Stewart JJ. Drug excretion in human breast milk: principles, pharmacokinetics and projected consequences. Clin Pharmacokinet 1980;5:1–66.

Name: **PERPHENAZINE**

Class: **Tranquilizer**   Risk Factor: **C**

Fetal Risk Summary

Perphenazine is a piperazine phenothiazine in the same group as prochlorperazine (see Prochlorperazine). The phenothiazines readily cross the placenta (1). The Collaborative Perinatal Project monitored 50,282 mother-child pairs, 63 of which had 1st trimester exposure to perphenazine (2). For use anytime during pregnancy, 166 exposures were recorded. No evidence was found in either group to suggest a relationship to malformations, nor an effect on perinatal mortality rates, birth weight, or intelligence quotient scores at 4 years of age. Although occasional reports have attempted to link various phenothiazine compounds with congenital defects, the bulk of the evidence indicates that these drugs are safe for the mother and fetus (see also Chlorpromazine).

Breast Feeding Summary

No data available.

References

1. Moya F, Thorndike V. Passage of drugs across the placenta. Am J Obstet Gynecol 1962;84:1778–98.
2. Slone D, Siskind V, Heinonen OP, Monson RR, Kaufman DW, Shapiro S. Antenatal exposure to the phenothiazines in relation to congenital malformations, perinatal mortality rate, birth weight, and intelligence quotient score. Am J Obstet Gynecol 1977;128:486–8.

Name: **PHENACETIN**

Class: **Analgesic/Antipyretic**   Risk Factor: **B**

Fetal Risk Summary

Phenacetin, in combination products, is routinely used during pregnancy. It is metabolized mainly to acetaminophen (see also Acetaminophen). The Collaborative Perinatal Project monitored 50,282 mother-child pairs, 5,546 of which had 1st trimester exposure to phenacetin (1). Although no evidence was found to suggest a relationship to large categories of major or minor malformations, possible associations were found with several individual defects (2). The statistical significance of these associations is unknown and independent confirmation is required. Further, phenacetin is rarely used alone, being consumed usually in combination with aspirin and caffeine.

Craniosynostosis (6 cases)
Adrenal syndromes (5 cases)
Anal atresia (7 cases)
Accessory spleen (5 cases)

For use anytime during pregnancy, 13,031 exposures were recorded (3). With the same qualifications, possible associations with individual defects were found (4).

Musculoskeletal malformations (6 cases)
Hydronephrosis (8 cases)
Adrenal anomalies (8 cases)

Breast Feeding Summary

Phenacetin is excreted into breast milk, appearing along with its major metabolite, acetaminophen (5). A patient who consumed two tablets of Empirin Compound with Codeine No. 3 (aspirin-phenacetin-caffeine-codeine) produced an average phenacetin milk concentration of 71 ng/ml (5). Milk:plasma ratios in this and a second patient varied from 0.16 to 0.90 (5).

References

1. Heinonen OP, Slone D, Shapiro S. *Birth Defects and Drugs in Pregnancy*. Littleton:Publishing Sciences Group, 1977:286–95.
2. *Ibid*, 471.
3. *Ibid*, 434.
4. *Ibid*, 483.
5. Findlay JWA, DeAngelis RL, Kearney MF, Welch RM, Findlay JM. Analgesic drugs in breast milk and plasma. Clin Pharmacol Ther 1981;29:625–33.

Name: **PHENAZOCINE**

Class: **Narcotic Analgesic**   Risk Factor: **B***

Fetal Risk Summary

No reports linking the use of phenazocine with congenital defects have been located. The drug is not commercially available in the United States. Withdrawal could theoretically occur in infants exposed *in utero* to prolonged maternal ingestion of phenazocine. Phenazocine may cause neonatal respiratory depression when used in labor (1, 2).

[* Risk Factor D if used for prolonged periods or in high doses at term.]

Breast Feeding Summary

No data available.

References

1. Sadove M, Balagot R, Branion J Jr, Kobak A. Report on the use of a new agent, phenazocine, in obstetric analgesia. Obstet Gynecol 1960;16:448–53.
2. Corbit J, First S. Clinical comparison of phenazocine and meperidine in obstetric analgesia. Obstet Gynecol 1961;18:488–91.

Name: **PHENAZOPYRIDINE**

Class: **Urinary Tract Analgesic**   Risk Factor: **B$_M$**

Fetal Risk Summary

No reports linking the use of phenazopyridine with congenital defects have been located. The Collaborative Perinatal Project monitored 50,282 mother-child pairs, 219 of which had 1st trimester exposure to phenazopyridine (1). For use anytime during pregnancy, 1,109 exposures were recorded (2). In neither case was evidence found to suggest a relationship to large categories of major or minor malformations or to individual defects.

Breast Feeding Summary

No data available.

References

1. Heinonen OP, Slone D, Shapiro S. *Birth Defects and Drugs in Pregnancy*. Littleton:Publishing Sciences Group, 1977:299–308.
2. *Ibid*, 435.

Name: **PHENCYCLIDINE**

Class: **Hallucinogenic**   Risk Factor: **X**

Fetal Risk Summary

Phencyclidine (PCP) is an illicit drug used for its hallucinogenic effects. Transfer to the fetus has been demonstrated in humans with placental metabolism of the drug (1–7). Qualitative analysis of the urine from two newborns discovered phencyclidine levels of 75 ng/ml or greater up to 3 days after birth (2). In 24 (12%) of 200 women evaluated at a Los Angeles hospital, cord blood PCP levels ranged from 0.10 to 5.80 ng/ml (3). Cord blood concentrations were twice as high as maternal serum—1215 vs 514 pg/ml in one woman who allegedly consumed her last dose 53 days before delivery (4). PCP in the newborn's urine measured 5,841 pg/ml (4).

Relatively few studies have appeared on the use of phencyclidine during pregnancy, but fetal exposure may be more common than this lack of reporting indicates. During a 9-month period in 1980 to 1981 in a Cleveland hospital, 30 of 519 (5.8%) consecutively screened pregnant patients were discovered to have PCP exposure (8). In a subsequent report from this same hospital, 2,327 pregnant patients were screened for PCP exposure between 1981 and 1982 (6). Only 19 patients (0.8%) had positive urine samples, but up to 256 (11%) or more may have tested positive with more frequent checking (6). In the Los Angeles study cited above, 12% were exposed (3). However, the specificity of the chemical screening methods used in this latter report have been questioned (7).

Most pregnancies in which the mother used phencyclidine apparently end with healthy newborns (3, 4, 9). However, case reports involving four newborns indicate the use of this agent may result in long-term damage (2, 9, 10):

Depressed at birth, jittery, hypertonic, poor feeding (2) (2 infants)
Irritable, poor feeding and sucking reflex (9) (1 infant)
Triangular shaped face with pointed chin, narrow mandibular angle, antimongo-loid slanted eyes, poor head control, nystagmus, inability to track visually, respiratory distress, hypertonic, jitteriness (10) (1 infant)

Irritability, jitteriness, hypertonicity, and poor feeding were common features in the affected infants. In three of the neonates, most of the symptoms had persisted at the time of the report. In the case with the malformed child, no causal relationship with PCP could be established. Marijuana was also taken, and it is a known teratogen in some animal species (11). Human teratogenicity secondary to marijuana has been suspected, but the evidence is weak, since the case reports also involved exposure to lysergic acid diethylamide (LSD) (12, 13).

Breast Feeding Summary

PCP is excreted into breast milk (14). One lactating mother, who took her last dose 40 days previously, excreted 3.90 ng/ml in her milk. In animal studies, milk concentrations of PCP were 10 times that of plasma (1). Women consuming PCP should not breast-feed.

References

1. Nicholas JM, Lipshitz J, Schreiber EC. Phencyclidine: its transfer across the placenta as well as into breast milk. Am J Obstet Gynecol 1982;143:143–6.

2. Strauss AA, Modanlou HD, Bosu SK. Neonatal manifestations of maternal phencyclidine (PCP) abuse. Pediatrics 1981;68:550–2.
3. Kaufman KR, Petrucha RA, Pitts FN Jr, Kaufman ER. Phencyclidine in umbilical cord blood: preliminary data. Am J Psychiatry 1983;140:450–2.
4. Petrucha RA, Kaufman KR, Pitts FN. Phencyclidine in pregnancy: a case report. J Reprod Med 1982;27:301–3.
5. Rayburn WF, Holsztynska EF, Domino EF. Phencyclidine: biotransformation by the human placenta. Am J Obstet Gynecol 1984;148:111–2.
6. Golden NL, Kuhnert BR, Sokol RJ, Martier S, Bagby BS. Phencyclidine use during pregnancy. Am J Obstet Gynecol 1984;148:254–9.
7. Lipton MA. Phencyclidine in umbilical cord blood: some cautions. Am J Psychiatry 1983;140:449.
8. Golden NL, Sokol RJ, Martier S, Miller SI. A practical method for identifying angel dust abuse during pregnancy. Am J Obstet Gynecol 1982;142:359–61.
9. Lerner SE, Burns RS. Phencyclidine use among youth: history, epidemiology, and acute and chronic intoxication. In Petersen R, Stillman R, eds. Phencyclidine (PCP) Abuse: An Appraisal. National Institute on Drug Abuse Research Monograph No. 21, US Government Printing Office, 1978.
10. Golden NL, Sokol RJ, Rubin IL. Angel dust: possible effects on the fetus. Pediatrics 1980;65:18–20.
11. Persaud TVN, Ellington AC. Teratogenic activity of cannabis resin. Lancet 1968;2:406–7.
12. Hecht F, Beals RK, Lees MH, Jolly H, Roberts P. Lysergic-acid-diethylamide and cannabis as possible teratogens in man. Lancet 1968;2:1087.
13. Carakushansky G, Neu RL, Gardner LI. Lysergide and cannabis as possible teratogens in man. Lancet 1969;1:150–1.
14. Kaufman KR, Petrucha RA, Pitts FN Jr, Weekes ME. PCP in amniotic fluid and breast milk: case report. J Clin Psychiatry 1983;44:269–70.

Name: **PHENDIMETRAZINE**

Class: **Central Stimulant/Anorectant**   Risk Factor: **C**

Fetal Risk Summary

No data available (see Phentermine or Dextroamphetamine).

Breast Feeding Summary

No data available.

Name: **PHENELZINE**

Class: **Antidepressant**   Risk Factor: **C**

Fetal Risk Summary

Phenelzine is a monoamine oxidase inhibitor. The Collaborative Perinatal Project monitored 21 mother-child pairs exposed to these drugs during the 1st trimester, 3 of which were exposed to phenelzine (1). An increased risk of malformations was found. Details of the three cases with phenelzine exposure are not available.

Breast Feeding Summary

No data available.

References

1. Heinonen OP, Slone D, Shapiro S. *Birth Defects and Drugs in Pregnancy*. Littleton:Publishing Sciences Group, 1977:336–7.

Name: **PHENINDIONE**

Class: **Anticoagulant**   Risk Factor: **D**

Fetal Risk Summary

See Coumarin Derivatives.

Breast Feeding Summary

See Coumarin Derivatives.

Name: **PHENIRAMINE**

Class: **Antihistamine**   Risk Factor: **C**

Fetal Risk Summary

The Collaborative Perinatal Project monitored 50,282 mother-child pairs, 831 of whom were exposed to pheniramine during the 1st trimester (1). A possible relationship between this use and respiratory malformations and eye/ear defects was found, but the statistical significance of these findings is unknown. Independent confirmation is required to determine the actual risk. For use anytime during pregnancy, 2,442 exposures were recorded (2). No evidence was found in this group to suggest a relationship to congenital anomalies.

Breast Feeding Summary

No data available.

References

1. Heinonen OP, Slone D, Shapiro S. *Birth Defects and Drugs in Pregnancy*. Littleton:Publishing Sciences Group, 1977:322–34.
2. *Ibid*, 436–7.

Name: **PHENOBARBITAL**

Class: **Sedative/Anticonvulsant**   Risk Factor: **D**

Fetal Risk Summary

Phenobarbital has been used widely in clinical practice as a sedative and anticonvulsant since 1912 (1). The potential teratogenic effects of phenobarbital were recognized in 1964 along with phenytoin (2). Since this report, there have been numerous reviews and studies on the teratogenic effects of phenobarbital either alone or in combination with phenytoin and other anticonvulsants. Based on this literature, the epileptic pregnant woman taking phenobarbital in combination with other antiepileptics has a two to three times greater risk for delivering a child with congenital defects over the general population (3–10). It is not known if this increased risk is due to antiepileptic drugs, the disease itself, genetic factors, or a combination of these, although some evidence indicates that drugs are the causative factor (10). A phenotype, as described for phenytoin in the fetal hydantoin syndrome (FHS), apparently does not occur with phenobarbital (see Phenytoin for details of FHS). However, as summarized by Janz (11), some of the minor malformations composing the FHS have been occasionally observed in infants of epileptic mothers treated only with phenobarbital.

The Collaborative Perinatal Project monitored 50,282 mother-child pairs, 1,415 of which had 1st trimester exposure to phenobarbital (12). For use anytime during pregnancy, 8,037 exposures were recorded (13). In neither case was evidence found to suggest a relationship to large categories of major or minor malformations, although a possible association with Down's syndrome was shown statistically.

Phenobarbital and other anticonvulsants (e.g., phenytoin) may cause early hemorrhagic disease of the newborn (14–23). Hemorrhage occurs during the first 24 hours after birth and may be severe or even fatal. The exact mechanism of the defect is unknown but may involve phenobarbital induction of fetal liver microsomal enzymes that deplete the already low reserves of fetal vitamin K (23). This results in suppression of the vitamin K-dependent coagulation factors, II, VII, IX, and X. In a 1985 review, Lane and Hathaway (23) summarized the various prophylactic treatment regimens that have been proposed (see Phenytoin for details).

Barbiturate withdrawal has been observed in newborns exposed to phenobarbital *in utero* (24). The average onset of symptoms in 15 addicted infants was 6 days (range 3–14 days). These infants had been exposed during gestation to doses varying from 64 to 300 mg/day with unknown amounts in four patients.

Phenobarbital may induce folic acid deficiency in the pregnant woman (25–27). A discussion of this effect and the possible consequences for the fetus are presented under Phenytoin.

High-dose phenobarbital, contained in an anti-asthmatic preparation, was reported in a mother giving birth to a stillborn full-term female infant with complete triploidy (28). The authors speculated on the potential phenobarbital-induced chromosome damage, but an earlier *in vitro* study found no effect of the drug on the incidence of chromosome gaps, breaks, or abnormal forms (29).

Phenobarbital and/or cholestyramine have been used to treat cholestasis of pregnancy (30, 31). Although no drug-induced fetal complications were noted, the therapy was ineffective for this condition.

In summary, phenobarbital therapy in the epileptic pregnant woman presents a risk to the fetus in terms of minor congenital defects, hemorrhage at birth, and addiction. The risk to the mother, however, is greater if the drug is withheld and seizure control is lost. The benefit:risk ratio, in this case, favors continued use of the drug during pregnancy at the lowest possible level to control seizures. Use of the drug in nonepileptic patients does not seem to pose a significant risk for congenital defects, but hemorrhage and addiction in the newborn are still concerns.

Breast Feeding Summary

Phenobarbital is excreted into breast milk (32–36). The milk:plasma ratio varies between 0.4 and 0.6 (33, 34). The amount of phenobarbital ingested by the nursing infant has been estimated to reach 2–4 mg/day (35). The pharmacokinetics of phenobarbital during lactation have been reviewed by Nau and co-workers (34). Due to slower elimination in the nursing infant, accumulation may occur to the point that blood levels in the infant may actually exceed those of the mother (34). Phenobarbital-induced sedation has been observed in three nursing infants, probably caused by this accumulation (32). Women consuming phenobarbital during breast-feeding, especially those on high doses, should be instructed to observe their infants for sedation. Phenobarbital levels in the infant should also be monitored to avoid toxic concentrations (34). The American Academy of Pediatrics considers the drug compatible with breast-feeding (37).

References

1. Hauptmann A. Luminal bei epilepsie. Muench Med Wochenschr 1912;59:1907–8.
2. Janz D, Fuchs V. Are anti-epileptic drugs harmful when given during pregnancy? German Med Monogr 1964;9:20–3.
3. Hill RB. Teratogenesis and anti-epileptic drugs. N Engl J Med 1973;289:1089–90.
4. Bodendorfer TW. Fetal effects of anticonvulsant drugs and seizure disorders. Drug Intell Clin Pharm 1978;12:14–21.
5. Committee on Drugs, American Academy of Pediatrics. Anticonvulsants and pregnancy. Pediatrics 1977;63:331–3.
6. Nakane Y, Okoma T, Takahashe R, et al. Multi-institutional study of the teratogenicity and fetal toxicity of anti-epileptic drugs: a report of a collaborative study group in Japan. Epilepsia 980;21:633–80.
7. Andermann E, Dansky L, Andermann F, Loughnan PM, Gibbons J. Minor congenital malformations and dermatoglyphic alterations in the offspring of epileptic women; a clinical investigation of the teratogenic effects of anticonvulsant medication. In *Epilepsy, Pregnancy and the Child*. Proceedings of a Workshop in Berlin, September 1980. New York:Raven Press, 1981.
8. Dansky L, Andermann E, Andermann F. Major congenital malformations in the offspring of epileptic patients. *Ibid.*
9. Janz D. The teratogenic risks of antiepileptic drugs. Epilepsia 1975;16:159–69.
10. Hanson JW, Buehler BA. Fetal hydantoin syndrome: current status. J Pediatr 1982;101:816–8.
11. Janz D. Antiepileptic drugs and pregnancy: altered utilization patterns and teratogenesis. Epilepsia 1982;23(Suppl 1):S53–S63.
12. Heinonen OP, Slone D, Shapiro S. *Birth Defects and Drugs in Pregnancy*. Littleton:Publishing Sciences Group, 1977:336–9.
13. *Ibid*, 438.
14. Spiedel BD, Meadow SR. Maternal epilepsy and abnormalities of the fetus and the newborn. Lancet 1972;2:839–43.
15. Bleyer WA, Skinner AL. Fatal neonatal hemorrhage after maternal anticonvulsant therapy. JAMA 1976;235:826–7.
16. Lawrence A. Anti-epileptic drugs and the foetus. Br Med J 1963;2:1267.
17. Kohler HG. Haemorrhage in the newborn of epileptic mothers. Lancet 1966;1:267.

18. Mountain KR, Hirsh J, Gallus AS. Neonatal coagulation defect due to anticonvulsant drug treatment in pregnancy. Lancet 1970;1:265–8.
19. Evans AR, Forrester RM, Discombe C. Neonatal haemorrhage during anticonvulsant therapy. Lancet 1970;1:517–8.
20. Margolin FG, Kantor NM. Hemorrhagic disease of the newborn. An unusual case related to maternal ingestion of an anti-epileptic drug. Clin Pediatr (Phila) 1972;11:59–60.
21. Srinivasan G, Seeler RA, Tiruvury A, Pildes RS. Maternal anticonvulsant therapy and hemorrhagic disease of the newborn. Obstet Gynecol 1982;59:250–2.
22. Payne NR, Hasegawa DK. Vitamin K deficiency in newborns: a case report in α-1-antitrypsin deficiency and a review of factors predisposing to hemorrhage. Pediatrics 1984;73:712–6.
23. Lane PA, Hathaway WE. Vitamin K in infancy. J Pediatr 1985;106:351–9.
24. Desmond MM, Schwanecke RP, Wilson GS, Yasunaga S, Burgdorff I. Maternal barbiturate utilization and neonatal withdrawal symptomatology. J. Pediatr 1972;80:190–7.
25. Pritchard JA, Scott DE, Whalley PJ. Maternal folate deficiency and pregnancy wastage. IV. Effects of folic acid supplements, anticonvulsants, and oral contraceptives. Am J Obstet Gynecol 1971;109:341–6.
26. Hiilesmaa VK, Teramo K, Granstrom ML, Bardy AH. Serum folate concentrations during pregnancy in women with epilepsy: relation to antiepileptic drug concentrations, number of seizures, and fetal outcome. Br Med J 1983;287:577–9.
27. Biale Y, Lewenthal H. Effect of folic acid supplementation on congenital malformations due to anticonvulsive drugs. Eur J Obstet Reprod Biol 1984;18:211–6.
28. Halbrecht I, Komlos L, Shabtay F, Solomon M, Book JA. Triploidy 69, XXX in a stillborn girl. Clin Genet 1973;4:210–2.
29. Stenchever MA, Jarvis JA. Effect of barbiturates on the chromosomes of human cells in vitro—a negative report. J Reprod Med 1970;5:69–71.
30. Heikkinen J, Maentausta O, Ylostalo P, Janne O. Serum bile acid levels in intrahepatic cholestasis of pregnancy during treatment with phenobarbital or cholestyramine. Eur J Obstet Reprod Biol 1982;14:153–62.
31. Shaw D, Frohlich J, Wittmann BAK, Willms M. A prospective study of 18 patients with cholestasis of pregnancy. Am J Obstet Gynecol 1982;142:621–5.
32. Tyson RM, Shrader EA, Perlman HN. Drugs transmitted through breast-milk. II. Barbiturates. J Pediatr 1938;13:86–90.
33. Kaneko S, Sata T, Suzuki K. The levels of anticonvulsants in breast milk. Br J Clin Pharmacol 1979;7:624–7.
34. Nau H, Kuhnz W, Egger HJ, Rating D, Helge H. Anticonvulsants during pregnancy and lactation: transplacental, maternal and neonatal pharmacokinetics. Clin Pharmacokinet 1982;7:508–43.
35. Horning MG, Stillwell WG, Nowling J, Lertratanangkoon K, Stillwell RN, Hill RM. Identification and quantification of drugs and drug metabolites in human breast milk using GC-MS-COM methods. Mod Probl Paediatr 1975;15:73–9.
36. Reith H, Schafer H. Antiepileptic drugs during pregnancy and the lactation period. Pharmacokinetic data. Dtsch Med Wochenschr 1979;104:818–23.
37. Committee on Drugs, American Academy of Pediatrics. The transfer of drugs and other chemicals into human breast milk. Pediatrics 1983;72:375–83.

Name: **PHENPROCOUMON**

Class: **Anticoagulant**   Risk Factor: **D**

Fetal Risk Summary

See Coumarin Derivatives.

Breast Feeding Summary

See Coumarin Derivatives.

Name: **PHENSUXIMIDE**

Class: **Anticonvulsant**   Risk Factor: **D**

Fetal Risk Summary

The use of phensuximide, the first succinimide anticonvulsant used in the treatment of petit mal epilepsy, has been reported in three pregnancies (1, 2). Due to multiple drug therapy and difference in study methodology, conclusions linking the use of phensuximide with congenital defects are difficult. Fetal abnormalities identified with the three pregnancies include: ambiguous genitalia, inquinal hernia, and pyloric stenosis. Phensuximide has a much lower teratogenic potential than the oxozolidinedione class of anticonvulsants (see Trimethadione) (3, 4). Due to a high incidence of toxic effects, the new succinimides should be considered in favor of phensuximide for the treatment of petit mal epilepsy (see Ethosuximide, Methsuximide) (5).

Breast Feeding Summary

No data available.

References

1. Fedrick J. Epilepsy and pregnancy: a report from the Oxford Record Linkage Study. Br Med J 1973;2:442–8.
2. McMullin GP. Teratogenic effects of anticonvulsants. Br Med J 1971;2:430.
3. Fabro S, Brown NA. Teratogenic potential of anticonvulsants. N Engl J Med 1979;300:1280–1.
4. The National Institutes of Health. Anticonvulsants found to have teratogenic potential. JAMA 1981;241:36.
5. Schmidt RP, Wilder BJ. Epilepsy. In *Contemporary Neurology Series*: No. 2. Philadelphia: FA Davis Co, 1968;159.

Name: **PHENTERMINE**

Class: **Central Stimulant**   Risk Factor: **C**

Fetal Risk Summary

No data available (see Diethylpropion or Dextroamphetamine).

Breast Feeding Summary

No data available.

Name: **PHENYLBUTAZONE**

Class: **Nonsteroidal Anti-Inflammatory Analgesic**   Risk Factor: **D**

Fetal Risk Summary

Two reports have been located that describe congenital defects in the offspring of mothers consuming phenylbutazone during pregnancy (1, 2). A cause-and-effect relationship was not established in either case. Possible embryotoxicity has been demonstrated in animals, and the drug crosses the placenta to the human fetus (3–6). Theoretically, phenylbutazone, a prostaglandin synthetase inhibitor, could cause constriction of the ductus arteriosus *in utero* (7). Persistent pulmonary hypertension of the newborn should also be considered (7). Drugs in this class have been shown to inhibit labor and prolong pregnancy (8). The manufacturer recommends that the drug not be used in pregnancy (3).

Breast Feeding Summary

Phenylbutazone is excreted into breast milk in low concentrations, although some investigators failed to detect the drug 3 hours after maternal administration (7–9). The drug has been measured in infant serum after breast-feeding, but no adverse effects in the nursing infant have been reported. The American Academy of Pediatrics considers phenylbutazone compatible with breast-feeding (10).

References

1. Tuchmann-Duplessis H. Medication in the course of pregnancy and teratogenic malformation. Concours Med 1967;89:2119–20.
2. Kullander S, Kallen B. A prospective study of drugs in pregnancy. Acta Obstet Gynecol Scand 1976;55:289–95.
3. Product information. Butazolidin. Geigy Pharmaceuticals, 1985.
4. Leuxner E, Pulver R. Verabreichung von irgapryin bei schwangeren und wochnerinnen. Muench Med Wochenschr 1956;98:84–6.
5. Strobel S, Leuxner E. Uber die zullassigkeit der verabreichung von butazolidin bei schwangeren und wochnerinnen. Med Klin 1957;39:1708–10.
6. Akbaraly R, Leng JJ, Brachet-Liermain A, White P, Laclau-Lacrouts B. Trans-placental transfer of four anti-inflammatory agents. A study carried out by in vitro perfusion. J Gynecol Obstet Biol Reprod 1981;10:7–11.
7. Levin DL. Effects of inhibition of prostaglandin synthesis on fetal development, oxygenation, and the fetal circulation. Semin Perinatol 1980;4:35–44.
8. Fuchs F. Prevention of prematurity. Am J Obstet Gynecol 1976;126:809–20.
9. Wilson JT. Milk/plasma ratios and contraindicated drugs. In Wilson JT, ed. *Drugs in Breast Milk.* Balgowlah, Australia:ADIS Press, 1981:78–9.
10. Committee on Drugs, American Academy of Pediatrics. The transfer of drugs and other chemicals into human breast milk. Pediatrics 1983;72:375–83.

Name: **PHENYLEPHRINE**

Class: **Sympathomimetic (Adrenergic)**   Risk Factor: **C**

Fetal Risk Summary

Phenylephrine is a sympathomimetic used in emergency situations to treat hypotension and to alleviate allergic symptoms of the eye and ear. Uterine vessels are normally maximally dilated, and they have only α-adrenergic receptors (1). Use of the predominantly α-adrenergic stimulant, phenylephrine, could cause constriction of these vessels and reduce uterine blood flow, thereby producing fetal hypoxia (bradycardia). Phenylephrine may also interact with oxytocics or ergot derivatives to produce severe persistent maternal hypertension (1). Rupture of a cerebral vessel is possible. If a pressor agent is indicated, other drugs such as ephedrine should be considered. Sympathomimetic amines are teratogenic in some animal species, but human teratogenicity has not been suspected (2, 3). Recent data may require a reappraisal of this opinion. The Collaborative Perinatal Project monitored 50,282 mother-child pairs, 1,249 of which had 1st trimester exposure to phenylephrine (4). For use anytime during pregnancy, 4,194 exposures were recorded (5). An association was found between 1st trimester use of phenylephrine and malformations; minor defects were greater than major (4). For individual malformations, several possible associations were found (4, 6, 7):

First trimester:
   Eye and ear defects (8 cases)
   Syndactyly (6 cases)
   Preauricular skin tag (4 cases)
   Clubfoot (3 cases)
Anytime use:
   Congenital dislocation of hip (15 cases)
   Other musculoskeletal malformations (4 cases)
   Umbilical hernia (6 cases)

The statistical significance of these associations is not known and independent confirmation is required. For the sympathomimetic class of drugs as a whole, an association was found between 1st trimester use and minor malformations (not life-threatening or major cosmetic defects), inguinal hernia, and clubfoot (4).

Sympathomimetics are often administered in combination with other drugs to alleviate the symptoms of upper respiratory infections. Thus, the fetal effects of sympathomimetics, other drugs, and viruses cannot be totally separated. However, indiscriminate use of this class of drugs, especially in the 1st trimester, is not without risk.

Phenylephrine has been used as a stress test to determine fetal status in high-risk pregnancies (8). In the United States, however, this test is normally conducted with oxytocin.

Breast Feeding Summary

No data available.

References

1. Smith NT, Corbascio AN. The use and misuse of pressor agents. Anesthesiology 1970;33:58–101.
2. Nashimura H, Tanimura T. *Clinical Aspects of the Teratogenicity of Drugs*. Amsterdam:Excerpta Medica, 1976:231.
3. Shepard TH. *Catalog of Teratogenic Agents*, ed 3. Baltimore:The Johns Hopkins University Press, 1980:134–5.
4. Heinonen OP, Slone D, Shapiro S. *Birth Defects and Drugs in Pregnancy*. Littleton:Publishing Sciences Group, 1977:345–56.
5. *Ibid*, 439.
6. *Ibid*, 476.
7. *Ibid*, 491.
8. Eguchi K, Yonezawa M, Hagegawa T, Lin TT, Ejiri K, Kudo T, Sekiba K, Takeda Y. Fetal activity determination and Neosynephrine test for evaluation of fetal well-being in high risk pregnancies. Nippon Sanka Fujinka Gakkai Zasshi 1980;32:663–8.

Name: **PHENYLPROPANOLAMINE**

Class: **Sympathomimetic (Adrenergic)**   Risk Factor: **C**

Fetal Risk Summary

Phenylpropanolamine is a sympathomimetic used for anorexia and to alleviate the symptoms of allergic disorders or upper respiratory infections. Uterine vessels are normally maximally dilated and they have only α-adrenergic receptors (1). Use of the α- and β-adrenergic stimulant, phenylpropanolamine, could cause constriction of these vessels and reduce uterine blood flow, thereby producing fetal hypoxia (bradycardia). This drug is a common component of proprietary mixtures containing antihistamines and other drugs. Thus, it is difficult to separate the effects of phenylpropanolamine on the fetus from other drugs, disease states, and viruses.

Sympathomimetic amines are teratogenic in some animal species, but human teratogenicity has not been suspected (2, 3). Recent data may require a reappraisal of this opinion. The Collaborative Perinatal Project monitored 50,282 mother-child pairs, 726 of which had 1st trimester exposure to phenylpropanolamine (4). For use anytime during pregnancy, 2,489 exposures were recorded (5). An association was found between 1st trimester use of phenylpropanolamine and malformations; minor defects were greater than major (4). For individual malformations, several possible associations were found (4, 6, 7):

First trimester:
  Hypospadias (4 cases)
  Eye and ear defects (7 cases) (statisically significant)
  Polydactyly (6 cases)
  Cataract (3 cases)
  Pectus excavatum (7 cases)
Anytime use:
  Congenital dislocation of hip (12 cases)

Except for eye and ear defects, the statistical significance of these associations is not known, and independent confirmation is required. For the sympathomimetic class of drugs as a whole, an association was found between 1st trimester use and minor malformations (not life-threatening or major cosmetic defects), inguinal hernia, and clubfoot (4). Indiscriminate use of this class of drugs, especially in the 1st trimester, is not without risk.

A case of infantile malignant osteopetrosis was described in a 4-month-old boy exposed *in utero* on several occasions to Contac (chlorpheniramine, phenylpropanolamine, and belladonna alkaloids), but this is a known genetic defect (8). The infant also had a continual "stuffy" nose.

Breast Feeding Summary

No data available.

References

1. Smith NT, Corbascio AN. The use and misuse of pressor agents. Anesthesiology 1970;33:58–101.
2. Nishimura H, Tanimura T. *Clinical Aspects of the Teratogenicity of Drugs*. Amsterdam:Excerpta Medica, 1976:231.
3. Shepard TH. *Catalog of Teratogenic Drugs*, ed 3. Baltimore:The Johns Hopkins University Press, 1980:134–5.
4. Heinonen OP, Slone D, Shapiro S. *Birth Defects and Drugs in Pregnancy*. Littleton:Publishing Sciences Group, 1977:345–56.
5. *Ibid*, 439.
6. *Ibid*, 477.
7. *Ibid*, 491.
8. Golbus MS, Koerper MA, Hall BD. Failure to diagnose osteopetrosis in utero. Lancet 1976;2:1246.

Name: **PHENYLTOLOXAMINE**

Class: **Antihistamine**   Risk Factor: **C**

Fetal Risk Summary

No data available.

Breast Feeding Summary

No data available.

Name: **PHENYTOIN**

Class: **Anticonvulsant**   Risk Factor: **D**

Fetal Risk Summary

Phenytoin is a hydantoin anticonvulsant introduced in 1938. The teratogenic effects of phenytoin were recognized in 1964 (1). Since this report there have been numerous reviews and studies on the teratogenic effects of phenytoin and other anticonvulsants. Based on this literature, the epileptic pregnant woman taking phenytoin, either alone or in combination with other anticonvulsants, has a two to three times greater risk for delivering a child with congenital defects over the general population (2–9). It is not known if this increased risk is due to antiepileptic drugs, the disease itself, genetic factors, or a combination of these, although some evidence indicates that drugs are the causative factor (9). Fifteen epidemiologic studies cited by Hanson and Buehler in 1982 (9) found an incidence of defects in treated epileptics varying from 2.2 to 26.1%. In each case, the rate for treated patients was higher than that for untreated epileptics or normal controls. Animal studies have also implicated drugs and have suggested that a dose-related response may occur (9).

A recognizable pattern of malformations, now known as the fetal hydantoin syndrome (FHS), was partially described in 1968 when Meadow (10) observed distinct facial abnormalities in infants exposed to phenytoin and other anticonvulsants (10). In 1973, Loughnan and co-workers (11) and Hill and co-workers (12), in independent reports, described unusual anomalies of fingers and toes in exposed infants. The basic syndrome consists of variable degrees of hypoplasia and ossification of the distal phalanges and craniofacial abnormalities. Clinical features of the FHS, not all of which are apparent in every infant, are (10–12):

Craniofacial:
  Broad nasal bridge
  Wide fontanel
  Low set hairline
  Broad alveolar ridge
  Metopic ridging
  Short neck
  Ocular hypertelorism
  Microcephaly
  Cleft lip/palate
  Abnormal or low-set ears
  Epicanthal folds
  Ptosis of eyelids
  Coloboma
  Coarse scalp hair
Limbs:
  Small or absent nails
  Hypoplasia of distal phalanges
  Altered palmar crease
  Digital thumb
  Dislocated hip

Impaired growth, both physical and mental, congenital heart defects, and cleft lip and/or palate are often observed in conjunction with the FHS.

Numerous other defects have been reported to occur after phenytoin exposure in pregnancy. Janz, in a 1982 review (13), stated that nearly all possible types of malformations may be observed in the offspring of epileptic mothers. This statement is supported by the large volume of literature describing various anomalies that have been attributed to phenytoin with or without other anticonvulsants (1–49).

Eleven case reports have been located that, taken in sum, suggest that phenytoin is a human transplacental carcinogen (14–24). Tumors reported to occur in infants after *in utero* exposure to phenytoin include:

Neuroblastoma (5 cases) (14–18)
Ganglioneuroblastoma (1 case) (19)

Melanotic neuroectodermal tumor (1 case) (20)
Extrarenal Wilms' tumor (1 case) (21)
Mesenchymoma (1 case) (22)
Lymphangioma (1 case) (23)
Ependymoblastoma (1 case) (24)

Children exposed *in utero* to phenytoin should be closely observed for several years since tumor development may take that long to express itself.

Phenytoin and other anticonvulsants (e.g., phenobarbital) may cause early hemorrhagic disease of the newborn (14, 50–64). Hemorrhage occurs during the first 24 hours after birth and may be severe or even fatal. The exact mechanism of the defect is unknown but may involve phenytoin-induction of fetal liver microsomal enzymes that deplete the already low reserves of fetal vitamin K (64). This results in suppression of the vitamin K-dependent coagulation factors, II, VII, IX, and X. Phenytoin-induced thrombocytopenia has also been reported as a mechanism for hemorrhage in the newborn (61). In a 1985 review, Lane and Hathaway (64) summarized the various prophylactic treatment regimens that have been proposed:

Administering 10 mg orally of vitamin K daily during the last 2 months of pregnancy
Administering 20 mg orally of vitamin K daily during the last 2 weeks of pregnancy
Avoiding salicylates and administering vitamin K during labor
Cesarean section if a difficult or traumatic delivery is anticipated
Administering intravenous vitamin K to the newborn in the delivery room plus cord blood clotting studies

Although all of the above suggestions are logical, none has been tested in controlled trials (64). Lane and Hathaway (64) recommend immediate intramuscular vitamin K and close observation of the infant (see also Phytonadione).

Liver damage was observed in an infant exposed during gestation to phenytoin and valproic acid (65). Although they were unable to demonstrate which anticonvulsant caused the injury, the authors concluded that valproic acid was the more likely offending agent.

Phenytoin may induce folic acid deficiency in the epileptic patient by impairing gastrointestinal absorption or by increasing hepatic metabolism of the vitamin (66–68). Whether phenytoin also induces folic acid deficiency in the fetus is less certain since the fetus seems to be efficient in drawing on available maternal stores of folic acid (see Folic Acid). Low maternal folate levels, however, have been proposed as one possible mechanism for the increased incidence of defects observed in infants exposed *in utero* to phenytoin. Biale and Leventhal (66) conducted research on the relationship between folic acid, anticonvulsants, and fetal defects. In the retrospective part of this study, a group of 24 women treated with phenytoin and other anticonvulsants produced 66 infants, 10 (15%) with major anomalies. Two of the mothers with affected infants had markedly low red blood cell folate concentrations. A second group of 22 epileptic women were then given supplements of folic acid daily, 2.5–5.0 mg, starting before conception in 26 pregnancies and within the first 40 days in six. This group produced 33 newborns (32 pregnancies; 1 set of twins) with no defects, a significant difference from the unsupplemented group. Loss of seizure control caused by folic acid lowering of phenytoin serum levels, which is known to occur, was not a problem in this small series.

Negative associations between phenytoin-induced folate deficiency have been reported by Pritchard and co-workers (67) and Hiilesmaa and co-workers (68). In the study of Hiilesmaa *et al.* (68), mothers were given supplements with an average folic acid dose of 0.5 mg/day from the 6th to 16th week of gestation until delivery. Defects were observed in 20 infants (15%) from the 133 women taking anticonvulsants, which is similar to the reported frequency in pregnant patients not given supplements. Folate levels were usually within the normal range for pregnancy.

The pharmacokinetics and placental transport of phenytoin have been extensively studied and reviewed (69–71). Plasma concentrations of phenytoin may fall during pregnancy. Animal studies and recent human reports suggest a dose-related teratogenic effect of phenytoin (72, 73). While these results are based on a small series of patients, it is reasonable to avoid excessively high plasma concentrations of phenytoin. Close monitoring of plasma phenytoin concentrations is recommended to maintain adequate seizure control and prevent potential fetal hypoxia.

Placental function in women taking phenytoin has been evaluated (74). No effect was detected from phenytoin as measured by serum human placental lactogen, 24-hour urinary total estriol excretion, placental weight, and birth weight.

In a study evaluating thyroid function, no differences were found between treated epileptic pregnant women and normal pregnant controls (75). Thyroxine levels in the cord blood of anticonvulsant exposed infants were significantly lower than those of controls, but this was shown to be due to altered protein binding and not to altered thyroid function. Other parameters studied, levels of thyrotropin, free thyroxine, and triiodothyronine, were similar in both groups.

The effect of phenytoin on maternal and fetal vitamin D metabolism was examined in a 1984 study (76). In comparison to normal controls, several significant differences were found in the level of various vitamin D compounds and in serum calcium, but the values were still within normal limits. No alterations were found in alkaline phosphatase and phosphate concentrations. The authors doubted if the observed differences were of major clinical significance.

In summary, the use of phenytoin during pregnancy involves significant risk to the fetus in terms of major and minor congenital abnormalities and hemorrhage at birth. The risk to the mother, however, is also great if the drug is not used to control her seizures. The benefit:risk ratio, in this case, favors continued use of the drug during pregnancy. Frequent determinations of phenytoin levels are recommended to maintain the lowest level required to prevent seizures and to possibly lessen the likelihood of fetal anomalies. Based on recent research, consideration should also be given to monitoring folic acid levels simultaneously with phenytoin determinations and administering folic acid very early in pregnancy or before conception to those women shown to have low folate concentrations.

Breast Feeding Summary

Phenytoin is excreted into breast milk. Milk:plasma ratios range from 0.18 to 0.54 (69,77–80). Nau reviewed the pharmacokinetics of phenytoin during lactation and concluded that little risk to the nursing infant was present if maternal levels were kept in the therapeutic range (69). However, methemoglobinenemia, drowsiness and decreased sucking activity have been reported in one infant (81). Except for this one case, no other reports of adverse effects with the use of phenytoin during lactation have been located. The American Academy of Pediatrics considers the drug compatible with breast feeding (82).

References

1. Janz D, Fuchs V. Are anti-epileptic drugs harmful when given during pregnancy? German Med Monogr 1964;9:20–3.
2. Hill RB. Teratogenesis and antiepileptic drugs. N Engl J Med 1973;289:1089–90.
3. Janz D. The teratogenic risk of antiepileptic drugs. Epilepsia 1975;16:159–69.
4. Bodendorfer TW. Fetal effects of anticonvulsant drugs and seizure disorders. Drug Intell Clin Pharm 1978;12:14–21.
5. Committee on Drugs, American Academy of Pediatrics. Anticonvulsants and pregnancy. Pediatrics 1977;63:331–3.
6. Nakane Y, Okuma T, Takahashi R, et al. Multi-institutional study of the teratogenicity and fetal toxicity of antiepileptic drugs: a report of a collaborative study group in Japan. Epilepsia 1980;21:663–80.
7. Andermann E, Dansky L, Andermann F, Loughnan PM, Gibbons J. Minor congenital malformations and dermatoglyphic alterations in the offspring of epileptic women: a clinical investigation of the teratogenic effects of anticonvulsant medication. In *Epilepsy, Pregnancy and the Child*. Proceedings of a Workshop in Berlin, September 1980. New York:Raven Press, 1981.
8. Dansky L, Andermann E, Andermann F. Major congenital malformations in the offspring of epileptic patients. *Ibid*.
9. Hanson JW, Buehler BA. Fetal hydantoin syndrome: current status. J Pediatr 1982;101:816–8.
10. Meadow SR. Anticonvulsant drugs and congenital abnormalities. Lancet 1968;2:1296.
11. Loughnan PM, Gold H, Vance JC. Phenytoin teratogenicity in man. Lancet 1973;1:70–2.
12. Hill RM, Horning MG, Horning EC. Antiepileptic drugs and fetal well-being. In Boreus L, ed. *Fetal Pharmacology*. New York:Raven Press, 1973:375–9.
13. Janz D. Antiepileptic drugs and pregnancy: altered utilization patterns and teratogenesis. Epilepsia 1982;23(Suppl 1):S53–S63.
14. Allen RW Jr, Ogden B, Bentley FL, Jung AL. Fetal hydantoin syndrome, neuroblastoma, and hemorrhagic disease in a neonate. JAMA 1980;244:1464–5.
15. Ramilo J, Harris VJ. Neuroblastoma in a child with the hydantoin and fetal alcohol syndrome. The radiographic features. Br J Radiol 1979;52:993–5.
16. Pendergrass TW, Hanson JW. Fetal hydantoin syndrome and neuroblastoma. Lancet 1976;2:150.
17. Sherman S, Roizen N. Fetal hydantoin syndrome and neuroblastoma. Lancet 1976;2:517.
18. Ehrenbard LT, Chagantirs K. Cancer in the fetal hydantoin syndrome. Lancet 1981;1:197.
19. Seeler RA, Israel JN, Royal JE, Kaye CI, Rao S, Abulaban M. Ganglioneuroblastoma and fetal hydantoin-alcohol syndromes. Pediatrics 1979;63:524–7.
20. Jimenez JF, Seibert RW, Char F, Brown RE, Seibert JJ. Melanotic neuroectodermal tumor of infancy and fetal hydantoin syndrome. Am J Pediatr Hematol Oncol 1981;3:9–15.
21. Taylor WF, Myers M, Taylor WR. Extrarenal Wilms' tumour in an infant exposed to intrauterine phenytoin. Lancet 1980;2:481–2.
22. Blattner WA, Hanson DE, Young EC, Fraumeni JF. Malignant mesenchymoma and birth defects. JAMA 1977;238:334–5.
23. Kousseff BG. Subcutaneous vascular abnormalities in fetal hydantoin syndrome. Birth Defects 1982;18:51–4.
24. Lipson A. Bale P. Ependymoblastoma associated with prenatal exposure to diphenylhydantoin and methylphenobarbitone. Cancer 1985;55:1859–62.
25. Corcoran R, Rizk MW. VACTERL congenital malformation and phenytoin therapy? Lancet 1976;2:960.
26. Pinto W Jr, Gardner LI, Rosenbaum P. Abnormal genitalia as a presenting sign in two male infants with hydantoin embryopathy syndrome. Am J Dis Child 1977;131:452–5.
27. Hoyt CS, Billson FA. Maternal anticonvulsants and optic nerve hypoplasia. Br J Ophthalmol 1978;62:3–6.
28. Wilson RS, Smead W, Char F. Diphenylhydantoin teratogenicity: ocular manifestations and related deformities. J Pediatr Ophthalmol Strabismus 1970;15:137–40.
29. Dabee V, Hart AG, Hurley RM. Teratogenic effects of diphenylhydantoin. Can Med Assoc J 1975;112:75–7.
30. Anderson RC. Cardiac defects in children of mothers receiving anticonvulsant therapy during pregnancy. J Pediatr 1976;89:318–9.
31. Hill RM, Verniaud WM, Horning MG, McCulley LB, Morgan NF. Infants exposed in utero to antiepileptic drugs. A prospective study. Am J Dis Child 1974;127:645–53.

32. Stankler L, Campbell AGM. Neonatal acne vulgaris: a possible feature of the fetal hydantoin syndrome. Br J Dermatol 1980;103:453-5.
33. Ringrose CAD. The hazard of neurotropic drugs in the fertile years. Can Med Assoc J 1972;106:1058.
34. Pettifor JM, Benson R. Congenital malformations associated with the administration of oral anticoagulants during pregnancy. J Pediatr 1975;86:459-61.
35. Biale Y, Lewenthal H, Aderet NB. Congenital malformations due to anticonvulsant drugs and congenital abnormalities. Obstet Gynecol 1975;45:439-42.
36. Aase JM. Anticonvulsant drugs and congenital abnormalities. Am J Dis Child 1974;127:758.
37. Lewin PK. Phenytoin associated congenital defects with Y-chromosome variant. Lancet 1973 I:559.
38. Yang TS, Chi CC, Tsai CJ, Chang MJ. Diphenylhydantoin teratogenicity in man. Obstet Gynecol 1978;52:682-4.
39. Mallow DW, Herrick MK, Gathman G. Fetal exposure to anticonvulsant drugs. Arch Pathol Lab Med 1980;104:215-8.
40. Hirschberger M, Kleinberg F. Maternal phenytoin ingestion and congenital abnormalities: report of a case. Am J Dis Child 1975;129:984.
41. Hanson JW, Myrianthopoulos NC, Sedgwick Harvey MA, Smith DW. Risks to the offspring of women treated with hydantoin anticonvulsants, with emphasis on the fetal hydantoin syndrome. J Pediatr 1976;89:662-8.
42. Shakir RA, Johnson RH, Lambie DG, Melville ID, Nanda RN. Comparison of sodium valproate and phenytoin as single drug treatment in epilepsy. Epilepsia 1981;22:27-33.
43. Michalodimitrakis M, Parchas S, Coutselinis A. Fetal hydantoin syndrome: congenital malformation of the urinary tract – a case report. Clin Toxicol 1981;18:1095-7.
44. Phelan MC, Pellock JM, Nance WE. Discordant expression of fetal hydantoin syndrome in hetero-paternal dizygotic twins. N Engl J Med 1982;307:99-101.
45. Kousseff BG, Root ER. Expanding phenotype of fetal hydantoin syndrome. Pediatrics 1982;70:328-9.
46. Wilker R, Nathenson G. Combined fetal alcohol and hydantoin syndromes. Clin Pediatr (Phila) 1982;21:331-4.
47. Kogutt MS. Fetal hydantoin syndrome. South Med J 1984;77:657-8.
48. Krauss CM, Holmes LB, VanLang, QN, Keith DA. Four siblings with similar malformations after exposure to phenytoin and primidone. J Pediatr 1984;105:750-5.
49. Pearl KN, Dickens S, Latham P. Functional palatal incompetence in the fetal anticonvulsant syndrome. Arch Dis Child 1984;59:989-90.
50. Lawrence A. Antiepileptic drugs and the foetus. Br Med J 1963;2:1267.
51. Kohler HG. Haemorrhage in newborn of epileptic mothers. Lancet 1966;1:267.
52. Douglas H. Haemorrhage in the newborn. Lancet 1966;1:816-7.
53. Monnet P, Rosenberg D, Bovier-Lapierre M. Terapeutique anticomitale administree pendant la grosses et maladie hemorragique du nouveau-ne. In Bleyer WA, Skinner AL. Fetal neonatal hemorrhage after maternal anticonvulsant therapy. JAMA 1976;235:626-7.
54. Davis PP. Coagulation defect due to anticonvulsant drug treatment in pregnancy. Lancet 1970;1:413.
55. Evans AR, Forrester RM, Discombe C. Neonatal hemorrhage following maternal anticonvulsant therapy. Lancet 1970;1:517-8.
56. Stevensom MM, Bilbert EF. Anticonvulsants and hemorrhagic diseases of the newborn infant. J Pediatr 1970;77:516.
57. Speidel BD, Meadow SR. Maternal epilepsy and abnormalities of the fetus and newborn. Lancet 1972;2:839-40.
58. Truog WE, Feusner JH, Baker DL. Association of hemorrhagic disease and the syndrome of persistent fetal circulation with the fetal hydantoin syndrome. J Pediatr 1980;96:112-4.
59. Solomon GE, Hilgartner MW, Kutt H. Coagulation defects caused by diphenylhydantoin. Neurology 1972;22:1165-71.
60. Griffiths AD. Neonatal haemorrhage associated with maternal anticonvulsant therapy. Lancet 1981;2:1296-7.
61. Page TE, Hoyme HE, Markarian M, Jones KL. Neonatal hemorrhage secondary to thrombocyto-penia: an occasional effect of prenatal hydantoin exposure. Birth Defects 1982;18:47-50.
62. Srinivasan G, Seeler RA, Tiruvury A, Pildes RS. Maternal anticonvulsant therapy and hemorrhagic disease of the newborn. Obstet Gynecol 1982;59:250-2.

63. Payne NR, Hasegawa DK. Vitamin K deficiency in newborns: a case report in α-1-antitrypsin deficiency and a review of factors predisposing to hemorrhage. Pediatrics 1984;73:712–6.
64. Lane PA, Hathaway WE. Vitamin K in infancy. J Pediatr 1985;106:351–9.
65. Felding I, Rane A. Congenital liver damage after treatment of mother with valproic acid and phenytoin? Acta Paediatr Scand 1984;73:565–8.
66. Biale Y, Lewenthal H. Effect of folic acid supplementation on congenital malformations due to anticonvulsive drugs. Eur J Obstet Reprod Biol 1984;18:211–6.
67. Pritchard JA, Scott DE, Whalley PJ. Maternal folate deficiency and pregnancy wastage. IV. Effects of folic acid supplements, anticonvulsants, and oral contraceptives. Am J Obstet Gynecol 1971;109:341–6.
68. Hiilesmaa VK, Teramo K, Granstrom ML, Bardy AH. Serum folate concentrations during pregnancy in women with epilepsy: relation to antiepileptic drug concentrations, number of seizures, and fetal outcome. Br Med J 1983;287:577–9.
69. Nau H, Kuhnz W, Egger HJ, Rating D, Helge H. Anticonvulsants during pregnancy and lactation: transplacental, maternal and neonatal pharmacokinetics. Clin Pharmacokinet 1982;7:508–43.
70. Chen SS, Perucca E, Lee JN, Richens A. Serum protein binding and free concentrations of phenytoin and phenobarbitone in pregnancy. Br J Clin Pharmacol 1982;13:547–52.
71. van der Klign E, Schobben F, Bree TB. Clinical pharmacokinetics of antiepileptic drugs. Drug Intell Clin Pharm 1980;14:674–85.
72. Dansky L, Andermann E, Sherwin AL, Andermann F. Plasma levels of phenytoin during pregnancy and the puerperium. In *Epilepsy, Pregnancy and the Child*. Proceedings of a Workshop held in Berlin, September 1980. New York:Raven Press, 1981.
73. Dansky L, Andermann E, Andermann F, Sherwin AL, Kinch RA. Maternal epilepsy and congenital malformatioin: correlation with maternal plasma anticonvulsant levels during pregnancy. *Ibid*.
74. Hiilesmaa VK. Evaluation of placental function in women on antiepileptic drugs. J Perinat Med 1983;11:187–92.
75. Carriero R, Andermann E, Chen MF, Eeg-Oloffson O, Kinch RAH, Klein G, Pearson Murphy BE. Thyroid function in epileptic mothers and their infants at birth. Am J Obstet Gynecol 1985;151:641–4.
76. Markestad T, Ulstein M, Strandjord RE, Aksnes L, Aarskog D. Anticonvulsant drug therapy in human pregnancy: effects on serum concentrations of vitamin D metabolites in maternal and cord blood. Am J Obstet Gynecol 1984;150:254–8.
77. Horning MG, Stillwell WG, Nowling J, Lertratanangkoon K, Stillwell RN, Hill RM. Identification and quantification of drugs and drug metabolites in human breast milk using GC-MS-COM methods. Mod Probl Paediatr 1975;15:73–9.
78. Svensmark O, Schiller PJ. 5-5-Diphenylhydantoin (Dilantin) blood level after oral or intravenous dosage in man. Acta Pharmacol Toxicol 1960;16:331–46.
79. Kok THHG, Taitz LS, Bennett MJ, Holt DW. Drowsiness due to clemastine transmitted in breast milk. Lancet 1982;1:914–5.
80. Steen B, Rane A, Lonnerholm G, Falk O, Elwin CE, Sjoqvist F. Phenytoin excretion in human breast milk and plasma levels in nursed infants. Ther Drug Monit 1982;4:331–4.
81. Finch E, Lorber J. Methaemoglobinaemia in the newborn. Probably due to phenytoin excreted in human milk. J Obstet Gynaecol Br Emp 1954;61:833.
82. Committee on Drugs, American Academy of Pediatrics. The transfer of drugs and other chemicals into human breast milk. Pediatrics 1983;72:375–83.

Name: **PHYSOSTIGMINE**

Class: **Parasympathomimetic (Cholinergic)**   Risk Factor: **C**

Fetal Risk Summary

Physostigmine is rarely used in pregnancy. No reports linking its use with congenital defects have appeared. One report described its use in 15 women at term to reverse scopolamine-induced twilight sleep (1). Apgar scores of 14 of the newborns ranged from 7 to 9 at 1 minute and 8 to 10 at 5 minutes. One infant was depressed at birth and required resuscitation, but the mother had also received meperidine and diazepam. No other effects in the infants were mentioned.

Physostigmine is an anticholinesterase, but it does not contain a quaternary ammonium element. It crosses the blood-brain barrier and should be expected to cross the placenta (2). Transient muscular weakness has been observed in about 20% of newborns of mothers with myasthenia (3–5). The neonatal myasthenia is due to transplacental passage of anti-acetylcholine receptor immunoglobulin G antibodies (5).

Breast Feeding Summary

No data available.

References

1. Smiller BG, Bartholomew EG, Sivak BJ, Alexander GD, Brown EM. Physostigmine reversal of scopolamine delirium in obstetric patients. Am J Obstet Gynecol 1973;116:326–9.
2. Taylor P. Anticholinesterase agents. In Gilman AG, Goodman LS, Gilman A, eds. *The Pharmacological Basis of Therapeutics*, ed 6. New York:Macmillan Publishing Co, 1980:100–19.
3. McNall PG, Jafarnia MR. Management of myasthenia gravis in the obstetrical patient. Am J Obstet Gynecol 1965;92:518–25.
4. Blackhall MI, Buckley GA, Roberts DV, Roberts JB, Thomas BH, Wilson A. Drug-induced neonatal myasthenia. J Obstet Gynaecol Br Commonw 1969;76:157–62.
5. Plauche WG. Myasthenia gravis in pregnancy: an update. Am J Obstet Gynecol 1979;135:691–7.

Name: **PHYTONADIONE**

Class: **Vitamin**   Risk Factor: **C**

Fetal Risk Summary

Phytonadione is a synthetic, fat-soluble substance identical to vitamin K_1, the natural vitamin found in a variety of foods (1). It is used for the prevention and treatment of hypoprothrombinemia due to vitamin K deficiency (1).

The use of phytonadione (vitamin K_1) during pregnancy and in the newborn has been the subject of several large reviews (2–5). Administration of vitamin K during pregnancy is usually not required due to the abundance of natural sources in food and the synthesis of the vitamin by the normal intestinal flora. Vitamin K_1 is indicated for maternal hypoprothrombinemia and for the prevention of hemorrhagic disease of the newborn (HDN) induced by maternal drugs such as anticonvulsants, warfarin, rifampin, and isoniazid (2–5).

The placental transfer of vitamin K_1 is poor. A 1982 study found no detectable vitamin K (<0.10 ng/ml) in the cord blood of nine term infants although adequate levels (mean 0.20 ng/ml) were present in eight of the nine mothers (6). Vitamin K_1, 1 mg intravenously, was then given to six additional mothers shortly before delivery (11–47 minutes), resulting in plasma K_1 values of 45–93 ng/ml. K_1 was detected in only four of the six cord blood samples (ranging from 0.10 to 0.14 ng/ml) and its appearance did not seem to be time dependent.

Vitamin K_1 is nontoxic in doses less than 20 mg (3). In a double blind trial, 933 women at term were given 20 mg of either K_1 or K_2, the naturally occurring vitamins

(7). No toxicity from either vitamin was found, including no association with low birth weight, asphyxia, neonatal jaundice, or perinatal mortality.

Oral vitamin K_1 has been suggested during the last 2 weeks of pregnancy for women taking anticonvulsants to prevent hypoprothrombinemia and hemorrhage in their newborns, but the effectiveness of this therapy has not been proven (2, 3). In a group of mothers receiving phenindione, an oral anticoagulant, 10–30 mg of K_1 was given either intravenously or intra-amniotically 2–4 days prior to delivery (8). In a separate group, 2.5–3.0 mg of K_1 was injected intramuscularly into the fetuses at the same interval before delivery. Only in this latter group were coagulation factors significantly improved.

In summary, phytonadione (vitamin K_1) is the treatment of choice for maternal hypoprothrombinemia and for the prevention of HDN. Maternal supplements are not needed except for those patients deemed at risk for vitamin K deficiency.

Breast Feeding Summary

Levels of phytonadione (vitamin K_1) in breast milk are naturally low with most samples having less than 20 ng/ml and many less than 5 ng/ml (2, 3). In 20 lactating women, colostrum and mature milk concentrations were 2.3 and 2.1 ng/ml, less than half that found in cows' milk (9). Administration of a single 20-mg oral dose of phytonadione to one mother produced a concentration of 140 ng/ml at 12 hours with levels at 48 hours still about double normal values (9). In another study, 40 mg orally of K_1 or K_3 (menadione) were given to mothers within 2 hours after delivery (10). Effects from either vitamin on the prothrombin time of the breast-fed newborns were nil to slight during the first 3 days.

Natural levels of K_1 or K_2 in milk will not provide adequate supplies of the vitamin for the breast-fed infant (2, 3). The vitamin K_1-dependent coagulation factors, II, VII, IX, and X, are dependent on gestational age (2). In the newborn, these factors are approximately 30–60% of normal and do not reach adult levels until about 6 weeks (2). While not all newborns are vitamin K_1-deficient, many are, due to poor placental transfer of the vitamin. Exclusive breast-feeding will not prevent further decline of these already low stores and the possible development of deficiency in 48–72 hours (2, 3). In addition, the intestinal flora of breast-fed infants may produce less vitamin K than the flora of formula-fed infants (2). The potential consequences of this deficiency is hemorrhagic disease of the newborn (HDN).

The American Academy of Pediatrics has suggested that HDN be defined as "a hemorrhagic disorder of the first days of life caused by a deficiency of vitamin K and characterized by deficiency of prothrombin and proconvertin (stable factor, factor VII), and probably of other factors" (11). The hemorrhage is frequently life-threatening, with intracranial bleeding common. In a 1985 review, Lane and Hathaway (2) identified three types of HDN:

Early HDN (onset 0–24 hours)
Classic HDN (onset 2–5 days)
Late HDN (onset 1–12 months)

The maternal ingestion of certain drugs, such as anticonvulsants, warfarin, or antituberculous agents, is one of the known causes of early and classic HDN, while breast-feeding has been shown to be a cause of classic and late HDN (2). The administration of phytonadione to the newborn prevents HDN by preventing further decline of factors II, VII, IX, and X (2).

The use of prophylactic vitamin K_1 in all newborns is common in the United States but is controversial in other countries (2). The Committee on Nutrition of the American Academy of Pediatrics recommended in 1961 and again in 1980 that all newborns receive 0.5–1.0 mg of parenteral vitamin K_1 (11, 12). The Committee recommended that administration to the mother prenatally should not be substituted for newborn prophylaxis (11). The bleeding risk in breast-fed infants who did not receive prophylactic K_1 is 15–20 times greater than in infants fed cows' milk, given K_1, or both (2). In spite of this evidence, new cases of HDN are still reported (3, 13). In a recent report, 10 breast-fed infants with intracranial hemorrhage due to vitamin K deficiency were described (13). Onset of the bleeding was between 27 and 47 days of age with three infants dying and three having permanent brain injury. Milk levels of total vitamin K (K_1 + K_2) varied between 1.36 and 9.17 ng/ml. None of the infants had been given prophylactic therapy at birth.

In summary, the natural vitamin K content of breast milk is too low to protect the newborn from vitamin K deficiency and resulting hemorrhagic disease. The administration of vitamin K to the mother to increase milk concentrations may be possible but needs further study. All newborns should receive parenteral prophylactic therapy at birth consisting of 0.5–1.0 mg of phytonadione. Larger and/or repeat doses may be required for infants whose mothers are consuming anticonvulsants or oral anticoagulants (2, 11).

References

1. American Hospital Formulary Service. *Drug Information 1985*. Bethesda:American Society of Hospital Pharmacists, 1985:1709–10.
2. Lane PA, Hathaway WE. Vitamin K in infancy. J Pediatr 1985;106:351–9.
3. Payne NR, Hasegawa DK. Vitamin K deficiency in newborns: a case report in α-1-antitrypsin deficiency and a review of factors predisposing to hemorrhage. Pediatrics 1984;73:712–6.
4. Wynn RM. The obstetric significance of factors affecting the metabolism of bilirubin, with particular reference to the role of vitamin K. Obstet Gynecol Surv 1963;18:333–54.
5. Finkel MJ. Vitamin K_1 and the vitamin K analogues. J Clin Pharmacol Ther 1961;2:795–814.
6. Shearer MJ, Rahim S, Barkhan P, Stimmler L. Plasma vitamin K_1 in mothers and their newborn babies. Lancet 1982;2:460–3.
7. Blood Study Group of Gynecologists. Effect of vitamins K_2 and K_1 on the bleeding volume during parturition and the blood coagulation disturbance of newborns by a double blind controlled study. Igaku no Ayumi 1971;76:818. As cited in Nishimura H, Tanimura T. *Clinical Aspects of the Teratogenicity of Drugs*. New York:American Elsevier, 1976:253.
8. Larsen JF, Jacobsen B, Holm HH, Pedersen JF, Mantoni M. Intrauterine injection of vitamin K before delivery during anticoagulant therapy of the mother. Acta Obstet Gynecol Scand 1978;57:227–30.
9. Haroon Y, Shearer MJ, Rahim S, Gunn WG, McEnery G, Barkhan P. The content of phylloquinone (vitamin K_1) in human milk, cows' milk and infant formula foods determined by high-performance liquid chromatography. J Nutr 1982;112:1105–17.
10. Dyggve HV, Dam H, Sondergaard E. Influence on the prothrombin time of breast-fed newborn babies of one single dose of vitamin K_1 or Synkavit given to the mother within 2 hours after birth. Acta Obstet Gynecol Scand 1956;35:440–4.
11. Committee on Nutrition, American Academy of Pediatrics. Vitamin K compounds and the water-soluble analogues. Pediatrics 1961;28:501–7.
12. Committee on Nutrition, American Academy of Pediatrics. Vitamin and mineral supplement needs in normal children in the United States. Pediatrics 1980;66:1015–21.
13. Motohara K, Matsukura M, Matsuda I, Iribe K, Ikeda T, Kondo Y, Yonekubo A, Yamamoto Y, Tsuchiya F. Severe vitamin K deficiency in breast-fed infants. J Pediatr 1984;105:943–5.

Name: **PILOCARPINE**

Class: **Parasympathomimetic (Cholinergic)**   Risk Factor: **C**

Fetal Risk Summary

Pilocarpine is used in the eye. No reports of its use in pregnancy have been located.

Breast Feeding Summary

No data available.

Name: **PINDOLOL**

Class: **Sympatholytic (β-adrenergic Blocker)**   Risk Factor: **B$_M$**

Fetal Risk Summary

Pindolol, a nonselective β-adrenergic blocking agent, has been used for the treatment of hypertension occurring during pregnancy (1–4). The drug crosses the placenta to the fetus with maternal serum levels higher than cord concentrations (5). Cord:maternal serum ratios at 2 and 6 hours after the last dose were 0.37 and 0.67, respectively. Elimination half-lives in fetal and maternal serum were 1.6 and 2.2 hours, respectively.

No fetal malformations attributable to pindolol have been reported but experience in the 1st trimester is lacking. In a study comparing three β-blockers for the treatment of hypertension during pregnancy, the mean birth weight of pindolol-exposed babies was slightly higher than that of the acebutolol group and much higher than that of the offspring of atenolol-treated mothers (3,375 g vs 3,160 g vs 2,745 g) (2). It is not known if these differences were due to the degree of maternal hypertension, the potency of the drugs used, or a combination of these and other factors.

The preliminary results of another study found over a third of the infants delivered from hypertensive women treated with pindolol were of low birth weight, but the authors thought this incidence did not differ significantly from the expected rate for this population (3). In mothers treated with pindolol or atenolol, a decrease in the basal fetal heart rate was noted only in the atenolol-exposed fetuses (4).

β-Blockade in the newborn has not been reported in the offspring of pindolol-treated mothers. However, since this complication has been observed in infants exposed to other β-blockers (see Acebutolol, Atenolol, and Nadolol), close observation of the newborn is recommended during the first 24 to 48 hours after birth. Long-term effects of *in utero* exposure to β-blockers have not been studied but warrant evaluation.

Breast Feeding Summary

No reports have been located describing the excretion of pindolol into breast milk. Other members of this class are excreted into milk and the passage of pindolol should be anticipated. Although milk levels of other β-blockers are apparently to small to produce adverse reactions, nursing infants should be closely observed for bradycardia and other symptoms of β-blockade. Long-term effects of exposure to β-blockers from milk have not been studied but warrant evaluation.

References

1. Dubois D, Petitcolas J, Temperville B, Klepper A. Beta blockers and high-risk pregnancies. Int J Biol Res Pregnancy 1980;1:141–5.
2. Dubois D, Petitcolas J, Temperville B, Klepper A, Catherine Ph. Treatment of hypertension in pregnancy with B-adrenoceptor antagonists. Br J Clin Pharmacol 1982;13(Suppl):375S–8S.
3. Sukerman-Voldman E. Pindolol therapy in pregnant hypertensive patients. Br J Clin Pharmacol 1982;13(Suppl):379S.
4. Ingemarsson I, Liedholm H, Montan S, Westgren M, Melander A. Fetal heart rate during treatment of maternal hypertension with beta-adrenergic antagonists. Acta Obstet Gynecol Scand 1984;118(Suppl):95–7.
5. Grunstein S, Ellenbogen A, Anderman S, Davidson A, Jaschevatsky O. Transfer of pindolol across the placenta in hypertensive pregnant women. Curr Ther Res 1985;37:587–91.

Name: **PIPERACETAZINE**

Class: **Tranquilizer**   Risk Factor: **C**

Fetal Risk Summary

Piperacetazine is a piperidyl phenothiazine. The phenothiazines readily cross the placenta (1). No specific information on the use of piperacetazine in pregnancy has been located. Although occasional reports have attempted to link various phenothiazine compounds with congential malformations, the bulk of the evidence indicates that these drugs are safe for the mother and fetus (see also Chlorpromazine).

Breast Feeding Summary

No reports describing the excretion of piperacetazine into breast milk have been located. The American Academy of Pediatrics considers the drug compatible with breast-feeding (2).

References

1. Moya F, Thorndike V. Passage of drugs across the placenta. Am J Obstet Gynecol 1962;84:1778–98.
2. Committee on Drugs, American Academy of Pediatrics. The transfer of drugs and other chemicals into human breast milk. Pediatrics 1983;72:375–83.

Name: **PIPERAZINE**

Class: **Anthelmintic**   Risk Factor: **B**

Fetal Risk Summary

No reports linking the use of piperazine with congenital defects have been located. Animal data have also failed to demonstrate any teratogenic effect. The Collaborative Perinatal Project monitored 50,282 mother-child pairs, 3 of which had 1st trimester exposure to piperazine. No evidence was found to suggest a relationship to malformations (1).

Breast Feeding Summary

No data available.

References

1. Heinonen OP, Slone D, Shapiro S. *Birth Defects and Drugs in Pregnancy*. Littleton:Publishing Sciences Group, 1977:299.

Name: **PIPERIDOLATE**

Class: **Parasympatholytic (Anticholinergic)**   Risk Factor: **C**

Fetal Risk Summary

Piperidolate is an anticholinergic agent. In a large prospective study, 2,323 patients were exposed to this class of drugs during the 1st trimester, 16 of whom took piperadolate (1). A possible association was found between the total group and minor malformations.

Breast Feeding Summary

No data available (see also Atropine).

References

1. Heinonen OP, Slone D, Shapiro S. *Birth Defects and Drugs in Pregnancy*. Littleton:Publishing Sciences Group, 1977:346–53.

Name: **POLYMYXIN B**

Class: **Antibiotic**   Risk Factor: **B**

Fetal Risk Summary

No reports linking the use of polymyxin B with congenital defects have been located. Although available for injection, polymyxin B is used almost exclusively by topical administration. In one study, seven exposures were recorded in the 1st trimester (1). No association with congenital defects was observed.

Breast Feeding Summary

No data available.

References

1. Heinonen OP, Slone D, Shapiro S. *Birth Defects and Drugs in Pregnancy*. Littleton:Publishing Sciences Group, 1977:297.

Name: **POLYTHIAZIDE**

Class: **Diuretic**   Risk Factor: **D**

Fetal Risk Summary

See Chlorothiazide.

Breast Feeding Summary

See Chlorothiazide.

Name: **POTASSIUM CHLORIDE**

Class: **Electrolyte**   Risk Factor: **A**

Fetal Risk Summary

Potassium chloride is a natural constituent of human tissues and fluids. Exogenous potassium chloride may be indicated as replacement therapy for pregnant women with low potassium serum levels, such as those receiving diuretics. Since high or low levels are detrimental to maternal and fetal cardiac function, serum levels should be closely monitored.

Breast Feeding Summary

Human milk is naturally low in potassium (1). If maternal serum levels are maintained in a physiologic range, no harm will result in the nursing infant from the administration of potassium chloride to the mother.

References

1. Wilson JT. Production and characteristics of breast milk. In Wilson JT, ed. *Drugs in Breast Milk.* Balgowlah, Australia:ADIS Press, 1981:12.

Name: **POTASSIUM CITRATE**

Class: **Electrolyte**   Risk Factor: **A**

Fetal Risk Summary

See Potassium Chloride.

Breast Feeding Summary

See Potassium Chloride.

Name: **POTASSIUM GLUCONATE**

Class: **Electrolyte**   Risk Factor: **A**

Fetal Risk Summary

See Potassium Chloride.

Breast Feeding Summary

See Potassium Chloride.

Name: **POTASSIUM IODIDE**

Class: **Expectorant**   Risk Factor: **D**

Fetal Risk Summary

The primary concern with the use of potassium iodide during pregnancy relates to the effect of iodide on the fetal thyroid gland. Since aqueous solutions of iodine are in equilibrium with the ionized form, all iodide or iodine products are considered as one group.

Iodide readily crosses the placenta to the fetus (1). When used for prolonged periods or close to term, iodide may cause hypothyroidism and goiter in the fetus and newborn. Short-term use, such as a 10-day preparation course for maternal thyroid surgery, does not carry this risk and is apparently safe (2, 3). In a 1983 review, Mehta et al. (4) tabulated 49 cases of cogenital iodide goiter dating back to 1940 (66 references) (4). In 14 cases, the goiter was large enough to cause tracheal compression, resulting in death. Cardiomegaly was present in three surviving newborns and in one of the fatalities. In a majority of the cases, exposure to the iodide was due to maternal asthma treatment.

Three recent studies have shown the potential hazard resulting from the use of povidone-iodine during pregnancy (5–7). In each case, significant absorption of iodine occurred in the mother and fetus following vaginal or perineal use before delivery. Transient hypothyroidism was demonstrated in some newborns (5).

Since a large number of prescription and over-the-counter medications contain iodide or iodine, pregnant patients should consult with their physician prior to using these products. The American Academy of Pediatrics considers the use of iodides as expectorants during pregnancy to be contraindicated (8).

Breast Feeding Summary

Iodide is concentrated in breast milk (4, 9). In one report, a breast feeding mother used povidone-iodine vaginal gel daily for 6 days without douching (9). Two days after stopping the gel, the mother noted an odor of iodine on the 7½-month-old baby. The free iodide serum:milk ratio 1 day later was approximately 23:1. By day 7, the ratio had fallen to about 4:1 but then rose again on day 8 to 10:1. Serum and urine iodide levels in the infant were grossly elevated. No problems or alterations in thyroid tests were noted in the baby.

The normal iodine content of human milk has been recently assessed (10). Mean iodide levels in 37 lactating women were 178 μg/L. This is approximately four times the RDA for infants. The RDA for iodine was based on the amount of iodine found in breast milk in earlier studies (10). The higher levels now are probably due to dietary supplements of iodine (e.g., salt, bread, cow's milk). The significance to the nursing infant from the chronic ingestion of higher levels of iodine is not known. The American Academy of Pediatrics recommends decreasing or stopping the use of iodides as expectorants during lactation (8).

References

1. Wolff J. Iodide goiter and the pharmacologic effects of excess iodide. Am J Med 1969;47:101–24.
2. Herbst AL, Selenkow HA. Hyperthyroidism during pregnancy. N Engl J Med 1965;273:627–33.
3. Selenkow HA, Herbst AL. Hyperthyroidism during pregnancy. N Engl J Med 1966;274:165–6.
4. Mehta PS, Mehta SJ, Vorherr H. Congenital iodide goiter and hypothyroidism: a review. Obstet Gynecol Surv 1983;38:237–47.
5. l'Allemand D, Gruters A, Heidemann P, Schurnbrand P. Iodine-induced alterations of thyroid function in newborn infants after prenatal and perinatal exposure to povidone iodine. J Pediatr 1983;102:935–8.
6. Bachrach LK, Burrow GN, Gare DJ. Maternal-fetal absorption of povidone-iodine. J Pediatr 1984;104:158–9.
7. Jacobson JM, Hankins GV, Young RL, Hauth JC. Changes in thyroid function and serum iodine levels after prepartum use of a povidone-iodine vaginal lubricant. J Reprod Med 1984;29:98–100.
8. Committee on Drugs, American Academy of Pediatrics. Adverse reactions to iodide therapy of asthma and other pulmonary diseases. Pediatrics 1976;57:272–4.
9. Postellon DC, Aronow R. Iodine in mother's milk. JAMA 1982;247:463.
10. Gushurst CA, Mueller JA, Green JA, Sedor F. Breast milk iodide: reassessment in the 1980s. Pediatrics 1984;73:354–7.

Name: **PRAZOSIN**

Class: **Antihypertensive**   Risk Factor: **C**

Fetal Risk Summary

Prazosin is an α-adrenergic blocking agent used for hypertension. In two studies, prazosin was combined with oxprenolol or atenolol, β-adrenergic blockers, in the treatment of pregnant women with severe essential hypertension or pregnancy-induced hypertension (1, 2). The combinations were effective in the first group but less so in the patients with pregnancy-induced hypertension. No adverse effects attributable to the drugs were noted.

Prazosin has been used during the 3rd trimester in a patient with pheochromocytoma (3). Blood pressure was well controlled but maternal tachycardia required the addition of a β-blocker. A healthy male infant was delivered by cesarean section.

Breast Feeding Summary

No data available.

References

1. Lubbe WF, Hodge JV. Combined alpha- and beta-adrenoceptor antagonism with prazosin and oxprenolol in control of severe hypertension in pregnancy. NZ Med J 1981;94:169–72.
2. Lubbe WF. More on beta-blockers in pregnancy. N Engl J Med 1982;307:753.

3. Venuto R, Burstein P, Schneider R. Pheochromocytoma: antepartum diagnosis and management with tumor resection in the puerperium. Am J Obstet Gynecol 1984;150:431–2.

Name: **PREDNISOLONE**

Class: **Corticosteroid**   Risk Factor: **B**

Fetal Risk Summary

Prednisolone is the biologically active form of prednisone (see Prednisone). The placenta can oxidize prednisolone to inactive prednisone or less active cortisone (see Cortisone).

Breast Feeding Summary

See Prednisone.

Name: **PREDNISONE**

Class: **Corticosteroid**   Risk Factor: **B**

Fetal Risk Summary

Prednisone is metabolized to prednisolone. There are a number of studies in which pregnant patients received either prednisone or prednisolone (see also various antineoplastic agents for additional references) (1–14). These corticosteroids apparently have little, if any, effect on the developing fetus.

Immunosuppression was observed in a newborn exposed to high doses of prednisone with azathioprine throughout gestation (15). The newborn had lymphopenia, decreased survival of lymphocytes in culture, absence of IgM, and reduced levels of IgG. Recovery occurred at 15 weeks of age. However, these effects were not observed in a larger group of similarly exposed newborns (16). A 1968 study reported an increase in the incidence of stillbirths following prednisone therapy during pregnancy (7). Increased fetal mortality has not been confirmed by other investigators.

An infant exposed to prednisone throughout pregnancy was born with congenital cataracts (1). The eye defect was consistent with reports of subcapsular cataracts observed in adults receiving corticosteroids.

In a 1970 case report, a female infant with multiple deformities was described (17). Her father had been treated several years prior to conception with prednisone, azathioprine and radiation for a kidney transplant. The authors speculated that the child's defects may have been related to the father's immunosuppressive therapy. A relationship to prednisone seems remote since previous studies have shown that the drug has no effect on chromosome number or morphology (18). High, prolonged doses of prednisolone (30 mg/day for at least 4 weeks) may damage spermatogenesis (19). Recovery may require 6 months after the drug is stopped.

Prednisone has been used to successfully prevent neonatal respiratory distress syndrome when premature delivery occurs between 28 and 36 weeks of gestation (20). Therapy between 16 and 25 weeks of gestation had no effect on lecithin/sphingomyelin ratios (21).

In summary, prednisone and prednisolone apparently pose a very small risk to the developing fetus. The available evidence supports their use to control various maternal diseases.

Breast Feeding Summary

Trace amounts of prednisone and prednisolone have been measured in breast milk (22–24). Following a 10 mg oral dose of prednisone, milk concentrations of prednisone and prednisolone at 2 hours were 0.03 and 0.002 μg/ml, respectively (22). In a second study utilizing radioactive-labeled prednisolone in seven patients, a mean of 0.14% of a 5-mg oral dose was recovered per liter of milk over 48–61 hours (23). This is equivalent to 0.007 μg/ml.

In six lactating women, prednisolone doses of 10–80 mg/day resulted in milk concentrations ranging from 5 to 25% of maternal serum levels (24). The milk:plasma ratio increased with increasing serum concentrations. For maternal doses of 20 mg once or twice daily, the authors concluded that the nursing infant would be exposed to minimal amounts of steroid. At higher doses, they recommended waiting at least 4 hours after a dose before nursing was performed. However, even at 80 mg/day, the nursing infant would ingest <0.1% of the dose, which corresponds to <10% of the infant's endogenous cortisol production (24).

Although nursing infants were not involved in either study, it is doubtful if these amounts are clinically significant. The American Academy of Pediatrics considers prednisone and prednisolone compatible with breast-feeding (25).

References

1. Kraus AM. Congenital cataract and maternal steroid injection. J Pediatr Ophthalmol 1975;12:107–8.
2. Durie BGM, Giles HR. Successful treatment of acute leukemia during pregnancy: combination therapy in the third trimester. Arch Intern Med 1977;137:90–1.
3. Nolan GH, Sweet RL, Laros RK, Roure CA. Renal cadaver transplantation followed by successful pregnancies. Obstet Gynecol 1974;43:732–9.
4. Grossman JH III, Littner MR. Severe sarcoidosis in pregnancy. Obstet Gynecol 1977;50(Suppl):81s–4s.
5. Cutting HO, Collier TM. Acute lymphocytic leukemia during pregnancy: report of a case. Obstet Gynecol 1964;24:941–5.
6. Hanson GC, Ghosh S. Systemic lupus erythematosus and pregnancy. Br Med J 1965;2:1227–8.
7. Warrell DW, Taylor R. Outcome for the foetus of mothers receiving prednisolone during pregnancy. Lancet 1968;1:117–8.
8. Walsh SD, Clark FR. Pregnancy in patients on long-term corticosteroid therapy. Scott Med J 1967;12:302–6.
9. Zulman JI, Talal N, Hoffman GS, Epstein WV. Problems associated with the management of pregnancies in patients with systemic lupus erythematosus. J Rheumatol 1980;7:37–49.
10. Hartikainen-Sorri AL, Kaila J. Systemic lupus erythematosus and habitual abortion: case report. Br J Obstet Gynaecol 1980;87:729–31.
11. Minchinton RM, Dodd NJ, O'Brien H, Amess JAL, Waters AH. Autoimmune thrombocytopenia in pregnancy. Br J Haematol 1980;44:451–9.
12. Tozman ECS, Urowitz MB, Gladman DD. Systemic lupus erythematosus and pregnancy. J Rheumatol 1980;7:624–32.
13. Karpatkin M, Porges RF, Karpatkin S. Platelet counts in infants of women with autoimmune thrombocytopenia: effect of steroid administration to the mother. N Engl J Med 1981;305:936–9.
14. Pratt WR. Allergic diseases in pregnancy and breast feeding. Ann Allergy 1981;47:355–60.

15. Cote CJ, Meuwissen HJ, Pickering RJ. Effects on the neonate of prednisone and azathioprine administered to the mother during pregnancy. J Pediatr 1974;85:324–8.
16. Cederqvist LL, Merkatz IR, Litwin SD. Fetal immunoglobin synthesis following maternal immuno-suppression. Am J Obstet Gynecol 1977;129:687–90.
17. Tallent MB, Simmons RL, Najarian JS. Birth defects in child of male recipient of kidney transplant. JAMA 1970;211:1854–5.
18. Jensen MK. Chromosome studies in patients treated with azathioprine and amethopterin. Acta Med Scand 1967;182:445–55.
19. Mancini RE, Larieri JC, Muller F, Andrada JA, Saraceni DJ. Effect of prednisolone upon normal and pathologic human spermatogenesis. Fertil Steril 1966;17:500–13.
20. Szabo I, Csaba I, Novak P, Drozgyik I. Single-dose glucocorticoid for prevention of respiratory-distress syndrome. Lancet 1977;2:243.
21. Szabo I, Csaba I, Bodis J, Novak P, Drozgyik J, Schwartz J. Effect of glucocorticoid on fetal lecithin and sphingomyelin concentrations. Lancet 1980;1:320.
22. Katz FH, Duncan BR. Entry of prednisone into human milk. N Engl J Med 1975;293:1154.
23. McKenzie SA, Selley JA, Agnew JE. Secretion of prednisone into breast milk. Arch Dis Child 1975;50:894–6.
24. Ost L, Wettrell G, Bjorkhem I, Rane A. Prednisolone excretion in human milk. J Pediatr 1985;106:1008–11.
25. Committee on Drugs, American Academy of Pediatrics. The transfer of drugs and other chemicals into human breast milk. Pediatrics 1983;72:375–83.

Name: **PRIMAQUINE**

Class: **Plasmodicide**   Risk Factor: **C**

Fetal Risk Summary

No reports linking the use of primaquine with congenital defects have been located. Primaquine may cause hemolytic anemia in patients with glucose-6-phosphate dehydrogenase deficiency. Pregnant patients at risk for this disorder should be tested accordingly (1). If possible, the drug should be withheld until after delivery (2). However, if prophylaxis or treatment is required, primaquine should not be withheld (3).

Breast Feeding Summary

No data available.

References

1. Trenholme GM, Parson PE. Therapy and prophylaxis of malaria. JAMA 1978;240:2293–5.
2. Anonymous. Chemoprophylaxis of malaria. MMWR 1978;27:81–90.
3. Diro M, Beydoun SN. Malaria in pregnancy. South Med J 1982;75:959–62.

Name: **PRIMIDONE**

Class: **Anticonvulsant**   Risk Factor: **D**

Fetal Risk Summary

Primidone, a structural analog of phenobarbital, is effective against generalized convulsive seizures and psychomotor attacks. It is clear that the epileptic patient on anticonvulsant medication is at a higher risk for having a child with congenital defects than the general population (1–7). The difficulty in evaluating the increased malformation rate in epileptic patients lies in attempting to disentangle the effects of multiple drug therapy, the effects of the disease itself on the fetal outcome and any pattern of malformations associated with the drug. The literature describes 323 infants who were exposed to primidone during the 1st trimester (4, 8–17). Of the 41 malformed infants described in these reports, only three infants were exposed to primidone and no other anticonvulsants during gestation (8, 15, 16). The anomalies observed in these three infants were similar to those observed in the fetal hydantoin syndrome (see Phenytoin).

There are other potential complications associated with the use of primidone during pregnancy. Neurologic manifestations in the newborn such as overactivity and tumors have been associated with use of primidone in pregnancy (16, 18). Neonatal hemorrhagic disease with primidone alone or in combination with other anticonvulsants has been reported (14, 19–23). Suppression of vitamin K_1-dependent clotting factors is the proposed mechanism of the hemorrhagic effect (14, 19). Administration of prophylatic vitamin K_1 to the infant immediately after birth is recommended (see Phytonadione, Phenytoin, and Phenobarbital).

Breast Feeding Summary

Primidone is excreted into breast milk (24). Because primidone undergoes limited conversion to phenobarbital, breast milk concentrations of phenobarbital should also be anticipated (see Phenobarbital). A milk:plasma ratio of 0.8 for primidone has been reported (24). The amount of primidone available to the nursing infant is small with milk concentrations of 2.3 μg/ml. No reports linking adverse effects to the nursing infant have been located; however, patients that breast-feed should be instructed to watch for potential sedative effects in the infant. The American Academy of Pediatrics considers primidone compatible with breast-feeding (25).

References

1. Hill RB. Teratogenesis and antiepileptic drugs. N Engl J Med 1973;289:1089–90.
2. Bodendorfer TW. Fetal effect of anticonvulsant drugs and seizure disorders. Drug Intell Clin Pharm 1978;12:14–21.
3. Committee on Drugs, American Academy of Pediatrics. Anticonvulsants and pregnancy. Pediatrics 1977;63:331–3.
4. Nakane Y, Okoma T, Takahashe R, et al. Multiple-institutional study of the teratogenicity and fetal toxicity of antiepileptic drugs: a report of a collaborative study group in Japan. Epilepsia 1980;21:663–80.
5. Andermann E, Dansky L, Andermann F, Loughnan PM, Gibbons J. Minor congenital malformations and dermatoglyphic alterations in the offspring of epileptic women: a clinical investigation of the teratogenic effects of anticonvulsant medication. In *Epilepsy, Pregnancy and the Child*. Proceedings of a Workshop, Berlin, September 1980. New York:Raven Press, 1981.
6. Danksy L, Andermann F. Major congenital malformations in the offspring of epileptic patients. *Ibid*.
7. Janz D. The teratogenic risks of antiepileptic drugs. Epilepsia 1975;16:159–69.

8. Lowe CR. Congenital malformations among infants born to epileptic women. Lancet 1973;1:9–10.
9. Lander CM, Edwards BE, Eadie MJ, Tyrer JH. Plasma anticonvulsants concentrations during pregnancy. Neurology 1977;27:128–31.
10. Speidel BD, Meadow SR. Maternal epilepsy and abnormalities of the fetus and newborn. Lancet 1972;2:839–43.
11. McMullin GP. Teratogenic effects of anticonvulsants. Br Med J 1971;4:430.
12. Fedrick J. Epilepsy and pregnancy: a report from the Oxford Record Linkage Study. Br Med J 1973;2:442–8.
13. Biale Y, Lewenthal H, Aderet NB. Congenital malformations due to anticonvulsant drugs. Obstet Gynecol 1975;45:439–42.
14. Thomas P, Buchanan N. Teratogenic effect of anticonvulsants. J Pediatr 1981;99:163.
15. Myhree SA, Williams R. Teratogenic effects associated with maternal primidone therapy. J Pediatr 1981;99:160–2.
16. Rudd NL, Freedom RM. A possible primidone embryopathy. J Pediatr 1979;94:835–7.
17. Heinonen OP, Slone D, Shapiro S. Birth Defects and Drugs in Pregnancy. Littleton:Publishing Sciences Group, 1977:358.
18. Martinez G, Snyder RD. Transplacental passage of primidone. Neurology 1973;23:381–3.
19. Kohler HG. Haemorrhage in the newborn of epileptic mothers. Lancet 1966;1:267.
20. Bleyer WA, Skinner AL. Fatal neonatal hemorrhage after maternal anticonvulsant therapy. JAMA 1976;235:826–7.
21. Mountain KR, Hirsh J, Gallus AS. Neonatal coagulation defect due to anticonvulsant drug treatment in pregnancy. Lancet 1970;1:265–8.
22. Evans AR, Forrester RM, Discombe C. Neonatal hemorrhage following maternal anticonvulsant therapy. Lancet 1970;1:517–8.
23. Margolin DO, Kantor NM. Hemorrhagic disease of the newborn: an unusual case related to maternal ingestion of antiepileptic drug. Clin Pediatr (Phila) 1972;11:59–60.
24. Kaneko S, Sato T, Suzuki K. The levels of anticonvulsants in breast milk. Br J Clin Pharmacol 1979;7:624–7.
25. Committee on Drugs, American Academy of Pediatrics. The transfer of drugs and other chemicals into human breast milk. Pediatrics 1983;72:375–83.

Name: **PROBENECID**

Class: **Uricosuric/Renal Tubular Blocking Agent**   Risk Factor: **B**

Fetal Risk Summary

No reports linking the use of probenecid with congenital defects have been located. Probenecid has been used during pregnancy without producing adverse effects in the fetus or in the infant (1–3).

Breast Feeding Summary

No data available.

References

1. Beidleman B. Treatment of chronic hypoparathyroidism with probenecid. Metabolism 1958;7:690–8.
2. Lee FI, Loeffler FE. Gout and pregnancy. J Obstet Gynaecol Br Commonw 1962;69:299.
3. Batt RE, Cirksena WJ, Lebhertz TB. Gout and salt-wasting renal disease during pregnancy. Diagnosis, management and follow-up. JAMA 1963;186:835–8.

Name: **PROCARBAZINE**

Class: **Antineoplastic**   Risk Factor: **D**

Fetal Risk Summary

The use of procarbazine during pregnancy has been described in seven patients, five during the 1st trimester (1–6). Pregnancy in one of the 1st trimester exposures was electively terminated, but no details on the fetus were given (5). Congenital malformations were observed in the remaining four 1st trimester exposures (1–4):

Multiple hemangiomas (1)

Oligodactyly of both feet with webbing of 3rd and 4th toes, 4 metatarsals on left, 3 on right, bowing of right tibia, cerebral hemorrhage, spontaneously aborted at 24 weeks gestation (2)

Malformed kidneys—markedly reduced size and malposition (3)

Small secundum atrial septal defect, intrauterine growth retardation (4)

A patient in the early 2nd trimester received procarbazine, 50 mg daily, in error for 30 days when she was given the drug instead of an iron/vitamin supplement (6). An apparently normal male infant was delivered.

Long-term studies of growth and mental development in offspring exposed to procarbazine during the 2nd trimester, the period of neuroblast multiplication, have not been conducted (7). Data from one review indicated that 40% of the infants exposed to anticancer drugs were of low birth weight (8). This finding was not related to the timing of exposure.

Procarbazine is mutagenic and carcinogenic in animals (9). In combination with other antineoplastic drugs, procarbazine may produce gonadal dysfunction in males and females (10–14). Ovarian and testicular function may return to normal, with successful pregnancies possible, depending on the patient's age at the time of therapy and the total dose of chemotherapy received (14–17).

Breast Feeding Summary

No data available.

References

1. Wells JH, Marshall JR, Carbone PP. Procarbazine therapy for Hodgkin's disease in early pregnancy. JAMA 1968;205:935–7.
2. Garrett MJ. Teratogenic effects of combination chemotherapy. Ann Intern Med 1974;80:667.
3. Mennuti MT, Shepard TH, Mellman WJ. Fetal renal malformation following treatment of Hodgkin's disease during pregnancy. Obstet Gynecol 1975;46:194–6.
4. Thomas PRM, Peckham MJ. The investigation and management of Hodgkin's disease in the pregnant patient. Cancer 1976;38:1443–51.
5. Daly H, McCann SR, Hanratty TD, Temperley IJ. Successful pregnancy during combination chemotherapy for Hodgkin's disease. Acta Haematol (Basel) 1980;64:154–6.
6. Daw EG. Procarbazine in pregnancy. Lancet 1970;2:984.
7. Dobbing J. Pregnancy and leukaemia. Lancet 1977;1:1155.
8. Nicholson HO. Cytotoxic drugs in pregnancy: review of reported cases. J Obstet Gynecol Br Commonw 1968;75:307–12.
9. Lee IP, Dixon RL. Mutagenicity, carcinogenicity and teratogenicity of procarbazine. Mutat Res 1978;55:1–14.
10. Sherins RJ, DeVita VT Jr. Effect of drug treatment for lymphoma on male reproductive capacity: studies of men in remission after therapy. Ann Intern Med 1973;79:216–20.

11. Sherins RJ, Olweny CLM, Ziegler JL. Gynecomastia and gonadal dysfunction in adolescent boys treated with combination chemotherapy for Hodgkin's disease. N Engl J Med 1978;299:12–6.
12. Johnson SA, Goldman JM, Hawkins DF. Pregnancy after chemotherapy for Hodgkin's disease. Lancet 1979;2:93.
13. Card RT, Holmes IH, Sugarman RG, Storb R, Thomas ED. Successful pregnancy after high dose chemotherapy and marrow transplantation for treatment of aplastic anemia. Exp Hematol 1980;8:57–60.
14. Schilsky RL, Sherins RJ, Hubbard SM, Wesley MN, Young RC, DeVita VT Jr. Long-term follow-up of ovarian function in women treated with MOPP chemotherapy for Hodgkin's disease. Am J Med 1981;71:552–6.
15. Whitehead E, Shalet SM, Blackledge G, Todd I, Crowther D, Beardwell CG. The effect of combination chemotherapy on ovarian function in women treated for Hodgkin's disease. Cancer 1983;52:988–93.
16. Andrieu JM, Ochoa-Molina ME. Menstrual cycle, pregnancies and offspring before and after MOPP therapy for Hodgkin's disease. Cancer 1983;52:435–8.
17. Schapira DV, Chudley AE. Successful pregnancy following continuous treatment with combination chemotherapy before conception and throughout pregnancy. Cancer 1984;54:800–3.

Name: **PROCHLORPERAZINE**

Class: **Tranquilizer**   Risk Factor: **C**

Fetal Risk Summary

Prochlorperazine is a piperazine phenothiazine. The drug readily crosses the placenta (1). Prochlorperazine has been used to treat nausea and vomiting of pregnancy. Most studies have found the drug to be safe for this indication (see also Chlorpromazine) (2–4). The Collaborative Perinatal Project monitored 50,282 mother-child pairs, 877 of which had 1st trimester exposure to prochlorperazine (4). For use anytime during pregnancy, 2,023 exposures were recorded. No evidence was found in either group to suggest a relationship to malformations or an effect on perinatal mortality rate, birth weight, or intelligence quotient scores at 4 years of age. Two infants exposed to prochlorperazine during the 1st trimester are described below:

> Cleft palate, micrognathia, congenital heart defects, skeletal defects (5)
> Thanatophoric dwarfism (short limb anomaly) (6)

The relationship between prochlorperazine and the above defects is unknown. The case of dwarfism may be due to genetic factors. A third report provided brief data on 14 infants, one half of whom were exposed to the drug before embryologic timing of their malformations (7).

In summary, although there are isolated reports of congenital defects in children exposed to prochlorperazine *in utero*, the majority of the evidence indicates that this drug and the general class of phenothiazines are safe for both mother and fetus if used occasionally in low doses. Other reviewers have also concluded that the phenothiazines are not teratogenic (8, 9).

Breast Feeding Summary

No reports describing the excretion of prochlorperazine into breast milk have been located. The American Academy of Pediatrics considers the drug compatible with breast-feeding (10).

References

1. Moya F, Thornidke V. Passage of drugs across the placenta. Am J Obstet Gynecol 1962;84:1778–98.
2. Reider RO, Rosenthal D. Wender P, Blumenthal H. The offspring of schizophrenics. Fetal and neonatal deaths. Arch Gen Psychiatry 1975; 32:200–11.
3. Milkovich L, Van den Berg BJ. An evaluation of the teratogenicity of certain antinauseant drugs. Am J Obstet Gynecol 1976;125:244–8.
4. Slone D, Siskind V, Heinonen OP, Monson RR, Kaufman DW, Shapiro S. Antenatal exposure to the phenothiazines in relation to congenital malformations, perinatal mortality rate, birth weight, and intelligence quotient score. Am J Obstet Gynecol 1977;128:486–8.
5. Ho CK, Kaufman RL, McAlister WH. Congenital malformations. Cleft palate, congenital heart disease, absent tibiae, and polydactyly. Am J Dis Child 1975;129:714–6.
6. Farag RA, Ananth J. Thanatophoric dwarfism associated with prochlorperazine administration. NY State J Med 1978;78:279–82.
7. Mellin GW. Report of prochlorperazine during pregnancy from the fetal life study bank. Teratology 1975;11:28A (Abstr).
8. Ayd FJ Jr. Children born of mothers treated with chlorpromazine during pregnancy. Clin Med 1964;71:1758–63.
9. Ananth J. Congenital malformations with psychopharmacologic agents. Compr Psychiatry 1975;16:437–45.
10. Committee on Drugs, American Academy of Pediatrics. The transfer of drugs and other chemicals into human breast milk. Pediatrics 1983;72:375–83.

Name: **PROCYCLIDINE**

Class: **Parasympatholytic (Anticholinergic)**   Risk Factor: **C**

Fetal Risk Summary

Procyclidine is an anticholinergic agent used in the treatment of parkinsonism. No reports of its use in pregnancy have been located (see also Atropine).

Breast Feeding Summary

No data available. See also Atropine.

Name: **PROMAZINE**

Class: **Tranquilizer**   Risk Factor: **C**

Fetal Risk Summary

Promazine is a propylamino phenothiazine structurally related to chlorpromazine. The drug readily crosses the placenta (1, 2). A possible relationship between the use of promazine (100 mg or more) in labor and neonatal hyperbilirubinemia was reported in 1975 (3). The Collaborative Perinatal Project monitored 50,282 mother-child pairs, 50 of which had 1st trimester exposure to promazine (4). For use anytime during pregnancy, 347 exposures were recorded. No evidence was found in either group to suggest a relationship to malformations or an effect on perinatal mortality rate, birth weight, or intelligence quotient scores at 4 years of age. Although occasional reports have attempted to link various phenothiazine compounds with congenital defects, the bulk of the evidence indicates that these drugs are safe for mother and fetus (see also Chlorpromazine).

Breast Feeding Summary

No data available.

References

1. Moya F, Thorndike V. Passage of drugs across the placenta. Am J Obstet Gynecol 1962;84:1778–98.
2. O'Donoghue SEF. Distribution of pethidine and chlorpromazine in maternal, foetal and neonatal biological fluids. Nature 1971;229:124–5.
3. John E. Promazine and neonatal hyperbilirubinemia. Med J Aust 1975;2:342–4.
4. Slone D, Siskind V, Heinonen OP, Monson RR, Kaufman DW, Shapiro S. Antenatal exposure to the phenothiazines in relation to congenital malformations, perinatal mortality rate, birth weight, and intelligence quotient score. Am J Obstet Gynecol 1977;128:486–8.

Name: **PROMETHAZINE**

Class: **Antihistamine**   Risk Factor: **C**

Fetal Risk Summary

Promethazine is a phenothiazine antihistamine that is sometimes used as an antiemetic in pregnancy and as an adjunct to narcotic analgesics during labor. The Collaborative Perinatal Project monitored 50,282 mother-child pairs, 114 of which had promethazine exposure in the 1st trimester (1). For use anytime during pregnancy, 746 exposures were recorded (2). In neither case was evidence found to suggest a relationship to large categories of major or minor malformations or to individual defects. A 1964 report also failed to show an association between 165 cases of promethazine exposure in the 1st trimester and malformations (3). Finally, in a 1971 reference, infants of mothers who had ingested antiemetics during the 1st trimester actually had significantly fewer abnormalities when compared to controls (4). Promethazine was the most commonly used antiemetic in this latter study.

At term, the drug rapidly crosses the placenta, appearing in cord blood within 1½ minutes of an intravenous dose (5). Fetal and maternal blood concentrations are at equilibrium in 15 minutes with infant levels persisting for at least 4 hours.

Several investigators have studied the effect of promethazine on labor and the newborn (6–13). Significant neonatal respiratory depression was seen in a small group of patients (6). However, in three large series, no clinical evidence of promethazine-induced respiratory depression was found (7–9). In a series of 33 mothers at term, 28 received either promethazine alone (1 patient) or a combination of meperidine with promethazine or phenobarbital (27 patients). Transient behavioral and electroencephalographic changes, persisting for less than 3 days, were seen in all newborns (11).

Maternal tachycardia due to promethazine (mean increase 30 beats/min) or promethazine-meperidine (mean increase 42 beats/min) was observed in one series (10). The maximum effect occurred about 10 minutes after injection. The fetal heart rate did not change significantly.

Fatal shock was reported in a pregnant woman with an undiagnosed pheochromocytoma given promethazine (14). A precipitous drop in blood pressure resulted from administration of the drug, probably secondary to unmasking of hypovolemia (14).

Effects on the uterus have been mixed, with both increases and decreases in uterine activity reported (9, 10, 12).

Promethazine used during labor has been shown to markedly impair platelet aggregation in the newborn but less so in the mother (13, 15). While the clinical significance of this is unknown, the degree of impairment in the newborn is comparable to those disorders associated with a definite bleeding state.

Promethazine has been used to treat hydrops fetalis in cases of anti-erythrocytic isoimmunization (16). Six patients were treated with 150 mg orally per day between the 26th and 34th week of gestation while undergoing intraperitoneal transfusions. No details on the infants' conditions were given except that all were born alive. Other authors have reported similarly successful results in Rh-sensitized pregnancies (17, 18). As described by Gusdon (17), doses up to 6.5 mg/kg/day may be required.

Two female anencephalic infants were born to mothers after ovulatory stimulation with clomiphene (19). One of the mothers had taken promethazine for morning sickness. No association between promethazine and this defect has been suggested.

Breast Feeding Summary

Available laboratory methods for the accurate detection of promethazine in breast milk are not clinically useful due to the rapid metabolism of phenothiazines (20).

References

1. Heinonen OP, Slone D, Shapiro S. *Birth Defects and Drugs in Pregnancy*. Littleton:Publishing Sciences Group, 1977:323–4.
2. *Ibid*, 437.
3. Wheatley D. Drugs and the embryo. Br Med J 1964;1:630.
4. Nelson MM, Forfar JO. Association between drugs administered during pregnancy and congenital abnormalities of the fetus. Br Med J 1971;1:523–7.
5. Moya F, Thorndike V. The effects of drugs used in labor on the fetus and newborn. Clin Pharmacol Ther 1963;4:628–53.
6. Crawford JS, as quoted by Moya F, Thorndike V. The effects of drugs used in labor on the fetus and newborn. Clin Pharmacol Ther 1963;4:628–53.
7. Powe CE, Kiem IM, Fromhagen C, Cavanagh D. Propiomazine hydrochloride in obstetrical analgesia. JAMA 1962;181:290–4.
8. Potts CR, Ullery JC. Maternal and fetal effects of obstetric analgesia. Am J Obstet Gynecol 1961;81:1253–9.
9. Carroll JJ, Moir RS. Use of promethazine (Phenergan) hydrochloride in obstetrics. JAMA 1958;168:2218–24.
10. Riffel HD, Nochimson DJ, Paul RH, Hon EH. Effects of meperidine and promethazine during labor. Obstet Gynecol 1973;42:738–45.
11. Borgstedt AD, Rosen MG. Medication during labor correlated with behavior and EEG of the newborn. Am J Dis Child 1968;115:21–4.
12. Zakut H, Mannor SM, Serr DM. Effect of promethazine on uterine contractions. Harefuah 1970;78:61–2. As reported in JAMA 1970; 211:1572.
13. Corby DG, Shulman I. The effects of antenatal drug administration on aggregation of platelets of newborn infants. J Pediatr 1971;79:307–13.
14. Montminy M, Teres D. Shock after phenothiazine administration in a pregnant patient with a pheochromocytoma: a case report and literature review. J Reprod Med 1983;28:159–62.

15. Whaun JM, Smith GR, Sochor VA. Effect of prenatal drug administration on maternal and neonatal platelet aggregation and PF₄ release. Haemostasis 1980;9:226–37.
16. Bierme S, Bierme R. Antihistamines in hydrops foetalis. Lancet 1967;1:574.
17. Gusdon JP Jr. The treatment of erythroblastosis with promethazine hydrochloride. J Reprod Med 1981;26:454–8.
18. Charles AG, Blumenthal LS. Promethazine hydrochloride therapy in severely Rh-sensitized pregnancies. Obstet Gynecol 1982;60:627–30.
19. Dyson JL, Kohler HC. Anecephaly and ovulation stimulation. Lancet 1973;1:1256–7.
20. Lipshutz M, Assistant to Director, Medical Communications, Wyeth Laboratories, 1981. Personal communication.

Name: **PROPANTHELINE**

Class: **Parasympatholytic (Anticholinergic)**   Risk Factor: C_M

Fetal Risk Summary

Propantheline is an anticholinergic quaternary ammonium bromide. The Collaborative Perinatal Project monitored 50,282 mother-child pairs, 33 of which used propantheline in the 1st trimester (1). No evidence was found for an association with congenital malformations. However, when the group of parasympatholytics were taken as a whole (2,323 exposures), a possible association with minor malformations was found (1).

Breast Feeding Summary

No data available (see also Atropine).

References

1. Heinonen OP, Slone D, Shapiro S. *Birth Defects and Drugs in Pregnancy*. Littleton:Publishing Sciences Group, 1977:346–53.

Name: **PROPOXYPHENE**

Class: **Analgesic**   Risk Factor: **C***

Fetal Risk Summary

Three case reports, involving four patients, have linked the use of propoxyphene during pregnancy to congenital abnormalties (1–3). However, other drugs were used in each case and any association may be fortuitous:

Pierre Robin syndrome, arthrogryposis, severe mental and growth retardation (1) (1 infant)

Absence of left forearm and radial 2 digits, syndactyly of ulnar 3 digits and left 4th and 5th toes, hypoplastic left femur (2) (1 infant)

Omphalocele, defective anterior left wall, diaphragmatic defect, congenital heart disease with partial ectopic cordis due to sternal cleft, dysplastic hips (2) (1 infant)

Micrognathia, widely spaced sutures, beaked nose, bifid uvula, defects of toes, withdrawal seizures (3) (1 infant)

The Collaborative Perinatal Project monitored 50,282 mother-child pairs, 686 of which had 1st trimester exposure to propoxyphene (4). For use anytime during pregnancy, 2,914 exposures were recorded (5). No evidence was found in either case to suggest a relationship to large categories of major or minor malformations or, in the 1st trimester, to individual defects. Five possible associations with individual defects after anytime use were observed (6). The statistical significance of these associations is unknown and independent confirmation is required:

Microcephaly (6 cases)
Ductus arteriosus persistens (5 cases)
Cataract (5 cases)
Benign tumors (12 cases)
Clubfoot (18 cases)

Neonatal withdrawal has been reported in five infants (3, 7–10). The relationship between heavy maternal ingestion of this drug and neonatal withdrawal seems clear. The infants were asymptomatic with normal Apgar scores until 3½–14 hours after delivery. Withdrawal was marked by the onset of irritability, tremors, diarrhea, fever, high-pitched cry, hyperactivity, hypertonicity, diaphoresis, and, in two cases, seizures. Symptoms began to subside by day 4, usually without specific therapy. Examinations after 2–3 months were normal.

Propoxyphene has been used in labor without causing neonatal respiratory depression (11). However, a significant shortening of the first stage of labor occurred without an effect on uterine contractions.

[* Risk Factor D if used for prolonged periods.]

Breast Feeding Summary

Propoxyphene passes into breast milk, but the amounts and clinical significance are unknown. In one case, a nursing mother attempted suicide with propoxyphene (12). The concentration of the drug in her breast milk was found to be 50% of her plasma level. By calculation, the authors predicted that a mother consuming a maximum daily dose of the drug would provide her infant with 1 mg/day. The American Academy of Pediatrics considers propoxyphene compatible with breast-feeding (13).

References

1. Barrow MV, Souder DE. Propoxyphene and congenital malformations. JAMA 1971;217:1551–2.
2. Ringrose CAD. The hazard of neurotrophic drugs in the fertile years. Can Med Assoc J 1972;106:1058.
3. Golden NL, King KC, Sokol RJ. Propoxyphene and acetaminophen: possible effects on the fetus. Clin Pediatr (Phila) 1982;21:752–4.
4. Heinonen OP, Slone D, Shapiro S. *Birth Defects and Drugs in Pregnancy*. Littleton:Publishing Sciences Group, 1977:287–95.
5. *Ibid*, 434.
6. *Ibid*, 484.
7. Tyson HK. Neonatal withdrawal symptoms associated with maternal use of propoxyphene hydrochloride (Darvon). J Pediatr 1974;85:684–5.
8. Klein RB, Blatman S, Little GA. Probable neonatal propoxyphene withdrawal: a case report. Pediatrics 1975;55:882–4.

9. Quillan WW, Dunn CA. Neonatal drug withdrawal from propoxyphene. JAMA 1976;235:2128.
10. Ente G, Mehra MC. Neonatal drug withdrawal from propoxyphene hydrochloride. NY State J Med 1978;78:2084–5.
11. Eddy NB, Friebel H, Hahn KJ, Halbach H. Codeine and its alternatives for pain and cough relief. 2. Alternates for pain relief. Bull WHO 1969;40:1–53.
12. Catz C, Guiacoia G. Drugs and breast milk. Pediatr Clin North Am 1972;19:151–66.
13. Committee on Drugs, American Academy of Pediatrics. The transfer of drugs and other chemicals into human breast milk. Pediatrics 1983;72:375–83.

Name: **PROPRANOLOL**

Class: **Sympatholytic (β-Adrenergic Blocker)**   Risk Factor: **C$_M$**

Fetal Risk Summary

Propranolol, a nonselective β-adrenergic blocking agent, has been used for various indications in pregnancy:

Maternal hyperthyroidism (1–7)
Pheochromocytoma (8)
Maternal cardiac disease (6, 7, 9–20)
Fetal tachycardia/arrhythmia (21, 22)
Maternal hypertension (7, 20, 23–30)
Dysfunctional labor (31)
Termination of pregnancy (32)

The drug readily crosses the placenta (2, 6, 12, 16, 22, 29, 33, 34). Cord serum levels varying between 19 and 127% of maternal serum have been reported (2, 16, 22, 29). Oxytocic effects have been demonstrated following intravenous and extra-amniotic injections and high oral dosing (17, 31, 32, 35, 36). Intravenous propranolol has been shown to block or decrease the marked increase in maternal plasma progesterone induced by vasopressin or theophyllamine (37). The pharmacokinetics of propranolol in pregnancy have been described (38). Plasma levels and elimination were not significantly altered by pregnancy.

A number of fetal/neonatal adverse effects have been reported following the use of propranolol in pregnancy. Whether these effects are due to propranolol, maternal disease, other drugs consumed concurrently, or a combination of these factors is not always clear. Daily doses of 160 mg/day or higher seem to produce the more serious complications, but lower doses have also resulted in toxicity. Analysis of 23 reports involving 167 liveborn infants exposed to chronic propranolol *in utero* is shown below (1–4, 6, 7, 9, 11–14, 20, 22–24, 26–29, 39–42):

	No. Cases	%
Intrauterine growth retardation	23	14
Hypoglycemia	16	10
Bradycardia	12	7
Respiratory depression at birth	6	4
Hyperbilirubinemia	6	4
Small placenta (size not always noted)	4	2
Polycythemia	2	1
Thrombocytopenia (40,000/mm^3)	1	0.6

	No. Cases	%
Hyperirritability	1	0.6
Hypocalcemia with convulsions	1	0.6
Blood coagulation defect	1	0.6

Two infants were reported to have anomalies (pyloric stenosis; crepitus of hip), but the authors did not relate these to propranolol (27, 39). In another case, a malformed fetus was spontaneously aborted from a 30-year-old woman with chronic renovascular hypertension (43). The patient had been treated with propranolol, amiloride, and captopril for her severe hypertension. Malformations included absence of the left leg below the midthigh, and no obvious skull formation above the brain tissue. The authors attributed the defect either to captopril alone or to a combination effect of the three drugs.

Respiratory depression was noted in four of five infants whose mothers were given 1 mg of propranolol intravenously just prior to cesarean section (44). None of the five controls in the double-blind study were depressed at birth. The author suggested the mechanism may have been due to β-adrenergic blockade of the cervical sympathetic discharge which occurs at cord clamping.

Fetal bradycardia was observed in 2 of 10 patients treated with propranolol, 1 mg/min for 4 minutes, for dysfunctional labor (31). No lasting effects were seen in the babies. In a retrospective study, eight markedly hypertensive patients (nine pregnancies) treated with propranolol were compared with 15 hypertensive controls not treated with propranolol (25). Other antihypertensives were used in both groups. A significant difference was found between the perinatal mortality rates, with seven deaths in the propranolol group (78%) and only five deaths in the controls (33%). However, a possible explanation for the difference may have been the more severe hypertension and renal disease in the propranolol group than in the controls (45).

Intrauterine growth retardation may be related to propranolol. Several possible mechanisms for this effect, if indeed it is associated with the drug, have been reviewed by Redmond (46). Premature labor has been suggested as a possible complication of propranolol therapy in patients with pregnancy-induced hypertension (41). In nine women treated with propranolol for pregnancy-induced hypertension, three delivered prematurely. The author speculated that these patients were relatively hypovolumic and when a compensatory increase in cardiac output failed to occur, premature delivery resulted. However, another report on chronic propranolol use in fourteen women did not observe premature labor (42).

In a randomized, double-blind trial, 36 patients at term were given either 80 mg of propranolol or placebo (47). Fetal heart rate reaction to a controlled sound stimulus was then measured at 1, 2, and 3 hours. The heart rate reaction in the propranolol group was significantly depressed, compared to placebo, at all three time intervals.

The reactivity of nonstress tests (NST) was affected by propranolol in two hypertensive women in the 2nd and 3rd trimesters (48). One woman was taking 20 mg every 6 hours and the other 10 mg three times daily. Repeated NST were nonreactive in both women, but immediate follow-up contraction stress tests were negative. The NST became reactive 2 and 10 days, respectively, after propranolol was discontinued.

In summary, propranolol has been used during pregnancy for maternal and fetal indications. The drug is apparently not a teratogen, but fetal and neonatal toxicity may occur. Newborn infants of women consuming the drug near delivery should be closely observed during the first 24–48 hours after birth for bradycardia, hypoglycemia, and other symptoms of β-blockade. Long-term effects of *in utero* exposure to β-blockers have not been studied but warrant evaluation.

Breast Feeding Summary

Propranolol is excreted into breast milk. Peak concentrations occur 2–3 hours after a dose (12, 20, 42, 49). Milk levels have ranged from 4 to 64 ng/ml with milk:plasma ratios of 0.2 to 1.5 (12, 20, 29, 49). Although adverse effects such as respiratory depression, bradycardia, or hypoglycemia have not been reported, nursing infants exposed to propranolol in breast milk should be closely observed for these symptoms of β-blockade. Long-term effects of exposure to β-blockers from milk have not been studied but warrant evaluation. The American Academy of Pediatrics considers propranolol compatible with breast-feeding (50).

References

1. Jackson GL. Treatment of hyperthyroidism in pregnancy. Penn Med 1973;76:56–7.
2. Langer A, Hung CT, McA'Nulty JA, Harrigan JT, Washington E. Adrenergic blockade: a new approach to hyperthyroidism during pregnancy. Obstet Gynecol 1974;44:181–6.
3. Bullock JL, Harris RE, Young R. Treatment of thyrotoxicosis during pregnancy with propranolol. Am J Obstet Gynecol 1975;121:242–5.
4. Lightner ES, Allen HD, Loughlin G. Neonatal hyperthyroidism and heart failure: a different approach. Am J Dis Child 1977;131:68–70.
5. Levy CA, Waite JH, Dickey R. Thyrotoxicosis and pregnancy. Use of preoperative propranolol for thyroidectomy. Am J Surg 1977;133:319–21.
6. Habib A, McCarthy JS. Effects on the neonate of propranolol administered during pregnancy. J Pediatr 1977; 91:808–11.
7. Pruyn SC, Phelan JP, Buchanan GC. Long-term propranolol therapy in pregnancy: maternal and fetal outcome. Am J Obstet Gynecol 1979;135:485–9.
8. Leak D, Carroll JJ, Robinson DC, Ashworth EJ. Management of pheochromocytoma during pregnancy. Can Med Assoc J 1977;116:371–5.
9. Turner GM, Oakley CM, Dixon HG. Management of pregnancy complicated by hypertrophic obstructive cardiomyopathy. Br Med J 1968;4:281–4.
10. Barnes AB. Chronic propranolol administration during pregnancy: a case report. J Reprod Med 1970;5:79–80.
11. Schroeder JS, Harrison DC. Repeated cardioversion during pregnancy. Am J Cardiol 1971;27:445–6.
12. Levitan AA, Manion JC. Propranolol therapy during pregnancy and lactation. Am J Cardiol 1973;32:247.
13. Reed RL, Cheney CB, Fearon RE, Hook R, Hehre FW. Propranolol therapy throughout pregnancy: a case report. Anesth Analg 1974;53:214–8.
14. Fiddler GI. Propranolol pregnancy. Lancet 1974;2:722–3.
15. Kolibash AE, Ruiz DE, Lewis RP. Idiopathic hypertrophic subaortic stenosis in pregnancy. Ann Intern Med 1975;82:791–4.
16. Cottrill CM, McAllister RG Jr, Gettes L, Noonan JA. Propranolol therapy during pregnancy, labor, and delivery: evidence for transplacental drug transfer and impaired neonatal drug disposition. J Pediatr 1977;91:812–4.
17. Datta S, Kitzmiller JL, Ostheimer GW, Schoenbaum SC. Propranolol and parturition. Obstet Gynecol 1978;51:577–81.
18. Diaz JH, McDonald JS. Propranolol and induced labor: anesthetic implications. Anesth Rev 1979;6:29–32.
19. Oakley GDG, McGarry K, Limb DG, Oakley CM. Management of pregnancy in patients with hypertrophic cardiomyopathy. Br Med J 1979;1:1749–50.

20. Bauer JH, Pape B, Zajicek J, Groshong T. Propranolol in human plasma and breast milk. Am J Cardiol 1979;43:860–2.
21. Eibschitz I, Abinader EG, Klein A, Sharf M. Intrauterine diagnosis and control of fetal ventricular arrhythmia during labor. Am J Obstet Gynecol 1975;122:597–600.
22. Teuscher A, Boss E, Imhof P, Erb E, Stocker FP, Weber JW. Effect of propranolol on fetal tachycardia in diabetic pregnancy. Am J Cardiol 1978;42:304–7.
23. Gladstone GR, Hordof A, Gersony WM. Propranolol administration during pregnancy: effects on the fetus. J Pediatr 1975;86:962–4.
24. Tcherdakoff PH, Colliard M, Berrard E, Kreft C, Dupry A, Bernaille JM. Propranolol in hypertension during pregnancy. Br Med J 1978;2:670.
25. Lieberman BA, Stirrat GM, Cohen SL, Beard RW, Pinker GD, Belsey E. The possible adverse effect of propranolol on the fetus in pregnancies complicated by severe hypertension. Br J Obstet Gynaecol 1978;85:678–83.
26. Eliahou HE, Silverberg DS, Reisin E, Romen I, Mashiach S, Serr DM. Propranolol for the treatment of hypertension in pregnancy. Br J Obstet Gynaecol 1978;85:431–6.
27. Bott-Kanner G, Schweitzer A, Schoenfeld A, Joel-Cohen J, Rosenfeld JB. Treatment with propranolol and hydralazine throughout pregnancy in a hypertensive patient: a case report. Isr J Med Sci 1978;14:466–8.
28. Bott-Kanner G, Reisner SH, Rosenfeld JB. Propranolol and hydrallazine in the management of essential hypertension in pregnancy. Br J Obstet Gynaecol 1980;87:110–4.
29. Taylor EA, Turner P. Anti-hypertensive therapy with propranolol during pregnancy and lactation. Postgrad Med J 1981;57:427–30.
30. Serup J. Propranolol for the treatment of hypertension in pregnancy. Acta Med Scand 1979;206:333.
31. Mitrani A, Oettinger M, Abinader EG, Sharf M, Klein A. Use of propranolol in dysfunctional labour. Br J Obstet Gynaecol 1975;82:651–5.
32. Amy JJ, Karim SMM. Intrauterine administration of l-noradrenaline and propranolol during the second trimester of pregnancy. J Obstet Gynaecol Br Commonw 1974;81:75–83.
33. Smith MT, Livingstone I, Eadie MJ, Hooper WD, Triggs EJ. Metabolism of propranolol in the human maternal-placental-foetal unit. Eur J Clin Pharmacol 1983;24:727–32.
34. Erkkola R, Lammintausta R, Liukko P, Anttila M. Transfer of propranolol and sotalol across the human placenta. Acta Obstet Gynecol Scand 1982;61:31–4.
35. Barden TP, Stander RW. Myometrial and cardiovascular effects of an adrenergic blocking drug in human pregnancy. Am J Obstet Gynecol 1968;101:91–9.
36. Wansbrough H, Nakanishi H, Wood C. The effect of adrenergic receptor blocking drugs on the human fetus. J Obstet Gynaecol Br Commonw 1968;75:189–98.
37. Fylling P. Dexamethasone or propranolol blockade of induced increase in plasma progesterone in early human pregnancy. Acta Endocrinol (Copenh) 1973;72:569–72.
38. Smith MT, Livingstone I, Eadie MJ, Hooper WD, Triggs EJ. Chronic propranolol administration during pregnancy: maternal pharmacokinetics. Eur J Clin Pharmacol 1983;25:481–90.
39. O'Connor PC, Jick H, Hunter JR, Stergachis A, Madsen S. Propranolol and pregnancy outcome. Lancet 1981;2:1168.
40. Caldroney RD. Beta-blockers in pregnancy. N Engl J Med 1982;306:810.
41. Goodlin RC. Beta blocker in pregnancy-induced hypertension. Am J Obstet Gynecol 1982;143:237.
42. Livingstone I, Craswell PW, Bevan EB, Smith MT, Eadie MJ. Propranolol in pregnancy: three year prospective study. Clin Exp Hypertens [B] 1983;2:341–50.
43. Duminy PC, Burger P du T. Fetal abnormality associated with the use of captopril during pregnancy. S Afr Med J 1981;60:805.
44. Tunstall ME. The effect of propranolol on the onset of breathing at birth. Br J Anaesth 1969;41:792.
45. Rubin PC. Beta-blockers in pregnancy. N Engl J Med 1981;305:1323–6.
46. Redmond GP. Propranolol and fetal growth retardation. Semin Perinatol 1982;6:142–7.
47. Jensen OH. Fetal heart rate response to a controlled sound stimulus after propranolol administration to the mother. Acta Obstet Gynecol Scand 1984;63:199–202.
48. Margulis E, Binder D, Cohen AW. The effect of propranolol on the nonstress test. Am J Obstet Gynecol 1984;148:340–1.
49. Karlberg B, Lundberg O, Aberg H. Excretion of propranolol in human breast milk. Acta Pharmacol Toxicol (Copenh) 1974;34:222–4.
50. Committee on Drugs, American Academy of Pediatrics. The transfer of drugs and other chemicals into human breast milk. Pediatrics 1983;72:375–83.

Name: **PROPYLTHIOURACIL**

Class: **Antithyroid**   Risk Factor: **D**

Fetal Risk Summary

Propylthiouracil (PTU) has been used for the treatment of hyperthyroidism during pregnancy since its introduction in the 1940's (1–36). The drug prevents synthesis of thyroid hormones and inhibits peripheral deiodination of levothyroxine to liothyronine (37).

PTU crosses the placenta. Four patients undergoing therapeutic abortion were given a single 15-mg ^{35}S-labeled oral dose 2 hours before pregnancy termination (38). Serum could not be obtained from two 8-week-old fetuses, but 0.0016–0.0042% of the given dose was found in the fetal tissues. In two other fetuses at 12 and 16 weeks of age, the fetal:maternal serum ratios were 0.27 and 0.35, with 0.020 and 0.025% of the dose in the fetus.

The primary effect on the fetus from transplacental passage of PTU is the production of a mild hypothyroidism when the drug is used close to term. This usually resolves within a few days without treatment (33). Clinically, the hypothyroid state may be observed as a goiter in the newborn and is the result of increased levels of fetal pituitary thyrotropin (24). The incidence of fetal goiter after PTU treatment in reported cases is approximately 12% (28 goiters/240 patients) (1–36). Some of these cases may have been due to co-administration of iodides (9, 11, 18, 22). Use of PTU early in pregnancy does not produce fetal goiter since the fetal thyroid does not begin hormone production until approximately the 11th or 12th week of gestation (39). Goiters from PTU exposure are usually small and do not obstruct the airway as do iodide-induced goiters (see also Potassium Iodide) (39, 40). However, two reports have been located that described PTU-induced goiters in newborns that were sufficiently massive to produce tracheal compression, resulting in death in one infant and moderate respiratory distress in the second (7, 10). In two other PTU-exposed fetuses, clinical hypothyroidism was evident at birth with subsequent retarded mental and physical development (10–12). One of these infants was also exposed to high doses of iodide during gestation (12). PTU-induced goiters are not predictable or dose-dependent, but the smallest possible dose of PTU should be used, especially during the 3rd trimester (19, 32, 39–41). No effect on intellectual or physical development from PTU-induced hypothroxinemia was observed in comparison studies between exposed and nonexposed siblings (19, 42).

Congenital anomalies have been reported in seven newborns exposed to PTU *in utero* (14, 17, 21, 27, 33). This incidence is well within the expected rate of malformations. No association between PTU and defects is suggested. The reported defects are:

Congenital dislocation of hip (14)
Cryptorchidism (17)
Muscular hypotonicity (17)
Syndactyly of hand/foot (^{131}I also used) (21)
Hypospadias (27)
Aortic atresia (27)
Choanal atresia (33)

In a large prospective study, 25 patients were exposed to one or more noniodide thyroid suppressants during the 1st trimester, 16 of whom took PTU (43). From the total group, four children with nonspecified malformations were found, suggesting that this group of drugs may be teratogenic. However, since nine of the group took methimazole (a possible teratogen—see Methimazole) and two others were exposed to other thiouracil derivatives, the relationship between PTU and the anomalies cannot be determined.

In comparison with other antithyroid drugs, propylthiouracil is considered the drug of choice for the medical treatment of hyperthyroidism during pregnancy (see also Carbimazole, Methimazole, Potassium Iodide, ^{131}I) (33, 35, 39–41). Combination therapy with thyroid-antithyroid drugs was advocated at one time but is now considered inappropriate (25, 26, 33, 35, 39–41, 44). Two reasons contributed to this change: 1) use of thyroid hormones may require higher doses of PTU to be used, and 2) placental transfer of levothyroxine and liothyronine are minimal and not sufficient to reverse fetal hypothyroidism (see also Levothyroxine and Liothyronine).

Breast Feeding Summary

PTU is excreted into breast milk in low amounts. In a patient given 100 mg of radiolabeled PTU, the milk:plasma ratio was a constant 0.55 over a 24-hour period, representing about 0.077% of the given radioactive dose (45). In a second study, nine patients were given an oral dose of 400 mg (46). Mean serum and milk levels at 90 minutes were 7.7 and 0.7 μg/ml, respectively. The average amount excreted in milk during 4 hours was 99 μg, about 0.025% of the total dose. One mother took 200–300 mg daily while breast-feeding (46). No changes in any of the infant's thyroid parameters were observed.

Based on these two reports, PTU does not seem to pose a significant risk to the breast-fed infant. However, periodic evaluation of the infant's thyroid function may be prudent. The American Academy of Pediatrics considers propylthiouracil compatible with breast-feeding (47).

References

1. Astwood EB, VanderLaan WP. Treatment of hyperthyroidism with propylthiouracil. Ann Intern Med 1946;25:813–21.
2. Bain L. Propylthiouracil in pregnancy: report of a case. South Med J 1947;40:1020–1.
3. Lahey FH, Bartels EC. The use of thiouracil, thiobarbital and propylthiouracil in patients with hyperthyroidism. Ann Surg 1947;125:572–81.
4. Reveno WS. Propylthiouracil in the treatment of toxic goiter. J Clin Endocrinol Metab 1948;8:866–74.
5. Eisenberg L. Thyrotoxicosis complicating pregnancy. NY State J Med 1950;50:1618–9.
6. Astwood EB. The use of antithyroid drugs during pregnancy. J Clin Endocrinol Metab 1951;11:1045–56.
7. Aaron HH, Schneierson SJ, Siegel E. Goiter in newborn infant due to mother's ingestion of propylthiouracil. JAMA 1955;159:848–50.
8. Waldinger C, Wermer OS, Sobel EH. Thyroid function in infant with congenital goiter resulting from exposure to propylthiouracil. J Am Med Wom Assoc 1955;10:196–7.
9. Bongiovanni AM, Eberlein WR, Thomas PZ, Anderson WB. Sporadic goiter of the newborn. J Clin Endocrino Metab 1956;16:146–52.
10. Krementz ET, Hooper RG, Kempson RL. The effect on the rabbit fetus of the maternal administration of propylthiouracil. Surgery 1957;41:619–31.
11. Branch LK, Tuthill SW. Goiters in twins resulting from propylthio-uracil given during pregnancy. Ann Intern Med 1957;46:145–8.

12. Man EB, Shaver BA Jr, Cooke RE. Studies of children born to women with thyroid disease. Am J Obstet Gynecol 1958;75:728–41.
13. Becker WF, Sudduth PG. Hyperthyroidism and pregnancy. Ann Surg 1959;149:867–74.
14. Greenman GW, Gabrielson MO, Howard-Flanders J, Wessel MA. Thyroid dysfunction in pregnancy. N Engl J Med 1962;267:426–31.
15. Herbst AL, Selenkow HA. Combined antithyroid-thyroid therapy of hyperthyroidism in pregnancy. Obstet Gynecol 1963;21:543–50.
16. Reveno WS, Rosenbaum H. Observations on the use of antithyroid drugs. Ann Intern Med 1964;60:982–9.
17. Herbst AL, Selenkow HA. Hyperthyroidism during pregnancy. N Engl J Med 1965;273:627–33.
18. Burrow GN. Neonatal goiter after maternal propylthiouracil therapy. J Clin Endocrinol Metab 1965;25:403–8.
19. Burrow GN, Bartsocas C, Klatskin EH, Grunt JA. Children exposed in utero to propylthiouracil. Am J Dis Child 1968;116:161–5.
20. Talbert LM, Thomas CG Jr, Holt WA, Rankin P. Hyperthyroidism during pregnancy. Obstet Gynecol 1970;36:779–85.
21. Hollingsworth DR, Austin E. Thyroxine derivatives in amniotic fluid. J Pediatr 1971;79:923–9.
22. Ayromlooi J. Congenital goiter due to maternal ingestion of iodides. Obstet Gynecol 1972;39:818–22.
23. Worley RJ, Crosby WM. Hyperthyroidism during pregnancy. Am J Obstet Gynecol 1974;119:150–5.
24. Refetoff S, Ochi Y, Selenkow HA, Rosenfield RL. Neonatal hypothyroidism and goiter in one infant of each of two sets of twins due to maternal therapy with antithyroid drugs. J Pediatr 1974;85:240–4.
25. Mestman JH, Manning PR, Hodgman J. Hyperthyroidism and pregnancy. Arch Intern Med 1974;134:434–9.
26. Goluboff LG, Sisson JC, Hamburger JI. Hyperthyroidism associated with pregnancy. Obstet Gynecol 1974;44:107–16.
27. Mujtaba Q, Burrow GN. Treatment of hyperthyroidism in pregnancy with propylthiouracil and methimazole. Obstet Gynecol 1975;46:282–6.
28. Serup J, Petersen S. Hyperthyroidism during pregnancy treated with propylthiouracil. Acta Obstet Gynecol Scand 1977;56:463–6.
29. Serup J. Maternal propylthiouracil to manage fetal hyperthyroidism. Lancet 1978;2:896.
30. Wallace EZ, Gandhi VS. Triiodothyronine thyrotoxicosis in pregnancy. Am J Obstet Gynecol 1978;130:106–7.
31. Weiner S, Scharf JI, Bolognese RJ, Librizzi RJ. Antenatal diagnosis and treatment of a fetal goiter. J Reprod Med 1980;24:39–42.
32. Sugrue D, Drury MI. Hyperthyroidism complicating pregnancy: results of treatment by antithyroid drugs in 77 pregnancies. Br J Obstet Gynaecol 1980;87:970–5.
33. Cheron RG, Kaplan MM, Larsen PR, Selenkow HA, Crigler JF Jr. Neonatal thyroid function after propylthiouracil therapy for maternal Graves' disease. N Engl J Med 1981;304:525–8.
34. Check JH, Rezvani I, Goodner D, Hopper B. Prenatal treatment of thyrotoxicosis to prevent intrauterine growth retardation. Obstet Gynecol 1982;60:122–4.
35. Kock HCLV, Merkus JMWM. Graves' disease during pregnancy. Eur J Obstet Gynecol Reprod Biol 1983;14:323–30.
36. Hollingsworth DR, Austin E. Observations following I[131] for Graves disease during first trimester of pregnancy. South Med J 1969;62:1555–6.
37. American Hospital Formulary Service. Drug Information 84. Bethesda:American Society of Hospital Pharmacists,1984:1318.
38. Marchant B, Brownlie EW, Hart DM, Horton PW, Alexander WD. The placental transfer of propylthiouracil, methimazole and carbimazole. J Clin Endocrinol Metab 1977;45:1187–93.
39. Burr WA. Thyroid disease. Clin Obstet Gynecol 1981;8:341–51.
40. Burrow GN. Hyperthyroidism during pregnancy. N Engl J Med 1978; 298:150–3.
41. Burrow GN. Maternal-fetal considerations in hyperthyroidism. Clin Endocrinol Metab 1978;7:115–25.
42. Burrow GN, Klatskin EH, Genel M. Intellectual development in children whose mothers received propylthiouracil during pregnancy. Yale J Biol Med 1978;51:151–6.
43. Heinonen OP, Slone D, Shapiro S. Birth Defects and Drugs in Pregnancy. Littleton:Publishing Sciences Group,1977:388–400.

44. Anonymous. Transplacental passage of thyroid hormones. N Engl J Med 1967;277:486–7.
45. Low LCK, Lang J, Alexander WD. Excretion of carbimazole and propylthiouracil in breast milk. Lancet 1979;2:1011.
46. Kampmann JP, Johansen K, Hansen JM, Helweg J. Propylthiouracil in human milk. Lancet 1980;1:736–8.
47. Committee on Drugs, American Academy of Pediatrics. The transfer of drugs and other chemicals into human breast milk. Pediatrics 1983;72:375–83.

Name: **PROTAMINE**

Class: **Antiheparin** Risk Factor: **C**

Fetal Risk Summary

Protamine is used to neutralize the anticoagulant effect of heparin. No reports of its use in pregnancy have been located. Reproduction studies in animals have not been conducted (1).

Breast Feeding Summary

No data available.

References

1. Product information. Protamine sulfate. Eli Lilly & Co, 1985.

Name: **PROTRIPTYLINE**

Class: **Antidepressant** Risk Factor: **C**

Fetal Risk Summary

No data available.

Breast Feeding Summary

No data available.

Name: **PSEUDOEPHEDRINE**

Class: **Sympathomimetic (Adrenergic)** Risk Factor: **C**

Fetal Risk Summary

Pseudoephedrine is a sympathomimetic used to alleviate the symptoms of allergic disorders or upper respiratory infections. It is a common component of proprietary mixtures containing antihistamines and other ingredients. Thus, it is difficult to separate the effects of pseudoephedrine on the fetus from other drugs, disease states and viruses.

Sympathomimetic amines are teratogenic in some animal species, but human teratogenicity has not been suspected (1, 2). Recent data may require a reappraisal of this opinion. The Collaborative Perinatal Project monitored 50,282 mother-child pairs, 3,082 of which had 1st trimester exposure to sympathomimetic drugs (3). For use anytime during pregnancy, 9,719 exposures were recorded (4). An association in the 1st trimester was found between the sympathomimetic class of drugs as a whole and minor malformations (not life-threatening or major cosmetic defects), inguinal hernia, and clubfoot (3). These data are presented as a warning that indiscriminate use of pseudoephedrine, especially in the 1st trimester, is not without risk.

A 1981 report described a woman who consumed, throughout pregnancy, 480 to 840 ml per day of a cough syrup (5). The potential maximum daily doses based on 840 ml of syrup were 5.0 g pseudoephedrine, 16.8 g guaifenesin, 1.68 g dextromethorphan and 79.8 ml of ethanol. The infant had features of the fetal alcohol syndrome (see Ethanol) and displayed irritability, tremors and hypertonicity. It is not known if the ingredients, other than the ethanol, were associated with the adverse effects observed in the infant.

Breast Feeding Summary

No data available.

References

1. Nishimura H, Tanimura T. *Clinical Aspects of the Teratogenicity of Drugs*. Amsterdam:Excerpta Medica, 1976:231.
2. Shepard TH. *Catalog of Teratogenic Drugs*, ed 3. Baltimore:The Johns Hopkins University Press, 1980:134–5.
3. Heinonen OP, Slone D, Shapiro S. *Birth Defects and Drugs in Pregnancy*. Littleton:Publishing Sciences Group, 1977:345–56.
4. *Ibid*, 439.
5. Chasnoff IJ, Diggs G. Fetal alcohol effects and maternal cough syrup abuse. Am J Dis Child 1981;135:968.

Name: **PYRANTEL PAMOATE**

Class: **Anthelmintic**   Risk Factor: **C**

Fetal Risk Summary

No data available.

Breast Feeding Summary

No data available.

Name: **PYRETHRINS WITH PIPERONYL BUTOXIDE**

Class: **Pediculicide**   Risk Factor: **C**

Fetal Risk Summary

Pyrethrins with piperonyl butoxide is a synergistic combination product used topically for the treatment of lice infestations. It is not effective for the treatment of scabies (mite infestations). Pyrethrins with piperonyl butoxide is considered the drug of choice for lice (1). Although no reports of its use in pregnancy have been located, topical absorption is poor so potential toxicity should be less than lindane (see also Lindane) (2). For this reason, use of the combination is probably preferred over lindane in the pregnant patient.

Breast Feeding Summary

No data available.

References

1. Anonymous. Drugs for parasitic infections. In: *Handbook for Antimicrobial Therapy*. New Rochelle:The Medical Letter, Inc, 1984:100.
2. Robinson DH, Shepherd DA. Control of head lice in schoolchildren. Curr Ther Res 1980;27:1–6.

Name: **PYRIDOSTIGMINE**

Class: **Parasympathomimetic (Cholinergic)**   Risk Factor: **C**

Fetal Risk Summary

Pyridostigmine is a quaternary ammonium compound with anticholinesterase activity used in the treatment of myasthenia gravis. The drug has been used in pregnancy without producing fetal malformations (1–13). Because it is ionized at physiologic pH, pyridostigmine would not be expected to cross the placenta in significant amounts. Caution has been advised against the use in pregnancy of intravenous anticholinesterases since they may cause premature labor (1, 2). This effect on the pregnant uterus increases near term.

Transient muscular weakness has been observed in about 20% of newborns of mothers with myasthenia gravis (9). The neonatal myasthenia is due to transplacental passage of anti-acetylcholine receptor immunoglobulin G antibodies (9).

Breast Feeding Summary

Pyridostigmine is excreted into breast milk (13). Levels in two women receiving 120–300 mg/day were 2–25 ng/ml, representing milk:plasma ratios of 0.36–1.13. Because it is an ionized quaternary ammonium compound, these values were surprisingly high. The drug was not detected in the infants nor were any adverse effects noted. The authors estimated that the two infants were ingesting 0.1% or less of their mother's doses (13).

References

1. Foldes FF, McNall PG. Myasthenia gravis: a guide for anesthesiologists. Anesthesiology 1962;23:837–72.

2. McNall PG, Jafarnia MR. Management of myasthenia gravis in the obstetric patient. Am J Obstet Gynecol 1965;92:518–25.
3. Plauche WC. Myasthenia gravis in pregnancy. Am J Obstet Gynecol 1964;88:404–9.
4. Chambers DC, Hall JE, Boyce J. Myasthenia gravis and pregnancy. Obstet Gynecol 1967;29:597–603.
5. Hay DM. Myasthenia gravis and pregnancy. J Obstet Gynaecol Br Commonw 1969;76:323–9.
6. Heinonen OP, Slone D, Shapiro S. Birth Defects and Drugs in Pregnancy. Littleton:Publishing Sciences Group, 1977:345–56.
7. Blackhall MI, Buckley GA, Roberts DV, Roberts JB, Thomas BH, Wilson A. Drug-induced neonatal myasthenia. J Obstet Gynaecol Br Commonw 1969;76:157–62.
8. Rolbin SH, Levinson G, Shnider SM, Wright RG. Anesthetic considerations for myasthenia gravis and pregnancy. Anesth Analg 1978;57:441–7.
9. Plauche WC. Myasthenia gravis in pregnancy: an update. Am J Obstet Gynecol 1979;135:691–7.
10. Eden RD, Gall SA. Myasthenia gravis and pregnancy: a reappraisal of thymectomy. Obstet Gynecol 1983;62:328–33.
11. Cohen BA, London RS, Goldstein PJ. Myasthenia gravis and preeclampsia. Obstet Gynecol 1976;48(Suppl):35S–7S.
12. Catanzarite VA, McHargue AM, Sandberg EC, Dyson DC. Respiratory arrest during therapy for premature labor in a patient with myastenia gravis. Obstet Gynecol 1984;64:819–22.
13. Hardell LI, Lindstrom B, Lonnerholm G, Osterman PO. Pyridostigmine in human breast milk. Br J Clin Pharmacol 1982;14:565–7.

Name: **PYRIDOXINE**

Class: **Vitamin**   Risk Factor: **A***

Fetal Risk Summary

Pyridoxine (vitamin B_6), a water-soluble B complex vitamin, acts as an essential coenzyme involved in the metabolism of amino acids, carbohydrates, and lipids (1). The American RDA for pyridoxine in pregnancy is 2.4–2.6 mg (2).

Pyridoxine is actively transported to the fetus (3–5). Like other B complex vitamins, concentrations of pyridoxine in the fetus and newborn are higher than in the mother and are directly proportional to maternal intake (6–17). Actual pyridoxine levels vary from report to report due to the nutritional status of the populations studied and the microbiological assays used, but usually indicate an approximate newborn:maternal ratio of 2:1 with levels ranging from 22 to 87 ng/ml for newborns and 13 to 51 ng/ml for mothers (5, 15–17).

Pyridoxine deficiency without clinical symptoms is common during pregnancy (11, 17–34). Clinical symptoms consisting of oral lesions have been reported, however, in severe B_6 deficiency (35). Supplementation with multivitamin products reduces, but does not always eliminate, the incidence of pyridoxine hypovitaminemia (17).

Severe vitamin B_6 deficiency is teratogenic in experimental animals (36). No reports of human malformations linked to B_6 deficiency have been located. A brief report in 1976 described an anencephalic fetus resulting from a woman treated with high doses of pyridoxine and other vitamins and nutrients for psychiatric reasons but the relationship between the defect and the vitamins is unknown (37).

The effects on the mother and fetus resulting from pyridoxine deficiency or excess are controversial. These effects can be summarized as:

Pregnancy-induced hypertension (PIH, Toxemia, Preeclampsia, Eclampsia)
Gestational diabetes mellitus
Infantile convulsions
Hyperemesis gravidarum
Congenital malformations
Miscellaneous

Several researchers have claimed that pyridoxine deficiency is associated with the development of PIH (13, 38–40). Others have not found this relationship (11, 20, 41, 42). Sprince and co-workers (38) demonstrated that women with PIH excreted larger amounts of xanthurenic acid in their urine after a loading dose of dl-tryptophane than did normal pregnant women. Although the test was not totally specific for PIH, they theorized that it could be of value for early detection of the disease and was indicative of abnormal pyridoxine-niacin-protein metabolism. Wachstein and Graffeo (39) compared 410 women treated with 10 mg of pyridoxine daily to 410 controls. PIH occurred in 18 (4.4%) of the untreated controls and in 7 (1.7%) of the pyridoxine-supplemented patients, a significant difference. In an earlier report by this same author, no significant differences were found between women with PIH and normal controls in urinary excretion of 4-pyridoxic acid, a pyridoxine metabolite, after a loading dose of the vitamin (20). Brophy and Siiteri (13) measured lower levels of pyridoxine in mothers with PIH than in mothers without PIH (13). The difference in levels between the newborns of PIH and normal mothers was more than 2-fold and highly significant. In a 1961 Swedish report, Diding and Melander (41) compared pyridoxine levels in 10 women with PIH to 26 women with uncomplicated pregnancies. The difference between the mean levels of the two groups, 25 and 33 ng/ml, respectively, was not significant. Similarly. Heller and co-workers (11) and Hillman and co-workers (12) were unable to find a correlation between pyridoxine levels and PIH.

Coelingh Bennink (43) studied 14 pregnant women with an abnormal glucose tolerance test (GTT). Thirteen of these patients were shown to be pyridoxine-deficient. All were placed on a diet and given 100 mg of pyridoxine per day for 14 days, after which gestational diabetes mellitus was diagnosed in only two. The effect of the diet on the GTT was said to be negligible, although a control group was not used. Spellacy and co-workers (44) duplicated these results in 13 women using the same dose of pyridoxine but without mentioning any dietary manipulation and without controls. Perkins (45), however, was unable to demonstrate a beneficial effect in four patients with an abnormal GTT using 100 mg of B_6 for 21 days. Further, all of the mothers had large-for-gestational-age infants, an expected complication of diabetic pregnancies. Gillmer and Mazibuko (46) treated 13 diabetic women during gestation with the doses of pyridoxine described above and observed an improvement in the GTT in 2 patients, worsening in 6, and no significant change in the remaining 5.

An association between pyridoxine and infantile convulsions was first described in the mid 1950's (47–51). Some infants fed a diet deficient in this vitamin developed intractable seizures that responded only to pyridoxine. Scriver (52) has reviewed this complication in infants and differentiated between the states of pyridoxine deficiency and dependency. Whether or not these states can be induced in utero is open to question. As noted earlier, pyridoxine deficiency is common during pregnancy, even in well-nourished women, but the fetus accumulates the vitamin, although at lower levels, even in the face of maternal hypovitaminemia. Reports of seizures in newborn infants delivered from mothers with pyridoxine deficiency have not been located. On the other hand, high doses of pyridoxine early in gestation in one patient were suspected of altering the normal metabolism of pyridoxine leading to intractable convulsions in the newborn (53). Hunt and co-workers (53) described this patient in whom two pregnancies were complicated by hyperemesis gravidarum and were treated with frequent injections of pyridoxine and thiamine, 50 mg each. The first newborn began convulsing 4 hours after birth and died within 30 hours. Mild twitching began in the second infant at 3 hours of age and progressed to severe generalized convulsions on the 5th day. Successful treatment was eventually accomplished with pyridoxine but not before marked mental retardation had occurred. Hunt et al. postulated that the fetus, exposed to high doses of pyridoxine, developed an adaptive enzyme system that was capable of rapidly metabolizing the vitamin and following delivery, this adaptation was manifested by pyridoxine dependency and convulsions. Since this case, more than 50 additional cases of pyridoxine dependency have been reported, and the disease is now thought to be an inherited autosomal recessive disorder (54). In utero dependency-induced convulsions in three successive pregnancies has been reported in one woman (55). The first two newborns died—one during the 7th week and one on day 2—as a result of intractible convulsions. During the third pregnancy, in utero convulsions stopped after the mother was treated with 110 mg/day of pyridoxine 4 days before delivery. Following birth, the newborn was treated with pyridoxine. Convulsions occurred on three separate occasions when vitamin therapy was withheld and then abated when therapy was restarted.

The first use of pyridoxine for severe nausea and vomiting of pregnancy (hyperemesis gravidarum) was reported by Willis and co-workers in 1942 (56). Individual injections ranged from 10 to 100 mg with total doses up to 1,500 mg being given. Satisfactory relief was obtained in most cases. Weinstein and co-workers (57) successfully treated patients with intramuscular doses of 50–100 mg three times weekly. Hart and McConnell (58) described a single patient with hyperemesis that responded to an intravenous mixture of high dose B complex vitamins, including 50 mg of pyridoxine, each day for 3 days. Much smaller doses were used by Varas (59) in 17 patients. Intramuscular doses of 5 mg every 2–4 days were administered to these patients with an immediate response observed in 12 women and all responding by the second dose. Oral doses of 60–80 mg/day up to a total dose of 2,500 mg gave partial or complete relief from nausea and vomiting in 68 patients while an additional 10 patients required oral plus injectable pyridoxine (60). Dorsey (61) treated 62 cases with a combination of pyridoxine and suprarenal cortex, achieving successful results in 95% of the patients. None of the preceding six studies were double-blind or controlled, so it is difficult to judge the effectiveness of the vitamin in allaying the condition. The effect of pyridoxine on blood urea concentrations in hyperemesis was investigated by McGanity and co-workers (62). Blood urea was decreased below normal adult levels in pregnant women and even lower in patients with hyperemesis. Pyridoxine, 40 mg orally per day for 3 days, significantly increased blood urea only in women suffering from hyperemesis. In another measure of the effect of pyridoxine on hyperemesis, elevated serum glutamic acid levels observed with this condition were returned to normal pregnant values after pyridoxine therapy (63). Hesseltine (64) could not demonstrate any value from pyridoxine therapy in 16 patients. Placebos were used but the study was not blind. In addition, only 1 of 16 patients had hyperemesis gravidarum with the remaining 15 presenting with lesser degrees of nausea and vomiting.

A recent case report suggested a link between high doses of pyridoxine and phocomelia (65). The mother, who weighed only 47 kg, took 50 mg of pyridoxine daily plus unknown doses of lecithin and vitamin B_{12} through the first 7 months of pregnancy. The full-term female infant was born with a near-total amelia of her left leg at the knee. The relationship between the drug and defect is unknown. The combination of doxylamine and pyridoxine (Bendectin, others) has been the focus of considerable debate over the past few years. The debate centered on the question of whether or not the preparation was teratogenic. The combination had been used by millions of women for pregnancy-induced nausea and vomiting but was recently removed from the market by the manufacturer because of a number of large legal awards against the company. Jury decisions notwithstanding, the available scientific evidence indicates the combination is not teratogenic (see Doxylamine).

Among miscellaneous effects, two studies were unable to associate low maternal concentrations of pyridoxine with premature labor (39, 42). Similarly, no correlation was found between low levels and stillbirths (11, 39). However, 1-minute Apgar scores were significantly related to low maternal and newborn pyridoxine concentrations (15, 66). Swartwout and co-workers (67) studied the effect of pyridoxine in black pregnant women and observed lower maternal serum lipid level, fetal weight, and placental weight in women given supplements. Supplementation also reduced the frequency of placental vascular sclerosis. Others have not found a correlation between pyridoxine levels and birth weight (16, 42, 66). In an unusual report, pregnant women given daily 20-mg supplements of pyridoxine by either lozenges or capsules had less dental disease than untreated controls (68). The best cariostatic effect was seen in patients in the lozenge group.

In summary, pyridoxine deficiency during pregnancy is a common problem in unsupplemented women. Supplementation with oral pyridoxine reduces but does not eliminate the frequency of deficiency. No definitive evidence has appeared that indicates mild to moderate deficiency of this vitamin is a cause of maternal or fetal complications. Most of the studies with this vitamin have been open and uncontrolled. If a relationship does exist with poor pregnancy outcome, it is probable that a number of factors, of which pyridoxine is only one, contribute to the problem.

Severe deficiency or abnormal metabolism are related to fetal and infantile convulsions and possibly other conditions. High doses apparently pose little risk to the fetus. The available evidence does not support a teratogenic risk either alone or in combination with doxylamine. Double blind, randomized trials are needed to determine if pyridoxine is effective for severe nausea and vomiting of pregnancy.

Since pyridoxine is required for good maternal and fetal health and an increased demand for the vitamin occurs during pregnancy, supplementation of the pregnant woman with the RDA for pyridoxine is recommended.

[* Risk Factor C if used in doses above RDA.]

Breast Feeding Summary

Pyridoxine (vitamin B_6) is excreted in human breast milk (15, 69–75). Concentrations in milk are directly proportional to intake (69–75). In well nourished women, pyridoxine levels varied, depending on intake, from 123 to 314 ng/ml (69–71). Peak pyridoxine milk levels occurred 3–8 hours after ingestion of a vitamin supplement (69, 71, 72). A 1983 study measured pyridoxine levels in pooled human milk obtained from preterm (26 mothers: 29–34 weeks) and term (35 mothers: 39 weeks or longer) patients (73). Preterm milk level rose from 11.1 ng/ml (colostrum) to 62.2 ng/ml (16–196 days) while term milk level increased over the same period from 17.0 to 107.1 ng/ml. In a 1985 study, daily supplements of 0–20 mg resulted in milk concentrations of 93–413 ng/ml, corresponding to an infant intake of 0.06–0.28 mg/day (72). A significant correlation was found between maternal intake and infant intake. Most infants, however, did not receive the RDA for infants (0.3 mg) even when the mother was consuming eight times the RDA for lactating women (2.5 mg) (72). In lactating women with low nutritional status, supplementation with pyridoxine, 0.4–40.0 mg/day, resulted in mean milk concentrations of 80–158 ng/ml (74).

Convulsions have been reported in infants fed a pyridoxine-deficient diet (see discussion under "Fetal Risk Summary") (47–52). Bessey and co-workers (76) described seizures in two breast-fed infants, one of whom was receiving only 67 μg/day in the milk. Intake in the second infant was not determined. A similar report by Kirksey and Roepke (77) involved three infants whose mothers had levels less than 20 ng/ml (at 7 days postpartum) or less than 60 ng/ml (at 4 weeks) of pyridoxine in their milk. The convulsions responded promptly to B_6 therapy in all five of these infants.

Very large doses of pyridoxine have been reported to have a lactation-inhibiting effect (78). Using oral doses of 600 mg/day, lactation was successfully inhibited in 95% of patients within 1 week as compared to only 17% of placebo-treated controls. Very high intravenous doses of pyridoxine, 600 mg infused over 1 hour in healthy, nonlactating young adults, successfully suppressed the rise in prolactin induced by exercise (79). However, since use of this dose and method of administration in lactating women would be unusual, the relevance of these data to breast-feeding is limited. With dosage much closer to physiologic levels, such as 20 mg/day, no effect on lactation has been observed (72). In addition, two separate trials, utilizing 450 and 600 mg/day in divided oral doses, failed to reproduce the lactation-inhibiting effect observed earlier or to show any suppression of serum prolactin levels (80, 81). One writer, however, has suggested that pyridoxine be removed from multivitamin supplements intended for lactating women (82). This proposal has invoked sharp opposition from other correspondents who claimed that the available evidence does not support a milk-inhibiting property for pyridoxine (83, 84).

In summary, the American RDA for pyridoxine during lactation is 2.3–2.5 mg (2). If the diet of the lactating woman adequately supplies this amount, maternal supplementation with pyridoxine is not required (75). Supplementation with the RDA for pyridoxine is recommended for those women with inadequate nutritional intake.

References

1. American Hospital Formulary Service. *Drug Information 1985*. Bethesda:American Society of Hospital Pharmacists, 1985:1688–90.
2. *Recommended Dietary Allowances*, ed. 9. Washington, DC:National Academy of Sciences, 1980.
3. Frank O, Walbroehl G, Thomson A, Kaminetzky H, Kubes Z, Baker H. Placental transfer: fetal retention of some vitamins. Am J Clin Nutr 1970;23:662–3.
4. Hill EP, Longo LD. Dynamics of maternal-fetal nutrient transfer. Fed Proc 1980;39:239–44.
5. Baker H, Frank O, Deangelis B, Feingold S, Kaminetzky HA. Role of placenta in maternal-fetal vitamin transfer in humans. Am J Obstet Gynecol 1981;141:792–6.

6. Wachstein M, Moore C, Graffeo LW. Pyridoxal phosphate (B_6-al-PO_4) levels of circulating leukocytes in maternal and cord blood. Proc Soc Exp Biol Med 1957;96:326–8.

7. Wachstein M, Kellner JD, Ortiz JM. Pyridoxal phosphate in plasma and leukocytes of normal and pregnant subjects following B_6 load tests. Proc Soc Exp Biol Med 1960;103:350–3.

8. Brin M. Thiamine and pyridoxine studies of mother and cord blood. Fed Proc 1966;25:245.

9. Contractor SF, Shane B. Blood and urine levels of vitamin B_6 in the mother and fetus before and after loading of the mother with vitamin B_6. Am J Obstet Gynecol 1970;107:635–40.

10. Brin M. Abnormal tryptophan metabolism in pregnancy and with the oral contraceptive pill. II. Relative levels of vitamin B_6-vitamers in cord and maternal blood. Am J Clin Nutr 1971;24:704–8.

11. Heller S, Salkeld RM, Korner WF. Vitamin B_6 status in pregnancy. Am J Clin Nutr 1973;26:1339–48.

12. Kaminetzky HA, Baker H, Frank O, Langer A. The effects of intravenously administered water-soluble vitamins during labor in normovitaminemic and hypovitaminemic gravidas on maternal and neonatal blood vitamin levels at delivery. Am J Obstet Gynecol 1974;120:697–703.

13. Brophy MH, Siiteri PK. Pyridoxal phosphate and hypertensive disorders of pregnancy. Am J Obstet Gynecol 1975;121:1075–9.

14. Bamji MS. Enzymic evaluation of thiamin, riboflavin and pyridoxine status of parturient women and their newborn infants. Br J Nutr 1976;35:259–65.

15. Roepke JLB, Kirksey A. Vitamin B_6 nutriture during pregnancy and lactation. I. Vitamin B_6 intake, levels of the vitamin in biological fluids, and condition of the infant at birth. Am J Clin Nutr 1979;32:2249–56.

16. Baker H, Thind IS, Frank O, DeAngelis B, Caterini H, Louria DB. Vitamin levels in low-birth-weight newborn infants and their mothers. Am J Obstet Gynecol 1977;129:521–4.

17. Baker H, Frank O, Thomason AD, Langer A, Munves ED, De Angelis B, Kaminetzky HA. Vitamin profile of 174 mothers and newborns at parturition. Am J Clin Nutr 1975;28:59–65.

18. Wachstein M, Gudaitis A. Disturbance of vitamin B_6 metabolism in pregnancy. J Lab Clin Med 1952;40:550–7.

19. Wachstein M, Gudaitis A. Disturbance of vitamin B_6 metabolism in pregnancy. II. The influence of various amounts of pyridoxine hydrochloride upon the abnormal tryptophane load test in pregnant women. J Lab Clin Med 1953;42:98–107.

20. Wachstein M, Gudaitis A. Disturbance of vitamin B_6 metabolism in pregnancy. III. Abnormal vitamin B_6 load test. Am J Obstet Gynecol 1953;66:1207–13.

21. Wachstein M, Lobel S. Abnormal tryptophan metabolites in human pregnancy and their relation to deranged vitamin B_6 metabolism. Proc Soc Exp Biol Med 1954;86:624–7.

22. Zartman ER, Barnes AC, Hicks DJ. Observations on pyridoxine metabolism in pregnancy. Am J Obstet Gynecol 1955;70:645–9.

23. Turner ER, Reynolds MS. Intake and elimination of vitamin B_6 and metabolites by women. J Am Diet Assoc 1955;31:1119–20.

24. Page EW. The vitamin B_6 requirement for normal pregnancy. West J Surg Obstet Gynecol 1956;64:96–103.

25. Coursin DB, Brown VC. Changes in vitamin B_6 during pregnancy. Am J Obstet Gynecol 1961;82:1307–11.

26. Brown RR, Thornton MJ, Price JM. The effect of vitamin supplementation on the urinary excretion of tryptophan metabolites by pregnant women. J Clin Invest 1961;40:617–23.

27. Hamfelt A, Hahn L. Pyridoxal phosphate concentration in plasma and tryptophan load test during pregnancy. Clin Chim Acta 1969;25:91–6.

28. Rose DP, Braidman IP. Excretion of tryptophan metabolites as affected by pregnancy, contraceptive steroids, and steroid hormones. Am J Clin Nutr 1971;24:673–83.

29. Kaminetzky HA, Langer A, Baker H, Frank O, Thomson AD, Munves ED, Opper A, Behrle FC, Glista B. The effect of nutrition in teen-age gravidas on pregnancy and the status of the neonate. I. A nutritional profile. Am J Obstet Gynecol 1973;115:639–46.

30. Shane B, Contractor SF. Assessment of vitamin B_6 status. Studies on pregnant women and oral contraceptive users. Am J Clin Nutr 1975;28:739–47.

31. Cleary RE, Lumeng L, Li TK. Maternal and fetal plasma levels of pyridoxal phosphate at term: adequacy of vitamin B_6 supplementation during pregnancy. Am J Obstet Gynecol 1975;121:25–8.

32. Lumeng L, Cleary RE, Wagner R, Yu PL, Li TK. Adequacy of vitamin B_6 supplementation during pregnancy: a prospective study. Am J Clin Nutr 1976;29:1376–83.

33. Anonymous. Requirement of vitamin B_6 during pregnancy. Nutr Rev 1976;34:15–6.

34. Dostalova L. Correlation of the vitamin status between mother and newborn during delivery. Dev Pharmacol Ther 1982;4(Suppl I):45–57.

35. Bapurao S, Raman L, Tulpule PG. Biochemical assessment of vitamin B_6 nutritional status in pregnant women with orolingual manifestations. Am J Clin Nutr 1982;36:581–6.

36. Shepard TH. *Catalog of Teratogenic Agents*, ed 3. Baltimore:The Johns Hopkins University Press, 1980:279.

37. Averback P. Anencephaly associated with megavitamin therapy. Can Med Assoc J 1976;114:995.

38. Sprince H, Lowy RS, Folsome CE, Behrman J. Studies on the urinary excretion of "xanthurenic acid" during normal and abnormal pregnancy: a survey of the excretion of "xanthurenic acid" in normal nonpregnant, normal pregnant, pre-eclamptic, and eclamptic women. Am J Obstet Gynecol 1951;62:84–92.

39. Wachstein M, Graffeo LW. Influence of vitamin B_6 on the incidence of preeclampsia. Obstet Gynecol 1956;8:177–80.

40. Kaminetzky HA, Baker H. Micronutrients in pregnancy. Clin Obstet Gynecol 1977;20:363–80.

41. Diding NA, Melander SEJ. Serum vitamin B_6 level in normal and toxaemic pregnancy. Acta Obstet Gynecol Scand 1961;40:252–61.

42. Hillman RW, Cabaud PG, Nilsson DE, Arpin PD, Tufano RJ. Pyridoxine supplementation during pregnancy. Clinical and laboratory observations. Am J Clin Nutr 1963;12:427–30.

43. Coelingh Bennink HJT, Schreurs WHP. Improvement of oral glucose tolerance in gestational diabetes by pyridoxine. Br Med J 1975;3:13–5.

44. Spellacy WN, Buhi WC, Birk SA. Vitamin B_6 treatment of gestational diabetes mellitus. Studies of blood glucose and plasma insulin. Am J Obstet Gynecol 1977;127:599–602.

45. Perkins RP. Failure of pyridoxine to improve glucose tolerance in gestational diabetes mellitus. Obstet Gynecol 1977;50:370–2.

46. Gillmer MDG, Mazibuko D. Pyridoxine treatment of chemical diabetes in pregnancy. Am J Obstet Gynecol 1979;133:499–502.

47. Snyderman SE, Holt LE, Carretero R, Jacobs K. Pyridoxine deficiency in the human infant. J Clin Nutr 1953;1:200–7.

48. Molony CJ, Parmalee AH. Convulsions in young infants as a result of pyridoxine (vitamin B_6) deficiency. JAMA 1954;154:405–6.

49. Coursin DB. Vitamin B_6 deficiency in infants. Am J Dis Child 1955;90:344–8.

50. Coursin DB. Effects of vitamin B_6 on the central nervous activity in childhood. Am J Clin Nutr 1956;4:354–63.

51. Molony CJ, Parmelee AH. Convulsions in young infants as a result of pyridoxine (vitamin B_6) deficiency. JAMA 1954;154:405–6.

52. Scriver CR. Vitamin B_6 deficiency and dependency in man. Am J Dis Child 1967;113:109–14.

53. Hunt AD Jr, Stokes J Jr, McCrory WW, Stroud HH. Pyridoxine dependency: report of a case of intractable convulsions in an infant controlled by pyridoxine. Pediatrics 1954;13:140–5.

54. Bankier A, Turner M, Hopkins IJ. Pyridoxine dependent seizures—a wider clinical spectrum. Arch Dis Child 1983;58:415–8.

55. Bejsovec MIR, Kulenda Z, Ponca E. Familial intrauterine convulsions in pyridoxine dependency. Arch Dis Child 1967;42:201–7.

56. Willis RS, Winn WW, Morris AT, Newsom AA, Massey WE. Clinical observations in treatment of nausea and vomiting in pregnancy with vitamins B_1 and B_6. A preliminary report. Am J Obstet Gynecol 1942;44:265–71.

57. Weinstein BB, Mitchell GJ, Sustendal GF. Clinical experiences with pyridoxine hydrochloride in treatment of nausea and vomiting of pregnancy. Am J Obstet Gynecol 1943;46:283–5.

58. Hart BF, McConnell WT. Vitamin B factors in toxic psychosis of pregnancy and the puerperium. Am J Obstet Gynecol 1943;46:283.

59. Varas O. Treatment of nausea and vomiting of pregnancy with vitamin B_6. Bol Soc Chilena Obstet Ginecol 1943;8:404. As abstracted in Am J Obstet Gynecol 1945;50:347–8.

60. Weinstein BB, Wohl Z, Mitchell GJ, Sustendal GF. Oral administration of pyridoxine hydrochloride in the treatment of nausea and vomiting of pregnancy. Am J Obstet Gynecol 1944;47:389–94.

61. Dorsey CW. The use of pyridoxine and suprarenal cortex combined in the treatment of the nausea and vomiting of pregnancy. Am J Obstet Gynecol 1949;58:1073–8.

62. McGanity WJ, McHenry EW, Van Wyck HB, Watt GL. An effect of pyridoxine on blood urea in human subjects. J Biol Chem 1949;178:511–6.

63. Beaton JR, McHenry EW. Observations on plasma glutamic acid. Fed Proc 1951;10:161.

64. Hesseltine HC. Pyridoxine failure in nausea and vomiting of pregnancy. Am J Obstet Gynecol 1946;51:82–6.
65. Gardner LI, Welsh-Sloan J, Cady RB. Phocomelia in infant whose mother took large doses of pyridoxine during pregnancy. Lancet 1985;1:636.
66. Schuster K, Bailey LB, Mahan CS. Vitamin B6 status of low-income adolescent and adult pregnant women and the condition of their infants at birth. Am J Clin Nutr 1981;34:1731–5.
67. Swartwout JR, Unglaub WG, Smith RC. Vitamin B6, serum lipids and placental arteriolar lesions in human pregnancy. A preliminary report. Am J Clin Nutr 1960;8:434–44.
68. Hillman RW, Cabaud PG, Schenone RA. The effects of pyridoxine supplements on the dental caries experience of pregnant women. Am J Clin Nutr 1962;10:512–5.
69. West KD, Kirksey A. Influence of vitamin B6 intake on the content of the vitamin in human milk. Am J Clin Nutr 1976;29:961–9.
70. Thomas MR, Kawamoto J, Sneed SM, Eakin R. The effects of vitamin C, vitamin B6, and vitamin B12 supplementation on the breast milk and maternal status of well-nourished women. Am J Clin Nutr 1979;32:1679–85.
71. Sneed SM, Zane C, Thomas MR. The effects of ascorbic acid, vitamin B6, vitamin B12, and folic acid supplementation on the breast milk and maternal nutritional status of low socioeconomic lactating women. Am J Clin Nutr 1981;34:1338–46.
72. Styslinger L, Kirksey A. Effects of different levels of vitamin B-6 supplementation on vitamin B-6 concentrations in human milk and vitamin B-6 intakes of breastfed infants. Am J Clin Nutr 1985;41:21–31.
73. Ford JE, Zechalko A, Murphy J, Brooke OG. Comparison of the B vitamin composition of milk from mothers of preterm and term babies. Arch Dis Child 1983;58:367–72.
74. Deodhar AD, Rajalakshmi R, Ramakrishnan CV. Studies on human lactation. Part III. Effect of dietary vitamin supplementation vitamin contents of breast milk. Acta Pediatr 1964;53:42–8.
75. Thomas MR, Sneed SM, Wei C, Nail PA, Wilson M, Sprinkle EE III. The effects of vitamin C, vitamin B6, vitamin B12, folic acid, riboflavin, and thiamin on the breast milk and maternal status of well-nourished women at 6 months postpartum. Am J Clin Nutr 1980;33:2151–6.
76. Bessey OA, Adam DJD, Hansen AE. Intake of vitamin B6 and infantile convulsions: a first approximation of requirements of pyridoxine in infants. Pediatrics 1957;20:33–44.
77. Kirksey A, Roepke JLB. Vitamin B-6 nutriture of mothers of three breast-fed neonates with central nervous system disorders. Fed Proc 1981;40:864.
78. Foukas MD. An antilactogenic effect of pyridoxine. J Obstet Gynaecol Br Commonw 1973;80:718–20.
79. Moretti C, Fabbri A, Gnessi L, Bonifacio V, Fraioli F, Isidori A. Pyridoxine (B6) suppresses the rise in prolactin and increases the rise in growth hormone induced by exercise. N Engl J Med 1982;307:444–5.
80. MacDonald HN, Collins YD, Tobin MJW, Wijayaratne, DN. The failure of pyridoxine in suppression of puerperal lactation. Br J Obstet Gynaecol 1976;83:54–5.
81. Canales ES, Soria J, Zarate A, Mason M, Molina M. The influence of pyridoxine on prolactin secretion and milk production in women. Br J Obstet Gynaecol 1976;83:387–8.
82. Greentree LB.Dangers of vitamin B6 in nursing mothers. N Engl J Med 1979;300:141–2.
83. Lande NI. More on dangers of vitamin B6 in nursing mothers. N Engl J Med 1979;300:926–7.
84. Rivlin RS. Ibid, 927.

Name: PYRILAMINE

Class: **Antihistamine**   Risk Factor: **C**

Fetal Risk Summary

Pyrilamine is used infrequently during pregnancy. The Collaborative Perinatal Project monitored 50,282 mother-child pairs, 121 of which had pyrilamine exposure in the 1st trimester (1). No evidence was found to suggest a relationship to large categories of major or minor malformations. For use anytime during pregnancy,

392 exposures were recorded (2). A possible association with malformations was found based on 12 defects, 6 of which involved benign tumors (3).

Breast Feeding Summary

No data available.

References

1. Heinonen OP, Slone D, Shapiro S. *Birth Defects and Drugs in Pregnancy*. Littleton:Publishing Sciences Group, 1977:323–4.
2. *Ibid*, 436–7.
3. *Ibid*, 489.

Name: **PYRIMETHAMINE**

Class: **Antimalarial**   Risk Factor: **C**

Fetal Risk Summary

Pyrimethamine is a folic acid antagonist used as an antimalarial agent. Although some folic acid antagonists are teratogenic (see Methotrexate), no malformations attributable to pyrimethamine have been reported. One case report described gastroschisis in an infant exposed to the drug early in gestation (1). An association between the drug and the defect, however, is questionable (2, 3).

Most studies have found pyrimethamine to be safe during pregnancy (3–10). Folic acid supplementation should be given to prevent folate deficiency.

Breast Feeding Summary

Pyrimethamine is excreted into breast milk. Mothers treated with 25–75 mg orally produced peak concentrations of 3.1–3.3 μg/ml at 6 hours (11). The drug was detectable up to 48 hours after a dose. Malaria parasites were completely eliminated in infants up to 6 months of age who were entirely breast-fed. The American Academy of Pediatrics considers pyrimethamine compatible with breast-feeding (12).

References

1. Harpey J-P, Darbois Y, Lefebvre G. Teratogenicity of pyrimethamine. Lancet 1983;2:399.
2. Smithells RW, Sheppard S. Teratogenicity of Debendox and pyrimethamine. Lancet 1983;2:623–4.
3. Anonymous. Pyrimethamine combinations in pregnancy. Lancet 1983;2:1005–7.
4. Morley D, Woodland M, Cuthbertson WFJ. Controlled trial of pyrimethamine in pregnant women in an African village. Br Med J 1964;1:667–8.
5. Gilles HM, Lawson JB, Sibelas M, Voller A, Allan N. Malaria, anaemia and pregnancy. Ann Trop Med Parasitol 1969;63:245–63.
6. Heinonen OP, Slone D, Shapiro. *Birth Defects and Drugs in Pregnancy*. Littleton:Publishing Sciences Group, 1977;299,302.
7. Bruce-Chwatt LJ. Malaria and pregnancy. Br Med J 1983;286:1457–8.
8. Anonymous. Malaria in pregnancy. Lancet 1983;2:84–5.
9. Strang A, Lachman E, Pitsoe SB, Marszalek A, Philpott RH. Malaria in pregnancy with fatal complications. Case report. Br J Obstet Gynaecol 1984;91:399–403.
10. Main EK, Main DM, Krogstad DJ. Treatment of chloroquine-resistant malaria during pregnancy. JAMA 1983;249:3207–9.

11. Clyde DF, Shute GT, Press J. Transfer of pyrimethamine in human milk. J Trop Med Hyg 1956;59:277–84.
12. Committee on Drugs, American Academy of Pediatrics. The transfer of drugs and other chemicals into human breast milk. Pediatrics 1983;72:375–83.

Name: **PYRVINIUM PAMOATE**

Class: **Anthelmintic**   Risk Factor: **C**

Fetal Risk Summary

No data available.

Breast Feeding Summary

No data available.

Name: **QUINACRINE**

Class: **Antimalarial/Anthelmintic**   Risk Factor: **C**

Fetal Risk Summary

A newborn with renal agenesis, hydronephrosis, spina bifida, megacolon, and hydrocephalus whose mother received quinacrine, 0.1 g/day, during the 1st trimester has been reported (1). Animal data do not support a teratogenic effect. Topical application of solutions containing 125 mg/ml of quinacrine directly into the uterine cavity have resulted in tubal occlusion and infertility (2).

Breast Feeding Summary

No data available.

References

1. Vevera J, Zatlovkal F. Pfipad uruzenych malformact zpusobenych pravdepodobne atebrinem-ym uranem tehotenstui. In Nishmura H, Tanimura T, eds. *Clinical Aspects of the Teratogenicity of Drugs*. New York:American Elsevier, 1976:145.
2. Zipper JA, Stachetti E, Medel M. Human fertility control by transvaginal application of quinacrine on the fallopian tube. Fertil Steril 1970;21:581–9.

Name: **QUINETHAZONE**

Class: **Diuretic**   Risk Factor: **D**

Fetal Risk Summary

Quinethazone is structurally related to the thiazide diuretics. See Chlorothiazide.

Breast Feeding Summary

See Chlorothiazide.

Name: **QUINIDINE**

Class: **Antiarrthymic**   Risk Factor: **C**

Fetal Risk Summary

No reports linking the use of quinidine with congenital defects have been located. Eighth cranial nerve damage has been erroneously reported with high doses (1, 2). Quinine, the optical isomer of quinidine, was the actual drug suggested in the original reports (see Quinine) (3). Neonatal thrombocytopenia has been reported after maternal use of quinidine (4). Quinidine crosses the placenta and achieves fetal serum levels similar to maternal levels (1). Amniotic fluid levels may be in the toxic range (9–10 μg/ml), but the significance of this finding is unknown.

Quinidine has been in use as an antiarrhythmic drug since 1918. The drug has been used in combination with digoxin to treat fetal supraventricular and reciprocating atrioventricular tachycardia (5, 6). The authors of the latter report consider quinidine the second drug of choice after digoxin for the treatment of persistent fetal tachyarrhythmias (6).

The use of quinidine in pregnancy is relatively safe for the fetus (7, 8). The oxytocic properties of quinidine have not been observed in gravid patients, but high doses may produce this effect (9).

Breast Feeding Summary

Quinidine is excreted into breast milk (1). The milk:plasma ratio is approximately 1, based on measured milk concentrations of 6.4–8.2 μg/ml and maternal serum concentrations of 9.0 μg/ml (1). The American Academy of Pediatrics considers quinidine compatible with breast-feeding (10).

References

1. Hill LM, Malkasian GD Jr. The use of quinidine sulfate throughout pregnancy. Obstet Gynecol 1979;54:366–8.
2. Berkowitz RL, Coustan DR, Mochizuki TK. *Handbook for Prescribing Medications during Pregnancy*. Boston:Little, Brown, 1981:191.
3. Mendelson CL. Disorders of the heartbeat during pregnancy. Am J Obstet Gynecol 1956;72:1268–1301.
4. Domula VM, Weissach G, Lenk H. Uber die auswirkung medikamentoser behandlung in der schwangerschaft auf das gerennungspotential des neugeborenen. Zentralbl Gynaekol 1977;99:473.
5. Spinnato JA, Shaver DC, Flinn GS, Sibai BM, Watson DL, Marin-Garcia J. Fetal supraventricular tachycardia: in utero therapy with digoxin and quinidine. Obstet Gynecol 1984;64:730–5.
6. Guntheroth WG, Cyr DR, Mack LA, Benedetti T, Lenke RR, Petty CN. Hydrops from reciprocating atrioventricular tachycardia in a 27-week fetus requiring quinidine for conversion. Obstet Gynecol 1985;66(Suppl):29S–33S.
7. Rotmensch HH, Elkayam U, Frishman W. Antiarrhythmic drug therapy during pregnancy. Ann Intern Med 1983;98:487–97.
8. Tamari I, Eldar M, Rabinowitz B, Neufeld HN. Medical treatment of cardiovascular disorders during pregnancy. Am Heart J 1982;104:1357–63.
9. Bigger JT, Hoffman BF. Antiarrythmic drugs. In Gilman AG, Goodman LS, Gilman A, eds. *The Pharmacological Basis of Therapeutics*, ed 6. New York:Macmillan Publishing Co, 1980:768.
10. Committee on Drugs, American Academy of Pediatrics. The transfer of drugs and other chemicals into human breast milk. Pediatrics 1983;72:375–83.

Name: **QUININE**

Class: **Plasmodicide**   Risk Factor: **D***

Fetal Risk Summary

Nishimura and Tanimura (1) summarized the human case reports of teratogenic effects linked with quinine in 21 infants who were exposed during the 1st trimester after unsuccessful abortion attempts (some infants had multiple defects and are listed more than once):

Central nervous system anomalies (6 with hydrocephalus) (10 cases)
Limb defects (3 dysmelias) (8 cases)
Facial defects (7 cases)
Heart defects (6 cases)
Digestive organ anomalies (5 cases)
Urogenital anomalies (3 cases)
Hernias (3 cases)
Vertebral anomaly (1 case)

The malformations noted are varied, although central nervous system anomalies and limb defects were the most frequent. Auditory and optic nerve damage have also been reported (1–5). These reports usually concern the use of quinine in toxic doses as an abortifacient. Quinine has also been used for the induction of labor in women with intrauterine fetal death (6). Epidemiologic observations do not support an increased teratogenic risk or increased risk of congenital deafness over non-quinine-exposed patients (1, 7). Neonatal and maternal thrombocytopenia purpura and hemolysis in glucose-6-phosphate dehydrogenase-deficient newborns has been reported (8, 9).

Quinine has effectively been replaced by newer agents for the treatment of malaria. Although no increased teratogenic risk can be documented, its use during pregnancy should be avoided. One manufacturer considers the drug contraindicated in pregnancy (10). However, some investigators believe that quinine should be used for the treatment of chloroquine-resistant *Plasmodium falciparum* malaria (11).

[* Risk Factor X according to manufacturer—Merrell Dow, 1985.]

Breast Feeding Summary

Quinine is excreted into breast milk. Following 300- and 640-mg oral doses in six patients, milk concentrations varied up to 2.2 μg/ml with an average level of 1 μg/ml at 3 hours (12). No adverse effects were reported in the nursing infants. Patients at risk for glucose-6-phosphate dehydrogenase deficiency should not be breast-fed until this disease can be ruled out. The American Academy of Pediatrics considers quinine compatible with breast-feeding (13).

References

1. Nishimura H, Tanimura T. *Clinical Aspects of the Teratogenicity of Drugs*. Amsterdam:Excerpta Medica, 1976:140–3.
2. Robinson GC, Brummitt JR, Miller JR. Hearing loss in infants and preschool children. II. Etiological considerations. Pediatrics 1963;32:115–24.
3. West RA. Effect of quinine upon auditory nerve. Am J Obstet Gynecol 1938;36:241–8.
4. McKinna AJ. Quinine induced hypoplasia of the optic nerve. Can J Ophthalmol 1966;1:261.
5. Morgon A, Charachon D, Brinquier N. Disorders of the auditory apparatus caused by embryopathy or foetopathy. Prophylaxis and treatment. Acta Otolaryngol (Stockh) 1971;291(Suppl):5.
6. Mukherjee S, Bhose LN. Induction of labor and abortion with quinine infusion in intrauterine fetal deaths. Am J Obstet Gynecol 1968;101:853–4.
7. Heinonen OP, Slone D, Shapiro S. *Birth Defects and Drugs in Pregnancy*. Littleton:Publishing Sciences Group, 1977:299, 302, 333.
8. Mauer MA, DeVaux W, Lahey ME. Neonatal and maternal thrombocytopenic purpura due to quinine. Pediatrics 1957;19:84–7.
9. Glass L, Rajegowda BK, Bowne E, Evans HE. Exposure to quinine and jaundice in a glucose-6-phosphate dehydrogenase-deficient newborn infant. Pediatrics 1973;82:734–5.
10. Product information. Quinamm. Merrell Dow, 1985.

11. Strang A, Lachman E, Pitsoe SB, Marszalek A, Philpott RH. Malaria in pregnancy with fatal complications: case report. Br J Obstet Gynaecol 1984;91:399–403.
12. Terwilliger WG, Hatcher RA. The elimination of morphine and quinine in human milk. Surg Gynecol Obstet 1934;58:823–6.
13. Committee on Drugs, American Academy of Pediatrics. The transfer of drugs and other chemicals into human breast milk. Pediatrics 1983;72:375–83.

Name: **RANITIDINE**

Class: **Histamine (H₂) Receptor Antagonist**   Risk Factor: **B$_M$**

Fetal Risk Summary

The use of ranitidine in the 1st trimester has not been reported. Ranitidine crosses the placenta at term to produce a cord blood:maternal serum ratio of 0.9 (1). The drug has been used alone and with magnesium citrate to prevent gastric acid aspiration (Mendelson's syndrome) prior to vaginal delivery or cesarean section (1, 2). No effect was observed in the frequency and strength of uterine contractions, in fetal heart rate pattern, or in Apgar scores (1). Neonatal gastric acidity was not affected at 24 hours (1). No problems in the newborn attributable to ranitidine were reported in either study.

Breast Feeding Summary

Following a single oral dose of 150 mg in six subjects, ranitidine milk concentrations increased with time, producing mean milk:plasma ratios at 2, 4, and 6 hours of 1.9, 2.8, and 6.7, respectively (3). The effect of these concentrations on the nursing infant is not known. However, since ranitidine decreases gastric acidity, nursing should be avoided. Cimetidine, an agent with similar activity, is considered contraindicated during breast-feeding by the American Academy of Pediatrics (4).

References

1. McAuley DM, Moore J, Dundee JW, McCaughey W. Preliminary report on the use of ranitidine as an antacid in obstetrics. Ir J Med Sci 1982;151:91–2.
2. Gillett GB, Watson JD, Langford RM. Prophylaxis against acid aspiration syndrome in obstetric practice. Anesthesiology 1984;60:525.
3. Riley AJ, Crowley P, Harrison C. Transfer of ranitidine to biological fluids: milk and semen. In Misiewicz JJ, Wormsley KG, eds. *Proceedings of the 2nd International Symposium on Ranitidine*, Oxford: Medicine Publishing Foundation, 1981:78–81.
4. Committee on Drugs, American Academy of Pediatrics. The transfer of drugs and other chemicals into human breast milk. Pediatrics 1983;72:375–83.

Name: **RESERPINE**

Class: **Antihypertensive**   Risk Factor: **D**

Fetal Risk Summary

The Collaborative Perinatal Project monitored 50,282 mother-child pairs, 48 of which had 1st trimester exposure to reserpine (1). There were four defects with 1st trimester use. Although this incidence (8%) is greater than the expected frequency of occurrence, no major category or individual malformations were identified. For use anytime in pregnancy, 475 exposures were recorded (2). Malformations included:

Microcephaly (7 cases)
Hydronephrosis (3 cases)
Hydroureter (3 cases)
Inguinal hernia (12 cases)

Incidence of these latter malformations was not found to be statistically significant (3). Reserpine crosses the placenta. Use of reserpine near term has resulted in nasal discharge, retraction, lethargy, and anorexia in the newborn (4). Concern over the ability of reserpine to deplete catecholamine levels has appeared (5). The significance of this is not known.

Breast Feeding Summary

Reserpine is excreted into breast milk (6). No clinical reports of untoward effects in the nursing infant have been located. The American Academy of Pediatrics considers reserpine compatible with breast-feeding (7).

References

1. Heinonen OP, Slone D, Shapiro S. *Birth Defects and Drugs in Pregnancy*. Littleton:Publishing Sciences Group, 1977:376.
2. *Ibid*, 441.
3. *Ibid*, 495.
4. Budnick IS, Leikin S, Hoeck LE. Effect in the newborn infant to reserpine administration ante partum. Am J Dis Child 1955;90:286–9.
5. Towell ME, Hyman AI. Catecholamine depletion in pregnancy. J Obstet Gynaecol Br Commonw 1966;73:431–8.
6. Product information. Smith Kline & French Laboratories, 1980.
7. Committee on Drugs, American Academy of Pediatrics. The transfer of drugs and other chemicals into human breast milk. Pediatrics 1983;72:375–83.

Name: **RIBOFLAVIN**

Class: **Vitamin**   Risk Factor: **A***

Fetal Risk Summary

Riboflavin (vitamin B_2), a water-soluble B complex vitamin, acts as a coenzyme in humans and is essential for tissue respiration systems (1). The American RDA for riboflavin in pregnancy is 1.5–1.6 mg (2).

The vitamin is actively tansferred to the fetus, resulting in higher concentrations of riboflavin in the newborn than in the mother (3–11). The placenta converts flavin-adenine dinucleotide existing in the maternal serum to free riboflavin found in the fetal circulation (6, 7). This allows retention of the vitamin by the fetus since free riboflavin apparently cannot diffuse back to the mother (7). At term, mean riboflavin values in 174 mothers were 184 ng/ml (range 80–390) and in their newborns 318 ng/ml (range 136–665) (8).

The incidence of riboflavin deficiency in pregnancy is low (8, 12). In two studies, no correlation was discovered between the riboflavin status of the mother and the outcome of pregnancy even when riboflavin deficiency was present (13, 14). A 1977 study found no difference in riboflavin levels between infants of low and normal birth weight (11).

Riboflavin deficiency is teratogenic in animals (15). Although human teratogenicity has not been reported, low riboflavin levels were found in six mothers who had given birth to infants with neural tube defects (16). Other vitamin deficiencies present in these women were thought to be of more significance (see Folic Acid and Vitamin B$_{12}$).

Harpey and Charpentier (17) described a mother with multiple acylcoenzyme A dehydrogenase deficiency probably related to riboflavin metabolism. The mother had given birth to a healthy child followed by one stillbirth and six infants who had been breast-fed and died in early infancy after exhibiting a strong sweaty foot odor. In her 9th and 10th pregnancies, she was treated with 20 mg of riboflavin per day during the 3rd trimesters and delivered healthy infants. The authors thought the maternal symptoms were consistent with a mild form of acute fatty liver of pregnancy.

[* Risk Factor C if used in doses above the RDA.]

Breast Feeding Summary

Riboflavin (vitamin B$_2$) is excreted into human breast milk (18–22). Thomas and co-workers (18) gave well-nourished lactating women supplements of a multivitamin preparation containing 2.0 mg of riboflavin. At 6 months postpartum, milk concentrations of riboflavin did not differ significantly from those in control patients not receiving supplements. In a study of lactating women with low nutritional status, supplementation with riboflavin in doses of 0.10–10.0 mg/day resulted in mean milk concentrations of 200–740 ng/ml (19). Milk concentrations were directly proportional to dietary intake. A 1983 English study measured riboflavin levels in pooled human milk obtained from preterm (26 mothers: 29–34 weeks) and term (35 mothers: 39 weeks or longer) patients (20). Preterm milk rose from 276 ng/ml (colostrum) to 360 ng/ml (6–15 days) and then fell to 266 ng/ml (16–196 days). Over approximately the same time frame, term milk levels were 288, 279, and 310 ng/ml.

The American RDA for riboflavin during lactation is 1.7–1.8 mg (2). If the diet of the lactating woman adequately supplies this amount, supplementation with riboflavin is not needed (21). Maternal supplementation with the RDA for riboflavin is recommended for those women with inadequate nutritional intake.

References

1. American Hospital Formulary Service. *Drug Information 1985*. Bethesda:American Society of Hospital Pharmacists, 1985:1690–2.
2. *Recommended Dietary Allowances*, ed 9. Washington, DC:National Academy of Sciences, 1980.
3. Hill EP, Longo LD. Dynamics of maternal-fetal nutrient transfer. Fed Proc 1980;39:239–44.
4. Lust JE, Hagerman DD, Villee CA. The transport of riboflavin by human placenta. J Clin Invest 1954;33:38–40.
5. Frank O, Walbroehl G, Thomason A, Kaminetzky H, Kubes Z, Baker H. Placental transfer: fetal retention of some vitamins. Am J Clin Nutr 1970;23:662–3.
6. Kaminetzky HA, Baker H, Frank O, Langer A. The effects of intravenously administered water-soluble vitamins during labor in normovitaminemic and hypovitaminemic gravidas on maternal and neonatal blood vitamin levels at delivery. Am J Obstet Gynecol 1974;120:697–703.

7. Kaminetzky HA, Baker H. Micronutrients in pregnancy. Clin Obstet Gynecol 1977;20:363–80.
8. Baker H, Frank O, Thomason AD, Langer A, Munves ED, De Angelis B, Kaminetzky HA. Vitamin profile of 174 mothers and newborns at parturition. Am J Clin Nutr 1975;28:59–65.
9. Baker H, Frank O, Deangelis B, Feingold S, Kaminetzky HA. Role of placenta in maternal-fetal vitamin transfer in humans. Am J Obstet Gynecol 1981;141:792–6.
10. Bamji MS. Enzymic evaluation of thiamin, riboflavin and pyridoxine status of parturient women and their newborn infants. Br J Nutr 1976;35:259–65.
11. Baker H, Thind IS, Frank O, DeAngelis B, Caterini H, Lquria DB. Vitamin levels in low-birth-weight newborn infants and their mothers. Am J Obstet Gynecol 1977;129:521–4.
12. Dostalova L. Correlation of the vitamin status between mother and newborn during delivery. Dev Pharmacol Ther 1982;4(Suppl 1):45–57.
13. Vir SC, Love AHG, Thompson W. Riboflavin status during pregnancy. Am J Clin Nutr 1981;34:2699–2705.
14. Heller S, Salkeld RM, Korner WF. Riboflavin status in pregnancy. Am J Clin Nutr 1974;27:1225–30.
15. Shepard TH. *Catalog of Teratogenic Agents*, ed 3. Baltimore:The Johns Hopkins University Press, 1980:288–9.
16. Smithells RW, Sheppard S, Schorah CJ. Vitamin deficiencies and neural tube defects. Arch Dis Child 1976;51:944–50.
17. Harpey JP, Charpentier C. Acute fatty liver of pregnancy. Lancet 1983;1:586–7.
18. Thomas MR, Sneed SM, Wei C, Nail PA, Wilson M, Sprinkle EE III. The effects of vitamin C, vitamin B$_6$, vitamin B$_{12}$, folic acid, riboflavin, and thiamin on the breast milk and maternal status of well-nourished women at 6 months postpartum. Am J Clin Nutr 1980;33:2151–6.
19. Deodhar AD, Rajalakshmi R, Ramakrishnan CV. Studies on human lactation. Part III. Effect of dietary vitamin supplementation on vitamin contents of breast milk. Acta Paediatr Scand 1964;53:42–8.
20. Ford, JE, Zechalko A, Murphy J, Brooke OG. Comparison of the B vitamin composition of milk from mothers of preterm and term babies. Arch Dis Child 1983;58:367–72.
21. Nail PA, Thomas MR, Eakin R. The effect of thiamin and riboflavin supplementation on the level of those vitamins in human breast milk and urine. Am J Clin Nutr 1980;33:198–204.
22. Gunther M. Diet and milk secretion in women. Proc Nutr Soc 1968;27:77–82.

Name: **RIFAMPIN**

Class: **Antituberculosis Agent**   Risk Factor: **C**

Fetal Risk Summary

No controlled studies have linked the use of rifampin with congenital defects (1, 2). One report described 9 malformations in 204 pregnancies that went to term (3). This incidence, 4.4%, is similar to the expected frequency of defects in a healthy nonexposed population but higher than the 1.8% rate noted in other tuberculosis patients (3):

> Anencephaly (1 case)
> Hydrocephalus (2 cases)
> Limb malformations (4 cases)
> Renal tract defects (1 case)
> Congenital hip dislocation (1 case)

In a 1980 review, Snider and co-workers (4) evaluated the available treatment for tuberculosis during pregnancy. They concluded that rifampin was not a proven teratogen and recommended use of the drug with isoniazid and ethambutol if necessary.

Rifampin has been implicated as one of the agents responsible for hemorrhagic disease of the newborn (5). In one of the three infants affected, only laboratory evidence of hemorrhagic disease of newborn was present, but in the other two, clinically evident bleeding was observed. Prophylactic vitamin K_1 is recommended to prevent this serious complication (see Phytonadione).

Rifampin may interfere with oral contraceptives, resulting in unplanned pregnancies (see Oral Contraceptives) (6).

Breast Feeding Summary

Rifampin is excreted into breast milk in concentrations of 1–3 μg/ml (7). No reports describing adverse effects in nursing infants have been located. The American Academy of Pediatrics considers rifampin compatible with breast-feeding (8).

References

1. Reimers D. Missbildungen durch Rifampicin. Bericht ueber 2 faelle von normaler fetaler entwicklung nach rifampicin-therapie in der fruehsch wangerschaft. Muench Med Wochenschr 1971;113:1690.
2. Warkany J. Antituberculous drugs. Teratology 1979;20:133–8.
3. Steen JSM, Stainton-Ellis DM. Rifampicin in pregnancy. Lancet 1977;2:604–5.
4. Snider DE, Layde PM, Johnson MW, Lyle MA. Treatment of tuberculosis during pregnancy. Am Rev Respir Dis 1980;122:65–79.
5. Eggermont E, Logghe N, Van De Casseye W, Casteels-Van Daele M, Jaeken J, Cosemans J, Verstraete M, Renaer M. Haemorrhagic disease of the newborn in the offspring of rifampicin and isoniazid treated mothers. Acta Paediatr Belg 1976;29:87–90.
6. Gupta KC, Ali MY. Failure of oral contraceptives with rifampicin. Med J Zambia 1980;15:23.
7. Vorherr H. Drug excretion in breast milk. Postgrad Med J 1974;56:97–104.
8. Committee on Drugs, American Academy of Pediatrics. The transfer of drugs and other chemicals into human breast milk. Pediatrics 1983;72:375–83.

Name: **RITODRINE**

Class: **Sympathomimetic (Adrenergic)**   Risk Factor: **B*$_M$**

Fetal Risk Summary

Ritodrine is a β-sympathomimetic used to prevent premature labor. Its effects on the mother, fetus, and newborn have been reviewed in several publications (1–3). Ritodrine crosses the placenta, appearing in cord blood in amounts ranging from 20 to 100% of the maternal level (4). Although no congenital malformations have been observed, use of ritodrine prior to the 20th week of gestation has not been reported. The manufacturer considers ritodrine to be contraindicated before this time (5). Ritodrine increases fetal and maternal heart rates (6). Fetal rates up to 200 beats/min have been recorded (1–3, 5). Use of ritodrine may result in transient maternal and fetal hyperglycemia followed by increases in levels of serum insulin. If delivery occurs before these effects have terminated (usually 48–72 hours), low neonatal blood glucose levels may be observed (6). Ketoacidosis with fetal death has been reported (7). An insulin-dependent diabetic was treated with ritodrine for preterm labor at 28 weeks of gestation. Fetal heart patterns were normal prior to therapy. Maternal hyperglycemia with ketoacidosis developed, and 6 hours later fetal heart activity was undetectable. She was subsequently delivered of a stillborn fetus weighing 970 g. Ritodrine decreases the incidence of neonatal death and respiratory distress syndrome (8–10). Two-year follow-up studies of infants exposed to ritodrine *in utero* have failed to detect harmful effects on growth, incidence of disease, or development or functional maturation (5, 11).

[* Contraindicated before 20th week of gestation according to manufacturer—Astra, 1985.]

Breast Feeding Summary

No data available.

References

1. Barden TP, Peter JB, Merkatz IR. Ritodrine hydrochloride: a betamimetic agent for use in preterm labor. I. Pharmacology, clinical history, administration, side effects, and safety. Obstet Gynecol 1980;56:1–6.
2. Anonymous. Ritodrine for inhibition of preterm labor. Med Lett Drugs Ther 1980;22:89–90.
3. Finkelstein BW. Ritodrine (Yutopar, Merrell Dow Pharmaceuticals Inc.). Drug Intell Clin Pharm 1981;15:425–33.
4. Gandar R, De Zoeten LW, van der Schoot JB. Serum levels of ritodrine in man. Eur J Clin Pharmacol 1980;17:117–22.
5. Product information and clinical summary of Yutopar, Merrell-National Laboratories, Inc., Cincinnati, 1980.
6. Leake RD, Hobel CJ, Oh W, Thiebeault DW, Okada DM, Williams PR. A controlled, prospective study of the effects of ritodrine hydrochloride for premature labor. Clin Res 1980;28:90A (abstr).
7. Schilthius MS, Aarnoudse JG. Fetal death associated with severe ritodrine induced ketoacidosis. Lancet 1980;1:1145.
8. Boog G, Ben Brahim M, Gandar R. Beta-mimetic drugs and possible prevention of respiratory distress syndrome. Br J Obstet Gynaecol 1975;82:285–8.
9. Merkatz IR, Peter JB, Barden TP. Ritodrine hydrochloride: a betamimetic agent for use in preterm labor. II. Evidence of efficacy. Obstet Gynecol 1980;56:7–12.
10. Laursen NH, Merkatz IR, Tejani N, et al. Inhibition of premature labor: a multicenter comparison of ritodrine and ethanol. Am J Obstet Gynecol 1977;127:837–45.
11. Freysz H, Willard D, Lehr A, Messer J, Boog G. A long term evaluation of infants who received a beta-mimetic drug while in utero. J Perinat Med 1977;5:94–9.

S

Name: **SCOPOLAMINE**

Class: **Parasympatholytic (Anticholinergic)**   Risk Factor: **C**

Fetal Risk Summary

Scopolamine is an anticholinergic agent. The Collaborative Perinatal Project monitored 50,282 mother-child pairs, 309 of which used scopolamine in the 1st trimester (1). For anytime use, 881 exposures were recorded (2). In neither case was evidence found for an association with malformations. However, when the group of parasympatholytics were taken as a whole (2,323 exposures), a possible association with minor malformations was found (1). Scopolamine readily crosses the placenta (3). When administered to the mother at term, fetal effects include tachycardia, decreased heart rate variability, and decreased heart rate deceleration (4–6). Maternal tachycardia is comparable to that with other anticholinergic agents, such as atropine or glycopyrrolate (7). Scopolamine toxicity in a newborn has been described (8). The mother had received six doses of scopolamine (1.8 mg total) with several other drugs during labor. Symptoms in the female infant consisted of fever, tachycardia, and lethargy; she was also "barrel chested" without respiratory depression. Therapy with physostigmine reversed the condition.

Breast Feeding Summary

See Atropine.

References

1. Heinonen OP, Slone D, Shapiro S. *Birth Defects and Drugs in Pregnancy*. Littleton:Publishing Sciences Group, 1977:346–53.
2. *Ibid*, 439.
3. Moya F, Thorndike V. The effects of drugs used in labor on the fetus and newborn. Clin Pharmacol Ther 1963;4:628–53.
4. Shenker L. Clinical experiences with fetal heart rate monitoring of one thousand patients in labor. Am J Obstet Gynecol 1973;115:1111–6.
5. Boehm FH, Growdon JH Jr. The effect of scopolamine on fetal heart rate baseline variability. Am J Obstet Gynecol 1974;120:1099–1104.
6. Ayromlooi J, Tobias M, Berg P. The effects of scopolamine and ancillary analgesics upon the fetal heart rate recording. J Reprod Med 1980;25:323–6.
7. Diaz DM, Diaz SF, Marx GF. Cardiovascular effects of glycopyrrolate and belladonna derivatives in obstetric patients. Bull NY Acad Med 1980;56:245–8.
8. Evens RP, Leopold JC. Scopolamine toxicity in a newborn. Pediatrics 1980;329–30.

Name: **SECOBARBITAL**

Class: **Sedative/Hypnotic**   Risk Factor: **D$_M$**

Fetal Risk Summary

No reports linking the use of secobarbital with congenital defects have been located. The Collaborative Perinatal Project monitored 50,282 mother-child pairs, 378 of which had 1st trimester exposure to secobarbital (1). No evidence was found to suggest a relationship to large categories of major or minor malformations or to individual defects. Hemorrhagic disease of the newborn and barbiturate withdrawal are theoretical possibilities (see also Phenobarbital).

An *in vitro* study found no evidence of chromosome changes on exposure to secobarbital (3).

Breast Feeding Summary

Secobarbital is excreted into breast milk (2). The amount and effects on the nursing infant are not known. The American Academy of Pediatrics considers secobarbital compatible with breast-feeding (4).

References

1. Heinonen OP, Slone D, Shapiro S. *Birth Defects and Drugs in Pregnancy*. Littleton:Publishing Sciences Group, 1977:336–7.
2. Wilson JT, Brown RD, Cherek DR, Dailey JW, Hilman B, Jobe PC, Manno BR, Manno JE, Redetzki HM, Stewart JJ. Drug excretion in human breast milk: principles, pharmacokinetics and projected consequences. Clin Pharmacokinet 1980;5:1–66.
3. Stenchever MA, Jarvis JA. Effect of barbiturates on the chromosomes of human cells in vitro—a negative report. J Reprod Med 1970;5:69–71.
4. Committee on Drugs, American Academy of Pediatrics. The transfer of drugs and other chemicals into human breast milk. Pediatrics 1983;72:375–83.

Name: **SIMETHICONE**

Class: **Antiflatulent/Defoaming Agent**   Risk Factor: **C**

Fetal Risk Summary

Simethicone is a silicone product that is used as an antiflatulent. No reports linking the use of this agent with congenital defects have been located.

Breast Feeding Summary

No data available.

Name: SODIUM IODIDE

Class: **Expectorant**   Risk Factor: **D**

Fetal Risk Summary

See Potassium Iodide.

Breast Feeding Summary

See Potassium Iodide.

Name: SODIUM IODIDE I125

Class: **Radiopharmaceutical**   Risk Factor: **X**

Fetal Risk Summary

See Sodium Iodide I131

Breast Feeding Summary

See Sodium Iodide I131

Name: SODIUM IODIDE I131

Class: **Radiopharmaceutical**   Risk Factor: **X**

Fetal Risk Summary

Sodium iodide I131 (^{131}I) is a radiopharmaceutical agent used for diagnostic procedures and for therapeutic destruction of thyroid tissue. The diagnostic dose is approximately one-thousandth of the therapeutic dose. Like all iodides, the drug concentrates in the thyroid gland. ^{131}I readily crosses the placenta. The fetal thyroid is able to accumulate ^{131}I by about the 12th week of gestation (1–3). At term, the maternal serum:cord blood ratio is 1 (4).

As suggested by the above studies on uptake of ^{131}I in fetal thyroids, maternal treatment with radioiodine early in the 1st trimester should not pose a significant danger to the fetus. Two reports describing ^{131}I therapy at 4 and 8 weeks gestation resulting in normal infants seemingly confirmed the lack of risk (5, 6). However, Valensi and Nahum (7) described a newborn with a large head, exophthalmia, and thick, myxedematous-like skin who was exposed to ^{131}I at about 2 weeks gestation. The infant died shortly after birth. In another early report, Falk (8) attributed exposure to a diagnostic dose of ^{131}I during the middle of the 1st trimester to anomalies in the newborn, including microcephaly, hydrocephaly, dysplasia of the hip joints, and clubfoot. Finally, ^{131}I administered 1–3 days prior to conception was suggested as the cause of a spontaneous abortion at the end of the 1st trimester (9). All three of these latter reports must be viewed with caution due to the uniqueness of the effects and/or the timing of the exposure. Factors other than radioiodine may have been involved.

Therapeutic doses of radioiodine administered near the end of the 1st trimester (12 weeks) or beyond usually result in partial or complete abolition of the fetal thyroid gland (10–20). This effect is dose-dependent, as Hodges and co-workers (2) treated one mother at 19 weeks gestation with 6.1 mCi of ^{131}I apparently without causing fetal harm. In the pregnancies terminating with a hypothyroid infant, ^{131}I doses ranged from 10–225 mCi (10–20). Clinical features observed at or shortly after birth in 10 of the 12 newborns were consistent with congenital hypothyroidism. One of these infants was also discovered to have hypoparathyroidism (20). In one child, exposed *in utero* to repeated small doses over a 5-week period (total dose 12.2 mCi), hypothyroidism did not become evident until 4 years of age (17). Unusual anomalies observed in another infant included hydrocephaly, cardiopathy, genital hypotrophy, and a limb deformity (15).

In summary, sodium iodide I131 is a proven human teratogen. Because the effects of even small doses are not predictable, the use of the drug for diagnostic and therapeutic purposes should be avoided during pregnancy.

Breast Feeding Summary

Sodium iodide I131 is concentrated in breast milk (21–24). [125]I also appears in milk in significant quantities (25, 26). Uptake of ^{131}I contained in milk by an infant's thyroid gland has been observed (21). The time required for elimination of radioiodine from the milk may be as long as 14 days. Since this exposure may result in damage to the nursing infant's thyroid, including an increased risk of thyroid cancer, breast-feeding should be stopped until radioactivity is no longer present in the milk (27).

References

1. Chapman EM, Corner GW Jr, Robinson D, Evans RD. The collection of radioactive iodine by the human fetal thyroid. J Clin Endocrinol Metab 1948;8:717–20.
2. Hodges RE, Evans TC, Bradbury JT, Keettel WC. The accumulation of radioactive iodine by human fetal thyroids. J Clin Endocrinol Metab 1955;15:661–7.
3. Shepard TH. Onset of function in the human fetal thyroid: biochemical and radioautographic studies from organ culture. J Clin Endocrinol Metab 1967;27:945–58.
4. Kearns JE, Hutson W. Tagged isomers and analogues of thyroxine (their transmission across the human placenta and other studies). J Nucl Med 1963;4:453–61.
5. Hollingsworth DR, Austin E. Observations following I[131] for Graves disease during first trimester of pregnancy. South Med J 1969;62:1555–6.
6. Talbert LM, Thomas CG Jr, Holt WA, Rankin P. Hyperthyroidism during pregnancy. Obstet Gynecol 1970;36:779–85.
7. Valensi G, Nahum A. Action de l'iode radio-actif sur le foetus humain. Tunisie Med 1958;36:69. As cited in Nishimura H, Tanimura T. *Clinical Aspects of the Teratogenicity of Drugs*. New York:American Elsevier, 1976:260.
8. Falk W. Beitrag zur Frage der menschlichen Fruchtschadigung durch kunstliche radioaktive Isotope. Medizinische 1959;22:1480. As cited in Nishimura H, Tanimura T. *Clinical Aspects of the Teratogenicity of Drugs*. New York:American Elsevier, 1976:260.
9. Berger M, Briere J. Les dangers de la therapeutique par l'iode radioactif au debut d'une grossesse ignoree. Bull Med Leg Toxicol Med 1967;10:37. As cited in Nishimura H, Tanimura T. *Clinical Aspects of the Teratogenicity of Drugs*. New York:American Elsevier, 1976:260.
10. Russell KP, Rose H, Starr P. The effects of radioactive iodine on maternal and fetal thyroid function during pregnancy. Surg Gynecol Obstet 1957;104:560–4.
11. Ray EW, Sterling K, Gardner LI. Congenital cretinism associated with I[131] therapy of the mother. Am J Dis Child 1959;98:506–7.

12. Hamill GC, Jarman JA, Wynne MD. Fetal effects of radioactive iodine therapy in a pregnant woman with thyroid cancer. Am J Obstet Gynecol 1961;81:1018–23.

13. Fisher WD, Voorhess ML, Gardner LI. Congenital hypothyroidism in infant following maternal I[131] therapy. J Pediatr 1963;62:132–46.

14. Pfannenstiel P, Andrews GA, Brown DW. Congenital hypothyroidism from intrauterine ^{131}I damage. In: Cassalino C, Andreoli M, eds. *Current Topics in Thyroid Research*. New York:Academic Press, 1965:749. As cited in Nishimura H, Tanimura T. *Clinical Aspects of the Teratogenicity of Drugs*. New York:American Elsevier, 1976:260.

15. Sirbu P, Macarie E, Isaia V, Zugravesco A. L'influence de l'iode radio-actif sur le foetus. Bull Fed Soc Gynecol Obstet Lang Fr 1968;20:Suppl 314. As cited in Nishimura H, Tanimura T. *Clinical Aspects of the Teratogenicity of Drugs*. New York:American Elsevier, 1976:260.

16. Hollingsworth DR, Austin E. Thyroxine derivatives in amniotic fluid. J Pediatr 1971;79:923–9.

17. Green HG, Gareis FJ, Shepard TH, Kelley VC. Cretinism associated with maternal sodium iodide I 131 therapy during pregnancy. Am J Dis Child 1971;122:247–9.

18. Jafek BW, Small R, Lillian DL. Congenital radioactive iodine-induced stridor and hypothyroidism. Arch Otolaryngol 1974;99:369–71.

19. Exss R, Graewe B. Congenital athyroidism in the newborn infant from intra-uterine radioiodine action. Biol Neonate 1974;24:289–91.

20. Richards GE, Brewer ED, Conley SB, Saldana LR. Combined hypothyroidism and hypoparathyroidism in an infant after maternal ^{131}I administration. J Pediatr 1981;99:141–43.

21. Nurnberger CE, Lipscomb A. Transmission of radioiodine (I[131]) to infants through human maternal milk. JAMA 1952;150:1398–1400.

22. Miller H, Weetch RS. The excretion of radioactive iodine in human milk. Lancet 1955;2:1013.

23. Weaver JC, Kamm ML, Dobson RL. Excretion of radioiodine in human milk. JAMA 1960;173:872–5.

24. Karjalainen P, Penttila IM, Pystynen P. The amount and form of radioactivity in human milk after lung scanning, renography and placental localization by ^{131}I labelled tracers. Acta Obstet Gynecol Scand 1971;50:357–61.

25. Bland EP, Crawford JS, Docker MF, Farr RF. Radioactive iodine uptake by thyroid of breast-fed infants after maternal blood-volume measurements. Lancet 1969;2:1039–41.

26. Palmer KE. Excretion of ^{125}I in breast milk following administration of labelled fibinogen. Br J Radiol 1979;52:672–3.

27. Committee on Drugs, American Academy of Pediatrics. The transfer of drugs and other chemicals into human breast milk. Pediatrics 1983;72:375–83.

Name: **SODIUM NITROPRUSSIDE**

Class: **Antihypertensive**   Risk Factor: **C**

Fetal Risk Summary

No reports linking the use of sodium nitroprusside with congenital defects have been located. Nitroprusside has been used in pregnancy to produce deliberate hypotension during aneurysm surgery or to treat severe hypertension (1–7). Transient fetal bradycardia was the only adverse effect noted (1).

Sodium nitroprusside crosses the placenta and produces fetal cyanide concentrations higher than maternal levels in animals (8). This effect has not been studied in humans. A 1984 article reviewed the potential fetal toxicity of sodium nitroprusside (6). Avoidance of prolonged use and the monitoring of serum pH, plasma cyanide, red blood cell cyanide, and methemoglobin levels in the mother were recommended. Standard doses of sodium nitroprusside apparently do not pose a major risk of excessive cyanide accumulation in the fetal liver (6).

Breast Feeding Summary

No data available.

References

1. Donchin Y, Amirav B, Sahar A, Yarkoni S. Sodium nitroprusside for aneurysm surgery in pregnancy. Br J Anaesth 1978;50:849–51.
2. Paull J. Clinical report of the use of sodium nitroprusside in severe pre-eclampsia. Anaesth Intensive Care 1975;3:72.
3. Rigg D, McDonogh A. Use of sodium nitroprusside for deliberate hypotension during pregnancy. Br J Anaesth 1981;53:985–7.
4. Willoughby JS. Case reports: sodium nitroprusside, pregnancy and multiple intracranial aneurysms. Anaesth Intensive Care 1984;12:358–60.
5. Stempel JE, O'Grady JP, Morton MJ, Johnson KA. Use of sodium nitroprusside in complications of gestational hypertension. Obstet Gynecol 1982;60:533–8.
6. Shoemaker CT, Meyers M. Sodium nitroprusside for control of severe hypertensive disease of pregnancy: a case report and discussion of potential toxicity. Am J Obstet Gynecol 1984;149:171–3.
7. Willoughby JS. Review article: Sodium nitroprusside, pregnancy and multiple intracranial aneurysms. Anaesth Intens Care 1984;12:351–7.
8. Lewis PE, Cefalo RC. Naulty JS, Rodkey RL. Placental transfer and fetal toxicity of sodium nitroprusside. Gynecol Invest 1977;8:46.

Name: **SOMATOSTATIN**

Class: **Pituitary Hormone**   Risk Factor: **B**

Fetal Risk Summary

No data available.

Breast Feeding Summary

No data available.

Name: **SPECTINOMYCIN**

Class: **Antibiotic**   Risk Factor: **B**

Fetal Risk Summary

No reports linking the use of spectinomycin with congenital defects have been located. The drug has been used to treat gonorrhea in pregnant patients allergic to penicillin. Available data do not suggest a threat to mother or fetus (1, 2).

Breast Feeding Summary

No data available.

References

1. McCormack WM, Finland M. Spectinomycin. Ann Intern Med 1976;84:712–6.
2. Anonymous. Treatment of syphilis and gonorrhea. Med Lett Drugs Ther 1977;19:105–7.

Name: **SPIRONOLACTONE**

Class: **Diuretic**   Risk Factor: **D**

Fetal Risk Summary

Spironolactone is a potassium-conserving diuretic. No reports linking it with congenital defects have been located. Messina and co-workers (1) have commented, however, that spironolactone may be contraindicated during pregnancy, based on the known antiandrogenic effects in humans and the feminization observed in male rat fetuses. Other investigators consider diuretics in general contraindicated in pregnancy, except for patients with cardiovascular disorders, since they do not prevent or alter the course of toxemia, and they may decrease placental perfusion (2–4).

Breast Feeding Summary

It is not known if unmetabolized spironolactone is excreted in breast milk. Canrenone, the principal metabolite, was found, with milk:plasma ratios of 0.72 (2 hours) and 0.51 (14.5 hours) (5). These amounts would provide an estimated maximum of 0.2% of the mother's daily dose to the infant (5). The effects on the infant from this ingestion are unknown. The American Academy of Pediatrics considers spironolactone compatible with breast-feeding (6).

References

1. Messina M, Biffignandi P, Ghiga E, Jeantet MG, Molinatti GM. Possible contraindication of spironolactone during pregnancy. J Endocrinol Invest 1979;2:222.
2. Pitkin RM, Kaminetzky HA, Newton M, Pritchard JA. Maternal nutrition: a selective review of clinical topics. Obstet Gynecol 1972;40:773–85.
3. Lindheimer MD, Katz AI. Sodium and diuretics in pregnancy. N Engl J Med 1973;288:891–4.
4. Christianson R, Page EW. Diuretic drugs and pregnancy. Obstet Gynecol 1976;48:647–52.
5. Phelps DL, Karim A. Spironolactone: relationship between concentrations of dethioacetylated metabolite in human serum and milk. J Pharm Sci 1977;66:1203.
6. Committee on Drugs, American Academy of Pediatrics. The transfer of drugs and other chemicals into human breast milk. Pediatrics 1983;72:375–83.

Name: **STREPTOKINASE**

Class: **Thrombolytic**   Risk Factor: **C**

Fetal Risk Summary

No reports linking the use of streptokinase with congenital defects have been located. Only minimal amounts cross the placenta, and these are not sufficient to cause fibrinolytic effects in the fetus (1–7). Although the passage of streptokinase is blocked by the placenta, streptokinase antibodies do cross to the fetus (5). This passive sensitization would have clinical importance only if the neonate required streptokinase therapy. Ludwig (5) has treated 24 patients in the 2nd and 3rd trimesters without fetal complications. Use in the 1st trimester for maternal thrombophlebitis has also been reported (6). No adverse effects were observed in the infant born at term.

Breast Feeding Summary

No data available.

References

1. Pfeifer GW. Distribution and placental transfer of 131-I streptokinase. Aust Ann Med 1970;19(Suppl):17–8.
2. Hall RJC, Young C, Sutton GC, Campbell S. Treatment of acute massive pulmonary embolism by streptokinase during labour and delivery. Br Med J 1972;4:647–9.
3. McTaggart DR, Ingram TG. Massive pulmonary embolism during pregnancy treated with strepto-kinase. Med J Aust 1977;1:18–20.
4. Benz JJ, Wick A. The problem of fibrinolytic therapy in pregnancy. Schweiz Med Wochenschr 1973;103:1359–63.
5. Ludwig H. Results of streptokinase therapy in deep venous thrombosis during pregnancy. Postgrad Med J 1973;49(Suppl 5):65–7.
6. Walter C, Koestering H. Therapeutische thrombolyse in der neunten schwangerschalftswoche. Dtsch Med Wochenschr 1969;94:32–4.
7. Witchitz S, Veyrat C, Moisson P, Scheinman N, Rozenstajn L. Fibrinolytic treatment of thrombus on prosthetic heart valves. Br Heart J 1980;44:545–54.

Name: **STREPTOMYCIN**

Class: **Antibiotic**   Risk Factor: **D**

Fetal Risk Summary

Streptomycin is an aminoglycoside antibiotic. The drug rapidly crosses the placenta into the fetal circulation and amniotic fluid, obtaining concentrations usually less than 50% of the maternal serum level (1, 2). Early investigators, well aware of streptomycin-induced ototoxicity, were unable to observe this defect in infants exposed *in utero* to the agent (3–5). Eventually, ototoxicity was described in a 2½-month-old infant whose mother had been treated for tuberculosis with 30 g of streptomycin during the last month of pregnancy (6). The infant was deaf with a negative cochleopalpebral reflex. Several other case reports and small surveys describing similar toxicity followed this initial report (7, 8). In general, however, the incidence of congenital ototoxicity, cochlear or vestibular, from streptomycin is low, especially with careful dosage calculations and if the duration of fetal exposure is limited (9).

Except for eighth cranial nerve damage, no reports of congenital defects due to streptomycin have been located. The Collaborative Perinatal Project monitored 50,282 mother-child pairs, 135 of which had 1st trimester exposure to streptomycin (10). For use anytime during pregnancy, 355 exposures were recorded (11). In neither case was evidence found to suggest a relationship to large categories of major or minor malformations or to individual defects.

In a group of 1,619 newborns whose mothers were treated for tuberculosis during pregnancy with multiple drugs, including streptomycin, the incidence of congenital defects was the same as a healthy control group (2.34% vs 2.56%) (12). Other investigators had previously concluded that the use of streptomycin in pregnant tuberculosis patients was not teratogenic (13).

Breast Feeding Summary

Streptomycin is excreted into breast milk. Milk:plasma ratios of 0.5–1.0 have been reported (14). Since the oral absorption of this antibiotic is poor, ototoxicity in the infant would not be expected. However, three potential problems exist for the nursing infant: modification of bowel flora, direct effects on the infant, and interference with the interpretation of culture results if a fever work-up is required.

References

1. Woltz J, Wiley M. Transmission of streptomycin from maternal blood to the fetal circulation and the amniotic fluid. Proc Soc Exp Biol Med 1945;60:106–7.
2. Heilman D, Heilman F, Hinshaw H, Nichols D, Herrell W. Streptomycin: absorption, diffusion, excretion and toxicity. Am J Med Sci 1945;210:576–84.
3. Watson E, Stow R. Streptomycin therapy: effects on fetus. JAMA 1948;137:1599–1600.
4. Rubin A, Winston J, Rutledge M. Effects of streptomycin upon the human fetus. Am J Dis Child 1951;82:14–6.
5. Kistner R. The use of streptomycin during pregnancy. Am J Obstet Gynecol 1950;60:422–6.
6. Lerox M. Existe-t-il une surdite congenitale acquise due a la streptomycine? Am Otolaryngol 1950;67:194–6.
7. Nishimura H, Tanimura T. *Clinical Aspects of the Teratogenicity of Drugs*. Amsterdam:Excerpta Medica, 1976:130.
8. Donald PR, Sellars SL. Streptomycin ototoxicity in the unborn child. S Afr Med J 1981;60:316–8.
9. Mann J, Moskowitz R. Plaque and pregnancy. A case report. JAMA 1977;237:1854–5.
10. Heinonen OP, Slone D, Shapiro S. *Birth Defects and Drugs in Pregnancy*. Littleton:Publishing Sciences Group, 1977:297–301.
11. *Ibid*, 435.
12. Marynowski A, Sianozecka E. Comparison of the incidence of congenital malformations in neonates from healthy mothers and from patients treated because of tuberculosis. Ginekol Pol 1972;43:713–5.
13. Lowe C. Congenital defects among children born under supervision or treatment for pulmonary tuberculosis. Br J Prev Soc Med 1964;18:14–6.
14. Wilson JT. Milk/plasma ratios and contraindicated drugs. In Wilson JT, ed. *Drugs in Breast Milk*. Balgowlah, Australia:ADIS Press, 1981:79.

Name: **SULFASALAZINE**

Class: **Anti-infective**   Risk Factor: **B***

Fetal Risk Summary

Sulfasalazine is a compound composed of 5-aminosalicylic acid joined to sulfapyridine by an azo linkage (refer to Sulfonamides for a complete review of this class of agents). Sulfasalazine is used for the treatment of ulcerative colitis and Crohn's disease. No increase in congenital defects or newborn toxicity has been observed from its use in pregnancy (1–10). However, two reports, involving four infants (two stillborn), have described congenital malformations after exposure to this drug (11, 12). It cannot be determined if the observed defects were related to the therapy, to the disease, or to a combination of these or other factors:

Bilateral cleft lip/palate, severe hydrocephalus, death (11)
Coarctation of aorta, ventricular septal defect (12)
Potter-type IIa polycystic kidney, rudimentary left uterine cornu, stillborn (1st twin) (12)

Potter's facies, hypoplastic lungs, absent kidneys and ureters, talipes equino-varus, stillborn (2nd twin) (12)

Sulfasalazine and its metabolite, sulfapyridine, readily cross the placenta to the fetal circulation (5, 6). Fetal concentrations are approximately the same as maternal concentrations. Placental transfer of 5-aminosalicylic acid is limited since only negligible amounts are absorbed from the cecum and colon, and these are rapidly excreted in the urine (13).

At birth, concentrations of sulfasalazine and sulfapyridine in 11 infants were 4.6 and 18.2 μg/ml, respectively (6). Neither of these levels was sufficient to cause significant displacement of bilirubin from albumin (6). Kernicterus and severe neonatal jaundice have not been reported following maternal use of sulfasalazine, even when the drug was given up to the time of delivery (6, 7). Caution is advised, however, since other sulfonamides have caused jaundice in the newborn when given near term (see Sulfonamides).

Sulfasalazine may adversely affect spermatogenesis in male patients with inflammatory bowel disease (14, 15). Sperm counts and motility are both reduced and require 2 months or longer after the drug is stopped to return to normal levels (14).

[* Risk Factor D if administered near term.]

Breast Feeding Summary

Sulfapyridine is excreted into breast milk (see also Sulfonamides) (5, 13). Milk concentrations are approximately 50–60% of maternal serum levels. One infant's urine contained 3–4 μg/ml of the drug (1.2–1.6 mg/24 hr), representing about 30–40% of the total dose excreted in the milk. Unmetabolized sulfasalazine has been detected in only one study (milk:plasma ratio of 0.3) (5). Levels of 5-aminosalicylic acid were undetectable. No adverse effects were observed in the four infants exposed to the drug in milk (5, 13). The American Academy of Pediatrics considers sulfapyridine compatible with breast-feeding (16).

References

1. McEwan HP. Anorectal conditions in obstetric practice. Proc R Soc Med 1972;65:279–81.
2. Willoughby CP, Truelove SC. Ulcerative colitis and pregnancy. Gut 1980;21:469–74.
3. Levy N, Roisman I, Teodor I. Ulcerative colitis in pregnancy in Israel. Dis Colon Rectum 1981;24:351–4.
4. Mogadam M, Dobbins WO III, Korelitz BI, Ahmed SW. Pregnancy in inflammatory bowel disease: effect of sulfasalazine and corticosteroids on fetal outcome. Gastroenterology 1981;80:72–6.
5. Azad Khan AK, Truelove SC. Placental and mammary transfer of sulphasalazine. Br Med J 1979;2:1553.
6. Jarnerot G, Into-Malmberg MB, Esbjorner E. Placental transfer of sulphasalazine and sulphapyridine and some of its metabolites. Scand J Gastroenterol 1981;16:693–7.
7. Modadam M. Sulfasalazine, IBD, and pregnancy: reply. Gastroenterology 1981;81:194.
8. Fielding JF. Pregnancy and inflammatory bowel disease. J Clin Gastroenterol 1983;5:107–8.
9. Sorokin JJ, Levine SM. Pregnancy and inflammatory bowel disease: a review of the literature. Obstet Gynecol 1983;62:247–52.
10. Baiocco PJ, Korelitz BI. The influence of inflammatory bowel disease and its treatment on pregnancy and fetal outcome. J Clin Gastroenterol 1984;6:211–6.
11. Craxi A, Pagliarello F. Possible embryotoxicity of sulfasalazine. Arch Intern Med 1980;140:1674.
12. Newman NM, Correy JF. Possible teratogenicity of sulphasalazine. Med J Aust 1983;1:528–9.
13. Berlin CM Jr, Yaffe SJ. Disposition of salicylazosulfapyridine (Azulfidine) and metabolites in human breast milk. Dev Pharmacol Ther 1980;1:31–9.
14. Toovey S, Hudson E, Hendry WF, Levi AJ. Sulphasalazine and male infertility: reversibility and possible mechanism. Gut 1981;22:445–51.

15. Freeman JG, Reece VAC, Venables CW. Sulphasalazine and spermatogenesis. Digestion 1982;23:68–71.
16. Committee on Drugs, American Academy of Pediatrics. The transfer of drugs and other chemicals into human breast milk. Pediatrics 1983;72:375–83.

Name: **SULFONAMIDES**

Class: **Anti-infective**   Risk Factor: **B***

Fetal Risk Summary

Sulfonamides are a large class of antibacterial agents. While there are differences in their bioavailability, all share similar actions in the fetal and newborn periods, and they will be considered as a single group. The sulfonamides readily cross the placenta to the fetus during all stages of gestation (1–9). Equilibrium with maternal blood is usually established after 2–3 hours, with fetal levels averaging 70–90% of maternal. Significant levels may persist in the newborn for several days after birth when given near term. The primary danger of sulfonamide administration during pregnancy is manifested when these agents are given close to delivery. Toxicities that may be observed in the newborn include jaundice, hemolytic anemia, and, theoretically, kernicterus. Severe jaundice in the newborn has been related to maternal sulfonamide ingestion at term by several authors (10–15). Premature infants seem especially prone to development of hyperbilirubinemia (14). However, a study of 94 infants exposed to sulfadiazine *in utero* for maternal prophylaxis of rheumatic fever failed to show an increase in prematurity, hyperbilirubinemia, or kernicterus (16). Hemolytic anemia has been reported in two newborns and in a fetus following *in utero* exposure to sulfonamides (10, 11, 15). Both newborns survived. In the case involving the fetus, the mother had homozygous glucose-6-phosphate dehydrogenase deficiency (15). She was treated with sulfisoxazole for a urinary tract infection 2 weeks prior to delivery of a stillborn male infant. Autopsy revealed a 36-week infant with maceration, severe anemia, and hydrops fetalis.

Sulfonamides compete with bilirubin for binding to plasma albumin. *In utero*, the fetus clears free bilirubin by the placental circulation, but after birth, this mechanism is no longer available. Unbound bilirubin is free to cross the blood-brain barrier and may result in kernicterus. While this toxicity is well known when sulfonamides are administered directly to the neonate, kernicterus in the newborn following *in utero* exposure has not been reported. Most reports of sulfonamide exposure during gestation have failed to demonstrate an association with congenital malformations (9, 10, 17–23). Offspring of patients treated throughout pregnancy with sulfasalazine (sulfapyridine plus 5-aminosalicylic acid) for ulcerative colitis or Crohn's disease have not shown an increase in adverse effects (see also Sulfasalazine) (9, 20, 22). In contrast, a retrospective study of 1,369 patients found that significantly more mothers of 458 infants with congenital malformations took sulfonamides than did mothers in the control group (24). A 1975 study examined the *in utero* drug exposures of 599 children born with oral clefts (25). A significant difference ($p < 0.05$), as compared with matched controls, was found with 1st and 2nd trimester sulfonamide use only when other defects, in addition to the clefts, were present.

Sulfonamides are teratogenic in some species of animals, a finding which has prompted warnings of human teratogenicity (26, 27). In two reports, investigators associated *in utero* sulfonamide exposure with tracheoesophageal fistula and cataracts, but additional descriptions of these effects have not appeared (28, 29). A mother treated for food poisoning with sulfaguanidine in early pregnancy delivered a child with multiple anomalies (30). The author attributed the defects to use of the drug.

The Collaborative Perinatal Project monitored 50,282 mother-child pairs, 1,455 of which had 1st trimester exposure to sulfonamides (31). For use anytime during pregnancy, 5,689 exposures were reported (32). In neither case was evidence found to suggest a relationship to large categories of major or minor malformations. Several possible associations were found with individual defects after anytime use, but the statistical significance of these are not known (33). Independent confirmation is required.

Ductus arteriosus persistens (8 cases)
Coloboma (4 cases)
Hypoplasia of limb or part thereof (7 cases)
Miscellaneous foot defects (4 cases)
Urethral obstruction (13 cases)
Hypoplasia/atrophy of adrenal glands (6 cases)
Benign tumors (12 cases)

Taken in sum, sulfonamides do not appear to pose a significant teratogenic risk. Due to the potential toxicity to the newborn, these agents should be avoided near term.

[* Risk Factor D if administered near term.]

Breast Feeding Summary

Sulfonamides are excreted into breast milk in low concentrations. Milk levels of sulfanilamide (free and conjugated) are reported to range from 6 to 94 μg/ml (3, 34–39). Up to 1.6% of the total dose could be recovered from the milk (34, 37). Milk levels often exceeded serum levels and persisted for several days after maternal consumption of the drug was stopped. Milk:plasma (M:P) ratios during therapy with sulfanilamide were 0.5–0.6 (38). Reports of adverse effects in nursing infants are rare. Von Friesen (6) found reports of diarrhea and rash in breast-fed infants whose mothers were receiving sulfapyridine or sulfathiazole. Milk levels of sulfapyridine, the active metabolite of sulfasalazine, were 10.3 μg/ml, a M:P ratio of 0.5 (9). Based on these data, the nursing infant would receive approximately 3–4 mg/kg of sulfapyridine per day, an apparently nontoxic amount for a healthy neonate (16). Sulfisoxazole, a very water-soluble drug, was reported to produce a low M:P ratio of 0.06 (40). The conjugated form achieved a ratio of 0.22. The total amount of sulfisoxazole recovered in milk over 48 hours after a 4-g divided dose was only 0.45%. Although controversial, breast-feeding during maternal administration of sulfisoxazole seems to present a very low risk for the healthy neonate (41, 42).

In summary, sulfonamide excretion into breast milk apparently does not pose a significant risk for the healthy, full-term neonate. Exposure to sulfonamides via breast milk should be avoided in premature infants and in infants with hyperbilirubinemia or glucose-6-phosphate dehydrogenase deficiency. With these latter cautions, the American Academy of Pediatrics considers sulfonamides compatible with breast-feeding (43).

References

1. Barker RH. The placental transfer of sulfanilamide. N Engl J Med 1938;219:41.
2. Speert H. The passage of sulfanilamide through the human placenta. Bull Johns Hopkins Hosp 1938;63:337–9.
3. Stewart HL Jr, Pratt JP. Sulfanilamide excretion in human breast milk and effect on breast-fed babies. JAMA 1938;111:1456–8.
4. Speert H. The placental transmission of sulfanilamide and its effects upon the fetus and newborn. Bull Johns Hopkins Hosp 1940;66:139–55.
5. Speert H. Placental transmission of sulfathiazole and sulfadiazine and its significance for fetal chemotherapy. Am J Obstet Gynecol 1943;45:200–7.
6. von Freisen B. A study of small dose sulphamerazine prophylaxis in obstetrics. Acta Obstet Gynecol Scand 1951;31(Suppl):75–116.
7. Sparr RA, Pritchard JA. Maternal and newborn distribution and excretion of sulfamethoxypyridazine (Kynex). Obstet Gynecol 1958;12:131–4.
8. Nishimura H, Tanimura T. *Clinical Aspects of the Teratogenicity of Drugs*. Amsterdam:Excerpta Medica, 1976:88.
9. Azad Khan AK, Truelove SC. Placental and mammary transfer of sulphasalazine. Br Med J 1979;2:1553.
10. Heckel GP. Chemotherapy during pregnancy. Danger of fetal injury from sulfanilamide and its derivatives. JAMA 1941;117:1314–6.
11. Ginzler AM, Cherner C. Toxic manifestations in the newborn infant following placental transmission of sulfanilamide. With a report of 2 cases simulating erythroblastosis fetalis. Am J Obstet Gynecol 1942;44:46–55.
12. Lucey JF, Driscoll TJ Jr. Hazard to newborn infants of administration of long-acting sulfonamides to pregnant women. Pediatrics 1959;24:498–9.
13. Kantor HI, Sutherland DA, Leonard JT, Kamholz FH, Fry ND, White WL. Effect on bilirubin metabolism in the newborn of sulfisoxazole administration to the mother. Obstet Gynecol 1961;17:494–500.
14. Dunn PM. The possible relationship between the maternal administration of sulphamethoxypyridazine and hyperbilirubinaemia in the newborn. J Obstet Gynaecol Br Commonw 1964;71:128–31.
15. Perkins RP. Hydrops fetalis and stillbirth in a male glucose-6-phosphate dehydrogenase-deficient fetus possibly due to maternal ingestion of sulfisoxazole. Am J Obstet Gynecol 1971;111:379–81.
16. Baskin CG, Law S, Wenger NK. Sulfadiazine rheumatic fever prophylaxis during pregnancy: does it increase the risk of kernicterus in the newborn? Cardiology 1980;65:222–5.
17. Bonze EJ, Fuerstner PG, Falls FH. Use of sulfanilamide derivative in treatment of gonorrhea in pregnant and nonpregnant women. Am J Obstet Gynecol 1939;38:73–9.
18. Carter MP, Wilson F. Antibiotics and congenital malformations. Lancet 1963;1:1267–8.
19. Little PJ. The incidence of urinary infection in 5000 pregnant women. Lancet 1966;2:925–8.
20. McEwan HP. Anorectal conditions in obstetric patients. Proc R Soc Med 1972;65:279–81.
21. Williams JD, Smith EK. Single-dose therapy with streptomycin and sulfametopyrazine for bacteriuria during pregnancy. Br Med J 1970;4:651–3.
22. Mogadam M, Dobbins WO III, Korelitz BI, Ahmed SW. Pregnancy in inflammatory bowel disease: effect of sulfasalazine and corticosteroids on fetal outcome. Gastroenterology 1981;80:72–6.
23. Richards IDG. A retrospective inquiry into possible teratogenic effects of drugs in pregnancy. Adv Exp Med Biol 1972;27:441–55.
24. Nelson MM, Forfar JO. Association between drugs administered during pregnancy and congenital abnormalities of the fetus. Br Med J 1971;1:523–7.
25. Saxen I. Associations between oral clefts and drugs taken during pregnancy. Int J Epidemiol 1975;4:37–44.
26. Anonymous. Teratogenic effects of sulphonamides. Br Med J 1965;1:142.
27. Green KG. "Bimez" and teratogenic action. Br Med J 1963;2:56.
28. Ingalls TH, Prindle RA. Esophageal atresia with tracheoeosophageal fistula. Epidemiologic and teratologic implications. N Engl J Med 1949;240:987–95.
29. Harly JD, Farrar JF, Gray JB, Dunlop IC. Aromatic drugs and congenital cataracts. Lancet 1964;1:472–3.
30. Pogorzelska E. A case of multiple congenital anomalies in a child of a mother treated with sulfaguanidine. Patol Pol 1966;17:383–6.

31. Heinonen OP, Slone D, Shapiro S. *Birth Defects and Drugs in Pregnancy*. Littleton:Publishing Sciences Group, 1977:296–313.
32. *Ibid*, 435.
33. *Ibid*, 485–6.
34. Adair FL, Hesseltine HC, Hac LR. Experimental study of the behavior of sulfanilamide. JAMA 1938;111:766–70.
35. Hepburn JS, Paxson NF, Rogers AN. Secretion of ingested sulfanilamide in breast milk and in the urine of the infant. J Biol Chem 1938;123:liv–lv.
36. Pinto SS. Excretion of sulfanilamide and acetylsulfanilamide in human milk. JAMA 1938;111:1914–6.
37. Hac LR, Adair FL, Hesseltine HC. Excretion of sulfanilamide and acetylsulfanilamide in human breast milk. Am J Obstet Gynecol 1939;38:57–66.
38. Foster FP. Sulfanilamide excretion in breast milk: report of a case. Proc Staff Meet Mayo Clin 1939;14:153–5.
39. Hepburn JS, Paxson NF, Rogers AN. Secretion of ingested sulfanilamide in human milk and in the urine of the nursing infant. Arch Pediatr 1942;59:413–8.
40. Kauffman RE, O'Brien C, Gilford P. Sulfisoxazole secretion into human milk. J Pediatr 1980;97:839–41.
41. Elliott GT, Quinn SI. Sulfisoxazole in human milk. J Pediatr 1981;99:171–2.
42. Kauffman RE. Reply. J Pediatr 1981;99:172.
43. Committee on Drugs, American Academy of Pediatrics. The transfer of drugs and other chemicals into human breast milk. Pediatrics 1983;72:375–83.

Name: **SULINDAC**

Class: **Nonsteroidal Anti-inflammatory**   Risk Factor: **B***

Fetal Risk Summary

No reports linking the use of sulindac with congenital defects have been located. Theoretically, sulindac, a prostaglandin synthetase inhibitor, could cause constriction of the ductus arteriosus *in utero* (1). Persistent pulmonary hypertension of the newborn should also be considered (2). Drugs in this class have been shown to inhibit labor and prolong pregnancy (2). The manufacturer recommends that the drug not be used during pregnancy (3).

[* Risk Factor D if used in the 3rd trimester or near delivery.]

Breast Feeding Summary

No data available (4). The manufacturer recommends that the drug not be used when breast-feeding (3).

References

1. Levin DL. Effects of inhibition of prostaglandin synthesis on fetal development, oxygenation, and the fetal circulation. Semin Perinatol 1980;4:35–44.
2. Fuchs F. Prevention of prematurity. Am J Obstet Gynecol 1976;126:809–20.
3. Product information. Clinoril. Merck Sharp & Dohme, 1985.
4. Whalen JJ. Merck Sharp & Dohme, 1981. Personal communication.

Name: **TENIPOSIDE**

Class: **Antineoplastic**   Risk Factor: **D**

Fetal Risk Summary

Teniposide, a podophyllin derivative, has been used in the 2nd and 3rd trimesters of one pregnancy (1). An apparently normal infant was delivered at 37 weeks of gestation. Long-term studies of growth and mental development in offspring exposed to antineoplastic agents during the 2nd trimester, the period of neuroblast multiplication, have not been conducted (2).

Breast Feeding Summary

No data available.

References

1. Lowenthal RM, Funnell CF, Hope DM, Stewart IG, Humphrey DC. Normal infant after combination chemotherapy including teniposide for Burkitt's lymphoma in pregnancy. Med Pediatr Oncol 1982;10:165–9.
2. Dobbing J. Pregnancy and leukaemia. Lancet 1977;1:1155.

Name: **TERBUTALINE**

Class: **Sympathomimetic (Adrenergic)**   Risk Factor: **B**

Fetal Risk Summary

No reports linking the use of terbutaline with congenital defects have been located. Terbutaline, a β-sympathomimetic, has been used to prevent premature labor (see also parent compound Metaproterenol). Haller (1) has recently reviewed the use of this drug as a tocolytic agent. Terbutaline may cause fetal and maternal tachycardia (1–4). Fetal rates are usually less than 175 beats/min (3). Drops in maternal blood pressure may occur, but fetal distress as a consequence has not been observed (4, 5). Like all β-mimetics, terbutaline may cause transient maternal hyperglycemia followed by an increase in serum insulin levels (1, 6). Sustained neonatal hypoglycemia may be observed if maternal effects have not terminated prior to delivery (6). Terbutaline decreases the incidence of neonatal respiratory distress syndrome similar to other β-mimetics (7). Long-term evaluation of infants exposed to terbutaline *in utero* has been reported (8). No harmful effects in the infants (2–12 months) were found.

Breast Feeding Summary

No data available.

References

1. Haller DL. The use of terbutaline for premature labor. Drug Intell Clin Pharm 1980;14:757–64.
2. Andersson KE, Bengtsson LP, Gustafson I, Ingermarsson I. The relaxing effect of terbutaline on the human uterus during term labor. Am J Obstet Gynecol 1975;121:602–9.
3. Ingermarrson I. Effect of terbutaline on premature labor. A double-blind placebo-controlled study. Am J Obstet Gynecol 1976;125:520–4.
4. Ravindran R, Viegas OJ, Padilla LM, LaBlonde P. Anesthetic considerations in pregnant patients receiving terbutaline therapy. Anesth Analg 1980;59:391–2.
5. Vargas GC, Macedo GJ, Amved AR, Lowenberg FE. Terbutaline, a new uterine inhibitor. Ginecol Obstet Mex 1974;36:75–88.
6. Epstein MF, Nicholls RN, Stubblefield PG. Neonatal hypoglycemia after beta-sympathomimetic tocolytic therapy. J Pediatr 1979;94:449–53.
7. Bergman B, Hedner T. Antepartum administration of terbutaline and the incidence of hyaline membrane disease in preterm infants. Acta Obstet Gynecol Scand 1978;57:217–21.
8. Wallace R, Caldwell D, Ansbacher R, Otterson W. Inhibition of premature labor by terbutaline. Obstet Gynecol 1978;51:387–93.

Name: TETANUS/DIPHTHERIA TOXOIDS (ADULT)

Class: **Toxoid**   Risk Factor: **C**

Fetal Risk Summary

Tetanus/diphtheria toxoids for adult use are the specific toxoids of *Clostridium tetani* and *Corynebacterium diphtheriae* adsorbed onto aluminum compounds (1). Tetanus and diphtheria produce severe morbidity and mortality in the mother and a newborn tetanus mortality rate of 60% (2, 3). The risk to the fetus from tetanus/diphtheria toxoids is unknown (2, 3). The American College of Obstetricians and Gynecologists Technical Bulletin No. 64 recommends the use of tetanus/diphtheria toxoids in pregnancy for those women at risk who lack the primary series of immunizations or in whom no booster has been given within the past 10 years (2).

Breast Feeding Summary

No data available.

References

1. American Hospital Formulary Service. *Drug Information 1985*. Bethesda:American Society of Hospital Pharmacists, 1985:1527–9.
2. ACOG Technical Bulletin, No. 64, May 1982.
3. Amstey MS. Vaccination in pregnancy. Clin Obstet Gynaecol 1983;10:13–22.

Name: **TETRABENAZINE**

Class: **Tranquilizer**   Risk Factor: **C**

Fetal Risk Summary

Tetrabenazine has been used in pregnancy for the treatment of chorea gravidarum (1). Therapy was started late in the 2nd trimester in one patient. No drug-induced fetal or newborn effects were observed. A small ventricular septal defect was probably not due to tetrabenazine exposure.

Breast Feeding Summary

No data available.

References

1. Lubbe WF, Walker EB. Chorea gravidarum associated with circulating lupus anticoagulant: successful outcome of pregnancy with prednisone and aspirin therapy. Case report. Br J Obstet Gynaecol 1983;90:487–90.

Name: **TETRACYCLINE**

Class: **Antibiotic**   Risk Factor: **D**

Fetal Risk Summary

Tetracyclines are a class of antibiotics that should be used with extreme caution, if at all, in pregnancy. The following discussion, unless otherwise noted, applies to all members of this class. Problems attributable to the use of the tetracyclines during or around the gestational period can be classified into four areas:

  Adverse effects on fetal teeth and bones
  Maternal liver toxicity
  Congenital defects
  Miscellaneous effects

Placental transfer of a tetracycline was first demonstrated by Guilbeau and co-workers in 1950 (1). The tetracyclines were considered safe for the mother and fetus and were routinely used for maternal infections during the following decade (2–5). It was not until 1961 that Cohlan and co-workers (6) observed an intense yellow-gold fluorescence in the mineralized structures of a fetal skeleton whose mother had taken tetracycline just prior to delivery. Harcourt and co-workers (7) followed this report with the description of a 2-year-old child whose erupted deciduous teeth formed normally but were stained a bright yellow due to tetracycline exposure *in utero*. Fluorescence under ultraviolet light and yellow-colored deciduous teeth which eventually changed to yellow-brown were associated with maternal tetracycline ingestion during pregnancy by several other investigators (8–22). An increase in enamel hypoplasia and caries was initially suspected but later shown not to be related to *in utero* tetracycline exposure (14, 15, 22). Newborn growth and development were normal in all of these reports, although tetracycline has been shown to cause inhibition of fibula growth in premature infants (6). The characteristic dental defect produced by tetracycline is due to the potent chelating ability of the drug (13). Tetracycline forms a complex with calcium orthophosphate and becomes incorporated into bones and teeth undergoing calcification. In the latter structure, this complex causes a permanent discoloration, as remodeling and calcium exchange do not occur after calcification is completed. Since the deciduous teeth begin to calcify at around 5 or 6 months *in utero*, use of tetracycline after this time will result in staining.

The first case linking tetracycline with acute fatty metamorphosis of the liver in a pregnant woman was described by Schultz and co-workers in 1963 (23), although two earlier papers reported the disease without associating it with the drug (24, 25). This rare but often fatal syndrome usually follows intravenous dosing of more than 2 g/day. Many of the pregnant patients were being treated for pyelonephritis (24–37). Tetracycline-induced hepatotoxicity differs from acute fatty liver of pregnancy in that it is not unique to pregnant women, and reversal of the disease does not occur with pregnancy termination (38). The symptoms include jaundice, azotemia, acidosis, and terminal, irreversible shock. Pancreatitis and nonoliguric renal failure are often related findings. The fetus may not be affected directly, but as a result of the maternal pathology, stillborn infants and premature births are common. In an experimental study, Allen and Brown (39) demonstrated that increasing doses of tetracycline caused increasing fatty metamorphosis of the liver. The possibility that chronic maternal use of tetracycline before conception could result in fatal hepatotoxicity of pregnancy was recently raised (36). The authors speculated that tetracycline deposited in the bone of a 21-year-old patient was released during pregnancy, resulting in liver damage.

The Collaborative Perinatal Project monitored 50,282 mother-child pairs, 341 of which had 1st trimester exposure to tetracycline, 14 to chlortetracycline, 90 to demeclocycline, and 119 to oxytetracycline (40). For use anytime in pregnancy, 1,336 exposures were recorded for tetracycline, 0 for chlortetracycline, 280 for demeclocycline, and 328 for oxytetracycline (41). The findings of this study were:
Tetracycline: Evidence was found to suggest a relationship to minor, but not major, malformations. Three possible associations were found with individual defects, but the statistical significance of these is unknown (42). Independent confirmation is required to determine the actual risk.

Hypospadias (1st trimester only) (5 cases)
Inguinal hernia (25 cases)
Hypoplasia of limb or part thereof (6 cases)

Chlortetracycline: No evidence was found to suggest a relationship to large categories of major or minor malformations or to individual defects. However, the sample size is extremely small and safety should not be inferred from these negative results.

Demeclocycline: Evidence was found to suggest a relationship to major or minor malformations, but the sample size is small (40). Two possible associations were found with individual defects, but the statistical significance of these is unknown (42). Independent confirmation is required to determine the actual risk.

Clubfoot (1st trimester only) (3 cases)
Inguinal hernia (8 cases)

Oxytetracycline: Evidence was found to suggest a relationship to major and minor malformations (40). One possible association was found with individual defects, but the statistical significance of this is unknown (42). Independent confirmation is required to determine the actual risk.

Inguinal hernia (14 cases)

In 1962, a woman treated with tetracycline in the 1st trimester for acute bronchitis delivered an infant with congenital defects of both hands (43, 44). The mother had a history of minor congenital defects on her side of the family and doubt was cast on the role of the drug in this anomaly (45). A possible association between the use of tetracyclines in pregnancy or during lactation and congenital cataracts has been reported in four patients (46). The effects of other drugs, including several antibiotics and maternal infection, could not be determined and a causal relationship to the tetracyclines seems remote. An infant with multiple anomalies whose mother had been treated with clomocycline for acne daily during the first 8 weeks of pregnancy has been described (47). Some of the defects, particularly the incomplete fibrous ankylosis and bone changes, made the authors suspect this tetracycline as the likely cause.

Doxycycline has been used for 10 days very early in the 1st trimester for the treatment of mycoplasma infection in a group of previously infertile women (48). Dosage was based on the patient's weight, varying from 100 to 300 mg/day. All 43 of the exposed liveborn infants were normal at 1 year of age. Bubonic plague occurring in a woman at 22 weeks gestation was successfully treated with tetracycline and streptomycin (49). Long-term evaluation of the infant was not reported.

Under miscellaneous effects, two reports have appeared which, although they do not directly relate to effects on the fetus, do directly affect pregnancy. In 1974, Briggs (50) observed that a 1-week administration of 500 mg of chlortetracycline per day to male subjects was sufficient to produce sperm levels of the drug averaging 4.5 μg/ml. He theorized that tetracycline overdose could modify the fertilizing capacity of human sperm by inhibiting capacitation. Finally, a possible interaction between oral contraceptives and tetracycline resulting in pregnancy has been reported (51). The mechanism for this interaction may involve the interruption of enterohepatic circulation of contraceptive steroids by inhibition of gut bacterial hydrolysis of steroid conjugates, resulting in a lower concentration of circulating steroids.

Breast Feeding Summary

Tetracycline is excreted into breast milk in low concentrations. Milk:plasma ratios vary between 0.25 and 1.5 (4, 52, 53). Theoretically, dental staining and inhibition of bone growth could occur in breast-fed infants whose mothers were consuming tetracycline. However, this theoretical possibility seems remote, since tetracycline serum levels in infants exposed in such a manner were undectable (less than 0.05 μg/ml) (4). Three potential problems may exist for the nursing infant even though there are no reports in this regard: modification of bowel flora, direct effects on the infant, and interference with the interpretation of culture results if a fever work-up is required. The American Academy of Pediatrics considers tetracycline compatible with breast-feeding (54).

References

1. Guilbeau JA, Schoenbach EG, Schaub IG, Latham DV. Aureomycin in obstetrics: therapy and prophylaxis. JAMA 1950;143:520–6.
2. Charles D. Placental transmission of antibiotics. J Obstet Gynaecol Br Emp 1954;61:750–7.
3. Gibbons RJ, Reichelderfer TE. Transplacental transmission of demethylchlortetracycline and toxicity studies in premature and full term, newly born infants. Antibiot Med Clin Ther 1960;7:618–22.
4. Posner AC, Prigot A, Konicoff NG. Further observations on the use of tetracycline hydrochloride in prophylaxis and treatment of obstetric infections. In *Antibiotics Annual, 1954–55*. New York:Medical Encyclopedia, 594–8.
5. Posner AC, Konicoff NG, Prigot A. Tetracycline in obstetric infections. In *Antibiotics Annual, 1955–56*. New York:Medical Encyclopedia, 345–8.
6. Cohlan SQ, Bevelander G, Bross S. Effect of tetracycline on bone growth in the premature infant. Antimicrob Agents Chemother 1961:340–7.
7. Harcourt JK, Johnson NW, Storey E. In vivo incorporation of tetracycline in the teeth of man. Arch Oral Biol 1962;7:431–7.
8. Rendle-Short TJ. Tetracycline in teeth and bone. Lancet 1962;1:1188.
9. Douglas AC. The deposition of tetracycline in human nails and teeth: a complication of long term treatment. Br J Dis Chest 1963;57:44–7.
10. Kutscher AH, Zegarelli EV, Tovell HM, Hochberg B. Discoloration of teeth induced by tetracycline. JAMA 1963;184:586–7.
11. Kline AH, Blattner RJ, Lunin M. Transplacental effect of tetracyclines on teeth. JAMA 1964;188:178–80.
12. Macaulay JC, Leistyna JA. Preliminary observations on the prenatal administration of demethylchlortetracycline HCl. Pediatrics 1964;34:423–4.
13. Stewart DJ. The effects of tetracyclines upon the dentition. Br J Dermatol 1964;76:374–8.
14. Swallow JN. Discoloration of primary dentition after maternal tetracycline ingestion in pregnancy. Lancet 1964;2:611–2.
15. Porter PJ, Sweeney EA, Golan H, Kass EH. Controlled study of the effect of prenatal tetracycline on primary dentition. Antimicrob Agents Chemother 1965:668–71.
16. Toaff R, Ravid R. Tetracyclines and the teeth. Lancet 1966;2:281–2.
17. Kutscher AH, Zegarelli EV, Tovell HM, Hochberg B, Hauptman J. Discoloration of deciduous teeth induced by administrations of tetracycline antepartum. Am J Obstet Gynecol 1966;96:291–2.
18. Brearley LJ, Stragis AA, Storey E. Tetracycline-induced tooth changes. Part 1. Prevalence in pre-school children. Med J Aust 1968;2:653–8.
19. Brearley LJ, Storey E. Tetracycline-induced tooth changes. Part 2. Prevalence, localization and nature of staining in extracted deciduous teeth. Med J Aust 1968;2:714–9.
20. Baker KL, Storey E. Tetracycline-induced tooth changes. Part 3. Incidence in extracted first permanent molar teeth. Med J Aust 1970;1:109–13.
21. Anthony JR. Effect on deciduous and permanent teeth of tetracycline deposition in utero. Postgrad Med 1970;48:165–8.
22. Genot MT, Golan HP, Porter PJ, Kass EH. Effect of administration of tetracycline in pregnancy on the primary dentition of the offspring. J Oral Med 1970;25:75–9.
23. Schultz JC, Adamson JS Jr, Workman WW, Normal TD. Fatal liver disease after intravenous administration of tetracycline in high dosage. N Engl J Med 1963;269:999–1004.
24. Bruno M, Ober WB. Clinicopathologic conference: jaundice at the end of pregnancy. NY State J Med 1962;62:3792–800.
24. Lewis PL, Takeda M, Warren MJ. Obstetric acute yellow atrophy. Report of a case. Obstet Gynecol 1963;22:121–7.
26. Briggs RC. Tetracycline and liver disease. N Engl J Med 1963;269:1386.
27. Leonard GL. Tetracycline and liver disease. N Engl J Med 1963;269:1386.
28. Gough GS, Searcy RL. Additional case of fatal liver disease with tetracycline therapy. N Engl J Med 1964;270:157–8.
29. Whalley PJ, Adams RH, Combes B. Tetracycline toxicity in pregnancy. JAMA 1964;189:357–62.
30. Kunelis CT, Peters JL, Edmondson HA. Fatty liver of pregnancy and its relationship to tetracycline therapy. Am J Med 1965;38:359–77.
31. Lew HT, French SW. Tetracycline nephrotoxicity and nonoliguric acute renal failure. Arch Intern Med 1966;118:123–8.

32. Meihoff WE, Pasquale DN, Jacoby WJ Jr. Tetracycline-induced hepatic coma, with recovery. A report of a case. Obstet Gynecol 1967;29:260–5.
33. Aach R, Kissane J. Clinicopathologic conference: a seventeen year old girl with fatty liver of pregnancy following tetracycline therapy. Am J Med 1967;43:274–83.
34. Whalley PJ, Martin FG, Adams RH, Combes B. Disposition of tetracycline by pregnant women with acute pyelonephritis. Obstet Gynecol 1970;36:821–6.
35. Pride GL, Cleary RE, Hamburger RJ. Disseminated intravascular coagulation associated with tetracycline-induced hepatorenal failure during pregnancy. Am J Obstet Gynecol 1973;115:585–6.
36. Wenk RE, Gebhardt FC, Behagavan BS, Lustgarten JA, McCarthy EF. Tetracycline-associated fatty liver of pregnancy, including possible pregnancy risk after chronic dermatologic use of tetracycline. J Reprod Med 1981;26:135–41.
37. King TM, Bowe ET, D'Esopo DA. Toxic effects of the tetracyclines. Bull Sloane Hosp Women 1964;10:35–41.
38. Kaplan MM. Acute fatty liver of pregnancy. N Engl J Med 1985;313:367–70.
39. Allen ES, Brown WE. Hepatic toxicity of tetracycline in pregnancy. Am J Obstet Gynecol 1966;95:12–8.
40. Heinonen O, Slone D, Shaprio S. Birth Defects and Drugs in Pregnancy. Littleton:Publishing Sciences Group, 1977:297–313.
41. Ibid, 435.
42. Ibid, 472, 485.
43. Wilson F. Congenital defects in the newborn. Br Med J 1962;2:255.
44. Carter MP, Wilson F. Tetracycline and congenital limb abnormalities. Br Med J 1962;2:407–8.
45. Mennie AT. Tetracycline and congenital limb abnormalities. Br Med J 1962;2:480.
46. Harley JD, Farrar JF, Gray JB, Dunlop IC. Aromatic drugs and congenital cataracts. Lancet 1964;1:472.
47. Corcoran R, Castles JM. Tetracycline for acne vulgaris and possible teratogenesis. Br Med J 1977;2:807–8.
48. Horne HW Jr, Kundsin RB. The role of mycoplasma among 81 consecutive pregnancies: a prospective study. Int J Fertil 1980;25:315–7.
49. Coppes JB. Bubonic plague in pregnancy. J Reprod Med 1980;25:91–5.
50. Briggs M. Tetracycline and steroid hormone binding to human spermatozoa. Acta Endocrinol (Copenh) 1974;75:785–92.
51. Bacon JF, Shenfield GM. Pregnancy attributable to interaction between tetracycline and oral contraceptives. Br Med J 1980;1:283.
52. Knowles JA. Drugs in milk. Pediatr Curr 1972;21:28–32.
53. Graf VH, Reimann S. Untersuchungen uber die konzentration von pyrrolidino-methyl-tetracycline in der muttermilch. Dtsch Med Wochenschr 1959;84:1694.
54. Committee on Drugs, American Academy of Pediatrics. The transfer of drugs and other chemicals into human breast milk. Pediatrics 1983;72:375–83.

Name: **THEOPHYLLINE**

Class: **Spasmolytic/Vasodilator**   Risk Factor: **C**

Fetal Risk Summary

Theophylline is the bronchodilator of choice for asthma and chronic obstructive pulmonary disease in the pregnant patient (1–6). No reports linking the use of theophylline with congenital defects have been located.

Theophylline crosses the placenta, and newborn infants may have therapeutic serum levels (7–11). Transient tachycardia, irritability, and vomiting have been reported in newborns delivered from mothers consuming theophylline (7, 8). These effects are more likely to occur when maternal serum levels at term are in the high therapeutic range or above (therapeutic range 8–20 μg/ml) (9). Cord blood levels are approximately 100% of the maternal serum concentration (10, 11).

In patients at risk for premature delivery, aminophylline (theophylline ethylenediamine) was found to exert a beneficial effect by reducing the perinatal death rate and the frequency of respiratory distress syndrome (12, 13). In a nonrandomized study, aminophylline, 250 mg intramuscularly every 12 hours up to a maximum of 3 days, was compared to betamethasone, 4 mg intramuscularly every 8 hours for 2 days (13). Patients in the aminophylline group were excluded from receiving corticosteroids because of diabetes (4 patients), hypertension (10 patients), and ruptured membranes for more than 24 hours (4 patients). The aminophylline and steroid groups were comparable in length of gestation (32.5 weeks vs 32.1 weeks), male/female infant sex ratio (10/8 vs 8/8), Apgar scores (7.6 vs 7.7), birth weight (1,720 g vs 1,690 g), and hours between treatment and delivery (73 vs 68). Respiratory distress syndrome occurred in 11% of the aminophylline group (2 of 18) vs 0% of the corticosteroid group (0 of 16). The difference was not statistically significant. A significant difference ($p = 0.01$) was found in the incidence of neonatal infection with 8 of 16 (50%) of the betamethasone group having signs of infection and none in the aminophylline group. The mechanism proposed for aminophylline-induced fetal lung maturation is similar to that observed with betamethasone: enhancement of tissue cyclic AMP by inhibition of cyclic AMP phosphodiesterase and a corresponding increased production and/or release of phosphatidylcholine (13).

An intravenous infusion of aminophylline has been tested for its tocolytic effects on oxytocin-induced uterine contractions (14). A slight decrease in uterine activity occurred in the first 15 minutes, but this was due to the effect on contraction intensity, not frequency. The author conceded that aminophylline was a poor tocolytic agent.

The Collaborative Perinatal Project monitored 193 mother-child pairs with 1st trimester exposure to theophylline or aminophylline (15). No evidence was found for an association with malformations.

Concern over the depressant effects of methylxanthines on lipid synthesis in developing neural systems has been reported (16). Recent observations that infants treated with theophylline for apnea exhibit no overt neurologic deficits at 9–27 months of age are encouraging (17, 18). However, the long-term effects of these drugs on human brain development are not known (16).

Frequent, high-dose asthmatic medication containing theophylline, ephedrine, phenobarbital, and diphenhydramine was used by one woman throughout pregnancy who delivered a stillborn girl with complete triploidy (19). Although drug-induced chromosome damage could not be proven, theophylline has been shown in *in vitro* tests to cause breakage in chromosomes of human lymphocytes (20).

Theophylline withdrawal in a newborn exposed throughout gestation has been reported (10). Apneic spells developed at 28 hours after delivery and became progressively worse over the next 4 days. Therapy with theophylline resolved the spells.

Little is known about the pharmacokinetics of theophylline during pregnancy. A recent report suggests that plasma concentrations of theophylline fall during the 3rd trimester due to an increased maternal volume of distribution (21). Those patients that require theophylline during pregnancy should be monitored accordingly.

Breast Feeding Summary

Theophylline is excreted into breast milk (22, 23). A milk:plasma ratio of 0.7 has been measured (23). Estimates indicate that less than 1% of the maternal dose is excreted into breast milk (22, 23). However, one infant became irritable after a rapidly absorbed oral solution of aminophylline taken by the mother (22). Because very young infants may be more sensitive to levels which would be nontoxic in older infants, less rapidly absorbed theophylline preparations may be advisable for nursing mothers (8, 24).

References

1. Greenberger P, Patterson R. Safety of therapy for allergic symptoms during pregnancy. Ann Intern Med 1978;89:234–7.
2. Weinstein AM, Dubin BD, Podleski WK, Spector SL, Farr RS. Asthma and pregnancy. JAMA 1979;241:1161–5.
3. Hernandez E, Angell CS, Johnson JWC. Asthma in pregnancy: current concepts. Obstet Gynecol 1980;55:739–43.
4. Turner ES, Greenberger PA, Patterson R. Management of the pregnant asthmatic patient. Ann Intern Med 1980;93:905–18.
5. Pratt WR. Allergic diseases in pregnancy and breast feeding. Ann Allergy 1981;47:355–60.
6. Lalli CM, Raju L. Pregnancy and chronic obstructive pulmonary disease. Chest 1981;80:759–61.
7. Arwood LL, Dasta JF, Friedman C. Placental transfer of theophylline: two case reports. Pediatrics 1979;63:844–6.
8. Yeh TF, Pildes RS. Transplacental aminophylline toxicity in a neonate. Lancet 1977;1:910.
9. Labovitz E, Spector S. Placental theophylline transfer in pregnant asthmatics. JAMA 1982;247:786–8.
10. Horowitz DA, Jablonski W, Mehta KA. Apnea associated with theophylline withdrawal in a term neonate. Am J Dis Child 1982;136:73–4.
11. Ron M, Hochner-Celnikier D, Menczel J, Palti Z, Kidroni G. Maternal-fetal transfer of aminophylline. Acta Obstet Gynecol Scand 1984;63:217–8.
12. Hadjigeorgiou E, Kitsiou S, Psaroudakis A, Segos C, Nicolopoulos D, Kaskarelis D. Antepartum aminophylline treatment for prevention of the respiratory distress syndrome in premature infants. Am J Obstet Gynecol 1979;135:257–60.
13. Granati B, Grella PV, Pettenazzo A, Di Lenardo L, Rubaltelli FF. The prevention of respiratory distress syndrome in premature infants: efficacy of antenatal aminophylline treatment versus prenatal glucocorticoid administration. Pediatr Pharmacol 1984;4:21–4.
14. Lipshitz J. Uterine and cardiovasuclar effects of aminophylline. Am J Obstet Gynecol 1978;131:716–8.
15. Heinonen OP, Slone D, Shapiro S. *Birth Defects and Drugs in Pregnancy*. Littleton:Publishing Sciences Group, 1977:367, 370.
16. Volpe JJ. Effects of methylxanthines on lipid synthesis in developing neural systems. Semin Perinatol 1981;5:395–405.
17. Aranda JV, Dupont C. Metabolic effects of methylxanthines in premature infants. J Pediatr 1976;89:833–4.
18. Nelson RM, Resnick MB, Holstrum WJ, Eitzman DV. Development outcome of premature infants treated with theophylline. Dev Pharmacol Ther 1980;1:274–80.
19. Halbrecht I, Komlos L, Shabtay F, Solomon M, Book JA. Triploidy 69, XXX in a stillborn girl. Clin Genet 1973;4:210–2.
20. Weinstein D, Mauer I, Katz ML, Kazmer S. The effect of methylxanthines on chromosomes of human lymphocytes in culture. Mutat Res 1975;31:57–61.
21. Sutton PL, Koup JR, Rose JQ, Middleton E. The pharmacokinetics of theophylline in pregnancy. J Allergy Clin Immunol 1978;61:174.
22. Yurchak AM, Jusko WJ. Theophylline secretion into breast milk. Pediatrics 1976;57:518–25.
23. Stec GP, Greenberger P, Ruo TI, et al. Kinetics of theophylline transfer to breast milk. Clin Pharmacol Ther 1980;28:404–8.
24. Berlin CM. Excretion of methylxanthines in human milk. Semin Perinatol 1981;5:389–94.

Name: **THIAMINE**

Class: **Vitamin**   Risk Factor: **A***

Fetal Risk Summary

Thiamine (vitamin B$_1$), a water-soluble B complex vitamin, is an essential nutrient required for carbohydrate metabolism (1). The American RDA for thiamine in pregnancy is 1.4–1.5 mg (2).

Thiamine is actively transported to the fetus (3–6). Like other B complex vitamins, concentrations of thiamine in the fetus and newborn are higher than those in the mother (5–12).

Maternal thiamine deficiency is common during pregnancy (11–13). Supplementation with multivitamin products reduces the thiamine hypovitaminemia only slightly (10). Since 1938, several authors have attempted to link this deficiency to toxemia of pregnancy (14–17). In a 1945 paper, King and Ride (15) summarized the early work published in this area. All of the reported cases, however, involved patients with poor nutrition and pregnancy care in general. More recent investigations have failed to find any relationship between maternal thiamine deficiency and toxemia, fetal defects, or other outcome of pregnancy (9, 18).

No association was found between low birth weight and thiamine levels in a 1977 report (8). Roecklein and co-workers (19) have shown experimentally, though, that the characteristic intrauterine growth retardation of the fetal alcohol syndrome may be due to ethanol-induced thiamine deficiency.

Thiamine has been used to treat hyperemesis gravidarum although pyridoxine (vitamin B$_6$) was found to be more effective (see Pyridoxine) (20–22). In one early report, thiamine was effective in reversing severe neurologic complications associated with hyperemesis (20). A mother treated with frequent injections of thiamine and pyridoxine, 50 mg each per dose, for hyperemesis during the first half of two pregnancies delivered two infants with severe convulsions, one of whom died within 30 hours of birth (22). The convulsions in the mentally retarded second infant were eventually controlled with pyridoxine. Pyridoxine dependency-induced convulsions are rare. The authors speculated the defect was caused by *in utero* exposure to high circulating levels of the vitamin. Thiamine was not thought to be involved (see Pyridoxine).

An isolated case report has described an anencephalic fetus whose mother was under psychiatric care (23). She had been treated with very high doses of vitamins B$_1$, B$_6$, C, and folic acid. The relationship between the vitamins and the defect are unknown. Also unknown is the speculation by one writer than an association exists between thiamine deficiency and Down's syndrome (trisomy 21) or preleukemic bone marrow changes (24).

[* Risk Factor C if used in doses above the RDA.]

Breast Feeding Summary

Thiamine is excreted into breast milk (25–28). Thomas and co-workers (25) gave well-nourished lactating women supplements of a multivitamin preparation containing 1.7 mg of thiamine. At 6 months postpartum, milk concentrations of thiamine did not differ significantly from those of control patients not receiving supplements. In a study of lactating women with low nutritional status, supplementation with thiamine, 0.2–20.0 mg/day, resulted in mean milk concentrations of 125–268 ng/ml (26). Milk concentrations were directly proportional to dietary intake. A 1983 English study measured thiamine levels in pooled human milk obtained from preterm (26 mothers: 29–34 weeks) and term (35 mothers: 39 weeks or longer) patients (27). Preterm milk level rose from 23.7 ng/ml (colostrum) to 89.3 ng/ml (16–196 days), while term milk level increased over the same period from 28.4 to 183 ng/ml.

In Asian mothers with severe thiamine deficiency, including some with beriberi, infants have become acutely ill after breast-feeding, leading in some to convulsions and sudden death (29–32). Pneumonia was usually a characteristic finding. One author thought the condition was related to toxic intermediary metabolites, such as methylglyoxal, passing to the infant via the milk (29). Although a cause and effect relationship has not been proven, one report suggested that thiamine deficiency may aggravate the condition (30). Indian investigators measured very low thiamine milk levels in mothers of children with convulsions of unknown etiology (33). Mean milk thiamine concentrations in mothers of healthy children were 111 ng/ml while those in mothers of children with convulsions were 29 ng/ml. The authors were unable to establish an association between the low thiamine content in milk and infantile convulsions. (see Pyridoxine for correlation between low levels of vitamin B_6 and convulsions).

The American RDA for thiamine during lactation is 1.5–1.6 mg (2). If the diet of the lactating woman adequately supplies this amount, maternal supplementation with thiamine is not needed (28). Supplementation with the RDA for thiamine is recommended for those women with inadequate nutritional intake.

References

1. American Hospital Formulary Service. *Drug Information 1985*. Bethesda:American Society of Hospital Pharmacists, 1985:1692–3.
2. *Recommended Dietary Allowances*, ed 9. Washington, DC:National Academy of Sciences, 1980.
3. Frank O, Walbroehl G, Thomson A, Kaminetzky H, Kubes Z, Baker H. Placental transfer: fetal retention of some vitamins. Am J Clin Nutr 1970;23:662–3.
4. Hill EP, Longo LD. Dynamics of maternal-fetal nutrient transfer. Fed Proc 1980;39:239–44.
5. Kaminetzky HA, Baker H, Frank O, Langer A. The effects of intravenously administered water-soluble vitamins during labor in normovitaminemic and hypovitaminemic gravidas on maternal and neonatal blood vitamin levels at delivery. Am J Obstet Gynecol 1974;120:697–703.
6. Baker H, Frank O, Deangelis B, Feingold S, Kaminetzky HA. Role of placenta in maternal-fetal vitamin transfer in humans. Am J Obstet Gynecol 1981;141:792–6.
7. Slobody LB, Willner MM, Mestern J. Comparison of vitamin B_1 levels in mothers and their newborn infants. Am J Dis Child 1949;77:736–9.
8. Baker H, Thind IS, Frank O, DeAngelis B, Caterini H, Louria DB. Vitamin levels in low-birth-weight newborns infants and their mothers. Am J Obstet Gynecol 1977;129:521–4.
9. Heller S, Salkeld RM, Korner WF. Vitamin B_1 status in pregnancy. Am J Clin Nutr 1974;27:1221–4.
10. Baker H, Frank O, Thomson AD, Langer A, Munves ED, De Angelis B, Kaminetzky HA. Vitamin profile of 174 mothers and newborns at parturition. Am J Clin Nutr 1975;28:59–65.
11. Tripathy K. Erythrocyte transketolase activity and thiamine transfer across human placenta. Am J Clin Nutr 1968;21:739–42.
12. Bamji MS. Enzymic evaluation of thiamin, riboflavin and pyridoxine status of parturient women and their newborn infants. Br J Nutr 1976;35:259–65.
13. Dostalova L. Correlation of the vitamin status between mother and newborn during delivery. Dev Pharmacol Ther 1982;4(Suppl 1):45–57.
14. Siddall AC. Vitamin B_1 deficiency as an etiologic factor in pregnancy toxemias. Am J Obstet Gynecol 1938;35:662–7.

15. King G, Ride LT. The relation of vitamin B$_1$ deficiency to the pregnancy toxaemias: a study of 371 cases of beri-beri complicating pregnancy. J Obstet Gynaecol Br Emp 1945;52:130–47.
16. Chaudhuri SK, Halder K, Chowdhury SR, Bagchi K. Relationship between toxaemia of pregnancy and thiamine deficiency. J Obstet Gynaecol Br Commonw 1969;76:123–6.
17. Chaudhuri SK. Role of nutrition in the etiology of toxemia of pregnancy. Am J Obstet Gynecol 1971;110:46–8.
18. Thomson AM. Diet in pregnancy. 3. Diet in relation to the course and outcome of pregnancy. Br J Nutr 1959;13:509–25.
19. Roecklein B, Levin SW, Comly M, Mukherjee AB. Intrauterine growth retardation induced by thiamine deficiency and pyrithiamine during pregnancy in the rat. Am J Obstet Gynecol 1985;151:455–60.
20. Fouts PJ, Gustafson GW, Zerfas LG. Successful treatment of a case of polyneuritis of pregnancy. Am J Obstet Gynecol 1934;28:902–7.
21. Willis RS, Winn WW, Morris AT, Newsom AA, Massey WE. Clinical observations in treatment of nausea and vomiting in pregnancy with vitamins B$_1$ and B$_6$: a preliminary report. Am J Obstet Gynecol 1942;44:265–71.
22. Hunt AD Jr, Stokes J Jr, McCrory WW, Stroud HH. Pyridoxine dependency: report of a case of intractable convulsions in an infant controlled by pyridoxine. Pediatrics 1954;13:140–5.
23. Averback P. Anencephaly associated megavitamin therapy. Can Med Assoc J 1976;114:995.
24. Reading C. Down's syndrome, leukaemia and maternal thiamine deficiency. Med J Aust 1976;1:505.
25. Thomas MR, Sneed SM, Wei C, Nail P, Wilson M, Sprinkle EE III. The effects of vitamin C, vitamin B$_6$, vitamin B$_{12}$, folic acid, riboflavin, and thiamin on the breast milk and maternal status of well-nourished women at 6 months postpartum. Am J Clin Nutr 1980;33:2151–6.
26. Deodhar AD, Rajalakshmi R, Ramakrishnan CV. Studies on human lactation. Part III. Effect of dietary vitamin supplementation on vitamin contents of breast milk. Acta Paediatr Scand 1964;1964;53:42–8.
27. Ford JE, Zechalko A, Murphy J, Brooke OG. Comparison of the B vitamin composition of milk from mothers of preterm and term babies. Arch Dis Child 1983;58:367–72.
28. Nail PA, Thomas MR, Eakin R. The effect of thiamin and riboflavin supplementation on the level of those vitamins in human breast milk and urine. Am J Clin Nutr 1980;33:198–204.
29. Fehily L. Human-milk intoxication due to B$_1$ avitaminosis. Br Med J 1944;2:590–2.
30. Cruickshank JD, Trimble AP, Brown JAH. Interstitial mononuclear pneumonia: a cause of sudden death in Gurkha infants in the Far East. Arch Dis Child 1957;32:279–84.
31. Mayer J. Nutrition and lactation. Postgrad Med 1963;33:380–5.
32. Gunther M. Diet and milk secretion in women. Proc Nutr Soc 1968;27:77–82.
33. Rao RR, Subrahmanyam I. An investigation on the thiamine content of mother's milk in relation to infantile convulsions. Indian J Med Res 1964;52:1198–201.

Name: **THIOGUANINE**

Class: **Antineoplastic** Risk Factor: **D$_M$**

Fetal Risk Summary

The use of thioguanine in pregnancy has been reported in 16 patients, 4 during the 1st trimester (1–12). Use in the 1st and 2nd trimesters has been associated with congenital malformations and chromosomal abnormalities (1, 2):

Trisomy for group C autosomes with mosaicism (1)
Two medial digits of both feet missing, distal phalanges of both thumbs missing with hypoplastic remnant of right thumb (2)

Data from one review indicated that 40% of the infants exposed to anticancer drugs were of low birth weight (13). This finding was not related to the timing of exposure. Long-term studies of growth and mental development in offspring exposed to thioguanine during the 2nd trimester, the period of neuroblast multiplication, have not been conducted (14).

Although abnormal chromosomal changes were observed in one aborted fetus, karyotyping of cultured cells in two other newborns did not show anomalies (1, 4). Paternal use of thioguanine with other antineoplastic agents prior to conception may have been associated with congenital defects observed in three infants:

Anencephalic stillborn (15)
Tetralogy of Fallot with syndactyly of the 1st and 2nd toes (15)
Multiple anomalies (16)

Exposed men have also fathered normal children (16, 17).

Breast Feeding Summary

No data available.

References

1. Maurer LH, Forcier RJ, McIntyre OR, Benirschke K. Fetal group C trisomy after cytosine arabinoside and thioguanine. Ann Intern Med 1971;75:809–10.
2. Schafer AI. Teratogenic effects of antileukemic chemotherapy. Arch Intern Med 1981;141:514–5.
3. Au-Yong R, Collins P, Young JA. Acute myeloblastic leukaemia during pregnancy. Br Med J 1972;4:493–4.
4. Raich PC, Curet LB. Treatment of acute leukemia during pregnancy. Cancer 1975;36:861–2.
5. Gokal R, Durrant J, Baum JD, Bennett MJ. Successful pregnancy in acute monocytic leukaemia. Br J Cancer 1976;34:299–302.
6. Lilleyman JS, Hill AS, Anderton KJ. Consequences of acute myelogenous leukemia in early pregnancy. Cancer 1977;40:1300–3.
7. Moreno H, Castleberry RP, McCann WP. Cytosine arabinoside and 6-thioguanine in the treatment of childhood acute myeloblastic leukemia. Cancer 1977;40:998–1004.
8. Manoharan A, Leyden MJ. Acute non-lymphocytic leukaemia in the third trimester of pregnancy. Aust NZ J Med 1979;9:71–4.
9. Taylor G, Blom J. Acute leukemia during pregnancy. South Med J 1980;73:1314–5.
10. Tobias JS, Bloom HJG. Doxorubicin in pregnancy. Lancet 1980;1:776.
11. Pawliger DF, McLean FW, Noyes WD. Normal fetus after cytosine arabinoside therapy. Ann Intern Med 1971;74:1012.
12. Plows CW. Acute myelomonocytic leukemia in pregnancy: report of a case. Am J Obstet Gynecol 1982;143:41–3.
13. Nicholson HO. Cytotoxic drugs in pregnancy: review of reported cases. J Obstet Gynaecol Br Commonw 1968;75:307–12.
14. Dobbing J. Pregnancy and leukaemia. Lancet 1977;1:1155.
15. Russell JA, Powles RL, Oliver RTD. Conception and congenital abnormalities after chemotherapy of acute myelogenous leukaemia in two men. Br Med J 1976;1:1508.
16. Evenson DP, Arlin Z, Welt S, Claps ML, Melamed MR. Male reproductive capacity may recover following drug treatment with the L-10 protocol for acute lymphocytic leukemia. Cancer 1984;53:30–6.
17. Matthews JH, Wood JK. Male fertility during chemotherapy for acute leukemia. N Engl J Med 1980;303:1235.

Name: **THIOPROPAZATE**

Class: **Tranquilizer** Risk Factor: **C**

Fetal Risk Summary

Thiopropazate is a piperazine phenothiazine in the same group as prochlorperazine (see Prochlorperazine). Phenothiazines readily cross the placenta (1). No specific information on the use of thiopropazate in pregnancy has been located. Although occasional reports have attempted to link various phenothiazine compounds with congenital malformations, the bulk of the evidence indicates that these drugs are safe for the mother and fetus (see also Chlorpromazine).

Breast Feeding Summary

No data available.

References

1. Moya F, Thorndike V. Passage of drugs across the placenta. Am J Obstet Gynecol 1962;84:1778–98.

Name: **THIORIDAZINE**

Class: **Tranquilizer** Risk Factor: **C**

Fetal Risk Summary

Thioridazine is a piperidyl phenothiazine. The phenothiazines readily cross the placenta (1). Extrapyramidal symptoms were seen in a newborn exposed to thioridazine *in utero*, but the reaction was probably due to chlorpromazine (2). A case of a congenital heart defect was described in 1969 (3). However, Scanlan (4) found no anomalies in the offspring of 23 patients exposed throughout gestation to thioridazine. Twenty of the infants were evaluated for up to 13 years. Although occasional reports have attempted to link various phenothiazine compounds with congenital malformations, the bulk of the evidence indicates that these drugs are safe for the mother and fetus (see Chlorpromazine).

Breast Feeding Summary

No reports describing the excretion of thioridazine into breast milk have been located. The American Academy of Pediatrics considers the drug compatible with breast-feeding (5).

References

1. Moya F, Thorndike V. Passage of drugs across the placenta. Am J Obstet Gynecol 1962;84:1778–98.
2. Hill RM, Desmond MM, Kay JL. Extrapyramidal dysfunction in an infant of a schizophrenic mother. J Pediatr 1966;69:589–95.
3. Vince DJ. Congenital malformations following phenothiazine administration during pregnancy. Can Med Assoc J 1969;100:223.
4. Scanlan FJ. The use of thioridazine (Mellaril) during the first trimester. Med J Aust 1972;1:1271–2.
5. Committee on Drugs, American Academy of Pediatrics. The transfer of drugs and other chemicals into human breast milk. Pediatrics 1983;72:375–83.

Name: **THIOTEPA**

Class: **Antineoplastic**   Risk Factor: **D**

Fetal Risk Summary

Thiotepa has been used during the 2nd and 3rd trimesters in one patient without apparent fetal harm (1). Long-term studies of growth and mental development in offspring exposed to antineoplastic agents during the 2nd trimester, the period of neuroblast multiplication, have not been conducted (2).

Breast Feeding Summary

No data available.

References

1. Gililland J, Weinstein L. The effects of cancer chemotherapeutic agents on the developing fetus. Obstet Gynecol Surv 1983;38:6–13.
2. Dobbing J. Pregnancy and leukaemia. Lancet 1977;1:1155.

Name: **THIOTHIXENE**

Class: **Tranquilizer**   Risk Factor: **C**

Fetal Risk Summary

Thiothixene is structurally and pharmacologically related to trifluoperazine and chlorprothixene. No specific data on its use in pregnancy have been located (see also Trifluoperazine).

Breast Feeding Summary

No data available.

Name: **THIPHENAMIL**

Class: **Parasympatholytic (Anticholinergic)**   Risk Factor: **C**

Fetal Risk Summary

Thiphenamil is an anticholinergic agent used in the treatment of parkinsonism. No reports of its use in pregnancy have been located (see also Atropine).

Breast Feeding Summary

No data available (see also Atropine).

Name: **THYROGLOBULIN**

Class: **Thyroid** Risk Factor: **A**

Fetal Risk Summary

See Thyroid.

Breast Feeding Summary

See Thyroid.

Name: **THYROID**

Class: **Thyroid** Risk Factor: **A**

Fetal Risk Summary

Thyroid contains the two thyroid hormones levothyroxine (T_4) and liothyronine (T_3) plus other materials peculiar to the thyroid gland. It is used during pregnancy for the treatment of hypothyroidism. Neither T_4 or T_3 crosses the placenta when physiologic serum concentrations are present in the mother (see Levothyroxine and Liothyronine). In one report, however, two patients, each of whom had produced two cretins in previous pregnancies, were given huge amounts of thyroid, up to 1,600 mg or more per day (1). Both newborns were normal at birth even though one was found to be athyroid. The authors concluded that sufficient hormone was transported to the fetuses to prevent hypothyroidism.

Congenital defects have been reported with the use of thyroid but are thought to be due to maternal hypothyroidism or other factors (see Levothyroxine and Liothyronine).

Combination therapy with thyroid-antithyroid drugs was advocated at one time for the treatment of hyperthyroidism but is now considered inappropriate (see Propylthiouracil).

Breast Feeding Summary

See Levothyroxine and Liothyronine.

References

1. Carr EA Jr, Beierwaltes WH, Raman G, Dodson VN, Tanton J, Betts JS, Stambaugh RA. The effect of maternal thyroid function on fetal thyroid function and development. J Clin Endocrinol Metab 1959;19: 1–18.

Name: **THYROTROPIN**

Class: **Thyroid**   Risk Factor: C_M

Fetal Risk Summary

Thyrotropin (thyroid-stimulating hormone, TSH) does not cross the placenta (1). No correlation exists between maternal and fetal concentrations of TSH at any time during gestation (2).

Breast Feeding Summary

No reports describing the excretion of thyrotropin in human milk have been located. Levels of this hormone have been measured and compared in breast-fed and bottle-fed infants (3–7). Breast milk does not provide sufficient levothyroxine (T_4) or liothyronine (T_3) to prevent the effects of congenital hypothyroidism (see Levothyroxine and Liothyronine). As a consequence, serum levels of TSH in breast-fed hypothyroid infants are markedly elevated (3, 4). In euthyroid babies, no differences in TSH levels have been discovered between breast-fed and bottle-fed groups (5–7).

References

1. Cohlan SQ. Fetal and neonatal hazards from drugs administered during pregnancy. NY State J Med 1964;64:493–9.
2. Feely J. The physiology of thyroid function in pregnancy. Postgrad Med J 1979;55:336–9.
3. Abbassi V, Steinour TA. Successful diagnosis of congenital hypothyroidism in four breast-fed neonates. J Pediatr 1980;97:259–61.
4. Letarte J, Guyda H, Dussault JH, Glorieux J. Lack of protective effect of breast-feeding in congenital hypothyroidism: report of 12 cases. Pediatrics 1980;65:703–5.
5. Mizuta H, Amino N, Ichihara K, Harada T, Nose O, Tanizawa O, Miyai K. Thyroid hormones in human milk and their influence on thyroid function of breast-fed babies. Pediatr Res 1983;17:468–71.
6. Hahn HB Jr, Spiekerman M, Otto WR, Hossalla DE. Thyroid function tests in neonates fed human milk. Am J Dis Child 1983;137:220–2.
7. Franklin R, O'Grady C, Carpenter L. Neonatal thyroid function: comparison between breast-fed and bottle-fed infants. J Pediatr 1985;106:124–6.

Name: **TICARCILLIN**

Class: **Antibiotic**   Risk Factor: **B**

Fetal Risk Summary

Ticarcillin is a penicillin antibiotic. The drug rapidly crosses the placenta into the fetal circulation and amniotic fluid (1). Following a 1-g intravenous dose, single determinations of the amniotic fluid from six patients, 15–76 minutes after injection, yielded levels ranging from 1.0 to 3.3 μg/ml. Similar measurements of ticarcillin in cord serum ranged from 12.6 to 19.2 μg/ml.

No reports linking the use of ticarcillin with congenital defects have been located. The Collaborative Perinatal Project monitored 50,282 mother-child pairs, 3,546 of which had 1st trimester exposure to penicillin derivatives (2). For use anytime during pregnancy, 7,171 exposures were recorded (3). In neither case was evidence found to suggest a relationship to large categories of major or minor malformations or to individual defects.

Breast Feeding Summary

Ticarcillin is excreted into breast milk in low concentrations. After a 1-g intravenous dose given to five patients, only trace amounts of drug were measured at intervals up to 6 hours (1). Although these amounts are probably not significant, three potential problems exist for the nursing infant: modification of bowel flora, direct effects on the infant (e.g., allergic response), and interference with the interpretation of culture results if a fever work-up is required.

References

1. Cho N, Nakayama T, Vehara K, Kunii K. Laboratory and clinical evaluation of ticarcillin in the field of obstetrics and gynecology. Chemotherapy (Tokyo) 1977;25:2911–23.
2. Heinonen OP, Slone, D, Shapiro S. *Birth Defects and Drugs in Pregnancy*. Littleton:Publishing Sciences Group, 1977:297–313.
3. *Ibid*, 435.

Name: **TIMOLOL**

Class: **Sympatholytic (β-Adrenergic Blocker)**   Risk Factor: **C$_M$**

Fetal Risk Summary

Timolol is a nonselective β-adrenergic blocking agent. No reports of its use in pregnancy have been located. The use near delivery of some agents in this class has resulted in persistent β-blockade in the newborn (see Acebutolol, Atenolol, and Nadolol). Thus, newborns exposed *in utero* to timolol should be closely observed during the first 24–48 hours after birth for bradycardia and other symptoms. The long-term effects of *in utero* exposure to β-blockers have not been studied but warrant evaluation.

Breast Feeding Summary

Timolol is excreted into breast milk (1, 2). In nine lactating women given 5 mg orally three times daily, the mean milk concentration of timolol 105–135 minutes after a dose was 15.9 ng/ml (1). When a dose of 10 mg three times daily was given to four patients, mean milk levels of 41 ng/ml were measured. The milk:plasma ratios for the two regimens were 0.80 and 0.83, respectively.

A woman with elevated intraocular pressure applied ophthalmic 0.5% timolol drops to the right eye twice daily, resulting in excretion of the drug in her breast milk (2). Maternal timolol levels in milk and plasma were 5.6 and 0.93 ng/ml, respectively, about 1.5 hours after a dose. A milk sample taken 12 hours after the last dose contained 0.5 ng/ml of timolol. Assuming that the infant nursed every 4 hours and received 75 ml at each feeding, the daily dose would be below that expected to produce cardiac effects in the infant (2).

No adverse reactions were noted in the nursing infants described in the above reports. However, infants exposed to timolol via breast milk should be closely observed for bradycardia and other signs or symptoms of β-blockade. Long-term effects of exposure to β-blockers from milk have not been studied but warrant evaluation.

References

1. Fidler J, Smith V, DeSwiet M. Excretion of oxprenolol and timolol in breast milk. Br J Obstet Gynaecol 1983;90:961–5.
2. Lustgarten JS, Podos SM. Topical timolol and the nursing mother. Arch Ophthalmol 1983;101:1381–2.

Name: **TOBRAMYCIN**

Class: **Antibiotic**   Risk Factor: **D$_M$**

Fetal Risk Summary

Tobramycin is an aminoglycoside antibiotic. The drug crosses the placenta into the fetal circulation and amniotic fluid (1). Studies in patients undergoing elective abortions in the 1st and 2nd trimesters indicate that tobramycin distributes to most fetal tissues except the brain and cerebrospinal fluid. Amniotic fluid levels generally did not occur until the 2nd trimester. The highest fetal concentrations were found in the kidneys and urine. Reports measuring the passage of tobramycin in the 3rd trimester and at term are lacking.

No reports linking the use of tobramycin with congenital defects have been located. Ototoxicity, which is known to occur after tobramycin therapy, has not been reported as an effect of *in utero* exposure. However, eighth cranial nerve toxicity in the fetus is well known following exposure to other aminoglycosides (see Kanamycin and Streptomycin) and may potentially occur with tobramycin.

A potentially serious drug interaction may occur in newborns treated with aminoglycosides who were also exposed *in utero* to magnesium sulfate (see Gentamicin).

Breast Feeding Summary

Tobramycin is excreted into breast milk. Following an 80-mg intramuscular dose given to five patients, milk levels varied from trace to 0.52 μg/ml over 8 hours (2). Peak levels occurred at 4 hours postinjection. Since oral absorption of this antibiotic is poor, ototoxicity in the infant would not be expected. However, three potential problems exist for the nursing infant: modification of bowel flora, direct effects on the infant, and interference with the interpretation of culture results if a fever work-up is required.

References

1. Bernard B, Garcia-Cazares S, Ballard C, Thrupp L, Mathies A, Wehrle P. Tobramycin: maternal-fetal pharmacology. Antimicrob Agents Chemother 1977;11:688–94.
2. Takase Z. Laboratory and clinical studies on tobramycin in the field of obstetrics and gynecology. Chemotherapy (Tokyo) 1975;23:1402.

Name: **TOLAZAMIDE**

Class: **Oral Hypoglycemic**   Risk Factor: **D***

Fetal Risk Summary

Tolazamide is a sulfonylurea used for the treatment of adult-onset diabetes mellitus. It is not indicated for the pregnant diabetic since tolazamide will not provide good control in patients whose condition cannot be controlled by diet alone. Oral hypoglycemics may cause prolonged symptomatic hypoglycemia in newborns if exposed near term (see Chlorpropamide).

[* Risk Factor C according to manufacturer—The Upjohn Co, 1985.]

Breast Feeding Summary

No data available.

Name: **TOLAZOLINE**

Class: **Vasodilator**   Risk Factor: **C**

Fetal Risk Summary

Tolazoline is structurally and pharmacologically related to phentolamine (see also Phentolamine). Experience with tolazoline in pregnancy is limited. The Collaborative Perinatal Project monitored two 1st trimester exposures to tolazoline plus 13 other patients exposed to other vasodilators (1). From this small group of 15 patients, four malformed children were produced, a statisically significant incidence ($p <$ 0.02). It was not stated if tolazoline was taken by any of the mothers of the affected infants. Although the data serve as a warning, the number of patients is so small that conclusions as to the relative safety of this drug in pregnancy cannot be made.

Breast Feeding Summary

No data available.

References

1. Heinonen OP, Slone D, Shapiro S. *Birth Defects and Drugs in Pregnancy*. Littleton:Publishing Sciences Group, 1977:371–3.

Name: **TOLBUTAMIDE**

Class: **Oral Hypoglycemic**   Risk Factor: **D***

Fetal Risk Summary

Tolbutamide is a sulfonylurea used for the treatment of adult-onset diabetes mellitus. It is not indicated for the pregnant diabetic. When administered near term, the drug crosses the placenta (1, 2). Neonatal serum levels are higher than corresponding maternal concentrations. In one infant whose mother took 500 mg/day, serum levels at 27 hours were 7.2 mg/100 ml (maternal 2.7 mg/100 ml) (2). Prolonged symptomatic hypoglycemia has not been reported with tolbutamide but has been observed with other oral hypoglycemics (see also Acetohexamide and Chlorpropamide). If used during pregnancy, tolbutamide should be stopped at least 48 hours before delivery to avoid this potential complication (3).

Although teratogenic in animals, an increased incidence of congenital defects, other than those expected in diabetes mellitus, has not been found with tolbutamide (4–14). Four malformed infants have been attributed to tolbutamide, but the relationship is unclear (2, 15–17):

Hand/foot anomalies, finger/toe syndactyly, external ear defect, atresia of external auditory canal, gastrointestinal, heart, and renal anomalies (15)
Grossly malformed (16)
Severe talipes, absent left toe (17)
Right-sided preauricular skin tag, accessory right thumb, thrombocytopenia (nadir 19,000 mm^3 on 4th day) (2)

Maternal diabetes is known to increase the rate of malformations by 2–4-fold, but the mechanism(s) are not fully understood (see also Insulin). The neonatal thrombocytopenia, persisting for about 2 weeks, may have been induced by tolbutamide (2).

In spite of this relative lack of teratogenicity, tolbutamide should be avoided in pregnancy since the drug will not provide good control in patients whose condition cannot be controlled by diet alone (3). The manufacturer recommends it not be used in pregnancy (18).

[* Risk Factor C according to manufacturer—The Upjohn Co, 1985.]

Breast Feeding Summary

Tolbutamide is excreted into breast milk. Following long-term dosing with 500 mg orally twice daily, milk levels 4 hours after a dose in two patients averaged 3 and 18 μg/ml, respectively (19). Milk:plasma ratios were 0.09 and 0.40, respectively. The effect on an infant from these levels is unknown.

References

1. Miller DI, Wishinsky H, Thompson G. Transfer of tolbutamide across the human placenta. Diabetes 1962;11(Suppl):93–7.
2. Schiff D, Aranda J, Stern L. Neonatal thrombocytopenia and congenital malformation associated with administration of tolbutamide to the mother. J Pediatr 1970; 77:457–8.
3. Friend JR. Diabetes. Clin Obstet Gynaecol 1981;8:353–82.
4. Ghanem MH. Possible teratogenic effect of tolbutamide in the pregnant prediabetic. Lancet 1961;1:1227.
5. Dolger H, Bookman JJ, Nechemias C. The diagnostic and therapeutic value of tolbutamide in pregnant diabetics. Diabetes 1962;11(Suppl):97–8.
6. Jackson WPU, Campbell GD, Notelovitz M, Blumsohn D. Tolbutamide and chlorpropamide during pregnancy in human diabetes. Diabetes 1962;11(Suppl):98–101.
7. Campbell GD. Chlorpropamide and foetal damage. Br Med J 1963;1:59–60.
8. Macphail I. Chlorpropamide and foetal damage. Br Med J 1963; 1:192.
9. Jackson WPU, Campbell GD. Chlorpropamide and perinatal mortality. Br Med J 1963;2:1652.
10. Malins JM, Cooke AM, Pyke DA, Fitzgerald MG. Sulphonylurea drugs in pregnancy. Br Med J 1964;2:187.
11. Moss JM, Connor EJ. Pregnancy complicated by diabetes. Report of 102 pregnancies including eleven treated with oral hypoglycemic drugs. Med Ann DC 1965;34:253–60.

12. Adam PAJ, Schwartz R. Diagnosis and treatment: should oral hypoglycemic agents be used in pediatric and pregnant patients? Pediatrics 1968;42:819–23.
13. Dignan PSJ. Teratogenic risk and counseling in diabetes. Clin Obstet Gynecol 1981;24:149–59.
14. Burt RL. Reactivity to tolbutamide in normal pregnancy. Obstet Gynecol 1958;12:447–53.
15. Larsson Y, Sterky G. Possible teratogenic effect of tolbutamide in a pregnant prediabetic. Lancet 1960;2:1424–6.
16. Campbell GD. Possible teratogenic effect of tolbutamide in pregnancy. Lancet 1961;1:891–2.
17. Soler NG, Walsh CH, Malins JM. Congenital malformations in infants of diabetic mothers. QJ Med 1976;45:303–13.
18. Product information. Orinase. The Upjohn Co, 1985.
19. Moiel RH, Ryan JR. Tolbutamide (Orinase) in human breast milk. Clin Pediatr 1967;6:480.

Name: **TOLMETIN**

Class: **Nonsteroidal Anti-inflammatory**　　　　　　　　Risk Factor: **B***

Fetal Risk Summary

No reports linking the use of tolmetin with congenital defects have been located. Theoretically, tolmetin, a prostaglandin synthetase inhibitor, could cause constriction of the ductus arteriosus *in utero* (1). Persistent pulmonary hypertension of the newborn should also be considered (2). Drugs in this class have been shown to inhibit labor and prolong pregnancy (2). The manufacturer recommends that the drug not be used during pregnancy (3).

[* Risk Factor D if used in 3rd trimester or near delivery.]

Breast Feeding Summary

Tolmetin is excreted into breast milk (4). In the 4 hours following a single 400-mg oral dose, milk levels varied from 0.06 to 0.18 μg/ml with the highest concentration occurring at 0.67 hours. Milk:plasma ratios were 0.005–0.007. The significance of these levels to the nursing infant are unknown.

References

1. Levin DL. Effects of inhibition of prostaglandin synthesis on fetal development, oxygenation, and the fetal circulation. Semin Perinatol 1980;4:35–44.
2. Fuchs F. Prevention of prematurity. Am J Obstet Gynecol 1976;126:809–20.
3. Product information. Tolectin. McNeil Pharmaceutical, 1985.
4. Sagraves R, Waller ES, Goehrs HR. Tolmetin in breast milk. Drug Intell Clin Pharm 1985;19:55–6.

Name: **TRANYLCYPROMINE**

Class: **Antidepressant**　　　　　　　　　　　　　　　　Risk Factor: **C**

Fetal Risk Summary

Tranylcypromine is a monoamine oxidase inhibitor. The Collaborative Perinatal Project monitored 21 mother-child pairs exposed to these drugs during the 1st trimester, 13 of which were exposed to tranylcypromine (1). An increased risk of malformations was found. Details of the 13 cases with exposure to tranylcypromine are not available.

Breast Feeding Summary

No reports describing the excretion of tranylcypromine into breast milk have been located. The American Academy of Pediatrics considers the drug compatible with breast-feeding (2).

References

1. Heinonen OP, Slone D, Shapiro S. *Birth Defects and Drugs in Pregnancy*. Littleton:Publishing Sciences Group, 1977:336–7.
2. Committee on Drugs, American Academy of Pediatrics. The transfer of drugs and other chemicals into human breast milk. Pediatrics 1983;72:375–83.

Name: **TRIAMTERENE**

Class: **Diuretic**   Risk Factor: **D**

Fetal Risk Summary

Triamterene is a potassium-conserving diuretic. No reports linking it with congenital defects have been located. The drug crosses to the fetus in animals, but this has not been studied in humans (1). No defects were observed in five infants exposed to triamterene in the 1st trimester in one study (2). For use anytime during pregnancy, 271 exposures were recorded without an increase in malformations (3). Many investigators consider diuretics contraindicated in pregnancy, except for patients with heart disease, since they do not prevent or alter the course of toxemia, and they may decrease placental perfusion (4–6).

Breast Feeding Summary

Triamterene is excreted into cow's milk (1). Human data are not available.

References

1. Product information. Dyrenium. Smith Kline & French Laboratories, 1985.
2. Heinonen OP, Slone D, Shapiro S. *Birth Defects and Drugs in Pregnancy*. Littleton:Publishing Sciences Group, 1977:372.
3. *Ibid*, 441.
4. Pitkin RM, Kaminetzky HA, Newton M, Pritchard JA. Maternal nutrition: a selective review of clinical topics. Obstet Gynecol 1972;40:773–85.
5. Lindheimer MD, Katz AI. Sodium and diuretics in pregnancy. N Engl J Med 1973;288:891–4.
6. Christianson R, Page EW. Diuretic drugs and pregnancy. Obstet Gynecol 1976;48:647–52.

Name: **TRICHLORMETHIAZIDE**

Class: **Diuretic**   Risk Factor: **D**

Fetal Risk Summary

See Chlorothiazide.

Breast Feeding Summary

See Chlorothiazide.

Name: **TRIDIHEXETHYL**

Class: **Parasympatholytic (Anticholinergic)**   Risk Factor: **C**

Fetal Risk Summary

Tridihexethyl is an anticholinergic quaternary ammonium chloride. In a large prospective study, 2,323 patients were exposed to this class of drugs during the 1st trimester, 6 of whom took tridihexethyl (1). A possible association was found between the total group and minor malformations.

Breast Feeding Summary

No data available (see also Atropine).

References

1. Heinonen OP, Slone D, Shapiro S. *Birth Defects and Drugs in Pregnancy*. Littleton:Publishing Sciences Group, 1977:346–53.

Name: **TRIFLUOPERAZINE**

Class: **Tranquilizer**   Risk Factor: **C**

Fetal Risk Summary

Trifluoperazine is a piperazine phenothiazine. The drug readily crosses the placenta (1). Trifluoperazine has been used for the treatment of nausea and vomiting of pregnancy, but it is primarily used as a psychotropic agent. In 1962, the Canadian Food and Drug Directorate released a warning that eight cases of congenital defects had been associated with trifluoperazine therapy (2). This correlation was refuted in a series of articles from the medical staff of the manufacturer of the drug (3–5). In 480 trifluoperazine-treated pregnant women, the incidence of liveborn infants with congenital malformations was 1.1%, as compared to 8,472 nontreated controls with an incidence of 1.5% (4). Two reports of phocomelia appeared in 1962–63 and a case of a congenital heart defect in 1969 (6–8):

Twins, both with phocomelia of all four limbs (6)
Phocomelia of upper limbs (7)
Complete transposition of great vessels in heart (8)

In none of these cases is there a clear relationship between use of the drug and the defect. Extrapyramidal symptoms have been described in a newborn exposed to trifluoperazine *in utero*, but the reaction was probably due to chlorpromazine (see Chlorpromazine) (9).

The Collaborative Perinatal Project monitored 50,282 mother-child pairs, 42 of which had 1st trimester exposure to trifluoperazine (10). No evidence was found to suggest a relationship to malformations or an effect on perinatal mortality rate, birth weight, or intelligence quotient scores at 4 years of age.

In summary, although some reports have attempted to link trifluoperazine with congenital defects, the bulk of the evidence indicates that the drug is safe for mother and fetus. Other reviewers have also concluded that the phenothiazines are not teratogenic (11, 12).

Breast Feeding Summary

No reports describing the excretion of trifluoperazine into breast milk have been located. The American Academy of Pediatrics considers the drug compatible with breast-feeding (13).

References

1. Moya F, Thorndike V. Passage of drugs across the placenta. Am J Obstet Gynecol 1962;84:1778–98.
2. Canadian Department of National Health and Welfare, Food and Drug Directorate. Letter of notification to Canadian physicians. Ottawa, December 7, 1962.
3. Moriarity AJ. Trifluoperazine and congenital malformations. Can Med Assoc J 1963;88:97.
4. Moriarty AJ, Nance MR. Trifluoperazine and pregnancy. Can Med Assoc J 1963;88:375–6.
5. Schrire I. Trifluoperazine and foetal abnormalities. Lancet 1963;1:174.
6. Corner BD. Congenital malformations. Clinical considerations. Med J Southwest 1962;77:46–52.
7. Hall G. A case of phocomelia of the upper limbs. Med J Aust 1963;1:449–50.
8. Vince DJ. Congenital malformations following phenothiazine administration during pregnancy. Can Med Assoc J 1969;100:223.
9. Hill RM, Desmond MM, Kay JL. Extrapyramidal dysfunction in an infant of a schizophrenic mother. J Pediatr 1966;69:589–95.
10. Slone D, Siskind V, Heinonen OP, Monson RR, Kaufman DW, Shapiro S. Antenatal exposure to the phenothiazines in relation to congenital malformations, perinatal mortality rate, birth weight, and intelligence quotient score. Am J Obstet Gynecol 1977;128:486–8.
11. Ayd FJ Jr. Children born of mothers treated with chlorpromazine during pregnancy. Clin Med 1964;71:1758–63.
12. Ananth J. Congenital malformations with psychopharmacologic agents. Compr Psychiatry 1975;16:437–45.
13. Committee on Drugs, American Academy of Pediatrics. The transfer of drugs and other chemicals into human breast milk. Pediatrics 1983;72:375–83.

Name: **TRIFLUPROMAZINE**

Class: **Tranquilizer**   Risk Factor: **C**

Fetal Risk Summary

Triflupromazine is a propylamino phenothiazine in the same class as chlorpromazine. The phenothiazines readily cross the placenta (1). The Collaborative Perinatal Project monitored 50,282 mother-child pairs, 36 of which had 1st trimester exposure to triflupromazine (2). No evidence was found to suggest a relationship to malformations or an effect on perinatal mortality rates, birth weight, or intelligence quotient scores at 4 years of age. Although occasional reports have attempted to link various phenothiazine compounds with congenital defects, the bulk of the evidence indicates that these drugs are safe for the mother and fetus (see also Chlorpromazine).

Breast Feeding Summary

No data available.

References

1. Moya F, Thorndike V. Passage of drugs across the placenta. Am J Obstet Gynecol 1962;84:1778–98.
2. Slone D, Siskind V, Heinonen OP, Monson RR, Kaufman DW, Shapiro S. Antenatal exposure to the phenothiazines in relation to congenital malformations, perinatal mortality rate, birth weight, and intelligence quotient score. Am J Obstet Gynecol 1977;128:486–8.

Name: **TRIHEXYPHENIDYL**

Class: **Parasympatholytic (Anticholinergic)**   Risk Factor: **C**

Fetal Risk Summary

Trihexyphenidyl is an anticholinergic agent used in the treatment of parkinsonism. In a large prospective study, 2,323 patients were exposed to this class of drugs during the 1st trimester, 9 of whom took trihexyphenidyl (1). A possible association was found between the total group and minor malformations.

Breast Feeding Summary

No data available (see also Atropine).

References

1. Heinonen OP, Slone D, Shapiro S. *Birth Defects and Drugs in Pregnancy*. Littleton:Publishing Sciences Group, 1977:346–53.

Name: **TRIMEPRAZINE**

Class: **Antihistamine**   Risk Factor: **C**

Fetal Risk Summary

Trimeprazine is a phenothiazine antihistamine that is primarily used as an antipruritic. The Collaborative Perinatal Project monitored 50,282 mother-child pairs, 14 of which had 1st trimester exposure to trimeprazine (1). From this small sample, no evidence was found to suggest a relationship to large categories of major or minor malformations or to individual malformations. For use anytime in pregnancy, 140 exposures were recorded (2). Based on defects in five children, a possible association with malformations was found, but the significance of this is unknown.

In a 1971 study, infants of mothers who had ingested antihistamines during the 1st trimester actually had significantly fewer abnormalities when compared to controls (3). Trimeprazine was the eighth most commonly used antihistamine.

Breast Feeding Summary

Trimeprazine is excreted into human milk, but the levels are too low to produce effects in the infant (4). The American Academy of Pediatrics considers trimeprazine compatible with breast-feeding (5).

References

1. Heinonen OP, Slone D, Shapiro S. *Birth Defects and Drugs in Pregnancy*. Littleton:Publishing Sciences Group, 1977:323.
2. *Ibid*, 437.
3. Nelson MM, Forfar JO. Associations between drugs administered during pregnancy and congenital abnormalities. Br Med J 1971;1:523–7.
4. O'Brien TE. Excretion of drugs in human milk. Am J Hosp Pharm 1974; 31:844–54.
5. Committee on Drugs, American Academy of Pediatrics. The transfer of drugs and other chemicals into human breast milk. Pediatrics 1983;72:375–83.

Name: **TRIMETHADIONE**

Class: **Anticonvulsant**   Risk Factor: **D**

Fetal Risk Summary

Trimethadione is an oxazolidinedione anticonvulsant used in the treatment of petit mal epilepsy. Several case histories have suggested a phenotype for a fetal trimethadione syndrome of congenital malformations (1–7). The use of trimethadione in nine families was associated with a 69% incidence of congenital defects— 25 malformed children from 36 pregnancies. Three of these families reported five normal births after the anticonvulsant medication was stopped (1, 4). The incidence of fetal loss in these families was also increased over that seen in the general epileptic population. Because trimethadione has demonstrated both clinical and experimental fetal risk greater than other anticonvulsants, its use should be abandoned in favor of other medications used in the treatment of petit mal epilepsy (8–11).

Features of Fetal Trimethadione Syndrome (25 Cases)

Feature	No.*	%	Feature	No.*	%
Growth:			Cardiac:		
Prenatal deficiency	8	32	Septal defect	5	20
Postnatal deficiency	6	24	Not stated	4	16
Performance (19 cases):			Patent ductus arteriosus	4	16
Mental retardation	7	28	Limb:		
Vision (myopia)	5	20	Simian crease	7	28
Speech disorder	4	16	Malformed hand	2	8
Impaired hearing	2	8	Clubfoot	1	4
Craniofacial:			Genitourinary:		
Low-set, cupped or			Kidney and ureter		
abnormal ears	18	72	abnormalities	5	20
High arched or cleft			Inguinal hernia(s)	3	12
lip and/or palate	16	64	Hypospadias	3	12

Craniofacial, cont'd:			Genitourinary, cont'd:		
Microcephaly	6	24	Ambiguous genitalia	2	8
Irregular teeth	4	16	Clitoral hypertrophy	1	4
Epicanthic folds	3	12	Imperforate anus	1	4
Broad nasal bridge	3	12	Other:		
Strabismus	3	12	Tracheoesophageal		
Low hairline	2	8	fistula	3	12
Facial hemangiomata	1	4	Esophageal atresia	2	8
Unusual facies	3	12			
(details not given)			* Not mutually exclusive.		

Breast Feeding Summary

No data available.

References

1. German J, Kowan A, Ehlers KH. Trimethadione and human teratogenesis. Teratology 1970;3:349–62.
2. Zackae EH, Mellman WJ, Neiderer B, Hanson JW. The fetal trimethadione syndrome. J Pediatr 1975;87:280–4.
3. Nichols MM. Fetal anomalies following maternal trimethadione ingestion. J Pediatr 1973;82:885–6.
4. Feldman GL, Weaver DD, Lourien EW. The fetal trimethadione syndrome. Report of an additional family and further delineation of this syndrome. Am J Dis Child 1977;131:1389–92.
5. Rosen RC, Lightner ES. Phenotypic malformations in association with maternal trimethadione therapy. J Pediatr 1978;92:240–4.
6. Zellweger H. Anticonvulsants during pregnancy: a danger to the developing fetus? Clin Pediatr 1974;13:338–45.
7. Rischbieth RH. Troxidone (trimethadione) embryopathy: case report with review of the literature. Clin Exp Neurol 1979;16:251–6.
8. Fabro S, Brown NA. Teratogenic potential of anticonvulsants. N Engl J Med 1979;300:1280–1.
9. National Institutes of Health. Anticonvulsants found to have teratogenic potential. JAMA 1981;245:36.
10. Dansky L, Andermann E, Andermann F. Major congenital malformations in the offspring of epileptic patients. Genetic and environmental risk factors. In *Epilepsy, Pregnancy and the Child*. Proceedings of a Workshop, Berlin, September 1980. New York:Raven Press, 1981.
11. Nakane Y, Okuma T, Takahashi R, et al. Multi-institutional study on the teratogenicity and fetal toxicity of antiepileptic drugs: a report of a collaborative study group in Japan. Epilepsia 1980;21:663–80.

Name: # TRIMETHAPHAN

Class: **Antihypertensive** Risk Factor: **C**

Fetal Risk Summary

No reports linking the use of trimethaphan with congenital defects have been located. Trimethaphan, a short acting ganglionic blocker which requires continuous infusion for therapeutic effect, has been studied in pregnant patients (1, 2). It is not recommended for use in pregnancy because of adverse hemodynamic effects (3). The drug is not effective in the control of hypertension in toxemic patients (1–3).

Breast Feeding Summary

No data available.

References

1. Assali NS, Douglas RA Jr, Suyemoto R. Observations on the hemodynamic properties of a thiophanium derivative, Ro 2-2222 (Arfonad), in human subjects. Circulation 1953;8:62–9.
2. Assali NS, Suyemoto R. The place of the hydrazinophthalazine and thiophanium compounds in the management of hypertensive complications of pregnancy. Am J Obstet Gynecol 1952;64:1021–36.
3. Assali NS. Hemodynamic effects of hypotensive drugs used in pregnancy. Obstet Gynecol Surv 1954;9:776–94.

Name: **TRIMETHOBENZAMIDE**

Class: **Antiemetic**   Risk Factor: **C**

Fetal Risk Summary

Trimethobenzamide has been used in pregnancy to treat nausea and vomiting (1, 2). No adverse effects in the fetus were observed. In a third study, 193 patients were treated with trimethobenzamide in the 1st trimester (3). The incidence of severe congenital defects at 1 month, 1 year, and 5 years were 2.6, 2.6, and 5.8%, respectively. The 5.8% incidence was increased over that in nontreated controls (3.2%) ($p < 0.05$), but other factors, including the use of other antiemetics in some patients, may have contributed to the results. The authors concluded that the risk of congenital malformations with trimethobenzamide was low.

Breast Feeding Summary

No data available.

References

1. Breslow S, Belafsky HA, Shangold JE, Hirsch LM, Stahl MB. Antiemetic effect of trimethobenzamide in pregnant patients. Clin Med 1961;8:2153–5.
2. Winters HS. Antiemetics in nausea and vomiting of pregnancy. Obstet Gynecol 1961;18:753–6.
3. Milkovich L, van den Berg BJ. An evaluation of the teratogenicity of certain antinauseant drugs. Am J Obstet Gynecol 1976;125:244–8.

Name: **TRIMETHOPRIM**

Class: **Anti-infective**   Risk Factor: **C$_M$**

Fetal Risk Summary

Trimethoprim is available as a single agent and in combination with various sulfonamides (see also Sulfonamides). The drug crosses the placenta, producing similar levels in fetal and maternal serum and in amniotic fluid (1–3). Because trimethoprim is a folate antagonist, caution has been advocated for its use in pregnancy (4, 5). However, case reports and placebo-controlled trials involving several hundred patients have failed to demonstrate an increase in fetal abnormalities (6–11).

A case of Niikawa-Kuroki syndrome has been described in a non-Japanese girl whose mother had a viral and bacterial infection during the 2nd month of pregnancy (12). The bacterial infection was treated with trimethoprim-sulfamethoxazole. The syndrome is characterized by mental and growth retardation and craniofacial malformations (12). The etiology of the defects in this patient were not known, although the infections and/or the drug therapy may have played a role.

Sulfa-trimethoprim combinations have been shown to cause a drop in the sperm count after 1 month of continuous treatment in males (13). Decreases varied between 7 and 88%. The authors theorized that trimethoprim deprived the spermatogenetic cells of active folate by inhibiting dihydrofolate reductase.

No interaction between trimethoprim-sulfamethoxazole and oral contraceptives was found in one study (14). Short courses of the anti-infective combination are unlikely to affect contraceptive control.

Breast Feeding Summary

Trimethoprim is excreted into breast milk in low concentrations. Following doses of 160 mg twice daily for 5 days, milk concentrations varied between 1.2 and 2.4 μg/ml (average 1.8) with peak levels occurring at 2–3 hours (15). No adverse effects were reported in the infants. Nearly identical results were found in a study with 50 patients (16). Mean milk levels were 2.0 μg/ml, representing a milk:plasma ratio of 1.25. The authors concluded that these levels represented a negligible risk to the suckling infant. The American Academy of Pediatrics considers trimethoprim compatible with breast-feeding (17).

References

1. Ylikorkala O, Sjostedt E, Jarvinen PA, Tikkanen R, Raines T. Trimethoprim-sulfonamide combination administered orally and intravaginally in the 1st trimester of pregnancy: its absorption into serum and transfer to amniotic fluid. Acta Obstet Gynecol Scand 1973;52:229–34.
2. Reid DWJ, Caille G, Kaufmann NR. Maternal and transplacental kinetics of trimethoprim and sulfamethoxazole, separately and in combination. Can Med Assoc J 1975;112:67s–72s.
3. Reeves DS, Wilkinson PJ. The pharmacokinetics of trimethoprim and trimethoprim/sulfonamide combinations, including penetration into body tissues. Infection 1979;7(Suppl 4):S330–41.
4. McEwen LM. Trimethoprim/sulphamethoxazole mixture in pregnancy. Br Med J 1971;4:490–1.
5. Smithells RW. Co-trimoxazole in pregnancy. Lancet 1983;2:1142.
6. Williams JD, Condie AP, Brumfitt W, Reeves DS. The treatment of bacteriuria in pregnant women with sulphamethoxazole and trimethoprim. Postgrad Med J 1969;45(Suppl):71–6.
7. Ochoa AG. Trimethoprim and sulfamethoxazole in pregnancy. JAMA 1971;217:1244.
8. Brumfitt W, Pursell R. Double-blind trial to compare ampicillin, cephalexin, co-trimoxazole, and trimethoprim in treatment of urinary infection. Br Med J 1972;2:673–6.
9. Brumfitt W, Pursell R. Trimethoprim/sulfamethoxazole in the treatment of bacteriuria in women. J Infect Dis 1973;128(Suppl):S657–63.
10. Brumfitt W, Pursell R. Trimethoprim/sulfamethoxazole in the treatment of urinary infection. Med J Aust 1973;1(Suppl):44–8.
11. Bailey RR. Single-dose antibacterial treatment for bacteriuria in pregnancy. Drugs 1984;27:183–6.
12. Koutras A, Fisher S. Niikawa-Kuroki syndrome: a new malformation syndrome of postnatal dwarfism, mental retardation, unusual face, and protruding ears. J Pediatr 1982;101:417–9.
13. Murdia A, Mathur V, Kothari LK, Singh KP. Sulpha-trimethoprim combinations and male fertility. Lancet 1978;2:375–6.
14. Grimmer SFM, Allen WL, Back DJ, Breckenridge AM, Orme M, Tjia J. The effect of cotrimoxazole on oral contraceptive steroids in women. Contraception 1983;28:53–9.
15. Arnauld R, Soutoul JH, Gallier J, Borderon JC, Borderon E. A study of the passage of trimethoprim into the maternal milk. Quest Med 1972;25:959–64.
16. Miller RD, Salter AJ. The passage of trimethoprim/sulphamethoxazole into breast milk and its significance. In Daikos GK, ed., *Progress in Chemotherapy*, Proceedings of the Eighth International Congress of Chemotherapy, Athens, 1973. Athens:Hellenic Society for Chemotherapy, 1974:687–91.
17. Committee of Drugs, American Academy of Pediatrics. The transfer of drugs and other chemicals into human breast milk. Pediatrics 1983;72:375–83.

Name: **TRIPELENNAMINE**

Class: **Antihistamine**   Risk Factor: **B**

Fetal Risk Summary

The Collaborative Perinatal Project monitored 50,282 mother-child pairs, 100 of which were exposed to tripelennamine in the 1st trimester (1). For use anytime during pregnancy, 490 exposures were recorded (2). In neither case was evidence found to suggest a relationship to major or minor malformations.

A report from New Orleans described 24 infants born of mothers using the intravenous combination of pentazocine and tripelennamine ('T's and Blue's) (3). Doses were unknown but probably ranged from 200 to 600 mg of pentazocine and 100 to 250 mg of tripelennamine. Six of the newborns were exposed early in pregnancy. Birth weights for 11 of the infants were less than 2,500 g, nine of these were premature (less than 37 weeks) and two were small for gestational age. Daily or weekly exposure throughout pregnancy produced withdrawal symptoms, occurring within 7 days of birth, in 15 of 16 infants. Withdrawal was thought to be due to pentazocine, but antihistamine withdrawal has been reported (see Diphenhydramine). Thirteen of 15 infants became asymptomatic 3–11 days following onset of withdrawal but in two, symptoms persisted for up to 6 months.

Breast Feeding Summary

Tripelennamine is excreted into bovine milk, but human studies have not been reported (4). The manufacturer considers the drug contraindicated in the nursing mother, possibly due to the increased sensitivity of newborn or premature infants to antihistamines (5). However, the American Academy of Pediatrics considers tripelennamine compatible with breast-feeding (6).

References

1. Heinonen OP, Slone D, Shapiro S. *Birth Defects and Drugs in Pregnancy*. Littleton:Publishing Sciences Group 1977:323–4.
2. *Ibid*, 436–7.
3. Dunn DW, Reynolds J. Neonatal withdrawal symptoms associated with 'T's and Blue's (pentazocine and tripelennamine). Am J Dis Child 1982;136:644–5.
4. O'Brien TE. Excretion of drugs in human milk. Am J Hosp Pharm 1974;31:844–54.
5. Product information. PBZ. Geigy Pharmaceuticals, 1985.
6. Committee on Drugs, American Academy of Pediatrics. The transfer of drugs and other chemicals into human breast milk. Pediatrics 1983;72:375–83.

Name: **TRIPROLIDINE**

Class: **Antihistamine**   Risk Factor: **C$_M$**

Fetal Risk Summary

No reports linking the use of triprolidine with congenital defects have been located. The Collaborative Perinatal Project monitored 50,282 mother-child pairs, 16 of which had 1st trimester exposure to triprolidine (1). From this small sample, no evidence was found to suggest a relationship to large categories of major or minor malformations or to individual malformations.

In a 1971 study, infants and mothers who had ingested antihistamines during the 1st trimester actually had fewer abnormalities when compared to controls (2). Triprolidine was the third most commonly used antihistamine. The manufacturer claims that in over 20 years of marketing the drug they have not received any reports of triprolidine teratogenicity (3). Their animal studies have also been negative.

Breast Feeding Summary

No data available.

References

1. Heinonen OP, Slone D, Shapiro S. *Birth Defects and Drugs in Pregnancy*. Littleton:Publishing Sciences Group, 1977:323.
2. Nelson MM, Forfar JO. Associations between drugs administered during pregnancy and congenital abnormalities of the fetus. Br Med J 1971;1:523–7.
3. Frosolono MF, Burroughs Wellcome, 1980. Personal communication.

Name: **TROLEANDOMYCIN**

Class: **Antibiotic** Risk Factor: **C**

Fetal Risk Summary

Troleandomycin is the triacetyl ester of oleandomycin (see Oleandomycin).

Breast Feeding Summary

See Oleandomycin.

Name: **TYROPANOATE**

Class: **Diagnostic** Risk Factor: **D**

Fetal Risk Summary

Tyropanoate contains a high concentration of organically bound iodine. See Diatrizoate for possible effects on the fetus and newborn.

Breast Feeding Summary

See Potassium Iodide.

Name: **UREA**

Class: **Diuretic**   Risk Factor: **C**

Fetal Risk Summary

Urea is an osmotic diuretic that is used primarily to treat cerebral edema. Topical formulations for skin disorders are also available. No reports of its use in pregnancy following intravenous, oral, or topical administration have been located. Urea, given by intra-amniotic injection, has been used for the induction of abortion (1).

Breast Feeding Summary

No data available.

References

1. Ware A, ed. *Martindale: The Extra Pharmacopoeia*, ed 27. London:The Pharmaceutical Press, 1977:572.

Name: **UROKINASE**

Class: **Thrombolytic**   Risk Factor: **B$_M$**

Fetal Risk Summary

No reports of the use of urokinase in human pregnancy have been located. The drug is not teratogenic in rats or mice (1).

Breast Feeding Summary

No data available.

References

1. Shepard TH. *Catalog of Teratogenic Agents*, ed 3. Baltimore:The Johns Hopkins University Press, 1980:342.

Name: **VACCINE, BCG**

Class: **Vaccine**   Risk Factor: **C**

Fetal Risk Summary

BCG vaccine is a live, attenuated bacteria vaccine used to provide immunity to tuberculosis (1, 2). The risk to the fetus from maternal vaccination is unknown. However, since it is a live preparation, the vaccine should probably not be used during pregnancy (2).

Breast Feeding Summary

No data available.

References

1. American Hospital Formulary Service. *Drug Information 1985*. Bethesda:American Society of Hospital Pharmacists, 1985:1534–6.
2. Amstey MS. Vaccination in pregnancy. Clin Obstet Gynaecol 1983;10:13–22.

Name: **VACCINE, CHOLERA**

Class: **Vaccine**   Risk Factor: **C**

Fetal Risk Summary

Cholera vaccine is a killed bacteria vaccine (1, 2). Cholera during pregnancy may result in significant morbidity and mortality to the mother and the fetus, particularly during the 3rd trimester (1). The risk to the fetus from maternal vaccination is unknown. The American College of Obstetricians and Gynecologists Technical Bulletin No. 64 recommends the vaccine be given during pregnancy to meet international travel requirements (1).

Breast Feeding Summary

Maternal vaccination with cholera vaccine has increased specific IgA antibody titers in breast milk (3). In a second study, cholera vaccine (whole cell plus toxoid) was administered to six lactating mothers, resulting in a significant rise in milk anti-cholera toxin IgA titers in five of the patients (4). Milk from three of these five mothers also had a significant increase in anti-cholera toxin IgG titers.

References

1. ACOG Technical Bulletin, No. 64, May 1982.
2. Amstey MS. Vaccination in pregnancy. Clin Obstet Gynaecol 1983;10:13–22.

3. Svennerholm AM, Holmgren J, Hanson LA, Lindblad BS, Quereshi F, Rahimtoola RJ. Boosting of secretory IgA antibody responses in man by parenteral cholera vaccination. Scand J Immunol 1977;6:1345–49.
4. Merson MH, Black RE, Sack DA, Svennerholm AM, Holmgren J. Maternal cholera immunisation and secretory IgA in breast milk. Lancet 1980;1:931–2.

Name: **VACCINE, *ESCHERICHIA COLI***

Class: **Vaccine**   Risk Factor: **C**

Fetal Risk Summary

Escherichia coli vaccine is a nonpathogenic strain of bacteria used experimentally as a vaccine. Two reports of its use (strains O111 and 083) in pregnant women in labor or waiting for the onset of labor have been located (1, 2). The vaccines were given to these patients in an attempt to produce antimicrobial activity in their colostrum. No adverse effects in the newborn were noted.

Breast Feeding Summary

E. coli (strains O111 and 083) vaccines were given to mothers in labor or waiting for the onset of labor (1,2). Antibodies against *E. coli* were found in the colostrum of 7 of 47 (strain 0111) and 3 of 3 (strain 083) treated mothers but only in 1 of 101 controls. No adverse effects were noted in the nursing infants.

References

1. Dluholucky S, Siragy P, Dolezel P, Svac J, Bolgac A. Antimicrobial activity of colostrum after administering killed Escherichia coli O111 vaccine orally to expectant mothers. Arch Dis Child 1980;55:558–60.
2. Goldblum RM, Ahlstedt S, Carlsson B, Hanson LA, Jodal U, Lidin-Janson G, Sohl-Akerlund A. Antibody-forming cells in human colostrum after oral immunisation. Nature 1975;257:797–9.

Name: **VACCINE, HEPATITIS B**

Class: **Vaccine**   Risk Factor: **C$_M$**

Fetal Risk Summary

Hepatitis B vaccine is a killed virus (surface antigen HBsAg) vaccine (1, 2). The risk to the fetus from maternal vaccination is unknown. Preexposure prophylaxis is indicated for persons at high risk for exposure to the disease (1). Pregnancy probably does not change this recommendation.

Breast Feeding Summary

No data available.

References

1. American Hospital Formulary Service. *Drug Information 1985*. Bethesda:American Society of Hospital Pharmacists, 1985:1537–41.
2. Amstey MS. Vaccination in pregnancy. Clin Obstet Gynaecol 1983;10:13–22.

Name: **VACCINE, INFLUENZA**

Class: **Vaccine**
Risk Factor: **C**

Fetal Risk Summary

Influenza vaccine is an inactivated virus vaccine (1). Influenza during pregnancy may potentially result in an increased rate of spontaneous abortions (1). The risk to the fetus from maternal vaccination is unknown. The American College of Obstetricians and Gynecologists Technical Bulletin No. 64 recommends the vaccine be given only to pregnant women with serious underlying diseases (1). Public health officials should be consulted for current recommendations (1).

Breast Feeding Summary

No data available. Maternal vaccination is not thought to present any risk to the nursing infant (2).

References

1. ACOG Technical Bulletin, No. 64, May 1982.
2. Kilbourne ED. Questions and answers. Artificial influenza immunization of nursing mothers not harmful. JAMA 1973;226:87.

Name: **VACCINE, MEASLES**

Class: **Vaccine**
Risk Factor: **X**

Fetal Risk Summary

Measles (rubeola) vaccine is a live attenuated virus vaccine (1, 2). Measles occurring during pregnancy may result in significant maternal morbidity, an increased abortion rate, and congenital malformations (1). Although a fetal risk from the vaccine has not been confirmed, the vaccine should not be used during pregnancy because fetal infection with the attenuated viruses may occur (1, 2). The American College of Obstetricians and Gynecologists Technical Bulletin No. 64 lists the vaccine as contraindicated in pregnancy (1). (See also Vaccine, Rubella).

Breast Feeding Summary

No data available.

References

1. ACOG Technical Bulletin, No. 64, May 1982.
2. Amstey MS. Vaccination in pregnancy. Clin Obstet Gynaecol 1983;10:13–22.

Name: **VACCINE, MENINGOCOCCUS**

Class: **Vaccine**   Risk Factor: **C**

Fetal Risk Summary

Meningococcus vaccine is a killed bacteria (cell wall) vaccine (1, 2). The risk to the fetus from vaccination during pregnancy is unknown (1). In one study, vaccination resulted in transfer of maternal antibodies to the fetus, but the transfer was irregular and was not dependent on maternal titer or the period in pregnancy when vaccination occurred (3). The American College of Obstetricians and Gynecologists Technical Bulletin No. 64 recommends the vaccine be used during pregnancy only when the risk of maternal infection is high (1).

Breast Feeding Summary

No data available.

References

1. ACOG Technical Bulletin, No. 64, May 1982.
2. Amstey MS. Vaccination in pregnancy. Clin Obstet Gynaecol 1983;10:13–22.
3. Carvalho ADA, Giampaglia CMS, Kimura H, Pereira OADC, Farhat CK, Neves JC, Prandini R, Carvalho EDS, Zarvos AM. Maternal and infant antibody response to meningococcal vaccination in pregnancy. Lancet 1977;2:809–11.

Name: **VACCINE, MUMPS**

Class: **Vaccine**   Risk Factor: **X**

Fetal Risk Summary

Mumps vaccine is a live attenuated virus vaccine (1, 2). Mumps occurring during pregnancy may result in an increased rate of 1st trimester abortion, and there is a questionable association with fibroelastosis in the newborn (1). Although a fetal risk from the vaccine has not been confirmed, the vaccine should not be used during pregnancy because fetal infection with the attenuated viruses may occur (1, 2). The American College of Obstetricians and Gynecologists Technical Bulletin No. 64 lists the vaccine as contraindicated in pregnancy (1).

Breast Feeding Summary

No data available.

References

1. ACOG Technical Bulletin, No. 64, May 1982.
2. Amstey MS. Vaccination in pregnancy. Clin Obstet Gynaecol 1983;10:13–22.

Name: **VACCINE, PLAGUE**

Class: **Vaccine**   Risk Factor: **C**

Fetal Risk Summary

Plague vaccine is a killed bacteria vaccine (1, 2). The risk to the fetus from vaccination during pregnancy is unknown (1). The American College of Obstetricians and Gynecologists Technical Bulletin No. 64 recommends the vaccine be used in pregnancy only for exposed persons (1).

Breast Feeding Summary

No data available.

References

1. ACOG Technical Bulletin, No. 64, May 1982.
2. Amstey MS. Vaccination in pregnancy. Clin Obstet Gynaecol 1983;10:13–22.

Name: **VACCINE, PNEUMOCOCCAL POLYVALENT**

Class: **Vaccine**   Risk Factor: **C**

Fetal Risk Summary

Pneumococcal vaccine is a killed bacteria (cell wall) vaccine (1, 2). The risk to the fetus from vaccination during pregnancy is unknown (1). The American College of Obstetricians and Gynecologists Technical Bulletin No. 64 recommends the vaccine be used in pregnancy only for high-risk patients (1).

Breast Feeding Summary

No data available.

References

1. ACOG Technical Bulletin, No. 64, May 1982.
2. Amstey MS. Vaccination in pregnancy. Clin Obstet Gynaecol 1983;10:13–22.

Name: **VACCINE, POLIOVIRUS INACTIVATED**

Class: **Vaccine**   Risk Factor: **C**

Fetal Risk Summary

Poliovirus vaccine inactivated (Salk vaccine, IPV) is an inactivated virus vaccine administered by injection (1, 2). Although fetal damage may occur when the mother contracts the disease during pregnancy, the risk to the fetus from the vaccine is unknown (1). The American College of Obstetricians and Gynecologists Technical Bulletin No. 64 recommends use of the vaccine during pregnancy only if an increased risk of exposure exists (1). The oral vaccine (Sabin vaccine, OPV) is a live, attenuated virus strain and probably should not be used in the pregnant woman (2). However, if immediate protection against poliomyelitis is needed, the Immunization Practices Advisory Committee (ACIP) recommends the oral vaccine (3).

Breast Feeding Summary

No data available.

References

1. ACOG Technical Bulletin, No. 64, May 1982.
2. Amstey MS. Vaccination in pregnancy. Clin Obstet Gynaecol 1983;10:13–22.
3. Recommendation of the Immunization Practices Advisory Committee (ACIP); Poliomyelitis prevention. MMWR 1982;31:22–6, 31–4.

Name: **VACCINE, POLIOVIRUS LIVE**

Class: **Vaccine**   Risk Factor: **C**

Fetal Risk Summary

Poliovirus vaccine live (Sabin vaccine, OPV) is a live, attenuated virus strain vaccine administered orally (1, 2). Although fetal damage may occur when the mother contracts the disease during pregnancy, the risk to the fetus from the vaccine is unknown (1). If vaccination is required during pregnancy, one author has recommended use of the inactivated virus vaccine (Salk vaccine, IPV) to reduce the risk of potential fetal and neonatal infection (2). When immediate protection is needed, the Immunization Practices Advisory Committee (ACIP) recommends the oral (OPV) vaccine (3).

Breast Feeding Summary

Human milk contains poliovirus antibodies in direct relation to titers found in the mother's serum. When oral poliovirus vaccine (Sabin vaccine, OPV) is administered to the breast-fed infant in the immediate neonatal period, these antibodies, which are highest in colostrum, may prevent infection and development of subsequent immunity to wild poliovirus (4–15). To prevent inhibition of the vaccine, breast-feeding should not take place 6 hours before and after administration of the vaccine, although some authors recommend shorter times (10–14).

In the United States, the ACIP and the Committee on Infectious Diseases of the American Academy of Pediatrics do not recommend vaccination before 6 weeks of age (3, 16). At this age or older, the effect of the oral vaccine is not inhibited by breast-feeding, and no special instructions or planned feeding schedules are required (3, 16–20).

References

1. ACOG Technical Bulletin, No. 64, May 1982.
2. Amstey MS. Vaccination in pregnancy. Clin Obstet Gynaecol 1983;10:13–22.
3. Recommendation of the Immunization Practices Advisory Committee (ACIP); Poliomyelitis prevention. MMWR 1982;31:22–6, 31–4.

4. Lepow ML, Warren RJ, Gray N, Ingram VG, Robbins FC. Effect of Sabin type I poliomyelitis vaccine administered by mouth to newborn infants. N Engl J Med 1961;264:1071–8.
5. Holguin AH, Reeves JS, Gelfand HM. Immunization of infants with the Sabin oral poliovirus vaccine. Am J Public Health 1962;52:600–10.
6. Sabin AB, Fieldsteel AH. Antipoliomyelitic activity of human and bovine colostrum and milk. Pediatrics 1962;29:105–15.
7. Sabin AB, Michaels RH, Krugman S, Eiger ME, Berman PH, Warren J. Effect of oral poliovirus vaccine in newborn children. I. Excretion of virus after ingestion of large doses of type I or of mixture of all three types, in relation to level of placentally transmitted antibody. Pediatrics 1963;31:623–40.
8. Warren RJ, Lepow ML, Bartsch GE, Robbins FC. The relationship of maternal antibody, breast feeding, and age to the susceptibility of newborn infants to infection with attenuated polioviruses. Pediatrics 1964;34:4–13.
9. Plotkin SA, Katz M, Brown RE, Pagano JS. Oral poliovirus vaccination in newborn African infants. The inhibitory effect of breast feeding. Am J Dis Child 1966;111:27–30.
10. Katz M, Plotkin SA. Oral polio immunization of the newborn infant; a possible method for overcoming interference by ingested antibodies. J Pediatr 1968;73:267–70.
11. Adcock E, Greene H. Poliovirus antibodies in breast-fed infants. Lancet 1971;2:662–3.
12. Anonymous. Sabin vaccine in breast-fed infants. Med J Aust 1972;2:175.
13. John TJ. The effect of breast-feeding on the antibody response of infants to trivalent oral poliovirus vaccine. J Pediatr 1974;84:307.
14. Plotkin SA, Katz M. Administration of oral polio vaccine in relation to time of breast feeding. J Pediatr 1974;84:309.
15. Deforest A, Smith DS. Reply. J Pediatr 1974;84:308.
16. Kelein JO, Brunell PA, Cherry JD, Fulginiti VA, eds. Report of the Committee on Infectious Diseases, ed 19. Evanston:American Academy of Pediatrics, 1982:208.
17. Kim-Farley R, Brink E, Orenstein W, Bart K. Vaccination and breast-feeding. JAMA 1982;248:2451–2.
18. Deforest A, Parker PB, DiLiberti JH, Yates HT Jr, Sibinga MS, Smith DS. The effect of breast-feeding on the antibody response of infants to trivalent oral poliovirus vaccine. J Pediatr 1973;83:93–5.
19. John TJ, Devarajan LV, Luther L, Vijayarathnam P. Effect of breast-feeding on seroresponse of infants to oral poliovirus vaccination. Pediatrics 1976;57:47–53.
20. Welsh J, May JT. Breast-feeding and trivalent oral polio vaccine. J Pediatr 1979;95:333.

Name: **VACCINE, RABIES HUMAN**

Class: **Vaccine**   Risk Factor: **C**

Fetal Risk Summary

Rabies vaccine human is a killed virus vaccine (1, 2). Since rabies is nearly 100% fatal if contracted, the vaccine should be given for postexposure prophylaxis (1, 2). Fetal risk from the vaccine is unknown (1). Two reports that describe the use of the vaccine during pregnancy have been located (3, 4). Passive immunity was found in one newborn (titer >1:50) but was lost by 1 year of age (3). No adverse effects from the vaccine were noted in the newborn. The mother had not delivered at the time of the report in the second case (4).

Breast Feeding Summary

No data available.

References

1. ACOG Technical Bulletin, No. 64, May 1982.

2. Amstey MS. Vaccination in pregnancy. Clin Obstet Gynaecol 1983;10:13–22.
3. Varner MW, McGuinness GA, Galask RP. Rabies vaccination in pregnancy. Am J Obstet Gynecol 1982;143:717–8.
4. Klietmann W, Domres B, Cox JH. Rabies post-exposure treatment and side-effects in man using HDC (MRC 5) vaccine. Dev Biol Stand 1978;40:109–13.

Name: **VACCINE, RUBELLA**

Class: **Vaccine**   Risk Factor: **X**

Fetal Risk Summary

Rubella (German measles) vaccine is a live, attenuated virus vaccine (1, 2). Rubella occurring during pregnancy may result in the congenital rubella syndrome (CRS). The greatest risk period for viremia and fetal defects is 1 week prior to and 4 weeks after conception (3). The United States Department of Health and Human Services Centers for Disease Control (CDC) defines CRS as any two complications from list A or one complication from list A plus one from list B (3):

LIST A
      Cataracts/congenital glaucoma
      Congenital heart disease
      Loss of hearing
      Pigmentary retinopathy
LIST B
      Purpura
      Splenomegaly
      Jaundice (onset within 24 hours of birth)
      Microcephaly
      Mental retardation
      Meningoencephalitis
      Radiolucent bone disease

Prior to April 1979, the CDC collected data on 538 women vaccinated during pregnancy with either the Cendehill or HPV-77 vaccines (3). A total of 149 of these women were known to be susceptible at the time of vaccination and the outcome of pregnancy was known for 143 (96%). No evidence of CRS or other maternal/fetal complication was found in any of these cases or in an additional 196 infants exposed during pregnancy (3). Eight infants had serologic evidence of intrauterine infection after maternal vaccination, but follow-up for 2–7 years revealed no problems attributable to CRS.

Since January 1979, only RA 27/3 rubella vaccine has been available in the United States. In the United States between April 1979 and December 1984, a total of 592 women vaccinated during pregnancy with RA 27/3 have been reported to the CDC (4). The outcome of these pregnancies were:

Total Vaccinated (4/79–12/84)	592
Susceptible at vaccination	184
Live births	144 (2 sets of twins)
Spontaneous abortions/stillbirths	4

Induced abortions	28
Outcome unknown	10
Immune/unknown at vaccination	408
Live births	347 (1 set of twins)
Spontaneous abortions/stillbirths	9
Induced abortions	24
Outcome unknown	29

Evidence of subclinical infection was found in 1 of 33 fetuses/infants (3%) from susceptible mothers and in approximately 1% of fetuses/infants from 267 mothers with either immune or unknown immune status (4). As with the earlier strains of rubella vaccine, no defects compatible with CRS were found in any of fetuses/ infants where the outcome was known (4). Examinations up to 29 months after birth have revealed normal growth and development (4).

Although no defects attributable to rubella vaccine have been reported, the CDC calculates the theoretical risk of CRS following vaccination to be as high as 2.6%, still considerably lower than the 20% or greater risk associated with wild rubella virus infection during the 1st trimester (4). Because a risk does exist, the use of the vaccine in pregnancy is contraindicated (1–4). However, if vaccination does occur within 3 months of conception or during pregnancy, the actual risk is considered to be negligible and, in itself, should not be an indication to terminate the pregnancy (3, 4).

Breast Feeding Summary

Vaccination of susceptible women with rubella vaccine in the immediate postpartum period is recommended by the American College of Obstetricians and Gynecolo-gists Technical Bulletin No. 64 and the United States Public Health Service Immunization Practices Advisory Committee (1, 5). A large number of these women will breast-feed their newborns. Although two studies failed to find evidence of the attenuated virus in milk, subsequent reports have demonstrated transfer (6–10).

In one case, the mother noted rash and adenopathy 12 days after vaccination with the HPV-77 vaccine on the first postpartum day (8). Rubella virus was isolated from her breast milk and from the infant's throat (8). A significant level of rubella specific cell-mediated immunity was found in the infant, but no detectable serologic response as measured by rubella hemagglutination inhibition antibody titers (8). No adverse effects were noted in the infant. In a second case report, a 13-day-old breast-fed infant developed rubella about 11 days after maternal vaccination with HPV-77 (11). It could not be determined if the infant was infected by virus transmission via the milk (12, 13). Nine (69%) of 13 lactating women given either HPV-77 or RA 27/3 vaccine in the immediate postpartum period shed virus in their milk (9). In another report by these same researchers, 11 (68%) of 16 vaccinated women shed rubella virus or virus antigen in their milk (10). No adverse effects or symptoms of clinical disease were observed in the infants.

References

1. ACOG Technical Bulletin, No. 64, May 1982.
2. Amstey MS. Vaccination in pregnancy. Clin Obstet Gynaecol 1983;10:13–22.
3. Centers For Disease Control, U.S. Department of Health and Human Services. Rubella vaccination during pregnancy—United States, 1971–1982. MMWR 1983;32:429–32.
4. Preblud SR, Williams NM. Fetal risk associated with rubella vaccine: implications for vaccination of susceptible women. Obstet Gynecol 1985;66:121–3.

5. American Hospital Formulary Service. *Drug Information 1985*. Bethesda:American Society of Hospital Pharmacists, 1985:1560–3.
6. Isacson P, Kehrer AF, Wilson H, Williams S. Comparative study of live, attenuated rubella virus vaccines during the immediate puerperium. Obstet Gynecol 1971;37:332–7.
7. Grillner L, Hedstrom CE, Bergstrom H, Forssman L, Rigner A, Lycke E. Vaccination against rubella of newly delivered women. Scand J Infect Dis 1973;5:237–41.
8. Buimovici-Klein E, Hite RL, Byrne T, Cooper LZ. Isolation of rubella virus in milk after postpartum innumization. J Pediatr 1977;91:939–41.
9. Losonsky GA, Fishaut JM, Strussenberg J, Ogra PL. Effect of immunization against rubella on lactation products. I. Development and characterization of specific immunologic reactivity in breast milk. J Infect Dis 1982;145:654–60.
10. Losonsky GA, Fishaut JM, Strussenberg J, Ogra PL. Effect of immunization against rubella on lactation products. II. Maternal-neonatal interactions. J Infect Dis 1982;145:661–6.
11. Landes RD, Bass JW, Millunchick EW, Oetgen WJ. Neonatal rubella following postpartum maternal immunization. J Pediatr 1980;97:465–7.
12. Lerman SJ. Neonatal rubella following maternal immunization. J Pediatr 1981;98:668.
13. Bass JW, Landes RD. Neonatal rubella following maternal immunization. Reply. J Pediatr 1981;98:668–9.

Name: **VACCINE, SMALLPOX**

Class: **Vaccine**   Risk Factor: **X**

Fetal Risk Summary

Smallpox vaccine is a live, attenuated virus vaccine (1, 2). Although smallpox infection had a high mortality rate, the disease has been largely eradicated from the world (1, 3). Vaccination during pregnancy between 3 and 24 weeks has resulted in fetal death (2, 3). Based on the above information, smallpox vaccine is contraindicated during pregnancy (1–3).

Breast Feeding Summary

No data available.

References

1. Amstey MS. Vaccination in pregnancy. Clin Obstet Gynaecol 1983;10:13–22.
2. American Hospital Formulary Service. *Drug Information 1985*. Bethesda:American Society of Hospital Pharmacists, 1985:1563–5.
3. Hart RJC. Immunization. Clin Obstet Gynaecol 1981;8:421–30.

Name: **VACCINE, TULAREMIA**

Class: **Vaccine**   Risk Factor: **C**

Fetal Risk Summary

Tularemia vaccine is a live, attenuated bacteria vaccine (1, 2). Tularemia is a serious infectious disease occurring primarily in laboratory personnel, rabbit handlers, and forest workers (1). The risk to the fetus from the vaccine is unknown. One report described vaccination in a woman early in the 1st trimester (2). No adverse effects were observed in the term infant or at 1-year follow-up. Since tularemia is a severe disease, preexposure prophylaxis of indicated persons should occur regardless of pregnancy (1).

Breast Feeding Summary

No data available.

References

1. Amstey MS. Vaccination in pregnancy. Clin Obstet Gynaecol 1983;10:13–22.
2. Albrecht RC, Cefalo RC, O'Brien WF. Tularemia immunization in early pregnancy. Am J Obstet Gynecol 1980;138:1226–7.

Name: **VACCINE, TYPHOID**
Class: **Vaccine** Risk Factor: **C**

Fetal Risk Summary

Typhoid vaccine is a killed bacteria vaccine (1, 2). Typhoid is a serious infectious disease with high morbidity and mortality. The risk to the fetus from the vaccine is unknown (1). The American College of Obstetricians and Gynecologists Technical Bulletin No. 64 recommends vaccination during pregnancy only for close, continued exposure or travel to endemic areas (1).

Breast Feeding Summary

No data available.

References

1. ACOG Technical Bulletin, No. 64, May 1982.
2. Amstey MS. Vaccination in pregnancy. Clin Obstet Gynaecol 1983;10:13–22.

Name: **VACCINE, YELLOW FEVER**
Class: **Vaccine** Risk Factor: **D**

Fetal Risk Summary

Yellow fever vaccine is a live, attenuated virus vaccine (1, 2). Yellow fever is a serious infectious disease with high morbidity and mortality. The risk to the fetus from the vaccine is unknown (1, 2). The American College of Obstetricians and Gynecologists Technical Bulletin No. 64 lists the vaccine as contraindicated in pregnancy except if exposure is unavoidable (1).

Breast Feeding Summary

No data available.

References

1. ACOG Technical Bulletin, No. 64, May 1982.
2. Amstey MS. Vaccination in pregnancy. Clin Obstet Gynaecol 1983;10:13–22.

Name: **VALPROIC ACID**

Class: **Anticonvulsant**   Risk Factor: **D**

Fetal Risk Summary

Valproic acid is an anticonvulsant used in the treatment of seizure disorders. There are three cases of congenital abnormalities in which valproic acid was used (1–3). In two of these reports other anticonvulsants were also taken (1, 2). Malformations reported are similar to the fetal hydantoin syndrome:

Lumbosacral meningocele, sensory motor deficit, microcephaly (1)

Prolonged clotting abnormalities, hypoplastic nails, depressed nasal bridge, cleft lip, high arched palate, wide fontanel, abnormal palmar crease, tetralogy of Fallot (2)

Prenatal growth deficiency, microcephaly, bulging frontal eminences, hypoplastic nose and orbital edges, ptosis, low-set ears, small mandible, abnormal palmar creases, congenital dislocation of hip, cutaneous symphysis of toes (3)

Reports of normal births with *in utero* exposure to valproic acid have also been located (4–8).

Valproic acid crosses the placenta to achieve fetal serum concentrations 1.4 times maternal serum levels (6, 9).

Mclain (10) has reported a dose-related hepatoxic effect with serum levels exceeding 60 μg/ml. Because valproic acid is a potent teratogen in experimental studies and due to reports of possible association with human anomalies, it should be used with caution during pregnancy. If used, serum concentrations should be maintained below 60 μg/ml.

Breast Feeding Summary

Valproic acid is excreted into breast milk in small amounts (6, 11). Measured milk concentrations were 0.17–1.0 μg/ml, representing milk:plasma ratios of 0.01–0.07 (6, 9). No reports linking the use of valproic acid with adverse effects in the nursing infant have been located. The American Academy of Pediatrics considers valproic acid compatible with breast-feeding (12).

References

1. Gomez MR. Possible teratogenicity of valproic acid. J Pediatr 1981;98:508–9.
2. Thomas D, Buchanan N. Teratogenic effects of anticonvulsants. J Pediatr 1981;99:163.
3. Dalens B, Raymond EJ, Gaulme J. Teratogenicity of valproic acid. J Pediatr 1980;97:332–3.
4. Brown NA, Kao J, Fabro S. Teratogenic potential of valproic acid. Lancet 1980;1:660–1.
5. Alexander FW. Sodium valproate and pregnancy. Arch Dis Child 1979;54:240–2.
6. Dickenson RG, Harland RC, Lynn RK, Smith NB. Transmission of valproic acid (Depakene) across the placenta: half-life of the drug in mother and baby. J Pediatr 1979;94:832–5.
7. Hiilesmaa VK, Bardy AH, Granstrom ML, Teramo KAW. Valproic acid during pregnancy. Lancet 1980;1:883.

8. Nakane Y, Okuma T, Takahashi R, et al. Multi-institutional study on teratogenicity and fetal toxicity of antiepileptic drugs: a report of a collaborative study group in Japan. Epilepsia 1980;21:663–80.
9. Reith H, Schafer H. Antiepileptic drugs during pregnancy and the lactation period. Pharmacokinetic data. Dtsch Med Wochenschr 1979;104:818–23.
10. Mclain LW Jr. Teratogenic effects of valproic acid. JAMA 1979;242:1672.
11. Radd NL, Freedom RM. A possible primidone embryopathy. J Pediatr 1979;94:835.
12. Committee on Drugs, American Academy of Pediatrics. The transfer of drugs and other chemicals into human breast milk. Pediatrics 1983;72:375–83.

Name: **VANCOMYCIN**

Class: **Antibiotic**   Risk Factor: **C$_M$**

Fetal Risk Summary

Vancomycin has been used for subacute bacterial endocarditis prophylaxis in a penicillin-allergic woman at term with mitral valve prolapse (1). One hour prior to vaginal delivery, a 1-g intravenous dose was given over 3 minutes. Immediately after the dose, maternal blood pressure fell from 130/74 to 80/40 torr and then recovered in 3 minutes. Fetal bradycardia, 90 beats/min, persisted for 4 minutes. No adverse effects of the hypotension-induced fetal distress were observed in the newborn. The Apgar scores were 9 and 10 at 1 and 5 minutes, respectively (1).

Breast Feeding Summary

No data available.

References

1. Hill LM. Fetal distress secondary to vancomycin-induced maternal hypotension. Am J Obstet Gynecol 1985;153:74–5.

Name: **VASOPRESSIN**

Class: **Pituitary Hormone**   Risk Factor: **B**

Fetal Risk Summary

No reports linking the use of vasopressin with congenital defects have been located. Vasopressin and the structurally related synthetic polypeptides, desmopressin and lypressin, have been used during pregnancy to treat diabetes insipidus, a rare disorder (1–4). No adverse effects on the newborns were reported.

A 3-fold increase of circulating levels of endogenous vasopressin has been reported for women in the last trimester and in labor as compared to nonpregnant women (5). Although infrequent, the induction of uterine activity in the 3rd trimester has been reported after intramuscular and intranasal vasopressin (6). The intravenous use of desmopressin, which is normally given intranasally, has also been reported to cause uterine contractions (4).

Two investigators speculated that raised levels of vasopressin were the result of hypoxemia and acidosis and could produce signs of fetal distress (bradycardia and meconium staining) (7).

Breast Feeding Summary

Patients receiving vasopressin, desmopressin, or lypressin for diabetes insipidus have been reported to breast-feed without apparent problems in the infant (1, 2). Experimental work in lactating women suggests that suckling almost doubles the maternal blood concentration of vasopressin (5).

References

1. Hime MC, Richardson JA. Diabetes insipidus and pregnancy. Obstet Gynecol Surv 1978;33:375–9.
2. Hadi HA, Mashini IS, Devoe LD. Diabetes insipidus during pregnancy complicated by preeclampsia. A case report. J Reprod Med 1985;30:206–8.
3. Phelan JP, Guay AT, Newman C. Diabetes insipidus in pregnancy: a case review. Am J Obstet Gynecol 1978;130:365–6.
4. van der Wildt B, Drayer JIM, Eske TKAB. Diabetes insipidus in pregnancy as a first sign of a craniopharyngioma. Eur J Obstet Gynecol Reprod Biol 1980;10:269–74.
5. Robinson KW, Hawker RW, Robertson PA. Antidiuretic hormone (ADH) in the human female. J Clin Endocrinol Metab 1957;17:320–2.
6. Oravec D, Lichardus B. Management of diabetes insipidus in pregnancy. Br Med J 1972;4:114–5.
7. Gaffney PR, Jenkins DM. Vasopressin: mediator of the clinical signs of fetal distress. Br J Obstet Gynaecol 1983;90:987.

Name: **VERAPAMIL**

Class: **Cardiac**   Risk Factor: C_M

Fetal Risk Summary

Verapamil is a slow channel calcium inhibitor used as an antiarrhythmic agent. No reports linking its use with congenital defects have been located. Placental passage of verapamil was demonstrated in two of six patients given 80 mg orally at term (1). Cord levels were 15.4 and 24.5 ng/ml (17 and 26% of maternal serum) in two newborns delivered at 49 and 109 minutes, respectively. Verapamil could not be detected in the cord blood of four infants delivered 173–564 minutes after the dose. Intravenous (IV) verapamil was administered to patients in labor at a rate of 2 μg/kg/min for 60–110 minutes (2). The serum concentrations of the infants averaged 8.5 ng/ml (44% of maternal serum).

A 33-week fetus with a tachycardia of 240–280 beats/min was treated *in utero* for 6 weeks with β-acetyldigoxin and verapamil (80 mg three times daily) (1). The fetal heart rate returned to normal 5 days after initiation of therapy, but the authors could not determine if verapamil had produced the beneficial effect. At birth, no signs of cardiac hypertrophy or disturbances in repolarization were observed. Maternal supraventricular tachycardia in the 3rd trimester has been treated with a single 5-mg IV dose of verapamil (3). No adverse effects were noted in the fetus or newborn.

Verapamil has been used to lower blood pressure in a woman with severe pregnancy-induced hypertension in labor (4). Fifteen milligrams were given by rapid IV injection followed by an infusion of 185 mg over 6 hours. Fetal heart rate increase from 60 to 110 beats/min, and a normal infant was delivered without signs or symptoms of toxicity. Tocolysis with verapamil, either alone or in combination with β-mimetics, has also been described (5–9).

The manufacturer has reports of patients treated with verapamil during the 1st trimester without production of fetal problems (10). However, hypotension (systolic and diastolic) has been observed in 5–10% of patients after intravenous therapy (11, 12). Because of this, reduced uterine blood flow with fetal hypoxia (bradycardia) is a potential risk.

Breast Feeding Summary

Verapamil is excreted into breast milk (13). A daily dose of 240 mg produced milk levels that were approximately 23% of maternal serum. Serum levels in the infant were 2.1 ng/ml but could not be detected (<1 ng/ml) 38 hours after treatment was stopped. No effects of this exposure were observed in the infant.

References

1. Wolff F, Breuker KH, Schlensker KH, Bolte A. Prenatal diagnosis and therapy of fetal heart rate anomalies: with a contribution on the placental transfer of verapamil. J Perinat Med 1980;8:203–8.
2. Strigl R, Gastroph G, Hege HG, et al. Nachweis von verapamil in mutterlichen und fetalen blut des menschen. Geburtshilfe Frauenheilkd 1980;40:496–9.
3. Klein V, Repke JT. Supraventricular tachycardia in pregnancy: cardioversion with verapamil. Obstet Gynecol 1984;63:16S–8S.
4. Brittinger WD, Schwarzbeck A, Wittenmeier KW, et al. Klinisch-experimentelle untersuchungen uber die blutdruckendende wirkung von verapamil. Dtsch Med Wochenschr 1970;95:1871–7.
5. Mosler KH, Rosenboom HG. Neuere moglichkeiten einer tokolytischen behandlung in de geburt-schilfe. Z Geburtschilfe Perinatol 1972;176:85–96.
6. Gummerus M. Prevention of premature birth with nylidrin and verapamil. Z Geburtschilfe Perinatol 1975;179:261–6.
7. Gummerus M. Treatment of premature labor and antagonization of the side effects of tocolytic therapy with verapamil. Z Geburtschilfe Perinatol 1977;181:334–40.
8. Gummerus M. Prevention of premature birth with nylidrin and verapamil. Z Geburtschilfe Perinatol 1975;179:261–6.
9. Gummerus M. Treatment of premature labour and antagonization of the side effects of tocolytic therapy with verapamil. Z Geburtschilfe Perinatol 1977;181:334–40.
10. Anderson, MS, GD Searle & Co, 1981. Personal communication.
11. Product information. Calan. GD Searle & Co, 1985.
12. Product information. Isoptin. Knoll Pharmaceutical Co, 1985.
13. Andersen HJ. Excretion of verapamil in human milk. Eur J Clin Pharmacol 1983;25:279–80.

Name: **VIDARABINE**

Class: **Antiviral**   Risk Factor: **C$_M$**

Fetal Risk Summary

Vidarabine has not been studied in human pregnancy. The drug is teratogenic in some species of animals after topical and intramuscular administration (1, 2). Daily instillations of a 10% solution into the vaginas of pregnant rats in late gestation had no effect on the offspring.

Vidarabine was used for disseminated herpes simplex in one woman at about 28 weeks gestation (3, 4). Spontaneous rupture of the membranes occurred 48 hours after initiation of therapy and a premature infant was delivered. The infant died on the 13th day of life from complications of prematurity.

Breast Feeding Summary

No data available.

References

1. Pavan-Langston D, Buchanan RA, Alford CA Jr, eds. *Adenine Arabinoside: An Antiviral Agent*. New York:Raven Press, 1975:153.
2. Schardein JL, Hertz DL, Petretre JA, Fitzgerald JE, Kurtz SM. The effect of vidarabine on the development of the offspring of rats, rabbits and monkeys. Teratology 1977;15:213–42.
3. Hillard P, Seeds J, Cefalo R. Disseminated herpes simplex in pregnancy: two cases and a review. Obstet Gynecol Surv 1982;37:449–53.
4. Peacock JE Jr, Sarubbi FA. Disseminated herpes simplex virus infection during pregnancy. Obstet Gynecol 1983;61:13S–8S.

Name: **VINBLASTINE**

Class: **Antineoplastic**   Risk Factor: **D**

Fetal Risk Summary

Vinblastine is an antimitotic antineoplastic agent. The drug has been used in pregnancy, including the 1st trimester, without producing malformations (1–6). Two cases of malformed infants have been reported following 1st trimester exposure to vinblastine (7, 8). Garrett (7) reported a case of a 27-year-old woman with Hodgkin's disease who was given vinblastine, mechlorethamine, and procarbazine during the 1st trimester. At 24 weeks of gestation, she spontaneously aborted a male child with oligodactyly of both feet with webbing of the 3rd and 4th toes. These defects were attributed to mechlorethamine therapy. A mother with Hodgkin's disease treated with vinblastine, vincristine, and procarbazine in the 1st trimester (3 weeks after the last menstrual period) delivered a 1,900-g male infant at about 37 weeks of gestation who developed fatal respiratory distress syndrome (8). At autopsy, a small secundum atrial septal defect was found. Vinblastine in combination with other antineoplastic agents may produce ovarian dysfunction (9–11). Alkylating agents are the most frequent cause of this problem (11). Ovarian function may return to normal with successful pregnancies possible, depending on the patient's age at time of therapy and the total dose of chemotherapy received (10). Data from one review indicated that 40% of infants exposed to anticancer drugs were of low birth weight (12). This finding was not related to the timing of exposure. Long-term studies of growth and mental development in offspring exposed to vinblastine during the 2nd trimester, the period of neuroblast multiplication, have not been conducted (13).

Breast Feeding Summary

No data available.

References

1. Armstrong JG, Dyke RW, Fouts PJ, Jansen CJ. Delivery of a normal infant during the course of oral vinblastine sulfate therapy for Hodgkin's disease. Ann Intern Med 1964;61:106–7.

2. Rosenzweig AI, Crews QE Jr, Hopwood HG. Vinblastine sulfate in Hodgkin's disease in pregnancy. Ann Intern Med 1964;61:108–12.

3. Lacher MJ. Use of vinblastine sulfate to treat Hodgkin's disease during pregnancy. Ann Intern Med 1964;61:113–5.

4. Lacher MJ, Geller W. Cyclophosphamide and vinblastine sulfate in Hodgkin's disease during pregnancy. JAMA 1966;195:192–4.

5. Nordlund JJ, DeVita VT Jr, Carbone PP. Severe vinblastine-induced leukopenia during late pregnancy with delivery of a normal infant. Ann Intern Med 1968;69:581–2.

6. Goguei A. Hodgkin's disease and pregnancy. Nouv Presse Med 1970;78:1507–10.

7. Garrett MJ. Teratogenic effects of combination chemotherapy. Ann Intern Med 1974;80:667.

8. Thomas RPM, Peckham MJ. The investigation and management of Hodgkin's disease in the pregnant patient. Cancer 1976;38:1443–51.

9. Morgenfeld MC, Goldberg V, Parisier H, Bugnard SC, Bur GE. Ovarian lesions due to cytostatic agents during the treatment of Hodgkin's disease. Surg Gynecol Obstet 1972;134:826–8.

10. Ross GT. Congenital anomalies among children born of mothers receiving chemotherapy for gestational trophoblastic neoplasms. Cancer 1976;37:1043–7.

11. Schilsky RL, Lewis BJ, Sherins RJ, Young RC. Gonadal dysfunction in patients receiving chemotherapy for cancer. Ann Intern Med 1980;93:109–14.

12. Nicholson HO. Cytotoxic drugs in pregnancy: review of reported cases. J Obstet Gynaecol Br Commonw 1968;75:307–12.

13. Dobbing J. Pregnancy and leukaemia. Lancet 1977;1:1155.

Name: **VINCRISTINE**

Class: **Antineoplastic**   Risk Factor: **D**

Fetal Risk Summary

Vincristine is an antimitotic antineoplastic agent. Fifteen references have described the use of the drug in 20 pregnancies, six during the 1st trimester (1–15). A mother with Hodgkin's disease treated with vincristine, vinblastine, and procarbazine in the 1st trimester (3 weeks after the last menstrual period) delivered a 1,900-g male infant at about 37 weeks of gestation who developed fatal respiratory distress syndrome (9). At autopsy, a small secundum atrial septal defect was found. In a patient with Hodgkin's disease who was treated with vincristine, mechlorethamine, and procarbazine during the 1st trimester, the electively aborted fetus had malformed kidneys (markedly reduced size and malposition) (15). The only other apparent adverse effect observed following vincristine use in pregnancy was in a 1,000-g male infant born with pancytopenia who was exposed to six different antineoplastic agents in the 3rd trimester (1). Data from one review indicated that 40% of the infants exposed to anticancer drugs were of low birth weight (16). This finding was not related to the timing of exposure. Long-term studies of growth and mental development in offspring exposed to these drugs during the 2nd trimester, the period of neuroblast multiplication, have not been conducted (17). Vincristine, in combination with other antineoplastic agents, may produce gonadal dysfunction in men and women (18–25). Alkylating agents are the most frequent cause of this problem (22). Ovarian and testicular function may return to normal with successful pregnancies possible, depending on the patient's age at time of treatment and the total dose of chemotherapy received (18).

Breast Feeding Summary

No data available.

References

1. Pizzuto J, Aviles A, Noriega L, Niz J, Morales M, Romero F. Treatment of acute leukemia during pregnancy: presentation of nine cases. Cancer Treat Rep 1980;64:679–83.
2. Colbert N, Najman A, Gorin NC, et al. Acute leukaemia during pregnancy: favourable course of pregnancy in two patients treated with cytosine arabinoside and anthracyclines. Nouv Presse Med 1980;9:175–8.
3. Daly H, McCann SR, Hanratty TD, Temperley IJ. Successful pregnancy during combination chemotherapy for Hodgkin's disease. Acta Haematol (Basel) 1980;64:154–6.
4. Tobias JS, Bloom HJG. Doxorubicin in pregnancy. Lancet 1980;1:776.
5. Garcia V, San Miguel J, Borrasea AL. Doxorubicin in the first trimester of pregnancy. Ann Intern Med 1981;94:547.
6. Dara P, Slater LM, Armentrout SA. Successful pregnancy during chemotherapy for acute leukemia. Cancer 1981;47:845–6.
7. Burnier AM. Discussion. In Plows CW. Acute myelomonocytic leukemia in pregnancy: report of a case. Am J Obstet Gynecol 1982;143:41–3.
8. Lilleyman JS, Hill AS, Anderton KJ. Consequences of acute myelogenous leukemia in early pregnancy. Cancer 1977;40:1300–3.
9. Thomas PRM, Peckham MJ. The investigation and management of Hodgkin's disease in the pregnant patient. Cancer 1976;38:1443–51.
10. Pawliger DF, McLean FW, Noyes WD. Normal fetus after cytosine arabinoside therapy. Ann Intern Med 1971;74:1012.
11. Lowenthal RM, Funnell CF, Hope DM, Stewart IG, Humphrey DC. Normal infant after combination chemotherapy including teniposide for Burkitt's lymphoma in pregnancy. Med Pediatr Oncol 1982;10:165–9.
12. Sears HF, Reid J. Granulocytic sarcoma: local presentation of a systemic disease. Cancer 1976;37:1808–13.
13. Durie BGM, Giles HR. Successful treatment of acute leukemia during pregnancy: combination therapy in the third trimester. Arch Intern Med 1977;137:90–1.
14. Newcomb M, Balducci L, Thigpen JT, Morrison FS. Acute leukemia in pregnancy: successful delivery after cytarabine and doxorubicin. JAMA 1978;239:2691–2.
15. Mennuti MT, Shepard TH, Mellman WJ. Fetal renal malformation following treatment of Hodgkin's disease during pregnancy. Obstet Gynecol 1975;46:194–6.
16. Nicholson HO. Cytotoxic drugs in pregnancy: review of reported cases. J Obstet Gynaecol Br Commonw 1968;75:307–12.
17. Dobbing J. Pregnancy and leukaemia. Lancet 1977;1:1155.
18. Schilsky RL, Sherins RJ, Hubbard SM, Wesley MN, Young RC, DeVita VT Jr. Long-term follow-up of ovarian function in women treated with MOPP chemotherapy for Hodgkin's disease. Am J Med 1981;71:552–6.
19. Schwartz PE, Vidone RA. Pregnancy following combination chemotherapy for a mixed germ cell tumor of the ovary. Gynecol Oncol 1981;12:373–8.
20. Estiu M. Successful pregnancy in leukaemia. Lancet 1977;1:433.
21. Johnson SA, Goldman JM, Hawkins DF. Pregnancy after chemotherapy for Hodgkin's disease. Lancet 1979;2:93.
22. Schilsky RL, Lewis BJ, Sherins RJ, Young RC. Gonadal dysfunction in patients receiving chemotherapy for cancer. Ann Intern Med 1980;93:109–14.
23. Sherins RJ, DeVita VT Jr. Effect of drug treatment for lymphoma on male reproductive capacity. Ann Intern Med 1973;79:216–20.
24. Sherins RJ, Olweny CLM, Ziegler JL. Gynecomastia and gonadal dysfunction in adolescent boys treated with combination chemotherapy for Hodgkin's disease. N Engl J Med 1978;299:12–6.
25. Lendon PRM, Peckham MJ. The investigation and management of Hodgkin's disease in the pregnant patient. Cancer 1976;38:1944–51.

Name: **VITAMIN A**

Class: **Vitamin**   Risk Factor: **A***

Fetal Risk Summary

Vitamin A (retinol; vitamin A₁) is a fat-soluble essential nutrient that occurs naturally in a variety of foods. Vitamin A is required for the maintenance of normal epithelial tissue and for growth and bone development, vision, and reproduction (1). The RDA for normal pregnant women in America is 5,000 IU (2).

The teratogenicity of vitamin A in animals is well known. Both high and low levels of the vitamin result in defects (3–9). Various authors have speculated on the teratogenic effect of the vitamin in humans (10–12). In a 1983 case report, Bound (12) suggested that the vitamin A contained in a multivitamin product may have caused a cleft palate in one infant. The mother had a family history of cleft palate and had produced a previous infant with a malformation. In response to this report, Smithells (13) wrote that there was no acceptable evidence of human vitamin A teratogenicity and none at all with doses less than 10,000 IU/day. Isotretinoin, a synthetic isomer of vitamin A, has been shown to be a powerful human teratogen (see Isotretinoin). Although scarce and not conclusive, the available reports describing the effects of deficiencies and excesses of vitamin A (retinol) in human pregnancy are summarized below. Because of the experience with isotretinoin in humans and with vitamin A in animals, large doses or severe shortages of this vitamin in humans must be viewed as potentially harmful to the fetus.

Severe human vitamin A deficiency has been cited as the cause of three malformed infants (14–16). In the first case, a mother with multiple vitamin deficiencies produced a baby with congenital xerophthalmia and bilateral cleft lip (14). The defects may have been due to vitamin A deficiency because of their similarity to anomalies seen in animals deprived of this nutrient. The second report involved a malnourished pregnant woman with recent onset of blindness whose symptoms were the result of vitamin A deficiency (15). The mother gave birth to a premature male child with microcephaly and what appeared to be anophthalmia. The final case described a blind, mentally retarded girl with bilateral microphthalmia, coloboma of the iris and choroid, and retinal aplasia (16). During pregnancy, the mother was suspected of having vitamin A deficiency manifested by night blindness.

Excessive maternal vitamin A intake is suspected of producing malformations in at least three humans (17–19). Morriss and Thomson (20) mentioned personal knowledge of one or two other cases but gave no details. In all three of the known cases, defects of the urinary tract were prominant. In one report, the mother took 40,000 IU of vitamin A as well as 600,000 IU of vitamin D daily for 1 month of the 1st trimester (17). The infant had an anomaly of the urogenital system. Bernhardt and Dorsey (18) described a mother who consumed 25,000 IU daily during the 1st trimester then 50,000 IU the remainder of the pregnancy. She delivered an infant with congenital renal anomalies consisting of a double collecting system in the left kidney and resulting in a salt-losing obstructive uropathy. In a 1978 case, Stange and co-workers (19) reported a woman who was treated for acne with 150,000 IU daily on gestational days 19–40. The microcephalic infant, who died shortly after birth, had multiple anomalies of the central nervous system, very small adrenal glands, and hypoplastic kidneys.

Several investigators have studied maternal and fetal vitamin A levels during various stages of gestation (3, 21–32). Transport to the fetus is by passive diffusion (33). Maternal vitamin A concentrations are slightly greater than those found in either premature or term infants (21–23). In women with normal levels of vitamin A, maternal and newborn levels were 270 and 220 ng/ml, respectively (22). In 41 women not given supplements of vitamin A, a third of whom had laboratory evidence of hypovitaminemia A, mean maternal levels exceeded those in the newborn by almost a 2:1 ratio (22). In two reports, maternal serum levels were dependent on the length of gestation with concentrations decreasing during the 1st trimester, then increasing during the remainder of pregnancy until about the 38th week when they began to decrease again (3, 24). A more recent study found no difference in serum levels between 10 and 33 weeks gestation, although amniotic fluid vitamin A levels at 20 weeks onward were significantly greater than at 16–18 weeks (25). Premature infants (36 weeks or less) have significantly lower serum retinol and retinol-binding protein concentrations than do term neonates (21, 26–28).

Mild to moderate deficiency is common during pregnancy (22, 29). A 1984 report concluded that vitamin A deficiency in poorly nourished mothers was one of the features associated with an increased incidence of prematurity and intrauterine growth retardation (21). An earlier study, however, found no difference in vitamin A levels between low-birth-weight (<2,500 g) and normal-birth weight (>2,500 g) infants (23). Maternal concentrations of the low-birth-weight group were lower than those of the normal-weight group, 211 vs 273 ng/ml, but not significantly. An investigation in premature infants revealed that infants developing bronchopulmonary dysplasia had significantly lower serum retinol levels as compared to infants that did not develop this disease (28).

Relatively high liver vitamin A stores were found in the fetuses of women under 18 and greater than 40 years of age, two groups that produce a high incidence of fetal anomalies (3). Low fetal liver concentrations were measured in two infants with hydrocephalus and high levels in 14 infants with neural tube defects (NTD) (3). In another report relating to NTD, a high liver concentration occurred in an anencephalic infant (30). Significantly higher vitamin A amniotic fluid concentrations were discovered in 12 pregnancies from which infants with NTD were delivered as compared with 94 normal pregnancies (31). However, attempts to use this measurement as an indicator of anencephaly or other fetal anomalies failed because the values for abnormal and normal fetuses overlapped (25, 31).

Wild and co-workers (32) studied the effect of stopping oral contraceptives shortly before conception on vitamin A levels. Since oral contraceptives had been shown to increase serum levels of vitamin A, it was postulated that early conception might involve a risk of teratogenicity. However, no difference was found in early pregnancy vitamin A levels between users and nonusers. The results of this study have been challenged based on the methods used to measure vitamin A (34).

[* Risk Factor X if used in doses above the RDA.]

Breast Feeding Summary

Vitamin A is naturally present in breast milk. Deficiency of this vitamin in breast-fed infants is rare (35). The RDA of vitamin A during lactation is 6,000 IU (2). It is not known if high maternal doses of vitamin A present a danger to the nursing infant.

References

1. American Hospital Formulary Service. *Drug Information 1985*. Bethesda:American Society of Hospital Pharmacists, 1985:1681–3.
2. *Recommended Dietary Allowances*, ed 9. Washington, DC:National Academy of Sciences, 1980.
3. Gal I, Sharman IM, Pryse-Davies J. Vitamin A in relation to human congenital malformations. Adv Teratol 1972;5:143–58.
4. Cohlan SQ. Excessive intake of vitamin A as a cause of congenital anomalies in the rat. Science 1953;117:535–6.
5. Muenter MD. Hypervitaminosis A. Ann Intern Med 1974;80:105–6.
6. Morriss GM. Vitamin A and congenital malformations. Int J Vitam Nutr Res 1976;46:220–2.
7. Fantel AG, Shepard TH, Newell-Morris LL, Moffett BC. Teratogenic effects of retinoic acid in pigtail monkeys (Macaca nemestrina). Teratology 1977;15:65–72.
8. Vorhees CV, Brunner RL, McDaniel CR, Butcher RE. The relationship of gestational age to vitamin A induced postnatal dysfunction. Teratology 1978;17:271–6.
9. Ferm VH, Ferm RR. Teratogenic interaction of hyperthermia and vitamin A. Biol Neonate 1979;36:168–72.
10. Muenter MD. Hypervitaminosis A. Ann Intern Med 1974;80:105–6.
11. Read AP, Harris R. Spina bifida and vitamins. Br Med J 1983;286:560–1.
12. Bound JP. Spina bifida and vitamins. Br Med J 1983;286:147.
13. Smithells RW. Spina bifida and vitamins. Br Med J 1983;286:388–9.
14. Houet R, Ramioul-Lecomte S. Repercussions sur l'enfant des avitaminoses de la mere pendant la grossesse. Ann Paediat 1950;175:378. As cited in Warkany J. *Congenital Malformations. Notes and Comments*. Chicago:Year Book Medical Publishers, 1971:127–8.
15. Sarma V. Maternal vitamin A deficiency and fetal microcephaly and anophthalmia. Obstet Gynecol 1959;13:299–301.
16. Lamba PA, Sood NN. Congenital microphthalmus and colobomata in maternal vitamin A deficiency. J Pediatr Ophthalmol 1968;115–7. As cited in Warkany J. *Congenital Malformations. Notes and Comments*. Chicago:Year Book Medical Publishers, 1971:127–8.
17. Pilotti G, Scorta A. Ipervitaminosi A gravidica e malformazioni neonatali dell'apparato urinaria. Minerva Ginecol 1965;17:1103–8. As cited in Nishimura H, Tanimura T. *Clinical Aspects of the Teratogenicity of Drugs*. New York:American Elsevier, 1976:251–2.
18. Bernhardt IB, Dorsey DJ. Hypervitaminosis A and congenital renal anomalies in a human infant. Obstet Gynecol 1974;43:750–5.
19. Stange L, Carlstrom K, Eriksson M. Hypervitaminosis A in early human pregnancy and malformations of the central nervous system. Acta Obstet Gynecol Scand 1978;57:289–91.
20. Morriss GM, Thomson AD. Vitamin A and rat embryos. Lancet 1974;2:899–900.
21. Shah RS, Rajalakshmi R. Vitamin A status of the newborn in relation to gestational age, body weight, and maternal nutritional status. Am J Clin Nutr 1984;40:794–800.
22. Baker H, Frank O, Thomson AD, Langer A, Munves ED, De Angelis B, Kaminetzky HA. Vitamin profile of 174 mothers and newborns at parturition. Am J Clin Nutr 1975;28:59–65.
23. Baker H, Thind IS, Frank O, DeAngelis B, Caterini H, Louria DB. Vitamin levels in low-birth-weight newborn infants and their mothers. Am J Obstet Gynecol 1977;129:521–4.
24. Gal I, Parkinson CE. Effects of nutrition and other factors on pregnant women's serum vitamin A levels. Am J Clin Nutr 1974;27:688–95.
25. Wallingford JC, Milunsky A, Underwood BA. Vitamin A and retinol-binding protein in amniotic fluid. Am J Clin Nutr 1983;38:377–81.
26. Brandt RB, Mueller DG, Schroeder JR, Guyer KE, Kirkpatrick BV, Hutcher NE, Ehrlich FE. Serum vitamin A in premature and term neonates. J Pediatr 1978;92:101–4.
27. Shenai JP, Chytil F, Jhaveri A, Stahlman MT. Plasma vitamin A and retinol-binding protein in premature and term neonates. J Pediatr 1981;99:302–5.
28. Hustead VA, Gutcher GR, Anderson SA, Zachman RD. Relationship of vitamin A (retinol) status to lung disease in the preterm infant. J Pediatr 1984;105:610–5.
29. Kaminetzky HA, Langer A, Baker H, Frank O, Thomson AD, Munves ED, Opper A, Behrle FC, Glista B. The effect of nutrition in teen-age gravidas on pregnancy and the status of the neonate. I. A nutritional profile. Am J Obstet Gynecol 1973;115:639–46.
30. Gal I, Sharman IM, Pryse-Davies J, Moore T. Vitamin A as a possible factor in human teratology. Proc Nutr Soc 1969;28:9A–10A.
31. Parkinson CE, Tan JCY. Vitamin A concentrations in amniotic fluid and maternal serum related to neural-tube defects. Br J Obstet Gynaecol 1982;89:935–9.

32. Wild J, Schorah CJ, Smithells RW. Vitamin A, pregnancy, and oral contraceptives. Br Med J 1974;1:57–9.
33. Hill EP, Longo LD. Dynamics of maternal-fetal nutrient transfer. Fed Proc 1980;39:239–44.
34. Bubb FA. Vitamin A, pregnancy, and oral contraceptives. Br Med J 1974;1:391–2.
35. Committee on Nutrition, American Academy of Pediatrics. Vitamin and mineral supplement needs in normal children in the United States. Pediatrics 1980;66:1015–21.

Name: **VITAMIN B$_{12}$**

Class: **Vitamin**   Risk Factor: **A***

Fetal Risk Summary

Vitamin B$_{12}$ (cyanocobalamin), a water-soluble B complex vitamin, is an essential nutrient required for nucleoprotein and myelin synthesis, cell reproduction, normal growth, and the maintenance of normal erythropoiesis (1). The American RDA for vitamin B$_{12}$ in pregnancy is 4 μg (2).

Vitamin B$_{12}$ is actively transported to the fetus (3–7). This process is responsible for the progressive decline of maternal levels that occurs during pregnancy (7–15). Similar to other B complex vitamins, higher concentrations of B$_{12}$ are found in the fetus and newborn than in the mother (6–10, 17–25). At term, mean vitamin B$_{12}$ levels in 174 mothers were 115 pg/ml and in their newborns 500 pg/ml, a newborn:maternal ratio of 4.3 (17). Comparable values have been observed by others (6, 8, 22–24). Mean levels in 51 Brazilian women, in their newborns, and in the intervillous space of their placentas were approximately 340, 797, and 1074 pg/ml, respectively (25). The newborn:maternal ratio in this report was 2.3. The high levels in the placenta may indicate a mechanism by which the fetus can accumulate the vitamin against a concentration gradient. This study also found a highly significant correlation between vitamin B$_{12}$ and folate concentrations. This is in contrast to an earlier report that did not find such a correlation in women with megaloblastic anemia (26).

Maternal deficiency of vitamin B$_{12}$ is common during pregnancy (16–18, 27). Tobacco smoking reduces maternal levels of the vitamin even further (28). Megaloblastic anemia may result when the deficiency is severe, but the condition responds readily to therapy (29–32). On the other hand, tropical macrocytic anemia during pregnancy responds erratically to B$_{12}$ therapy and is better treated with folic acid (32, 34).

Megaloblastic (pernicious) anemia may be a cause of infertility (30, 31, 34). Varadi (30) described a mother with undiagnosed pernicious anemia who had lost her 3rd, 9th, and 10th pregnancies. A healthy child resulted from her 11th pregnancy following treatment with B$_{12}$. Jackson and co-workers (31) treated eight infertile women having pernicious anemia with B$_{12}$ and seven became pregnant within 1 year of therapy. One of three patients in a report by Parr and Ramsey (34) may have had infertility associated with very low B$_{12}$ levels.

Vitamin B$_{12}$ deficiency was associated with prematurity (as defined by a birth weight of 2,500 g or less) in a 1968 paper (10). However, many of the patients who delivered prematurely had normal or elevated B$_{12}$ levels. Streiff and Little (35, 36), in two reports, found no correlation between B$_{12}$ deficiency and abruptio placentae. Two reports found a positive association between low birth weight and low B$_{12}$ levels (22, 37). In both instances, folate levels were also low and iron was deficient in one. Others could not correlate low B$_{12}$ concentrations with the weight at delivery (12, 16).

In experimental animals, vitamin B$_{12}$ deficiency is teratogenic (8, 38). Schorah and associates (39), in their work on neural tube defects, measured very low B$_{12}$ levels in three of four mothers of anencephalic fetuses. Additional evidence led them to conclude that the low B$_{12}$ level resulted in depletion of maternal folic acid and involvement in the etiology of the defect. Two other reports have shown no relationship between low levels of vitamin B$_{12}$ and congenital malformations (10, 20).

No reports linking high doses of vitamin B$_{12}$ with maternal or fetal complications have been located. B$_{12}$ administration at term has produced maternal levels approaching 50,000 pg/ml with corresponding cord blood levels of approximately 15,000 pg/ml (5, 6). In fetal methylmalonic acidemia, large doses of B$_{12}$, 10 mg orally initially then changed to 5 mg intramuscularly, were administered daily to a mother to treat the affected fetus (40). On this dosage regimen, maternal levels rose as high as 18,000 pg/ml shortly after a dose. This metabolic disorder is not always treatable with B$_{12}$: Morrow and co-workers (41) reported a newborn with the B$_{12}$-unresponsive form of methylmalonic acidemia.

In summary, severe maternal vitamin B$_{12}$ deficiency may result in megaloblastic anemia with subsequent infertility and poor pregnancy outcome. Less severe maternal deficiency apparently is common and does not pose a significant risk to the mother or fetus. Ingestion of vitamin B$_{12}$ during pregnancy up to the RDA either via the diet or by supplementation is recommended.

[* Risk Factor C if used in doses above the RDA.]

Breast Feeding Summary

Vitamin B$_{12}$ is excreted into human breast milk. In the first 48 hours after delivery, mean colostrum levels were 2,431 pg/ml and then fell rapidly to concentrations comparable to those in normal serum (42). Luhby and co-workers (3) also observed very high colostrum levels ranging from 6 to 17.5 times that of milk. Milk:plasma ratios are approximately 1.0 during lactation (20). Reported milk concentrations of B$_{12}$ vary widely (43–46). Deodhar and co-workers (43) gave mothers supplements of daily doses of 1–200 μg and measured milk levels increasing from 79 to 100 pg/ml. Milk concentrations were directly proportional to dietary intake. Thomas and co-workers (44), using 8 μg/day supplements, measured mean levels of 1,650 pg/ml at 1 week and 1,100 pg/ml at 6 weeks. Corresponding levels in mothers not receiving supplements were significantly different at 1,220 and 610 pg/ml, respectively. Sneed and co-workers (45) also used 8 μg/day supplements and found significantly different levels compared to women not receiving supplements: 910 vs 700 pg/ml at 1 week and 790 vs 550 pg/ml at 6 weeks. In contrast, Sandberg and co-workers (46) found no difference between well-nourished women who were given supplements of 5–100 μg/day and those who received no supplements. The mean B$_{12}$ concentration in their patients was 970 pg/ml. A 1983 English study measured B$_{12}$ levels in pooled human milk obtained from preterm (26 mothers: 29–34 weeks) and term (35 mothers: 39 weeks or longer) patients (47). Preterm milk levels decreased from 920 pg/ml (colostrum) to 220 pg/ml (16–196 days) while term milk levels decreased over the same period from 490 to 230 pg/ml.

Vitamin B$_{12}$ deficiency in the lactating mother may cause severe consequences in the nursing infant. Several reports have described megaloblastic anemia in infants exclusively breast-fed by B$_{12}$-deficient mothers (48–52). Many of these mothers were vegetarians whose diets provided low amounts of the vitamin (49–52). The adequacy of vegetarian diets in providing sufficient B$_{12}$ has been debated (53–55). However, a recent report measured only 1.4 μg of B$_{12}$ intake per day in lactovegetarians (56). This amount is approximately 35% of the RDA for lactating women in America (2).

The American RDA for vitamin B$_{12}$ during lactation is 4 μg (2). If the diet of the lactating woman adequately supplies this amount, maternal supplementation with B$_{12}$ is not needed. Supplementation with the RDA for B$_{12}$ is recommended for those women with inadequate nutritional intake.

References

1. American Hospital Formulary Service. *Drug Information 1985*. Bethesda:American Society of Hospital Pharmacists, 1985:1693–7.
2. *Recommended Dietary Allowances*, ed 9. Washington, DC:National Academy of Sciences, 1980.
3. Luhby AL, Cooperman JM, Donnenfeld AM, Herrero JM, Teller DN, Wenig JB. Observations on transfer of vitamin B$_{12}$ from mother to fetus and newborn. Am J Dis Child 1958;96:532–3.
4. Hill EP, Longo LD. Dynamics of maternal-fetal nutrient transfer. Fed Proc 1980;39:239–44.
5. Kaminetzky HA, Baker H, Frank O, Langer A. The effects of intravenously administered water-soluble vitamins during labor in normovitaminemic and hypovitaminemic gravidas on maternal and neonatal blood vitamin levels at delivery. Am J Obstet Gynecol 1974;120:697–703.
6. Frank O, Walbroehl G, Thomson A, Kaminetzky H, Kubes Z, Baker H. Placental transfer: fetal retention of some vitamins. Am J Clin Nutr 1970;23:662–3.
7. Luhby AL, Cooperman JM, Stone ML, Slobody LB. Physiology of vitamin B$_{12}$ in pregnancy, the placenta, and the newborn. Am J Dis Child 1961;102:753–4.
8. Baker H, Ziffer H, Pasher I, Sobotka H. A comparison of maternal and foetal folic acid and vitamin B$_{12}$ at parturition. Br Med J 1958;1:978–9.
9. Boger WP, Bayne GM, Wright LD, Beck GD. Differential serum vitamin B$_{12}$ concentrations in mothers and infants. N Engl J Med 1957;256:1085–7.
10. Temperley IJ, Meehan MJM, Gatenby PBB. Serum vitamin B12 levels in pregnant women. J Obstet Gynaecol Br Commonw 1968;75:511–6.
11. Boger WP, Wright LD, Beck GD, Bayne GM. Vit. B$_{12}$: correlation of serum concentrations and pregnancy. Proc Soc Exp Biol Med 1956;92:140–3.
12. Martin JD, Davis RE, Stenhouse N. Serum folate and vitamin B12 levels in pregnancy with particular reference to uterine bleeding and bacteriuria. J Obstet Gynaecol Br Commonw 1967;74:697–701.
13. Ball EW, Giles C. Folic acid and vitamin B$_{12}$ levels in pregnancy and their relation to megaloblastic anaemia. J Clin Pathol 1964;17:165–74.
14. Izak G, Rachmilewitz M, Stein Y, Berkovici B, Sadovsky A, Aronovitch Y, Grossowicz N. Vitamin B$_{12}$ and iron deficiencies in anemia of pregnancy and puerperium. Arch Intern Med 1957;99:346–55.
15. Edelstein T, Metz J. Correlation between vitamin B12 concentration in serum and muscle in late pregnancy. J Obstet Gynaecol Br Commonw 1969;76:545–8.
16. Roberts PD, James H, Petrie A, Morgan JO, Hoffbrand AV. Vitamin B$_{12}$ status in pregnancy among immigrants to Britain. Br Med J 1973;3:67–72.
17. Baker H, Frank O, Thomson AD, Langer A, Munves ED, De Angelis B, Kaminetzky HA. Vitamin profile of 174 mothers and newborns at parturition. Am J Clin Nutr 1975;28:59–65.
18. Kaminetzky HA, Baker H. Micronutrients in pregnancy. Clin Obstet Gynecol 1977;20:363–80.
19. Lowenstein L, Lalonde M, Deschenes EB, Shapiro L. Vitamin B$_{12}$ in pregnancy and the puerperium. Am J Clin Nutr 1960;8:265–75.
20. Baker SJ, Jacob E, Rajan KT, Swaminathan SP. Vitamin-B$_{12}$ deficiency in pregnancy and the puerperium. Br Med J 1962;1:1658–61.
21. Killander A, Vahlquist B. The vitamin B$_{12}$ concentration in serum from term and premature infants. Nord Med 1954;51:777–9.
22. Baker H, Thind IS, Frank O, DeAngelis B, Caterini H, Louria DB. Vitamin levels in low-birth-weight newborn infants and their mothers. Am J Obstet Gynecol 1977;129:521–4.

23. Okuda K, Helliger AE, Chow BF. Vitamin B$_{12}$ serum level and pregnancy. Am J Clin Nutr 1956;4:440–3.
24. Baker H, Frank O, Deangelis B, Feingold S, Kaminetzky HA. Role of placenta in maternal-fetal vitamin transfer in humans. Am J Obstet Gynecol 1981;141:792–6.
25. Giugliani ERJ, Jorge SM, Goncalves AL. Serum vitamin B$_{12}$ levels in parturients, in the intervillous space of the placenta and in full-term newborns and their interrelationships with folate levels. Am J Clin Nutr 1985;41:330–5.
26. Giles C. An account of 335 cases of megaloblastic anaemia of pregnancy and the puerperium. J Clin Pathol 1966;19:1–11.
27. Dostalova L. Correlation of the vitamin status between mother and newborn during delivery. Dev Pharmacol Ther 1982;4(Suppl 1):45–57.
28. McGarry JM, Andrews J. Smoking in pregnancy and vitamin B$_{12}$ metabolism. Br Med J 1972;2:74–7.
29. Heaton D. Another case of megaloblastic anemia of infancy due to maternal pernicious anemia. N Engl J Med 1979;300:202–3.
30. Varadi S. Pernicious anaemia and infertility. Lancet 1967;2:1305.
31. Jackson IMD, Doig WB, McDonald G. Pernicious anaemia as a cause of infertility. Lancet 1967;2:1059–60.
32. Chaudhuri S. Vitamin B$_{12}$ in megaloblastic anaemia of pregnancy and tropical nutritional macrocytic anaemia. Br Med J 1951;2:825–8.
33. Patel JC, Kocher BR. Vitamin B$_{12}$ in macrocytic anaemia of pregnancy and the puerperium. Br Med J 1950;1:924–7.
34. Parr JH, Ramsay I. The presentation of osteomalacia in pregnancy. Case report. Br J Obstet Gynaecol 1984;91:816–8.
35. Streiff RR, Little AB. Folic acid deficiency as a cause of uterine hemorrhage in pregnancy. J Clin Invest 1965;44:1102.
36. Streiff RR, Little AB. Folic acid deficiency in pregnancy. N Engl J Med 1967;276:776–9.
37. Whiteside MG, Ungar B, Cowling DC. Iron, folic acid and vitamin B$_{12}$ levels in normal pregnancy, and their influence on birth-weight and the duration of pregnancy. Med J Aust 1968;1:338–42.
38. Shepard TH. *Catalog of Teratogenic Agents*, ed 3. Baltimore:The Johns Hopkins University Press, 1980:348–9.
39. Schorah CJ, Smithells RW, Scott J. Vitamin B$_{12}$ and anencephaly. Lancet 1980;1:880.
40. Ampola MG, Mahoney MJ, Nakamura E, Tanaka K. Prenatal therapy of a patient with vitamin-B$_{12}$-responsive methylmalonic acidemia. N Engl J Med 1975;293:313–7.
41. Morrow G III, Schwarz RH, Hallock JA, Barness LA. Prenatal detection of methylmalonic acidemia. J Pediatr 1970;77:120–3.
42. Samson RR, McClelland DBL. Vitamin B$_{12}$ in human colostrum and milk. Acta Paediatr Scand 1980;69:93–9.
43. Deodhar AD, Rajalakshmi R, Ramakrishnan CV. Studies on human lactation. Part III. Effect of dietary vitamin supplementation on vitamin contents of breast milk. Acta Paediatr Scand 1964;53:42–8.
44. Thomas MR, Kawamoto J, Sneed SM, Eakin R. The effects of vitamin C, vitamin B$_6$, and vitamin B$_{12}$ supplementation on the breast milk and maternal status of well-nourished women. Am J Clin Nutr 1979;32:1679–85.
45. Sneed SM, Zane C, Thomas MR. The effects of ascorbic acid, vitamin B$_6$, vitamin B$_{12}$, and folic acid supplementation on the breast milk and maternal nutritional status of low socioeconomic lactating women. Am J Clin Nutr 1981;34:1338–46.
46. Sandberg DP, Begley JA, Hall CA. The content, binding, and forms of vitamin B$_{12}$ in milk. Am J Clin Nutr 1981;34:1717–24.
47. Ford JE, Zechalko A, Murphy J, Brooke OG. Comparison of the B vitamin composition of milk from mothers of preterm and term babies. Arch Dis Child 1983;58:367–72.
48. Lampkin BC, Shore NA, Chadwick D. Megaloblastic anemia of infancy secondary to maternal pernicious anemia. N Engl J Med 1966;274:1168–71.
49. Jadhav M, Webb JKG, Vaishnava S, Baker SJ. Vitamin-B$_{12}$ deficiency in Indian infants: a clinical syndrome. Lancet 1962;2:903–7.
50. Lampkin BC, Saunders EF. Nutritional vitamin B$_{12}$ deficiency in an infant. J Pediatr 1969;75:1053–5.
51. Higginbottom MC, Sweetman L, Nyhan WL. A syndrome of methylmalonic aciduria, homocystinuria,

megaloblastic anemia and neurologic abnormalities in a vitamin B$_{12}$-deficient breast-fed infant of a strict vegetarian. N Engl J Med 1978;299:317–23.

52. Frader J, Reibman B, Turkewitz D. Vitamin B$_{12}$ deficiency in strict vegetarians. N Engl J Med 1978;299:1319.
53. Fleiss PM, Douglass JM, Wolfe L. *Ibid*.
54. Hershaft A. *Ibid*, 1319–20.
55. Nyhan WL. *Ibid*, 1320.
56. Abdulla M, Aly KO, Andersson I, Asp NG, Birkhed D, Denker I, Johansson CG, Jagerstad M, Kolar K, Nair BM, Nilsson-Ehle P, Norden A, Rassner S, Svensson S, Akesson B, Ockerman PA. Nutrient intake and health status of lactovegetarians: chemical analyses of diets using the duplicate portion sampling technique. Am J Clin Nutr 1984;40:325–38.

Name: **VITAMIN C**

Class: **Vitamin**   Risk Factor: **A***

Fetal Risk Summary

Vitamin C (ascorbic acid) is a water-soluble essential nutrient required for collagen formation, tissue repair, and numerous metabolic processes including the conversion of folic acid to folinic acid and iron metabolism (1). The American RDA for vitamin C in pregnancy is 70–80 mg (2).

Vitamin C is actively transported to the fetus (3–6). When maternal serum levels are high, placental transfer changes to simple diffusion (6). During gestation, maternal serum vitamin C progressively declines (7, 8). As a consequence of this process, newborn serum vitamin C level (9–22 µg/ml) is approximately 2–4 times that of the mother (4–10 µg/ml) (5–20).

Maternal deficiency of vitamin C without clinical symptoms is common during pregnancy (19–21). Most studies have found no association between this deficiency and maternal or fetal complications, including congenital malformations (12, 13, 22–25). When low vitamin C levels were found in women or fetuses with complications it was a consequence of the condition and not a cause. However, a 1971 retrospective study of 1,369 mothers found that deficiency of vitamin C may have a teratogenic effect, although the authors advised caution in the interpretation of their results (26). In a later investigation, low 1st trimester white blood cell vitamin C levels were discovered in six mothers who gave birth to infants with neural tube defects (27). Folic acid, vitamin B$_{12}$, and riboflavin levels were also low in serum or red blood cells. The low folic acid and B$_{12}$ levels were thought to be involved in the etiology of the defects (see also Folic Acid, Vitamin B$_{12}$, and Riboflavin).

Only one report has been found that potentially relates high doses of vitamin C with fetal anomalies. This was in a brief 1976 case report describing an anencephalic fetus delivered from a woman treated with high doses of vitamin C and other water-soluble vitamins and nutrients for psychiatric reasons (28). The relationship between the defect and the vitamins is unknown. In another study, no evidence of adverse effects was found with doses up to 2,000 mg/day (29).

In summary, mild to moderate vitamin C deficiency or excessive doses do not seem to pose a significant risk to the mother or fetus. Since vitamin C is required for good maternal and fetal health and an increased demand for the vitamin occurs during pregnancy, intake up to the RDA is recommended.

[* Risk Factor C if used in doses above the RDA.]

Breast Feeding Summary

Vitamin C (ascorbic acid) is excreted into human breast milk. Reported concentrations in milk vary from 24 to 158 μg/ml (30–38). In lactating women with low nutritional status, milk vitamin C level is directly proportional to intake (31, 32). Supplementation with 4–200 mg/day of vitamin C produced milk levels of 24–61 μg/ml (31). Similarly, in another group of women with poor vitamin C intake, supplementation with 34–103 mg/day resulted in levels of 34–55 μg/ml (32). In contrast, studies in well-nourished women consuming the RDA or more of vitamin C in their diets indicate that ingestion of greater amounts does not significantly increase levels of the vitamin in their milk (33–37). Even consumption of total vitamin C exceeding 1,000 mg/day, 10 times the RDA, did not significantly increase milk concentrations or vitamin C intake of the infants (36). However, maternal urinary excretion of the vitamin did increase significantly. These studies indicate that vitamin C excretion in human milk is regulated to prevent exceeding a saturation level (36).

Storage of human milk in the freezer for up to 3 months did not affect vitamin C concentrations of preterm milk but resulted in a significant decrease in concentration in term milk (39). Both types of milk, however, maintained sufficient vitamin C to meet the RDA for infants.

The RDA for vitamin C during lactation is 90–100 mg (2). Well-nourished lactating women consuming the RDA of vitamin C in their diets normally excrete sufficient vitamin C in their milk to reach a saturation level and additional supplementation is not required. Maternal supplementation up to the RDA is needed only in those women with poor nutritional status.

References

1. American Hospital Formulary Service. *Drug Information 1985*. Bethesda:American Society of Hospital Pharmacists, 1985:1697–9.
2. *Recommended Dietary Allowances*, ed 9. Washington, DC:National Academy of Sciences, 1980.
3. Hill EP, Longo LD. Dynamics of maternal-fetal nutrient transfer. Fed Proc 1980;39:239–44.
4. Streeter ML, Rosso P. Transport mechanisms for ascorbic acid in the human placenta. Am J Clin Nutr 1981;34:1706–11.
5. Hamil BM, Munks B, Moyer EZ, Kaucher M, Williams HH. Vitamin C in the blood and urine of the newborn and in the cord and maternal blood. Am J Dis Child 1947;74:417–33.
6. Kaminetzky HA, Baker H, Frank O, Langer A. The effects of intravenously administered water-soluble vitamins during labor in normovitaminemic and hypovitaminemic gravidas on maternal and neonatal blood vitamin levels at delivery. Am J Obstet Gynecol 1974;120:697–703.
7. Snelling CE, Jackson SH. Blood studies of vitamin C during pregnancy, birth, and early infancy. J Pediatr 1939;14:447–51.
8. Adlard BPF, De Souza SW, Moon S. Ascorbic acid in fetal human brain. Arch Dis Child 1974;49:278–82.
9. Braestrup PW. Studies of latent scurvy in infants. II. Content of ascorbic (cevitamic) acid in the blood-serum of women in labour and in children at birth. Acta Paediatr 1937;19:328–34.
10. Braestrup PW. The content of reduced ascorbic acid in blood plasma in infants, especially at birth and in the first days of life. J Nutr 1938;16:363–73.
11. Slobody LB, Benson RA, Mestern J. A comparison of the vitamin C in mothers and their newborn infants. J Pediatr 1946;29:41–4.
12. Teel HM, Burke BS, Draper R. Vitamin C in human pregnancy and lactation. I. Studies during pregnancy. Am J Dis Child 1938;56:1004–10.
13. Lund CJ, Kimble MS. Some determinants of maternal and plasma vitamin C levels. Am J Obstet Gynecol 1943;46:635–47.

14. Manahan CP, Eastman NJ. The cevitamic acid content of fetal blood. Bull Johns Hopkins Hosp 1938;62:478–81.
15. Raiha N. On the placental transfer of vitamin C. An experimental study on guinea pigs and human subjects. Acta Physiol Scand 1958;45:Suppl 155.
16. Khattab AK, Al Nagdy SA, Mourad KAH, El Azghal HI. Foetal maternal ascorbic acid gradient in normal Egyptian subjects. J Trop Pediatr 1970;16:112–5.
17. McDevitt E, Dove MA, Dove RF, Wright IS. Selective filtration of vitamin C by the placenta. Proc Soc Exp Biol Med 1942;51:289–90.
18. Sharma SC. Levels of total ascorbic acid, histamine and prostaglandins E_2 and F_{2a} in the maternal antecubital and foetal umbilical vein blood immediately following the normal human delivery. Int J Vitam Nutr Res 1982;52:320–5.
19. Dostalova L. Correlation of the vitamin status between mother and newborn during delivery. Dev Pharmacol Ther 1982;4(Suppl 1):45–57.
20. Baker H, Frank O, Thomson AD, Langer A, Munves ED, De Angelis B, Kaminetzky HA. Vitamin profile of 174 mothers and newborns at parturition. Am J Clin Nutr 1975;28:59–65.
21. Kaminetzky HA, Langer A, Baker H, Frank O, Thomson AD, Munves ED, Opper A, Behrle FC, Glista B. The effect of nutrition in teen-age gravidas on pregnancy and the status of the neonate. I. A nutritional profile. Am J Obstet Gynecol 1973;115:639–46.
22. Martin MP, Bridgforth E, McGanity WJ, Darby WJ. The Vanderbilt cooperative study of maternal and infant nutrition. X. Ascorbic acid. J Nutr 1957;62:201–24.
23. Chaudhuri SK. Role of nutrition in the etiology of toxemia of pregnancy. Am J Obstet Gynecol 1971;110:46–8.
24. Wilson CWM, Loh HS. Vitamin C and fertility. Lancet 1973;2:859–60.
25. Vobecky JS, Vobecky J, Shapcott D, Munan L. Vitamin C and outcome of pregnancy. Lancet 1974;1:630.
26. Nelson MM, Forfar JO. Associations between drugs administered during pregnancy and congenital abnormalities of the fetus. Br Med J 1971;1:523–7.
27. Smithells RW, Sheppard S, Schorah CJ. Vitamin deficiencies and neural tube defects. Arch Dis Child 1976;51:944–50.
28. Averback P. Anencephaly associated with megavitamin therapy. Can Med Assoc J 1976;114:995.
29. Korner WF, Weber F. Zur toleranz hoher Ascorbinsauredosen. Int J Vitam Nutr Res 1972;42:528–44.
30. Ingalls TH, Draper R, Teel HM. Vitamin C in human pregnancy and lactation. II. Studies during lactation. Am J Dis Child 1938;56:1011–19.
31. Deodhar AD, Rajalakshmi R, Ramakrishnan CV. Studies on human lactation. Part III. Effect of dietary vitamin supplementation on vitamin contents of breast milk. Acta Paediatr 1964;53:42–8.
32. Bates CJ, Prentice AM, Prentice A, Lamb WH, Whitehead RG. The effect of vitamin C supplementation on lactating women in Keneba, a West African rural community. Int J Vitam Nutr Res 1983;53:68–76.
33. Thomas MR, Kawamoto J, Sneed SM, Eakin R. The effects of vitamin C, vitamin B_6, and vitamin B_{12} supplementation on the breast milk and maternal status of well-nourished women. Am J Clin Nutr 1979;32:1679–85.
34. Thomas MR, Sneed SM, Wei C, Nail PA, Wilson M, Sprinkle EE III. The effects of vitamin C, vitamin B_6, vitamin B_{12}, folic acid, riboflavin, and thiamin on the breast milk and maternal status of well-nourished women at 6 months postpartum. Am J Clin Nutr 1980;33:2151–6.
35. Sneed SM, Zane C, Thomas MR. The effects of ascorbic acid, vitamin B_6, vitamin B_{12}. and folic acid supplementation on the breast milk and maternal nutritional status of low socioeconomic lactating women. Am J Clin Nutr 1981;34:1338–46.
36. Byerley LO, Kirksey A. Effects of different levels of vitamin C intake on the vitamin C concentration in human milk and the vitamin C intakes of breast-fed infants. Am J Clin Nutr 1985;41:665–71.
37. Salmenpera L. Vitamin C nutrition during prolonged lactation: optimal in infants while marginal in some mothers. Am J Clin Nutr 1984;40:1050–6.
38. Grewar D. Infantile scurvy. Clin Pediatr 1965;4:82–9.
39. Bank MR, Kirksey A, West K, Giacoia G. Effect of storage time and temperature on folacin and vitamin C levels in term and preterm human milk. Am J Clin Nutr 1985;41:235–42.

Name: **VITAMIN D**

Class: **Vitamin**   Risk Factor: **A***

Fetal Risk Summary

Vitamin D analogs are a group of fat-soluble nutrients essential for human life with antirachitic and hypercalcemic activity (1). The RDA for normal pregnant women in America is 400–600 IU (2).

The two natural biologically active forms of vitamin D are 1,25-dihydroxyergo-calciferol and calcitriol (1,25-dihydroxyvitamin D_3) (1). A third active compound, 25-hydroxydihydrotachysterol, is produced in the liver from the synthetic vitamin D analogue, dihydrotachysterol.

Ergosterol (provitamin D_2) and 7-dehydrocholesterol (provitamin D_3) are activated by ultraviolet light to form ergocalciferol (vitamin D_2) and cholecalciferol (vitamin D_3), respectively. These, in turn, are converted in the liver to 25-hydroxyergocalci-ferol and calcifediol (25-hydroxyvitamin D_3), the major transport forms of vitamin D in the body. Activation of the transport compounds by enzymes in the kidneys results in the two natural active forms of vitamin D.

The commercially available forms of vitamin D are ergocalciferol, cholecalciferol, calcifediol, calcitriol, and dihydrotachysterol. Although differing in potency, all of these products have the same result in the mother and fetus. Thus, only the term vitamin D, unless otherwise noted, will be used in this monograph.

High doses of vitamin D are known to be teratogenic in experimental animals, but direct evidence for this is lacking in humans. Because of its action to raise calcium levels, vitamin D has been suspected in the pathogenesis of the supraval-vular aortic stenosis syndrome, which is often associated with idiopathic hypercal-cemia of infancy (3–5). The full features of this rare condition are characteristic elfin facies, mental and growth retardation, strabismus, enamel defects, craniosy-nostosis, supravalvular aortic and pulmonary stenosis, inguinal hernia, cryptorchid-ism in men, and early development of secondary sexual characteristics in women (3). Excessive intake or retention of vitamin D during pregnancy by mothers of infants who develop supravalvular aortic stenosis syndrome has not been consist-ently found (3, 4, 6). While the exact cause is unknown, it is possible that the syndrome results from abnormal vitamin D metabolism either in the mother or fetus or both.

Very high levels of vitamin D have been used to treat maternal hypoparathyroid-ism during pregnancy (7–10). Goodenday and Gordon (7, 8) treated 15 mothers with doses averaging 107,000 IU/day throughout their pregnancies to maintain maternal calcium levels within the normal range. All of the 27 infants were normal at birth and during follow-up examinations ranging up to 16 years. Calcitriol, in doses up to 3 µg/day, was used to treat another mother with hypoparathyroidism (9). The high dose was required in the latter half of pregnancy to prevent hypocal-cemia. The infant had no apparent adverse effects from this exposure. In a similar case, a mother received 100,000 IU/day throughout gestation and delivered a healthy, full-term infant (10). In contrast, a 1965 case report described a woman who received 600,000 IU of vitamin D and 40,000 IU of vitamin A daily for 1 month early in pregnancy (11). The resulting infant had a defect of the urogenital system, but this was probably due to ingestion of excessive vitamin A (see Vitamin A).

Vitamin D deficiency can be induced by decreased dietary intake or lack of exposure to sunlight. The conversion of provitamin D_3 to vitamin D_3 is catalyzed by ultraviolet light striking the skin (1). Severe deficiency during pregnancy, resulting in maternal osteomalacia, leads to significant morbidity in the mother and fetus (12–22). Pitkin (23), in a 1985 article, reviewed the relationship between vitamin D and calcium metabolism in pregnancy.

Although rare in America, the peak incidence of vitamin D deficiency occurs in the winter and early spring when exposure to sunlight is at a minimum. Certain ethnic groups, such as Asians, seem to be at greater risk for developing this deficiency because of their dietary and sun-exposure habits (l2–22). In the pregnant woman, osteomalacia may cause, among other effects, decreased weight gain and pelvic deformities that prevent normal vaginal delivery (12, 13). For the fetus, vitamin D deficiency has been associated with:

Reduced fetal growth (12, 13)
Neonatal hypocalcemia without convulsions (13–15, 21)
Neonatal hypocalcemia with convulsions (tetany) (16–18)
Neonatal rickets (19, 20)
Defective tooth enamel (22, 24)

Long-term use of heparin may induce osteopenia by inhibiting renal activation of calcifediol to the active form of vitamin D_3 (calcitriol or 1,25-dihydroxyvitamin D_3) (23). The decreased levels of calcitriol prevent calcium uptake by bone and result in osteopenia [see Pitkin, 1985 (23), for detailed review of calcium metabolism in pregnancy]. Pitkin suggests these patients may benefit from treatment with supplemental calcitriol.

A number of investigators have measured vitamin D levels in the mother during pregnancy and in the newborn (25–35). Although not universal, most studies have found a significant correlation between maternal serum and cord blood levels (25–29). Markestad and co-workers (30) calculated a close association between both of the transport vitamin D forms in maternal and cord serum. No significant correlation could be demonstrated, however, between the two biologically active forms in maternal and cord blood.

Using a perfused human placenta, a 1984 report confirmed that calcifediol and calcitriol were transferred from the mother to the fetus, although at a very slow rate (36). Binding to vitamin D_3-binding protein was a major rate-limiting factor, especially for calcifediol, the transport form of vitamin D_3. The researchers concluded that placental metabolism of calcifediol was not a major source of fetal calcitriol (36).

Maternal levels at term are usually higher than those in the newborn since the fetus has no need for intestinal calcium absorption (25–31). Maternal levels are elevated in early pregnancy and continue to increase throughout pregnancy (33). During the winter months a weak correlation may exist between maternal vitamin D intake and serum levels with exposure to ultraviolet light the main determinant of maternal concentrations (34, 35). A Norwegian study, however, was able to significantly increase maternal concentrations of active vitamin D during all seasons with daily supplementation of 400 IU (30).

[* Risk Factor D if used in doses above the RDA.]

Breast Feeding Summary

Vitamin D is excreted into breast milk in limited amounts (37). A direct relationship exists between maternal serum levels of vitamin D and the concentration in breast milk (38). Chronic maternal ingestion of large doses may lead to greater than normal vitamin D activity in the milk and resulting hypercalcemia in the infant (39). In the lactating woman who is not receiving supplements, there is considerable controversy over whether or not her milk contains sufficient vitamin D to protect the infant from vitamin deficiency. Several studies have supported the need for infant supplementation during breast-feeding (13, 37, 40–42). Other investigators have concluded that supplementation is not necessary if maternal vitamin D stores are adequate (29, 43–45).

In a 1977 report, Lakdawala and Widdowson (46) measured high levels of a vitamin D metabolite in the aqueous phase of milk. Although two other studies supported these findings, the conclusions were in direct opposition to previous measurements and have been vigorously disputed (47, 48). The argument that human milk is low in vitamin D is supported by clinical reports of vitamin D deficiency-induced rickets and decreased bone mineralization in breast-fed infants (41, 42, 49–51). Reeve and co-workers (52) measured the vitamin D activity of human milk and failed to find any evidence for significant activity of water-soluble vitamin D metabolites. Vitamin D activity in the milk was 40–50 IU/L with 90% of this accounted for by the usual fat-soluble components.

The American RDA for vitamin D in the lactating woman is 400–600 IU (2). The Committee on Nutrition of the American Academy of Pediatrics, recommends vitamin D supplements for breast-fed infants if maternal vitamin D nutrition is inadequate or if the infant lacks sufficient exposure to ultraviolet light (53).

References

1. American Hospital Formulary Service. *Drug Information 1985*. Bethesda:American Society of Hospital Pharmacists, 1985:1699–1702.
2. *Recommended Dietary Allowances*, ed 9. Washington, DC:National Academy of Sciences, 1980.
3. Friedman WF, Mills LF. The relationship between vitamin D and the craniofacial and dental anomalies of the supravalvular aortic stenosis syndrome. Pediatrics 1969;43:12–8.
4. Rowe, RD, Cooke RE. Vitamin D and craniofacial and dental anomalies of supravalvular stenosis. Pediatrics 1969;43:1–2.
5. Taussig HB. Possible injury to the cardiovascular system from vitamin D. Ann Intern Med 1966;65:1195–1200.
6. Anita AU, Wiltse HE, Rowe RD, Pitt EL, Levin S, Ottesen OE, Cooke RE. Pathogenesis of the supravalvular aortic stenosis syndrome. J Pediatr 1967;71:431–41.
7. Goodenday LS, Gordan GS. Fetal safety of vitamin D during pregnancy. Clin Res 1971;19:200.
8. Goodenday LS, Gordan GS. No risk from vitamin D in pregnancy. Ann Intern Med 1971;75:807–8.
9. Sadeghi-Nejad A, Wolfsdorf JI, Senior B. Hypoparathyroidism and pregnancy: treatment with calcitriol. JAMA 1980;243:254–5.
10. Greer FR, Hollis BW, Napoli JL. High concentrations of vitamin D_2 in human milk associated with pharmacologic doses of vitamin D_2. J Pediatr 1984;105:61–4.
11. Pilotti G, Scorta A. Ipervitaminosi A gravidica e malformazioni neonatali dell'apparato urinario. Minerva Ginecol 1965;17:1103–8. As cited in Nishimura H, Tanimura T. *Clinical Aspects of the Teratogenicity of Drugs*. New York:American Elsevier, 1976:251–2.
12. Parr JH, Ramsay I. The presentation of osteomalacia in pregnancy. Case report. Br J Obstet Gynaecol 1984;91:816–8.
13. Brooke OG, Brown IRF, Bone CDM, Carter ND, Cleeve HJW, Maxwell JD, Robinson VP, Winder SM. Vitamin D supplements in pregnant Asian women: effects on calcium status and fetal growth. Br Med J 1980;280:751–4.
14. Rosen JF, Roginsky M, Nathenson G, Finberg L. 25-Hydroxyvitamin D: plasma levels in mothers and their premature infants with neonatal hypocalcemia. Am J Dis Child 1974;127:220–3.

15. Watney PJM, Chance GW, Scott P, Thompson JM. Maternal factors in neonatal hypocalcaemia: a study in three ethnic groups. Br Med J 1971;2:432–6.
16. Heckmatt JZ, Peacock M, Davies AEJ, McMurray J, Isherwood DM. Plasma 25-hydroxyvitamin D in pregnant Asian women and their babies. Lancet 1979;2:546–9.
17. Roberts SA, Cohen MD, Forfar JO. Antenatal factors associated with neonatal hypocalcaemic convulsions. Lancet 1973;2:809–11.
18. Purvis RJ, Barrie WJM, MacKay GS, Wilkinson EM, Cockburn F, Belton NR, Forfar JO. Enamel hypoplasia of the teeth associated with neonatal tetany: a manifestation of maternal vitamin-D deficiency. Lancet 1973;2:811–4.
19. Ford JA, Davidson DC, McIntosh WB, Fyfe WM, Dunnigan MG. Neonatal rickets in Asian immigrant population. Br Med J 1973;3:211–2.
20. Moncrieff M, Fadahunsi TO. Congenital rickets due to maternal vitamin D deficiency. Arch Dis Child 1974;49:810–1.
21. Watney PJM. Maternal factors in the aetiology of neonatal hypocalcaemia. Postgrad Med J 1975;51(Suppl 3):14–7.
22. Cockburn F, Belton NR, Purvis RJ, Giles MM, Brown JK, Turner TL, Wilkinson EM, Forfar JO, Barrie WJM, McKay GS, Pocock SJ. Maternal vitamin D intake and mineral metabolism in mothers and their newborn infants. Br Med J 1980;2:11–4.
23. Pitkin RM. Calcium metabolism in pregnancy and the perinatal period: a review. Am J Obstet Gynecol 1985;151:99–109.
24. Stimmler L, Snodgrass GJAI, Jaffe E. Dental defects associated with neonatal symptomatic hypocalcaemia. Arch Dis Child 1973;48:217–20.
25. Hillman LS, Haddad JG. Human perinatal vitamin D metabolism. I: 25-hydroxyvitamin D in maternal and cord blood. J Pediatr 1974;84:742–9.
26. Dent CE, Gupta MM. Plasma 25-hydroxyvitamin-D levels during pregnancy in caucasians and in vegetarian and non-vegetarian Asians. Lancet 1975;2:1057–60.
27. Weisman Y, Occhipinti M, Knox G, Reiter E, Root A. Concentrations of 24,25-dihydroxyvitamin D and 25-hydroxyvitamin D in paired maternal-cord sera. Am J Obstet Gynecol 1978;130:704–7.
28. Steichen JJ, Tsang RC, Gratton TL, Hamstra A, DeLuca HF. Vitamin D homeostasis in the perinatal period: 1,25-dihydroxyvitamin D in maternal, cord, and neonatal blood. N Engl J Med 1980;302:315–9.
29. Birkbeck JA, Scott HF. 25-Hydroxycholecalciferol serum levels in breast-fed infants. Arch Dis Child 1980;55:691–5.
30. Markestad T, Aksnes L, Ulstein M, Aarskog D. 25-Hydroxyvitamin D and 1,25-dihydroxyvitamin D of D_2 and D_3 origin in maternal and umbilical cord serum after vitamin D_2 supplementation in human pregnancy. Am J Clin Nutr 1984;40:1057–63.
31. Kumar R, Cohen WR, Epstein FH. Vitamin D and calcium hormones in pregnancy. N Engl J Med 1980;302:1143–5.
32. Hillman LS, Haddad JG. Perinatal vitamin D metabolism. II. Serial 25-hydroxyvitamin D concentrations in sera of term and premature infants. J Pediatr 1975;86:928–35.
33. Kumar R, Cohen WR, Silva P, Epstein FH. Elevated 1,25-dihydroxyvitamin D plasma levels in normal human pregnancy and lactation. J Clin Invest 1979;63:342–4.
34. Hillman LS, Haddad JG. Perinatal vitamin D metabolism. III. Factors influencing late gestational human serum 25-hydroxyvitamin D. Am J Obstet Gynecol 1976;125:196–200.
35. Turton CWG, Stanley P, Stamp TCB, Maxwell JD. Altered vitamin-D metabolism in pregnancy. Lancet 1977;1:222–5.
36. Ron M, Levitz M, Chuba J, Dancis J. Transfer of 25-hydroxyvitamin D_3 and 1,25-dihydroxyvitamin D_3 across the perfused human placenta. Am J Obstet Gynecol 1984;148:370–4.
37. Greer FR, Hollis BW, Cripps DJ, Tsang RC. Effects of maternal ultraviolet B irradiation on vitamin D content of human milk. J Pediatr 1984;105:431–3.
38. Rothberg AD, Pettifor JM, Cohen DF, Sonnendecker EWW, Ross FP. Maternal-infant vitamin D relationships during breast-feeding. J Pediatr 1982;101:500–3.
39. Goldberg LD. Transmission of a vitamin-D metabolite in breast milk. Lancet 1972;2:1258–9.
40. Greer FR, Ho M, Dodson D, Tsang RC. Lack of 25-hydroxyvitamin D and 1,25-dihydroxyvitamin D in human milk. J Pediatr 1981;99:233–5.
41. Greer FR, Searcy JE, Levin RS, Steichen JJ, Steichen-Asch PS, Tsang RC. Bone mineral content and serum 25-hydroxyvitamin D concentration in breast-fed infants with and without supplemental vitamin D. J Pediatr 1981;98:696–701.
42. Greer FR, Searcy JE, Levin RS, Steichen JJ, Steichen-Asche PS, Tsang RC. Bone mineral content

and serum 25-hydroxyvitamin D concentrations in breast-fed infants with and without supplemental vitamin D: one-year follow-up. J Pediatr 1982;100:919–22.

43. Fairney A, Naughten E, Oppe TE. Vitamin D and human lactation. Lancet 1977;2:739–41.
44. Roberts CC, Chan GM, Folland D, Rayburn C, Jackson R. Adequate bone mineralization in breast-fed infants. J Pediatr 1981;99:192–6.
45. Chadwick DW. Commentary. Water-soluble vitamin D in human milk: a myth. Pediatrics 1982;70:499.
46. Lakdawala DR, Widdowson EM. Vitamin-D in human milk. Lancet 1977;1:167–8.
47. Greer FR, Reeve LE, Chesney RW, DeLuca HF. Water-soluble vitamin D in human milk: a myth. Pediatrics 1982;69:238.
48. Greer FR, Reeve LE, Chesney RW, DeLuca HF. Commentary. Water-soluble vitamin D in human milk: a myth. Pediatrics 1982;70:499–500.
49. Bunker JWM, Harris RS, Eustis RS. The antirachitic potency of the milk of human mothers fed previously on "vitamin D milk" of the cow. N Engl J Med 1933;208:313–5.
50. O'Connor P. Vitamin D-deficiency rickets in two breast-fed infants who were not receiving vitamin D supplementation. Clin Pediatr (Phila) 1977;16:361–3.
51. Little JA. Commentary. Water-soluble vitamin D in human milk: a myth. Pediatrics 1982;70:499.
52. Reeve LE, Chesney RW, DeLuca HF. Vitamin D of human milk: identification of biologically active forms. Am J Clin Nutr 1982;36:122–6.
53. Committee on Nutrition, American Academy of Pediatrics. Vitamin and mineral supplement needs in normal children in the United States. Pediatrics 1980;66:1015.

Name: **VITAMIN E**

Class: **Vitamin**   Risk Factor: **A***

Fetal Risk Summary

Vitamin E (tocopherols) is a group of fat-soluble vitamins that are essential for human health, although their exact biologic function is unknown (1). The American RDA for vitamin E in pregnancy is 15 IU (about 15 mg) (2).

Vitamin E concentrations in mothers at term are approximately 4–5 times that of the newborn (3–9). Levels in the mother rise throughout pregnancy (4). Maternal blood vitamin E usually ranges between 9 and 19 μg/ml with corresponding newborn levels varying from 2 to 6 μg/ml (3–10). Supplementation of the mother with 15–30 mg/day had no effect on either maternal or newborn vitamin E concentrations at term (5). Use of 600 mg/day in the last 2 months of pregnancy produced about a 50% rise in maternal serum vitamin E (+8 μg/ml) but a much smaller increase in the cord blood (+1 μg/ml) (8). Although placental transfer is by passive diffusion, passage of vitamin E to the fetus is dependent upon plasma lipid concentrations (9–11). At term, cord blood is low in β-lipoproteins, the major carrier of vitamin E, in comparison to maternal blood, and as a consequence, it is able to transport less of the vitamin (9). Since vitamin E is transported in the plasma by these lipids, recent investigations have focused on the ratio of vitamin E (in milligrams) to total lipids (in grams) rather than on blood vitamin E concentrations alone (10). Ratios above about 0.6–0.8 are considered normal, depending on the author cited and the age of the patients (10, 12, 13).

Vitamin E deficiency is relatively uncommon in pregnancy, occurring in less than 10% of all patients (4, 5, 14). No maternal or fetal complications from deficiency or excess of the vitamin have been identified. Doses far exceeding the RDA have not proved harmful (8, 15, 16). Early studies used vitamin E in conjunction with other therapy in attempts to prevent abortion and premature labor, but no effect of the vitamin therapy was demonstrated (17, 18). Premature infants born with low vitamin E stores may develop hemolytic anemia, edema, reticulocytosis, and thrombocytosis if not given adequate vitamin E in the first months following birth (16, 19, 20). In two studies, supplementation of mothers with 500–600 mg of vitamin E during the last 1–2 months of pregnancy did not produce values significantly different from those of controls in the erythrocyte hemolysis test with hydrogen peroxide, a test used to determine adequate levels of vitamin E (8, 16).

In summary, neither deficiency nor excess of vitamin E has been associated with maternal or fetal complications during pregnancy. In well-nourished women, adequate vitamin E is consumed in the diet and supplementation is not required. If dietary intake is poor, supplementation up to the RDA for pregnancy is recommended.

[* Risk Factor C if used in doses above the RDA.]

Breast Feeding Summary

Vitamin E is excreted into human breast milk (12, 13, 21, 22). Human milk is more than five times richer in vitamin E than cows' milk and is more effective in maintaining adequate serum vitamin E and vitamin E/total lipid ratio in infants up to 1 year of age (12, 22). A 1985 study measured 2.3 μg/ml of the vitamin in mature milk (21). Preterm milk (gestational age 27–33 weeks) level was significantly higher, 8.5 μg/ml, during the first week and then decreased progressively over the next 6 weeks to 3.7 μg/ml (21). The authors concluded that preterm milk plus multivitamin supplements would provide adequate levels of vitamin E for very low-birth-weight infants (<1,500 g and appropriate for gestational age).

Japanese researchers examined the pattern of vitamin E analogs (α-, γ-, δ-, and β-tocopherols) in plasma and red blood cells from breast-fed and bottle-fed infants (23). Several differences were noted, but the significance of these findings to human health is unknown.

Vitamin E applied for 6 days to the nipples of breast-feeding women resulted in a significant rise in infant serum levels of the vitamin (24). The study group, composed of 10 women, applied the contents of one 400-IU vitamin E capsule to both areolae and nipples after each nursing. Serum concentrations of the vitamin rose from 4 to 17.5 μg/ml while those in a similar group of untreated controls rose from 3.4 to 12.2 μg/ml. The difference between the two groups was statistically significant ($p < 0.025$). Although no adverse effects were observed, the authors cautioned that the long-term effects were unknown.

The American RDA of vitamin E during lactation is 16 IU (about 16 mg) (2). Maternal supplementation is recommended only if the diet does not provide sufficient vitamin E to meet the RDA.

References

1. American Hospital Formulary Service. *Drug Information 1985*. Bethesda:American Society of Hospital Pharmacists, 1985:1705–7.
2. *Recommended Dietary Allowances*, ed 9. Washington, DC:National Academy of Sciences, 1980.
3. Moyer WT. Vitamin E levels in term and premature newborn infants. Pediatrics 1950;6:893–6.
4. Leonard PJ, Doyle E, Harrington W. Levels of vitamin E in the plasma of newborn infants and of the mothers. Am J Clin Nutr 1972;25:480–4.
5. Baker H, Frank O, Thomson AD, Langer A, Munves ED, De Angelis B, Kaminetzky HA. Vitamin profile of 174 mothers and newborns at parturition. Am J Clin Nutr 1975;28:59–65.

6. Dostalova L. Correlation of the vitamin status between mother and newborn during delivery. Dev Pharmacol Ther 1982;4(Suppl I):45–57.
7. Kaminetzky HA, Baker H. Micronutrients in pregnancy. Clin Obstet Gynecol 1977;20:363–80.
8. Mino M, Nishino H. Fetal and maternal relationship in serum vitamin E level. J Nutr Sci Vitaminol 1973;19:475–82.
9. Haga P, Ek J, Kran S. Plasma tocopherol levels and vitamin E/B-lipoprotein relationships during pregnancy and in cord blood. Am J Clin Nutr 1982;36:1200–4.
10. Martinez FE, Goncalves AL, Jorge SM, Desai ID. Vitamin E in placental blood and its interrelationship to maternal and newborn levels of vitamin E. J Pediatr 1981;99:298–300.
11. Hill EP, Longo LD. Dynamics of maternal-fetal nutrient transfer. Fed Proc 1980;39:239–44.
12. Martinez FE, Jorge SM, Goncalves AL, Desai ID. Evaluation of plasma tocopherols in relation to hematological indices of Brazilian infants on human milk and cows' milk regime from birth to 1 year of age. Am J Clin Nutr 1984;39:969–74.
13. Mino M, Kitagawa M, Nakagawa S. Red blood cell tocopherol concentrations in a normal population of Japanese children and premature infants in relation to the assessment of vitamin E status. Am J Clin Nutr 1985;41:631–8.
14. Kaminetzky HA, Langer A, Baker O, Frank O, Thomson AD, Munves ED, Opper A, Behrle FC, Glista B. The effect of nutrition in teen-age gravidas on pregnancy and the status of the neonate. I. A nutritional profile. Am J Obstet Gynecol 1973;115:639–46.
15. Hook EB, Healy KM, Niles AM, Skalko RG. Vitamin E: teratogen or anti-teratogen? Lancet 1974;1:809.
16. Gyorgy P, Cogan G, Rose CS. Availability of vitamin E in the newborn infant. Proc Soc Exp Biol Med 1952;81:536–8.
17. Kotz J, Parker E, Kaufman MS. Treatment of recurrent and threatened abortion. Report of two hundred and twenty-six cases. J Clin Endocrinol 1941;1:838–49.
18. Shute E. Vitamin E and premature labor. Am J Obstet Gynecol 1942;44:271–9.
19. Oski FA, Barness LA. Vitamin E deficiency: a previously unrecognized cause of hemolytic anemia in the premature infant. J Pediatr 1967;70:211–20.
20. Ritchie JH, Fish MB, McMasters V, Grossman M. Edema and hemolytic anemia in premature infants. A vitamin E deficiency syndrome. N Engl J Med 1968;279:1185–90.
21. Gross SJ, Gabriel E. Vitamin E status in preterm infants fed human milk or infant formula. J Pediatr 1985;106:635–9.
22. Friedman Z. Essential fatty acids revisited. Am J Dis Child 1980;134:397–408.
23. Mino M, Kijima Y, Nishida Y, Nakagawa S. Difference in plasma- and red blood cell-tocopherols in breast-fed and bottle-fed infants. J Nutr Sci Vitaminol 1980;26:103–12.
24. Marx CM, Izquierdo A, Driscoll JW, Murray MA, Epstein MF. Vitamin E concentrations in serum of newborn infants after topical use of vitamin E by nursing mothers. Am J Obstet Gynecol 1985;152:668–70.

Name: VITAMINS, MULTIPLE

Class: **Vitamins**   Risk Factor: **A***

Fetal Risk Summary

Vitamins are essential for human life. Preparations containing multiple vitamins (multivitamins) are routinely given to pregnant women. A typical product will contain the vitamins A, D, E, and C, plus the B complex vitamins thiamine (B_1), riboflavin (B_2), niacinamide (B_3), pantothenic acid (B_5), pyridoxine (B_6), B_{12}, and folic acid. Miscellaneous substances that may be included are iron, calcium, and other minerals. The practice of supplementation during pregnancy with multivitamins varies from country to country but is common in America. The American RDA for pregnant women are (1):

Vitamins, Multiple

Vitamin A	5,000 IU
Vitamin D	400–600 IU
Vitamin C	70–80 mg
Thiamine (B_1)	1.4–1.5 mg
Riboflavin (B_2)	1.5–1.6 mg
Niacinamide (B_3)	15–17 mg
Pyridoxine (B_6)	2.4–2.6 mg
Folic acid	0.8 mg
Vitamin B_{12}	4 μg
Vitamin E	15 IU

Although essential for health, vitamin K is normally not included in multivitamin preparations since it is adequately supplied from natural sources. The fat-soluble vitamins A, D, and E may be toxic or teratogenic in high doses. The water-soluble vitamins, C and the B complex group, are generally considered safe in amounts above the RDA, but there are exceptions. Deficiencies of vitamins may also be teratogenic. (See individual vitamin monographs for further details.)

The role of vitamins in the prevention of certain congenital defects continues to be a major area of controversy. Two different classes of anomalies, cleft lip and/or palate and neural tube defects, have been the focus of numerous investigations with multivitamins. An investigation into a third class of anomalies, limb reduction defects, has recently appeared. The following sections will summarize the reported work on these topics.

Animal research in the 1930's and 1940's had shown that both deficiencies and excesses of selected vitamins could result in fetal anomalies, but it was not until two papers by Douglas in 1958 (2, 3) that attention was turned to humans. Douglas examined the role of environmental factors, in particular the B complex vitamins, as agents for preventing the recurrence of cleft lip and/or palate (CLP). In that same year, Conway (4) published a study involving 87 women who had previously given birth to infants with CLP. Although the series was too small to draw statistical conclusions, 48 women given no vitamin supplements had 78 pregnancies, resulting in four infants with CLP. The treated group, composed of 39 women, received multivitamins plus injectable B complex vitamins during the 1st trimester. This group had 59 pregnancies with none of the infants having CLP. A similar study found a CLP incidence of 1.9% (3 of 156) in pregnancies in treated women compared to 5.7% (22 of 383) in controls (5). The difference was not statistically significant. Fraser and Warburton (6) found no evidence that vitamins offer protection against CLP in a 1964 survey. Also in 1964, Peer and co-workers (7) published research involving 594 pregnant women who had previously given birth to an infant with CLP. This work was further expanded, and the total group involving 645 pregnancies was presented in a 1976 paper (8). Of the total group, 417 women were not given supplements during pregnancy, and they gave birth to 20 infants (4.8%) with CLP. In the treated group, 228 women were given B complex vitamins plus vitamin C before or during the 1st trimester. From this latter group, seven infants (3.1%) with CLP resulted. Although suggestive of a positive effect, the difference between the two groups was not significant. Tolarova (9) found only one instance of CLP in his group of 85 pregnancies in women given supplements. These patients were given daily multivitamins plus 10 mg of folic acid. In 206 pregnancies in women not given supplements where the infants/fetuses were examined 15 instances of CLP resulted. The difference between the two groups was significant ($p = 0.023$). In contrast, one author suggested that the vitamin A in the supplements caused a cleft palate in his patient (10). However, the conclusion of this report has been disputed (11). Thus, the published studies involving the role of multivitamins in the prevention of cleft lip and/or palate are inconclusive. No decisive benefit (or risk) of multivitamin supplementation has emerged from any of the studies.

The second part of the controversy surrounding multivitamins and the prevention of congenital defects involves their role in preventing neural tube defects (NTD). In a series of articles from 1976 to 1983, Smithells and co-workers (12–16) examined the effect of multivitamin supplements on a group of women who had previously given birth to one or more children with NTD. They defined, for the purpose of their study, NTD to include anencephaly, encephalocele, cranial meningocele, iniencephaly, myelocele, myelomeningocele, and meningocele but excluded isolated hydrocephalus and spina bifida occulta (14). In their initial publication, they found that in six mothers who had given birth to infants with NTD, there were lower lst trimester levels of serum folate, red blood cell folate, white blood cell vitamin C, and riboflavin saturation index (12). The differences between the case mothers and the controls were significant for red blood cell folate ($p < 0.001$) and white blood cell vitamin C ($p < 0.05$). Serum vitamin A levels were comparable to those of controls. Based on this experience, a multicenter study was launched to compare mothers receiving full supplements with control patients not receiving supplements (13–16). The supplemented group received a multivitamin-iron-calcium preparation from 28 days before conception to the date of the second missed menstrual period, which is after the time of neural tube closure. The daily vitamin supplement provided:

Vitamin A	4,000 IU	Nicotinamide	15 mg
Vitamin D	400 IU	Pyridoxine	1 mg
Vitamin C	40 mg	Folic acid	0.36 mg
Thiamine	1.5 mg	Ferrous sulfate	75.6 mg (as Fe)
Riboflavin	1.5 mg	Calcium phosphate	480 mg

Their findings, summarized in 1983, are shown below for the infants and fetuses that were examined (16):

One Previous NTD
    Supplemented   385
        Recurrences   2* (0.5%)
    Unsupplemented   458
        Recurrences   19* (4.1%)   *$p = 0.0004$
Two or More Previous NTD
    Supplemented   44
        Recurrences   1* (2.3%)
    Unsupplemented   52
        Recurrences   5* (9.6%)   *$p = 0.145$
Total
    Supplemented   429
        Recurrences   3 (0.7%)
    Unsupplemented   510
        Recurrences   24 (4.7%)

Although the numbers are suggestive of a protective effect offered by multivitamins, at least three other explanations were offered by the investigators (13):

1. A low risk group had selected itself for supplementation
2. The study group aborted more NTD fetuses than did controls
3. Other factors were responsible for the reduction in NTD

In a 1980 report, Laurence and co-workers (17) found that women receiving well-balanced diets had a lower incidence and recurrence rate of infants with NTD than women receiving poor diets. Although multivitamin supplements were not studied, it can be assumed that those patients who consumed adequate diets also consumed more vitamins from their food compared to those with poor diets. This study, then, added credibility to the thesis that good nutrition can prevent some NTD. Holmes-Siedle and co-workers (18, 19), using Smithells' protocol, observed that fully supplemented mothers (83) had no recurrences while an unsupplemented group (141) had four recurrences of NTD. Interestingly, a short report that appeared 6 years before Smithells' work found that both vitamins and iron were consumed more by mothers who gave birth to infants with anencephalus and spina bifida (20).

The above investigations have generated a number of discussions, criticisms, and defenses (21–51). The primary criticism centered around the fact that the groups were not randomly assigned but were self-selected for supplementation or no supplementation. The need for a controlled randomized study was recognized by many of the discussants and summarized by Wald and Polani in 1984 (52). The randomized clinical trial, finalized in 1982 and currently underway, should eventually resolve the issue of whether multivitamins prevent recurrences of neural tube defects.

A recent investigation into a third class of anomalies, limb reduction defects, was opened by a report that multivitamins may have caused this malformation in an otherwise healthy boy (49). The mother was taking the preparation because of a previous birth of a child with NTD. A retrospective analysis of Finnish records, however, failed to show any association between 1st trimester use of multivitamins and limb reduction defects (53).

In summary, the use of multivitamins up to the RDA for pregnancy is recommended for the general good health of the mother and the fetus. Whether or not this supplementation can prevent certain congenital defects such as cleft lip and/or palate and neural tube defects is currently unknown. Recommendations for or against vitamins used for this purpose must await the outcome of current investigations.

[* Risk Factor varies for amounts exceeding RDA—see individual vitamins.]

Breast Feeding Summary

Vitamins are naturally present in breast milk (see individual vitamins). The RDAs of vitamins and minerals during lactation are (1):

Vitamin A	6,000 IU
Vitamin D	400–600 IU
Vitamin E	16 IU
Vitamin C	90–100 mg
Folic acid	500 μg

Thiamine (B₁)	1.5–1.6 mg
Riboflavin (B₂)	1.7–1.8 mg
Niacinamide (B₃)	18–20 mg
Pyridoxine (B₆)	2.3–2.5 mg
Cyanocobalamin (B₁₂)	4 μg
Calcium	1200–1600 mg
Phosphorus	1200–1600 mg
Iodine	200 μg
Iron	18 mg
Magnesium	450 mg
Zinc	25 mg

References

1. *Recommended Dietary Allowances*, ed 9. Washington, DC:National Academy of Sciences, 1980.
2. Douglas B. The role of environmental factors in the etiology of "so-called" congenital malformations. Plast Reconstr Surg 1958;22:94–108.
3. *Ibid*, 214–29.
4. Conway H. Effect of supplemental vitamin therapy on the limitation of incidence of cleft lip and cleft palate in humans. Plast Reconstr Surg 1958;22:450–3.
5. Peer LA, Gordon HW, Bernhard WG. Experimental production of congenital deformities and their possible prevention in man. J Int Coll Surg 1963;39:23–35.
6. Fraser FC, Warburton D. No association of emotional stress or vitamin supplement during pregnancy to cleft lip or palate in man. Plast Reconstr Surg 1964;33:395–9.
7. Peer LA, Gordon HW, Bernhard WG. Effect of vitamins on human teratology. Plast Reconstr Surg 1964;34:358–62.
8. Briggs RM. Vitamin supplementation as a possible factor in the incidence of cleft lip/palate deformities in humans. Clin Plast Surg 1976;3:647–52.
9. Tolarova M. Periconceptional supplementation with vitamins and folic acid to prevent recurrence of cleft lip. Lancet 1982;2:217.
10. Bound JP. Spina bifida and vitamins. Br Med J 1983;286:147.
11. Smithells RW. Spina bifida and vitamins. Br Med J 1983;286:388–9.
12. Smithells RW, Sheppard S, Schorah CJ. Vitamin deficiencies and neural tube defects. Arch Dis Child 1976;51:944–50.
13. Smithells RW, Sheppard S, Schorah CJ, Seller MJ, Nevin NC, Harris R, Read AP, Fielding DW. Possible prevention of neural-tube defects by periconceptional vitamin supplementation. Lancet 1980;1:339–40.
14. Smithells RW, Sheppard S, Schorah CJ, Seller MJ, Nevin NC, Harris R, Read AP, Fielding DW. Apparent prevention of neural tube defects by periconceptional vitamin supplementation. Arch Dis Child 1981;56:911–8.
15. Smithells RW, Sheppard S, Schorah CJ, Seller MJ, Nevin NC, Harris R, Read Ap, Fielding DW, Walker S. Vitamin supplementation and neural tube defects. Lancet 1981;2:1425.
16. Smithells RW, Nevin NC, Seller MJ, Sheppard S, Harris R, Read AP, Fielding DW, Walker S, Schorah CJ, Wild J. Further experience of vitamin supplementation for prevention of neural tube defect recurrences. Lancet 1983;1:1027–31.
17. Laurence KM, James N, Miller M, Campbell H. Increased risk of recurrence of pregnancies complicated by fetal neural tube defects in mothers receiving poor diets, and possible benefit of dietary counselling. Br Med J 1980;281:1592–4.
18. Holmes-Siedle M, Lindenbaum RH, Galliard A, Bobrow M. Vitamin supplementation and neural tube defects. Lancet 1982;1:276.
19. Holmes-Siedle M. Vitamin supplementation and neural tube defects. Lancet 1983;2:41.
20. Choi NW, Klaponski FA. On neural-tube defects: an epidemiological elicitation of etiological factors. Neurology 1970;20:399–400.
21. Stone DH. Possible prevention of neural-tube defects by periconceptional vitamin supplementation. Lancet 1980;1:647.
22. Smithells RW, Sheppard S. *Ibid*.
23. Fernhoff PM. *Ibid*, 648.

24. Elwood JH. *Ibid*.
25. Anonymous. Vitamins, neural-tube defects, and ethics committees. Lancet 1980;1:1061–2.
26. Kirke PN. Vitamins, neural tube defects, and ethics committees. Lancet 1980;1:1300–1.
27. Freed DLJ. *Ibid*, 1301.
28. Raab GM, Gore SM. *Ibid*.
29. Hume K. Fetal defects and multivitamin therapy. Med J Aust 1980;2:731–2.
30. Edwards JH. Vitamin supplementation and neural tube defects. Lancet 1982;1:275–6.
31. Renwick JH. Vitamin supplementation and neural tube defects. Lancet 1982;1:748.
32. Chalmers TC, Sacks H. Vitamin supplements to prevent neural tube defects. Lancet 1982;1:748.
33. Stirrat GM. Vitamin supplementation and neural tube defects. Lancet 1982;1:625–6.
34. Kanofsky JD. Vitamin supplements to prevent neural tube defects. Lancet 1982;1:1075.
35. Walsh DE. *Ibid*.
36. Meier P. Vitamins to prevent neural tube defects. Lancet 1982;1:859.
37. Smith DE, Haddow JE. *Ibid*, 859–60.
38. Smithells RW, Sheppard S, Schorah CJ, Seller MJ, Nevin NC, Harris R, Read AP, Fielding DW. Vitamin supplements and neural tube defects. Lancet 1982;1:1186.
39. Anonymous. Vitamins to prevent neural tube defects. Lancet 1982;2:1255–6.
40. Lorber J. Vitamins to prevent neural tube defects. Lancet 1982;2:1458–9.
41. Read AP, Harris R. Spina bifida and vitamins. Br Med J 1983;286:560–1.
42. Rose G, Cooke ID, Polani, Wald NJ. Vitamin supplementation for prevention of neural tube defect recurrences. Lancet 1983;1:1164–5.
43. Knox EG. Vitamin supplementation and neural tube defects. Lancet 1983;2:39.
44. Emanuel I. *Ibid*, 39–40.
45. Smithells RW, Seller MJ, Harris R, Fielding DW, Schorah CJ, Nevin NC, Sheppard S, Read AP, Walker S, Wild J. *Ibid*, 40.
46. Oakley GP Jr, Adams MJ Jr, James LM. Vitamins and neural tube defects. Lancet 1983;2:798–9.
47. Smithells RW, Seller MJ, Harris R, Fielding DW, Schorah CJ, Nevin NC, Sheppard S, Read AP, Walker S, Wild J. *Ibid*, 799.
48. Elwood JM. Can vitamins prevent neural tube defects? Can Med Assoc J 1983;129:1088–92.
49. David TJ. Unusual limb-reduction defect in infant born to mother taking periconceptional multivitamin supplement. Lancet 1984;1:507–8.
50. Blank CE, Kumar D, Johnson M. Multivitamins and prevention of neural tube defects: a need for detailed counselling. Lancet 1984;1:291.
51. Smithells RW. Can vitamins prevent neural tube defects? Can Med Assoc J 1984;131:273–6.
52. Wald NJ, Polani PE. Neural-tube defects and vitamins: the need for a randomized clinical trial. Br J Obstet Gynecol 1984;91:516–23.
53. Aro T, Haapakoski J, Heinonen OP, Saxen L. Lack of association between vitamin intake during early pregnancy and reduction limb defects. Am J Obstet Gynecol 1984;150:433.

Name: **WARFARIN**

Class: **Anticoagulant**   Risk Factor: **D**

Fetal Risk Summary

See Coumarin Derivatives.

Breast Feeding Summary

See Coumarin Derivatives.

APPENDIX

A. ANTIHISTAMINES

Antazoline (C)
Azatadine (B$_M$)
Bromodiphenhydramine (C)
Brompheniramine (C$_M$)
Buclizine (C)
Carbinoxamine (C)
Chlorcyclizine (C)
Chlorpheniramine (B)
Cimetidine (B)
Cinnarizine (C)
Clemastine (C)
Cyclizine (B)
Cyproheptadine (B)
Dexbrompheniramine (C)
Dexchlorpheniramine (B$_M$)
Dimenhydrinate (B$_M$)
Dimethindene (C)
Dimethothiazine (C)
Diphenhydramine (C)
Doxylamine (B)
Hydroxyzine (C)
Meclizine (B$_M$)
Methdilazine (C)
Pheniramine (C)
Phenyltoloxamine (C)
Promethazine (C)
Pyrilamine (C)
Ranitidine (B$_M$)
Trimeprazine (C)
Tripelennamine (B)
Triprolidine (C$_M$)

B. ANTI-INFECTIVES

1. Amebicide
Carbarsone (D)
Iodoquinol (C)

2. Anthelmintics
Gentian Violet (C)
Piperazine (B)
Pyrantel Pamoate (C)
Pyrvinium Pamoate (C)

3. Aminoglycosides
Amikacin (C)
Gentamicin (C)
Kanamycin (D)
Neomycin (C)
Streptomycin (D)
Tobramycin (D$_M$)

4. Antifungals
Amphotericin B (B)
Clotrimazole (B)
Flucytosine (C)
Griseofulvin (C)
Miconazole (B)
Nystatin (B)

5. Cephalosporins
Cefaclor (B$_M$)
Cefadroxil (B$_M$)
Cefamandole (B$_M$)
Cefatrizine (B$_M$)
Cefazolin (B$_M$)
Cefonicid (B$_M$)
Cefoperazone (B$_M$)
Ceforanide (B$_M$)
Cefotaxime (B$_M$)
Cefoxitin (B)
Ceftizoxime (B$_M$)
Ceftriaxone (B$_M$)
Cefuroxime (B$_M$)
Cephalexin (B$_M$)
Cephalothin (B$_M$)
Cephapirin (B$_M$)
Cephradine (B$_M$)
Moxalactam (C$_M$)

6. Penicillins
Amoxicillin (B)
Ampicillin (B)
Bacampicillin (B$_M$)
Carbenicillin (B)
Cloxacillin (B$_M$)

Cyclacillin (B_M)
Dicloxacillin (B_M)
Hetacillin (B)
Methicillin (B_M)
Nafcillin (B)
Oxacillin (B_M)
Penicillin G (B)
Penicillin G, Benzathine (B)
Penicillin G, Procaine (B)
Penicillin V (B)
Ticarcillin (B)

7. Tetracyclines
Chlortetracycline (D)
Clomocycline (D)
Demeclocycline (D)
Doxycycline (D)
Methacycline (D)
Minocycline (D)
Oxytetracycline (D)
Tetracycline (D)

8. Other Anti-infectives
Bacitracin (C)
Chloramphenicol (C)
Clindamycin (B)
Colistimethate (B)
Erythromycin (B)
Furazolidone (C)
Lincomycin (B)
Novobiocin (C)
Oleandomycin (C)
Polymyxin B (B)
Spectinomycin (B)
Trimethoprim (C_M)
Troleandomycin (C)
Vancomycin (C_M)

9. Antituberculosis
para-Aminosalicyclic Acid (C)
Ethambutol (B)
Isoniazid (C)
Rifampin (C)

10. Antivirals
Acyclovir (C_M)
Amantadine (C_M)
Idoxuridine (C)
Vidarabine (C_M)

11. Plasmodicides
Chloroquine (C)
Primaquine (C)
Pyrimethamine (C)
Quinacrine (C)
Quinine (D/X)

12. Sulfonamides
Sulfasalazine (B/D)

Sulfonamides (B/D)

13. Trichomonacides
Metronidazole (B_M)

14. Urinary Germicides
Cinoxacin (B_M)
Mandelic Acid (C)
Methenamine (C_M)
Methylene Blue (C_M/D)
Nalidixic Acid (B)
Nitrofurantoin (B)

15. Scabicide/Pediculicide
Lindane (C)
Pyrethrins with Piperonyl Butoxide (C)

16. Iodine
Iodine (D)

C. ANTINEOPLASTICS

Aminopterin (X)
Azathioprine (D)
Bleomycin (D)
Busulfan (D)
Chlorambucil (D_M)
Cisplatin (D)
Cyclophosphamide (D)
Cytarabine (D/C)
Dacarbazine (C_M)
Dactinomycin (C_M)
Daunorubicin (D_M)
Doxorubicin (D)
Fluorouracil (D)
Laetrile (C)
Mechlorethamine (D)
Melphalan (D_M)
Mercaptopurine (D)
Methotrexate (D)
Mithramycin (D)
Procarbazine (D)
Teniposide (D)
Thioguanine (D_M)
Thiotepa (D)
Vinblastine (D)
Vincristine (D)

D. AUTONOMICS

1. Parasympathomimetics (Cholinergics)
Acetylcholine (C)
Ambenonium (C)
Bethanechol (C_M)
Carbachol (C)
Demecarium (C)
Echothiophate (C)
Edrophonium (C)

Isoflurophate (C)
Neostigmine (C_M)
Physostigmine (C)
Pilocarpine (C)
Pyridostigmine (C)
2. Parasympatholytics (Anticholinergic)
Anisotropine (C)
Atropine (C)
Belladonna (C)
Benztropine (C)
Biperiden (C_M)
Clidinium (C)
Cycrimine (C)
Dicyclomine (B)
Diphemanil (C)
Ethopropazine (C)
Glycopyrrolate (B_M)
Hexocyclium (C)
Homatropine (C)
l-Hyoscyamine (C)
Isopropamide (C)
Mepenzolate (C)
Methantheline (C)
Methixene (C)
Methscopolamine (C)
Orphenadrine (C)
Oxyphencyclimine (C)
Oxyphenonium (C)
Piperidolate (C)
Procyclidine (C)
Propantheline (C_M)
Scopolamine (C)
Thiphenamil (C)
Tridihexethyl (C)
Trihexyphenidyl (C)
3. Sympathomimetics (Adrenergic)
Albuterol (C_M)
Cocaine (C)
Dobutamine (C)
Dopamine (C)
Ephedrine (C)
Epinephrine (C)
Fenoterol (B)
Isoetharine (C)
Isoproterenol (C)
Isoxsuprine (C)
Levarterenol (D)
Mephentermine (C)
Metaproterenol (C_M)
Metaraminol (D)
Methoxamine (D)
Phenylephrine (C)

Phenylpropanolamine (C)
Pseudoephedrine (C)
Ritodrine (B_M/X)
Terbutaline (B)
4. Sympatholytics
Acebutolol (B_M)
Atenolol (C_M)
Labetalol (C_M)
Mepindolol (C)
Metoprolol (B_M)
Nadolol (C_M)
Oxprenolol (C)
Pindolol (B_M)
Prazosin (C)
Propranolol (C_M)
Timolol (C_M)
5. Skeletal Muscle Relaxants
Chlorzoxazone (C)
Decamethonium (C)

E. COAGULANTS/ANTICOAGULANTS
1. Anticoagulants
Anisindione (D)
Coumarin Derivatives (D)
Diphenadione (D)
Ethyl Biscoumacetate (D)
Heparin (C)
Nicoumalone (D)
Phenindione (D)
Phenprocoumon (D)
Warfarin (D)
2. Antiheparin
Protamine (C)
3. Hemostatics
Aminocaproic Acid (C)
Aprotinin (C)
4. Thrombolytics
Streptokinase (C)
Urokinase (B_M)

F. CARDIOVASCULAR DRUGS
1. Cardiac Drugs
Acetyldigitoxin (C)
Amiodarone (C)
Bretylium (C)
Deslanoside (C)
Digitalis (C)
Digitoxin (C_M)
Digoxin (C_M)
Disopyramide (C)
Gitalin (C)
Lanatoside C (C)
Nifedipine (C_M)

Ouabain (B)
Quinidine (C)
Verapamil (C_M)
2. Antihypertensives
Acebutolol (B_M)
Atenolol (C_M)
Captopril (C_M)
Clonidine (C)
Diazoxide (C_M)
Hexamethonium (C)
Hydralazine (C)
Labetalol (C_M)
Mepindolol (C)
Methyldopa (C)
Metoprolol (B_M)
Minoxidil (C_M)
Nadolol (C_M)
Oxprenolol (C)
Pargyline (C_M)
Pindolol (B_M)
Prazosin (C)
Propranolol (C_M)
Reserpine (D)
Sodium Nitroprusside (C)
Timolol (C_M)
Trimethaphan (C)
3. Vasodilators
Amyl Nitrite (C)
Cyclandelate (C)
Dioxyline (C)
Dipyridamole (C)
Erythrityl Tetranitrate (C)
Isosorbide Dinitrate (C)
Isoxsuprine (C)
Nicotinyl Alcohol (C)
Nitroglycerin (C_M)
Nylidrin (C_M)
Pentaerythritol Tetranitrate (C)
Tolazoline (C)
4. Antilipemics
Cholestyramine (C)

G. **CENTRAL NERVOUS SYSTEM DRUGS**
1. Analgesics and Antipyretics
Acetaminophen (B)
Aspirin (C/D)
Aspirin, Buffered (C/D)
Ethoheptazine (C)
Phenacetin (B)
Propoxyphene (C/D)
2. Narcotic Analgesics
Alphaprodine (C_M/D)

Anileridine (B/D)
Butorphanol (B/D)
Codeine (C/D)
Dihydrocodeine Bitartrate (B/D)
Fentanyl (B/D)
Heroin (B/D)
Hydrocodone (B/D)
Hydromorphone (B/D)
Levorphanol (B/D)
Meperidine (B/D)
Methadone (B/D)
Morphine (B/D)
Nalbuphine (B/D)
Opium (B/D)
Oxycodone (B/D)
Oxymorphone (B/D)
Pentazocine (B/D)
Phenazocine (B/D)
3. Narcotic Antagonists
Cyclazocine (D)
Levallorphan (D)
Nalorphine (D)
Naloxone (B_M)
4. Nonsteroidal Anti-inflammatory Drugs
Fenoprofen (B/D)
Ibuprofen (B/D)
Indomethacin (B/D)
Meclofenamate (B/D)
Naproxen (B_M/D)
Oxyphenbutazone (D)
Phenylbutazone (D)
Sulindac (B/D)
Tolmetin (B/D)
5. Anticonvulsants
Aminoglutethimide (D_M)
Bromides (D)
Carbamazepine (C_M)
Clonazepam (C)
Ethosuximide (C)
Ethotoin (D)
Magnesium Sulfate (B)
Mephenytoin (C)
Mephobarbital (D)
Metharbital (B)
Methsuximide (C)
Paramethadione (D_M)
Phenobarbital (D)
Phensuximide (D)
Phenytoin (D)
Primidone (D)
Trimethadione (D)
Valproic Acid (D)

6. Antidepressants
Amitriptyline (D)
Amoxapine (C_M)
Butriptyline (D)
Clomipramine (D)
Desipramine (C)
Dibenzepin (D)
Dothiepin (D)
Doxepin (C)
Imipramine (D)
Iprindole (D)
Iproniazid (C)
Isocarboxazid (C)
Maprotiline (B_M)
Mebanazine (C)
Nialamide (C)
Nortriptyline (D)
Opipramol (D)
Phenelzine (C)
Protriptyline (C)
Tranylcypromine (C)

7. Tranquilizers
Acetophenazine (C)
Butaperazine (C)
Carphenazine (C)
Chlorpromazine (C)
Chlorprothixene (C)
Droperidol (C)
Flupenthixol (C)
Fluphenazine (C)
Haloperidol (C)
Hydroxyzine (C)
Lithium (D)
Loxapine (C)
Mesoridazine (C)
Molindone (C)
Perphenazine (C)
Piperacetazine (C)
Prochlorperazine (C)
Promazine (C)
Tetrabenazine (C)
Thiopropazate (C)
Thioridazine (C)
Thiothixene (C)
Trifluoperazine (C)
Triflupromazine (C)

8. Stimulants
Caffeine (B)
Dextroamphetamine (D/C)
Diethylpropion (B)
Fenfluramine (C_M)
Mazindol (C)
Methylphenidate (C)

Phendimetrazine (C)
Phentermine (C)

9. Sedatives and Hypnotics
Amobarbital (D/B)
Aprobarbital (C)
Butalbital (C/D)
Chloral Hydrate (C_M)
Chlordiazepoxide (D)
Diazepam (D)
Ethanol (D/X)
Ethchlorvynol (C_M)
Flunitrazepam (C)
Lorazepam (C)
Mephobarbital (D)
Meprobamate (D)
Methaqualone (D)
Metharbital (D)
Oxazepam (C)
Pentobarbital (D_M)
Phenobarbital (D)
Secobarbital (D_M)

H.   DIAGNOSTIC AGENTS
Diatrizoate (D)
Ethiodized Oil (D)
Evans Blue (C)
Indigo Carmine (B)
Iocetamic Acid (D)
Iodamide (D)
Iodipamide (D)
Iodoxamate (D)
Iopanoic Acid (D)
Iothalamate (D)
Ipodate (D)
Methylene Blue (C_M/D)
Metrizamide (D)
Sodium Iodide I125 (X)
Sodium Iodide I131 (X)
Tyropanoate (D)

I.   ELECTROLYTES
Potassium Chloride (A)
Potassium Citrate (A)
Potassium Gluconate (A)

J.   NUTRIENTS
Hyperalimentation, Parenteral (C)
Lipids (C)

K.   DIURETICS
Acetazolamide (C)
Amiloride (B_M)

Bendroflumethiazide (D/C)
Benzthiazide (D)
Chlorothiazide (D)
Chlorthalidone (D)
Cyclopenthiazide (D)
Cyclothiazide (D)
Ethacrynic Acid (D)
Furosemide (C_M)
Glycerin (C)
Hydrochlorothiazide (D)
Hydroflumethiazide (D)
Isosorbide (C)
Mannitol (C)
Methyclothiazide (D)
Metolazone (D)
Polythiazide (D)
Quinethazone (D)
Spironolactone (D)
Triamterene (D)
Trichlormethiazide (D)
Urea (C)

L. ACIDIFYING AGENTS
Ammonium Chloride (B)

M. ANTIDIARRHEALS
Diphenoxylate (C_M)
Loperamide (B_M)
Paregoric (B/D)

N. GASTROINTESTINAL AGENTS
1. Antiemetics
Buclizine (C)
Cyclizine (B)
Dimenhydrinate (B)
Doxylamine (B)
Meclizine (B_M)
Prochlorperazine (C)
Trimethobenzamide (C)
2. Laxatives/Purgatives
Casanthranol (C)
Cascara Sagrada (C)
Danthron (C)
Docusate Calcium (C)
Docusate Potassium (C)
Docusate Sodium (C)
Lactulose (C)
Mineral Oil (C)
3. Antiflatulents
Simethicone (C)

O. GOLD COMPOUNDS
Aurothioglucose (C)
Gold Sodium Thiomalate (C)

P. HEAVY METAL ANTAGONISTS
Deferoxamine (C)
Penicillamine (D)

Q. HORMONES
1. Adrenal
Betamethasone (C)
Cortisone (D)
Dexamethasone (C)
Prednisolone (B)
Prednisone (B)
2. Estrogens
Chlorotrianisene (X_M)
Clomiphene (X_M)
Dienestrol (X)
Diethylstilbestrol (X_M)
Estradiol (X)
Estrogens, Conjugated (X_M)
Estrone (X)
Ethinyl Estradiol (X)
Hormonal Pregnancy Test Tablets (X)
Mestranol (X)
Oral Contraceptives (X)
3. Progestogens
Ethisterone (D)
Ethynodiol (D)
Hydroxyprogesterone (D)
Lynestrenol (D)
Medroxyprogesterone (D)
Norethindrone (D)
Norethynodrel (D)
Norgestrel (D)
Oral Contraceptives (X)
4. Antidiabetic Agents
Acetohexamide (D)
Chlorpropamide (D/C)
Insulin (B)
Tolazamide (D/C)
Tolbutamide (D/C)
5. Pituitary
Corticotropin/Cosyntropin (C)
Desmopressin (B_M)
Lypressin (B)
Somatostatin (B)
Vasopressin (B)
6. Thyroid
Calcitonin (B)
Iodothyrin (A)

Levothyroxine (A_M)
Liothyronine (A)
Liotrix (A)
Thyroglobulin (A)
Thyroid (A)
Thyrotropin (C_M)
7. Antithyroid
Carbimazole (D)
Methimazole (D)
Propylthiouracil (D)
Sodium Iodide I131 (X)

R. SPASMOLYTICS
Aminophylline (C)
Dyphylline (C_M)
Oxtriphylline (C)
Theophylline (C)

S. ANTITUSSIVES   AND   EXPECTO-RANTS
1. Antitussives
Codeine (C/D)
2. Expectorants
Guaifenesin (C)
Hydriodic Acid (D)
Iodinated Glycerol (X_M)
Potassium Iodide (D)
Sodium Iodide (D)

T. SERUMS,   TOXOIDS,   AND   VAC-CINES
1. Serums
Immune Globulin, Hepatitis B (B)
Immune Globulin, Rabies (B)
Immune Globulin, Tetanus (B)
2. Toxoids
Tetanus/Diphtheria Toxoids (Adult) (C)
3. Vaccines
BCG (C)
Cholera (C)
Escherichia coli (C)
Hepatitis B (C_M)
Influenza (C)
Measles (X)
Meningococcus (C)
Mumps (X)

Plague (C)
Pneumococcal Polyvalent (C)
Poliovirus Inactivated (C)
Poliovirus Live (C)
Rabies Human (C)
Rubella (X)
Smallpox (X)
Tularemia (C)
Typhoid (C)
Yellow Fever (D)

U. VITAMINS
β-Carotene (C)
Calcifediol (A/D)
Calcitriol (A/D)
Cholecalciferol (A/D)
Dihydrotachysterol (A/D)
Ergocalciferol (A/D)
Folic Acid (A/C)
Isotretinoin (X)
Leucovorin (C_M)
Menadione (C/X)
Niacin (A/C)
Niacinamide (A/C)
Pantothenic Acid (A/C)
Phytonadione (C)
Pyridoxine (A/C)
Riboflavin (A/C)
Thiamine (A/C)
Vitamin A (A/X)
Vitamin B_{12} (A/C)
Vitamin C (A/C)
Vitamin D (A/D)
Vitamin E (A/C)
Vitamins, Multiple (A)

V. MISCELLANEOUS
Bromocriptine (C_M)
Camphor (C)
Clofibrate (C)
Colchicine (C_M)
Cyclamate (C)
Disulfiram (X)
Phenazopyridine (B_M)
Phencyclidine (X)
Probenecid (B)

INDEX

503